Systemic Effects of Antihypertensive Agents

Editor
Mohinder P. Sambhi, M.D., Ph.D.

Formal papers and selected edited discussions from The Effects of Antihypertensive Therapy Symposium organized by the Hypertension Division at Sepulveda VA Hospital, UCLA School of Medicine, Los Angeles, California, through an educational grant from Pennwalt Prescription Products.

Published by
Symposia Specialists
MEDICAL BOOKS

STRATTON INTERCONTINENTAL MEDICAL BOOK CORPORATION
381 Park Avenue South, New York, New York 10016

Library of Congress Catalog
Card No. 76-14018

ISBN 0-88372-048-5

Contents

IV EFFECTS OF ACUTE RECEPTOR BLOCKADE

Dedication

This work is dedicated

To the scientific investigators from all over the world who have contributed to the accumulation of knowledge on hypertension, one of modern mankind's most prevalent afflictions.

To the contributions, independent and shared by the industry, in all free democratic societies that have been vital in stimulating the expansion of the horizons of this knowledge and the spirit of man.

To salute a period in the history of man that nourished and preserved the interaction

1776 to 1976

Acknowledgments

It is a pleasure to express my sincere appreciation to Isaac R. McGraw, president of the Pharmaceutical Division of Pennwalt Corporation, not only for his essential, generous and unfailing support, but also for his equally important, and vital, collaboration at all phases of this project.

Preface

The past 25 years have seen unprecedented strides in unravelling the adrenally and renally mediated causes of secondary hypertension, followed by intensified search for the etiology of essential hypertension. It should be likewise recognized that during the preceding several decades the industrial research and development of antihypertensive drugs, better tolerated with fewer side effects, has contributed as much or more to the general acceptance of antihypertensive therapy as a lifelong preventive management than the informed zeal of the medical investigator diligently searching for means of preventing the ravages of a widely prevalent malady. This mutually supportive collaboration between academia and industry is certainly not unique to the area of hypertension, but historically it appears that medical thought has lagged behind drug development in providing a rational basis for aggressive long-term therapy designed to maintain the elevated blood pressure near normotensive levels. This contention is further supported by the fact that the crucial Veterans Administration cooperative study documenting the benefits of antihypertensive therapy was done as late as it was. To pursue the point, one only has to look back about 20 years, to the mid-1950s, when an authoritative book on hypertension started its chapter on "Management of Asymptomatic Cases of Essential Hypertension" as follows:

> At the outset, it is to be emphasized that many individuals with essential hypertension not only need no treatment whatsoever but are much better off without it. Many persons with asymptomatic hypertension would have been more fortunate if they had never learned of their hypertension. As things are, however, it is almost always necessary to tell the individual with hypertension that his blood pressure is elevated, for he is very apt to learn it from another source and then his confidence in the physician is destroyed. Or he feels that his condition must be serious if his devoted physician did not tell him about it. To be

sure, discretion must be used in the manner in which the patient is told the state of affairs. He may be told that his blood pressure is somewhat higher than that of most people of his age but that this is by no means a serious matter if he takes proper care of himself; *in fact in some respects high blood pressure is rather a sign of a vigorous constitution.* (Emphasis added.)

From an era of severely restricted therapeutic choice, too toxic for prolonged use and thus limited to handling the emergent and dire consequences of long-standing hypertension, antihypertensive therapy enjoys today a very wide field of choices with far-reaching goals. The nationally supported programs for mass screening and treatment aim at the prevention of target organ damage through lifelong treatment with minimum but conceded side effects. It is also clear that the ultimate goal lies in the future development of specific modes of rational treatment directed at the root cause. The use of specific antagonists, including those of aldosterone and angiotensin, is beginning to burrow into the hitherto impenetrable mantle of absolute empiricism.

The choice of a title for this symposium presented a challenge, greater than usual. The subject matter does not encompass the pharmacologic or therapeutic aspects of antihypertensive drugs nor is it a comprehensive treatment of one particular aspect, such as side effects of all or even most available antihypertensive agents. And it largely excludes, albeit not by design, a consideration of the effects of antihypertensive agents on the central nervous system.

This symposium was organized to bring together some of the available information on the subject and to stimulate future thought on the importance of studies on the mechanisms of therapeutic as well as nontherapeutic perturbations in homeostasis resulting from both the acute and the prolonged use of antihypertensive agents. The existing information in several areas is sparse and controversial. One of the most common errors on the part of the investigator in this area is to study the effects of antihypertensive drugs for an acute or relatively short period of time and then imply, tacitly or otherwise, that the findings apply to the long-term and chronic effects. This error is particularly dangerous when considering the effects of drugs on axial hormonal systems, such as renin-angiotensin-aldosterone.

The topics in the symposium were selected to emphasize several of these considerations. A summary of additional scheduled events at the conference is included in the last chapter. I wish to express my sincere appreciation to the contributors for generously allowing me the privilege of editorial deletions and alterations. It is a pleasure to express my personal gratitude to all who shared in the success of this symposium and the completion of this publication.

Mohinder P. Sambhi

Introduction: Whence and Whither?

It has been said that the functions of those who write prefaces and introduce symposia are several: (1) to give time for the stragglers to sit down and the narcoleptics to surface; (2) to avoid the awkward, jolting abruptness resulting when the speaker's only introduction to his audience is "show me the first slide"; likely as not he has not seen it; (3) to humor the old war horses who will give the same speech they gave five decades ago; (4) like the fan dancer, to get the audience's attention but not expose the subject; and (5) to say something portentous but innocent of all meaning, such as: "And would you fail to feel strongly against our refusal not to withdraw from Vietnam?"

I believe I can fulfill most of these specifications. In short, I am your man. My subject is "whither" and to foreshadow "whither" we must know "whence."

It will be agreed that serious work on the mechanisms and treatment of hypertension began about half a century ago. There were two schools of thought about whether arterial pressure should be lowered, which then would constitute "*treatment*." One maintained that to lower it would dangerously reduce the perfusion of organs because of the narrowed arteries and arterioles in the hypertensive. The other school believed reduction of blood pressure would relieve the work strain on the heart and blood vessels and so prove beneficial. It was not much of a problem at the time I became interested in hypertension because no one knew how to lower pressure reliably without severe side effects, nor were methods available for measuring blood flow in organs such as the kidney to determine whether ischemia had occurred as a result of the reduction.

Low salt diets had been tried in France at the turn of the century but created hardly a ripple of interest. Low salt diets were vigorously and belligerently revived in 1922 by Allen and Sherill and made simple, with a faint odor of masochism, by Kempner in 1948. Potassium thiocyanate was the other standby. It seems odd to some that those who wanted to make a profit — that is, the pharmaceutical manufacturers — were the first to enlarge upon these feeble efforts.

But the initial cadre of antihypertensive drugs included some strange aberrations, indeed. In quick succession, watermelon and cucumber seed, mistletoe, bismuth subnitrate, vitamin A, rutin and garlic were highly recommended. The crowning achievement was "whiffless garlic."

The next therapeutic phase took on quite a different hue. Ganglion-blocking agents, hydralazine, reserpine and guanethidine were the chief constituents. This was followed by several groups of drugs, some of them better, or just as good — methyldopa, triamterene, spironolactone, sodium nitroprusside, diazoxide. The big break came with the introduction of the thiazide diuretics and then in quick succession, bethanidine, debrisoquine, propranolol, clonidine and minoxidil.

Added to the drug treatments internists have had to fend off the usual inroads of the "cutting" surgeons, beginning with that form of mayhem called an "anterior nerve root section" and followed closely in time by splanchnicectomy. Then renal arterial vascular surgery had a fling along with nephrectomy, dialysis and transplantation. Who can forget the Alfred Adsons, Max Peets, Reg Smithwicks and George Heuers? But this is all "old hat"! By 1950, it was clear that we were on the right track. Surgical operation, by temporarily lowering blood pressure, had shown beyond doubt that malignant hypertension could be reversed and drug treatment, even with all the side effects, clearly had benefited patients with essential or renal hypertension! It was another of those examples where we know more about treatment than about mechanisms.

But enough of "whence." No one yet, I trust, has been tempted to disobey that wondrous sign stenciled over the door of the Ford Engineering Division: "Emergency exit — not to be used under any circumstances."

A *whither* report is not "futurism," science fiction or the empty lucubrations of the graduation ceremony speaker. It should have two characteristics: (1) brevity and (2) creativity. Brevity, I promise; creativity you must judge. To ensure the first I will merely list what in my view will be a few of the creative ventures ahead.

(1) The teaching of hypertension in medical schools will vastly improve in quality. (2) The problems of compliance of patients as regards treatment will be restudied and improved. (3) Smaller numbers of drugs will be used by practitioners, but with greater understanding, reserving the more complex problems for specialists. (4) Treatment of hypertension will go hand in hand with treatment of atherosclerosis. (5) The multifactorial — or faceted — nature of hypertension will be accepted and followed by suitable reclassification of hypertensives. (6) Hypertension will be treated in accord with the disturbed regulatory mechanisms involved. (7) The multiple, highly complex regulatory mechanism of hypertension will continue to be unraveled in depth. New mechanisms will be discovered: humoral, neural and hemodynamic. (8) Many of the terms describing, but not explaining, mechanisms will be clarified. Names such as "autoregulation," "cardiac efficiency" and "hypertensive vascular disease" will be understood in terms of why and how they occur. (9) A fresh start will be made to understand the mechanisms of atherogenesis. We have gotten stuck with risk factors, lipids and stress. We need a new approach to the understanding of the mechanisms that regulate fibrogenesis, cardiac hypertrophy and endothelial permeability among many other aspects. (10) So far, epidemiologic studies have not been singularly successful in providing leads regarding prevention of hypertension. Salt, soft water, pyelonephritis, autoimmunity, heredity and chronic stress have received some attention, but none have prevailed to the extent of being put to prospective tests.

And now a brief and perhaps gratuitous comment on the future of researchers themselves. How does the young crop look to us oldsters? On balance, quite good! There seems to be good leadership; they have the capability of research in depth and celebrity seeking and political ambition have not overwhelmed them. Their technology seems impeccable although they appear curiously unwilling to use double-blind controls.

On the less laudable side of the ledger are the quite understandable but too competitive efforts for more money, more technicians, more equipment and more postgraduate students. The "whirling dervish" syndrome has become a virulent infection. The infectious agent is the distant symposium, committee meeting or visiting firemanship. The field needs a period of benign neglect for investigators to think and recover the spirit and adventure of research itself. An old friend, Peyton Rous, once said, "Thought is the sharpest of tools; people are always cutting themselves with it." My particular anathema is committees, characterized by the aphorism, "I came, I saw, was seen and left." We have the dreadful example of over-organization and underachievement constantly before us in the many examples drawn from federal and state governments. For unknown reasons, legislators believe they know how to conduct research and spend research dollars better than do researchers. A senator recently said we should pay our taxes with a smile. Wish I had known that on April 15th. I sent cash!

I suspect, and almost hope, that the trend toward conservatism and belt tightening will have a salutary effect in restoring the enormous productivity and creativity of the recent past. It is not enough that people live within their incomes until they regain their confidence. Prudence and hard work should not be viewed as punishment but as an effective way of life. In my view, this country needs articulate citizens for the extreme middle.

In the past 50 years we have come a long way. A large variety of models of experimental hypertension are now available. A vast array of biochemical and physiological techniques have been developed. Indeed, such an abundance has come our way, we are in danger of being overwhelmed by the multiplicity of detail to the detriment of general principles.

The response of patients to treatment showed long ago that there was no single, uniform correct pattern. Fortunately, drugs and other therapeutic procedures ranging from the most powerful vasodilators like sodium nitroprusside to the gentle relaxant, transcendental meditation, all seem to have their place in our efforts to readjust the regulatory mechanisms controlling blood pressure and tissue perfusion.

Diseases of regulation such as hypertension are in some ways unique because their understanding can encompass such a variety of scientific disciplines. We have been fortunate in eliciting the abiding interest of people trained in what superficially might seem inapplicable disciplines — chemistry, molecular biology, mathematics and even engineering. By breadth of vision, research in hypertension has been made a truly cooperative venture, one far beyond what could possibly have been envisioned even 30 years ago. The idea of including under one rubric so diverse a body of knowledge as that of hypertension has been one of the major organizational achievements in biomedical research. This principle of multidisciplinary investigation in depth has made many medical societies, formerly dominant on the basis of descriptive classification of disease, largely obsolete. We may all be proud of the body of knowledge built by the many capable and far-seeing people.

Let me say, finally, that though I am long retired, I have no plans to turn my back on either the people or the field of cardiovascular disease. My affection for both is unflagging. I hope you will have to suffer me for some time to come. But I shall not forget that Socrates went about giving advice. They poisoned him!

Irvine H. Page, M.D.
Editor, Modern Medicine Publishing

I

Effects on Target Organs and Homeostasis

Antihypertensive Measures and Their Consequences in Malignant Hypertensive Rats

R. Dietz, M.D., H. Haebara, M.D., B. Lüth, M.D., G. J. Mast, M.D., A. Schömig, M.D. and F. Gross, M.D.

Malignant hypertension is characterized by the severity of the vascular lesions and the rapid progress of the disease. Fibrinoid necrosis of small arteries and arterioles, proliferative endarteritis and periarteritis may occur in various vascular beds, with the consequence of severe organ damage [1, 2]. In various types of hypertension, a malignant course may develop; in general, blood pressure has to pass a critical level before severe vascular lesions occur, the appearance of which may be favored by certain conditions. Among these, the administration of a high salt diet or of desoxycorticosterone and salt may be mentioned [3, 4], but also negative sodium balance may induce a malignant course of hypertension [5, 6]. Furthermore, the sudden exposure of a vascular bed to high blood pressure may cause vascular lesions that are indistinguishable from those seen in malignant hypertension [1].

Before discussing the procedures that may influence the course of malignant hypertension, it is necessary to give a short analysis of the pathogenic mechanisms responsible for the occurrence of changes that are characteristic of malignant hypertension.

R. Dietz, M.D., H. Haebara, M.D., B. Lüth, M.D., G. J. Mast, M.D., A. Schömig, M.D. and F. Gross, M.D., Department of Pharmacology, University of Heidelberg, Federal Republic of Germany.

Acute Malignant Phase Elicited by Negative Sodium Balance

In rats with unilateral renal artery stenosis and an untouched contralateral kidney, an acute malignant phase may develop when the blood pressure exceeds a critical systolic level of between 180 and 190 mm Hg [5, 6]. Negative salt and water balance, increased fluid consumption, reduced food intake, decrease in body weight and diminished plasma and extracellular fluid volume occur. The renin-angiotensin system is markedly stimulated, plasma concentrations of both renin and angiotensin II are elevated and aldosterone secretion is enhanced [7]. The activation of the renin-angiotensin-aldosterone system is the consequence of the negative salt and water balance, but in about half the animals, compensation is not achieved. In the contralateral, untouched kidney, arteriolar lesions, such as fibrinoid necrosis, thickening of the intima, media hypertrophy, and periarteriolar infiltration, are seen as characteristic signs of an acute malignant phase. No similar morphological changes were observed in other vascular beds.

Malignant Hypertension Induced by Salt Loading

In rats in which one renal artery was clamped and the contralateral kidney left untouched, 10 mg of desoxycorticosterone acetate (DOCA) in oily solution were injected daily, and 2% saline was offered, in addition to water, as drinking fluid. The rats drank increasing amounts of saline, and their blood pressure rose more rapidly than that of rats having no DOCA treatment and only water to drink. After 14 days, the blood pressure had reached a mean value of 176 mm Hg, which was in the same range as the mean seen in renal hypertensive rats without additional salt supply. Despite this fact, signs of malignant hypertension (reduced body-weight gain or body-weight loss, reduced food intake, further increase in water and saline consumption) developed, and characteristic severe arterial and arteriolar lesions occurred in various vascular beds, such as the contralateral, unclamped kidney, the mesenterium, the heart and the brain. In six of 15 rats, brain hemorrhages of different sizes were found. From these experiments it may be concluded that the administration of DOCA and salt aggravates the vascular lesions and induces a more severe state of malignant hypertension than that observed in animals with unilateral renal artery stenosis and having water only as drinking fluid. Since body-weight gain was similar in the two groups of renal hypertensive rats and independent of salt consumption, it may be presumed that the animals which received DOCA had an increased salt and fluid turnover. On the other hand, DOCA did not prevent the pressure-induced salt and fluid loss by the contralateral kidney, with the consequence of a negative sodium balance. Hence, an untouched contralateral kidney, fully exposed to high blood pressure, may become a sodium-losing kidney when the pressure exceeds a critical level, even if sodium consumption is abundant and DOCA is administered simultaneously.

Antihypertensive Measures

To obtain further information about the significance of various factors that may be responsible for the malignant course of hypertension, the effects of the following procedures were studied: (1) sodium supply during the acute malignant phase that had been induced by negative sodium balance; (2) elimination of the sodium-losing kidney; (3) correction of renal artery stenosis; and (4) antihypertensive drugs.

Sodium Supply

In former experiments, sodium was offered as 0.9% saline in addition to water as drinking fluid, so that the rats could choose according to their preference [5, 6]. When their sodium balance was negative, they drank copiously and almost exclusively saline, up to 150 ml/day. As a consequence of the increased sodium intake, the blood pressure may fall, the body weight rise and the general condition of the animal improve; the stimulation of the renin-angiotensin system is reduced, the aldosterone secretion diminished and the plasma volume as well as the extracellular fluid volume are restored to normal. However, such a beneficial effect of salt administration is transient, and after a few days, the blood pressure begins to rise again [8]. If sodium supply is continued or saline alone is given as drinking fluid, signs of malignant hypertension will reappear. Hence, salt supply as a means of affecting the malignant course of hypertension is only indicated in the presence of a negative sodium balance and only for a limited period.

Elimination of the Sodium-Losing Kidney

If the contralateral, untouched kidney were responsible for the negative sodium balance, the removal of this kidney or the placing of a clip on its artery should prevent sodium and fluid loss and consequently also the appearance of an acute malignant phase of hypertension. In several experiments, we found that in rats that had a clip on either of their renal arteries and in rats in which, after unilateral nephrectomy, the artery of the remaining kidney was clamped, the blood pressure rose to higher values than in rats with an untouched contralateral kidney (Fig. 1). However, despite the marked hypertension, no symptoms of an acute malignant phase, which could have been attributed to negative sodium balance, were observed. Food intake was not reduced, nor was body-weight gain; fluid consumption did not increase, and the renin-angiotensin system was only mildly stimulated, without a significant elevation of the plasma angiotensin II concentration (Table 1). Furthermore, serum urea did not increase significantly. The kidneys were free from vascular lesions, because they were protected by the clip, at least in part, from the elevated blood pressure. However, 24 days after the induction of renal artery stenosis, severe lesions were found in other vascular beds, such as the mesenterium, the liver and the heart. From these data it may be concluded that the hypertension after bilateral renal artery stenosis or after unilateral stenosis in the absence of a contralateral kidney is not caused by a stimulation of the renin-angiotensin system, since plasma concentrations of renin and of angiotensin II are at the upper normal limit. Furthermore, it is obvious that the marked stimulation of the renin-angiotensin-aldosterone system, seen in the presence of an untouched contralateral kidney, is the response to an acute sodium and fluid loss, which elicits the characteristic symptoms seen at the beginning of the acute malignant phase.

On the basis of the results of these studies it may be presumed that the acute malignant phase of renal hypertension is the consequence of a pressure-induced sodium loss by the

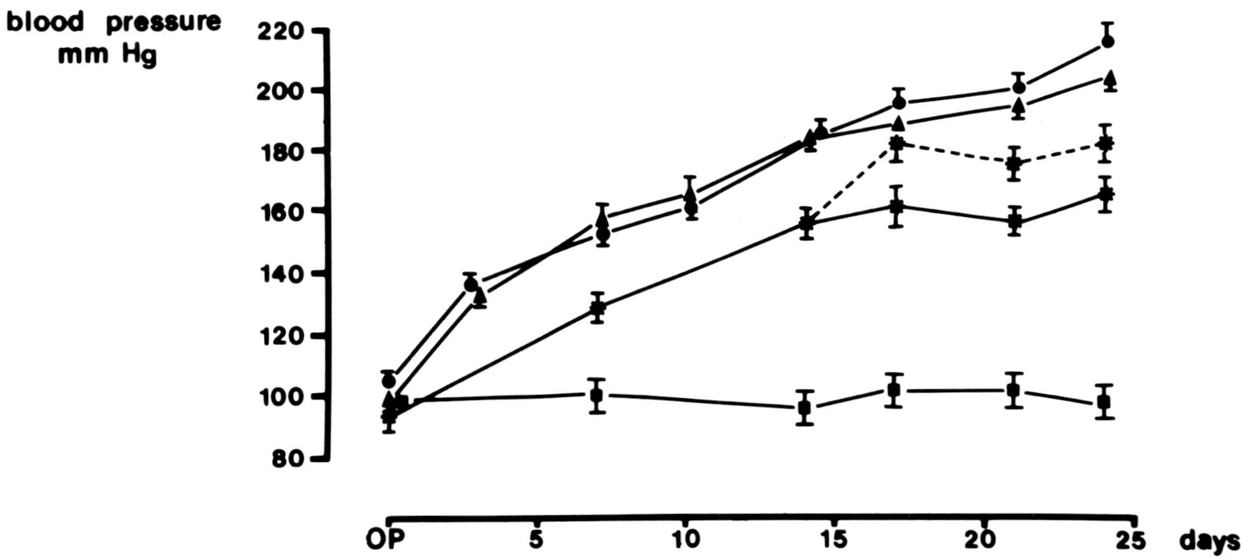

FIG. 1. Blood-pressure curves of the rats of groups A to D. Points are mean values with standard errors indicated by vertical lines. Group A: sham-operated controls (■—■); group B: unilateral renal artery stenosis in the presence of an untouched contralateral kidney (★—★); group C: unilateral nephrectomy and stenosis of the remaining renal artery (●—●); group D: bilateral renal artery stenosis (▲—▲). On the 14th day of the experiment, group B was subdivided into B_b and B_m.

Table 1.

GROUP	n	PCV %	Na^+ $mEq \cdot l^{-1}$	K^+ $mEq \cdot l^{-1}$	Urea $mmol \cdot l^{-1}$	AII $pg \cdot ml^{-1}$
A	10	45.7 ± 0.3	143.4 ± 0.5	4.09 ± 0.07	5.6 ± 0.2	112.4 ± 11.8
B_b	7	47.9** ± 0.6	143.6 ± 0.6	3.60*** ± 0.06	6.0 ± 0.2	221.9** ± 25.7
B_m	15	51.0*** ± 0.7	138.5*** ± 1.3	3.60*** ± 0.07	12.0*** ± 0.8	425.6*** ± 61.2
C	10	43.0** ± 0.7	143.7 ± 3.1	3.99 ± 0.10	6.9* ± 0.3	151.1 ± 21.5
D	10	42.6** ± 0.9	145.1 ± 1.1	3.88* ± 0.01	6.3* ± 0.2	177.2 ± 32.7

Packed cell volume (PCV), plasma sodium and potassium concentrations, serum urea and plasma angiotensin II (A II) concentrations in rats of groups A to D at the end of the experimental period. Values are means, with standard errors.

Group A – Controls (sham-operated)
Group B_b – Left renal artery stenosis, benign course
B_m – Left renal artery stenosis, malignant course
Group C – Left renal artery stenosis, right nephrectomy
Group D – Bilateral renal artery stenosis

n: Number of rats. The level of significance is indicated: $^*p < 0.05$; $^{**}p < 0.01$; $^{***}p < 0.001$ as compared with normotensive controls of group A.

contralateral kidney. On the other hand, excessive high blood pressure as such may induce severe lesions of the arterial and arteriolar wall in various vascular beds, such as that of the mesenteric artery, the heart or the brain, which are characteristic of the malignant type of hypertension.

Correction of Renal Artery Stenosis

Removal of the clip from the renal artery in the presence of an untouched contralateral kidney may result in a fall of blood pressure. The immediate effects of declamping on blood pressure, renal function and the renin-angiotensin system were studied in rats with hypertension induced by either unilateral (group 1) or bilateral (group 2) renal artery stenosis. In an additional group with bilateral renal artery stenosis, the ureter of the declamped kidney was ligated immediately after the clip had been removed (group 3). The animals were placed into individual cages and after the operation were deprived of food and water for six hours (Fig. 2). In all three experimental groups, the removal of one clip caused a similar fall in blood pressure of about 90 mm Hg. Urine volume and urinary sodium excretion increased in groups 1 and 2, but not in the rats in which the ureter of the declamped kidney was ligated. The increase in urine volume and sodium excretion was much more pronounced in the rats in which the contralateral renal artery remained clamped. Under these conditions, also the activity of the renin-angiotensin system was markedly stimulated, whereas it was reduced to normal after the removal of the sole clip (Figs. 3 and 4).

In rats with unilateral renal artery stenosis, a positive correlation between plasma angiotensin II concentration and serum urea was calculated ($r = 0.97$), whereas an inverse relationship existed between angiotensin II concentration and urine volume ($r = -0.79$) (Fig. 5). When the clip was removed, these relationships became less distinct, together with the reduction in activity of the renin-angiotensin system. In rats with bilateral renal artery stenosis, no correlation was demonstrable between plasma angiotensin II concentration and serum urea, but when one renal artery was declamped, serum urea concentration rose simultaneously with the increase in plasma angiotensin concentration, and a correlation became apparent ($r = 0.60$). It may be assumed that an elevated concentration of plasma angiotensin II may reduce glomerular filtration rate and urine output, and, as a consequence, serum urea may rise. However, in both experimental groups, no correlation was observed between the fall in blood pressure and the excretion of salt and water. An increased packed cell volume and a reduced plasma sodium concentration indicated the decrease in extracellular fluid volume under these experimental conditions (Fig. 6).

No satisfactory explanation can be given for the similar fall of blood pressure in all three groups of rats. Neither the reduction in the activity of the renin-angiotensin system nor the loss of sodium was correlated with the fall of blood pressure

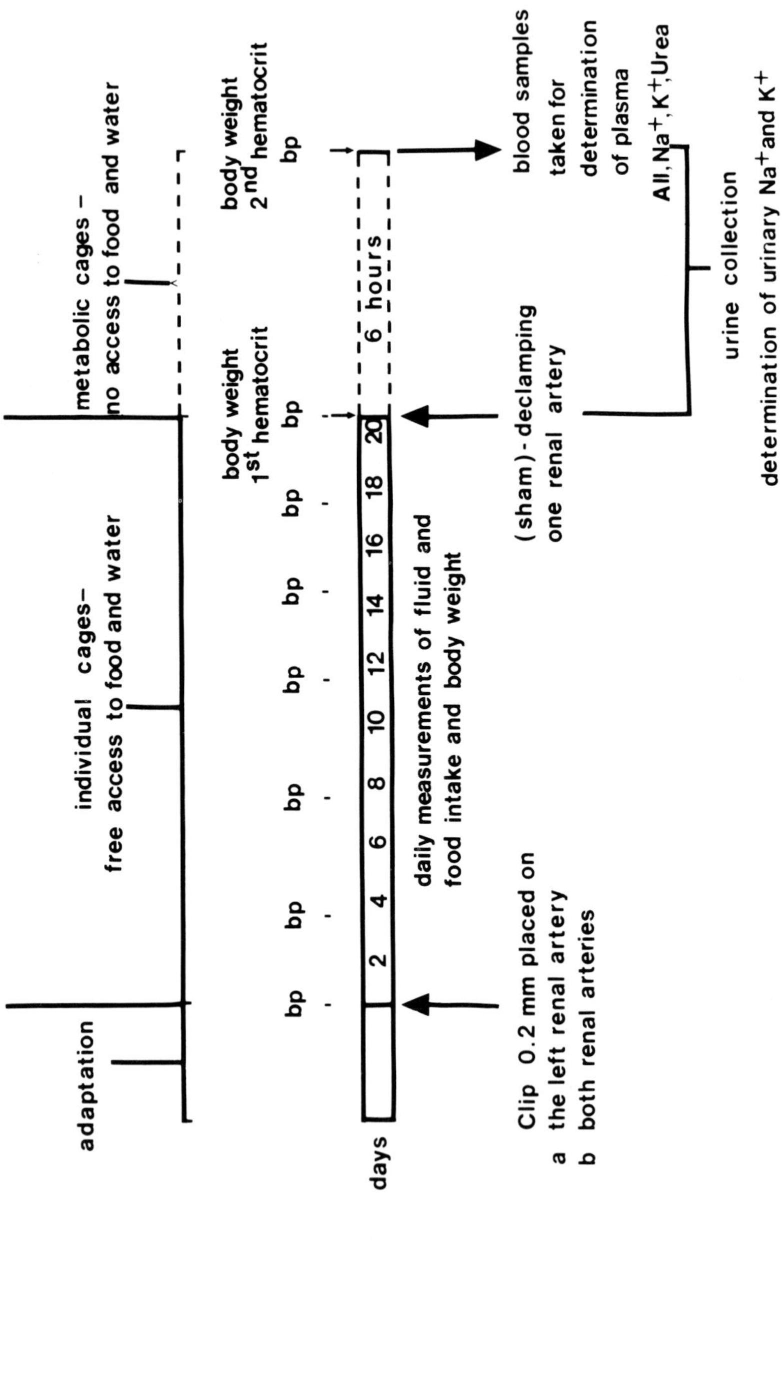

FIG. 2. Experimental protocol.

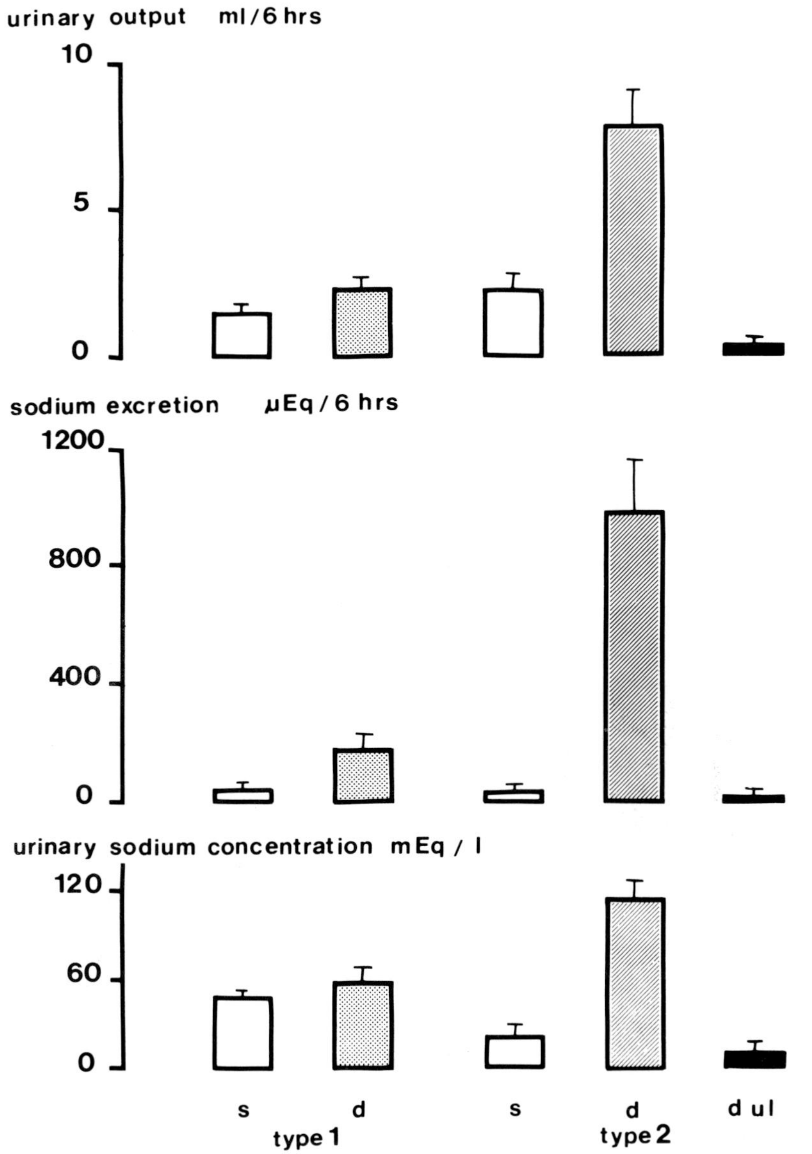

FIG. 3. Urine volume, urinary sodium excretion and urinary sodium concentration in all groups. Type 1: Rats with one renal artery stenosis and an untouched contralateral kidney. Type 2: Rats with bilateral renal artery stenosis. s: sham-declamped; d: declamped; d ul: declamped, ureter ligated.

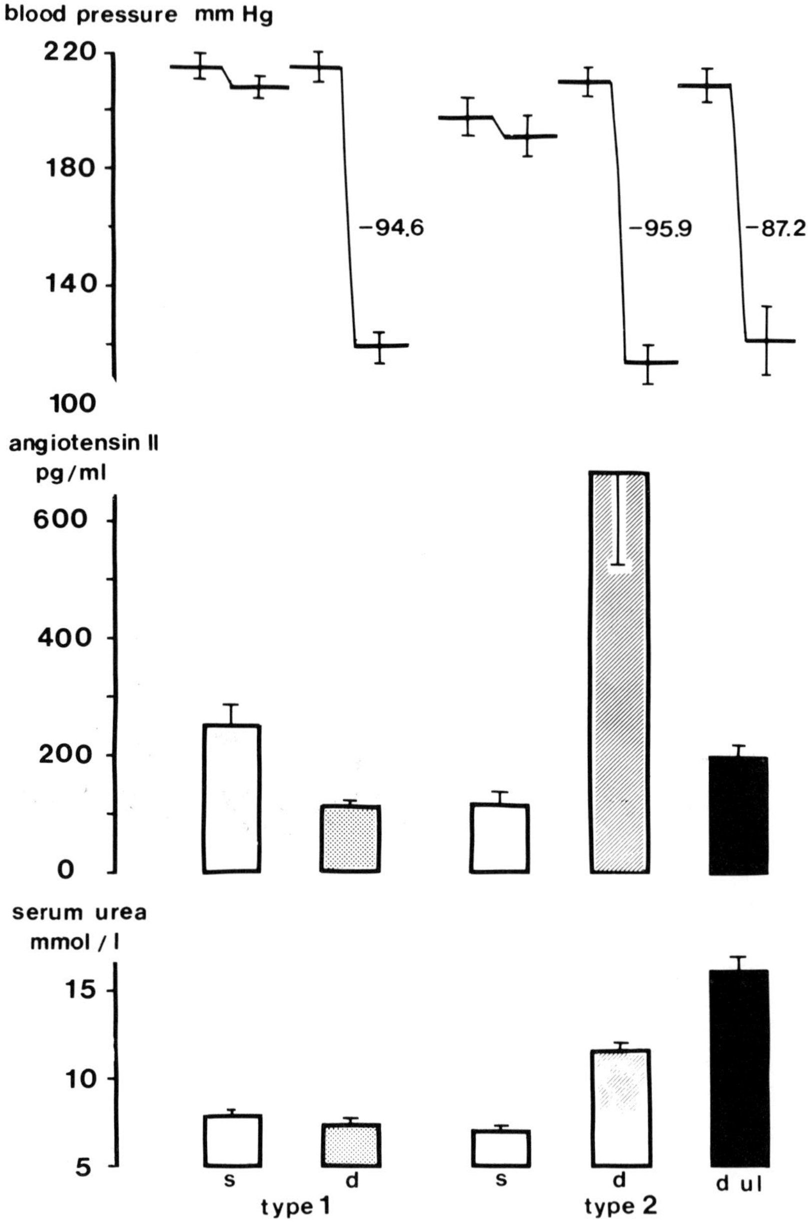

FIG. 4. Blood pressure, plasma angiotensin II concentration and serum urea before and after removal of one renal artery stenosis. Groups correspond to those in Figure 3.

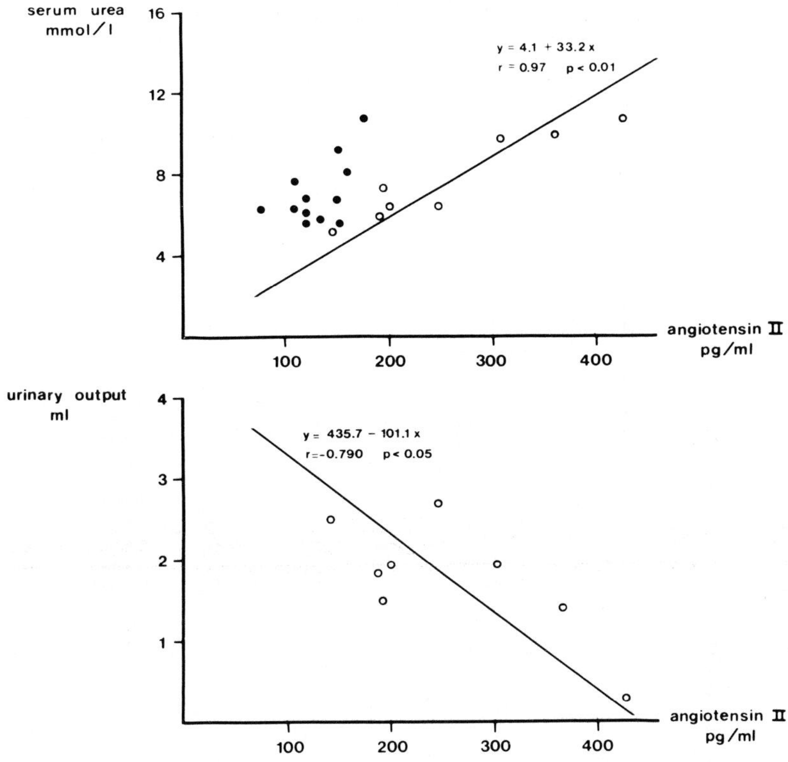

FIG. 5. Relationship between plasma angiotensin II concentration and serum urea (above) and between plasma angiotensin II concentration and urine output (below) in rats with one renal artery stenosis and an untouched contralateral kidney. Circles: sham-declamped; filled circles: declamped.

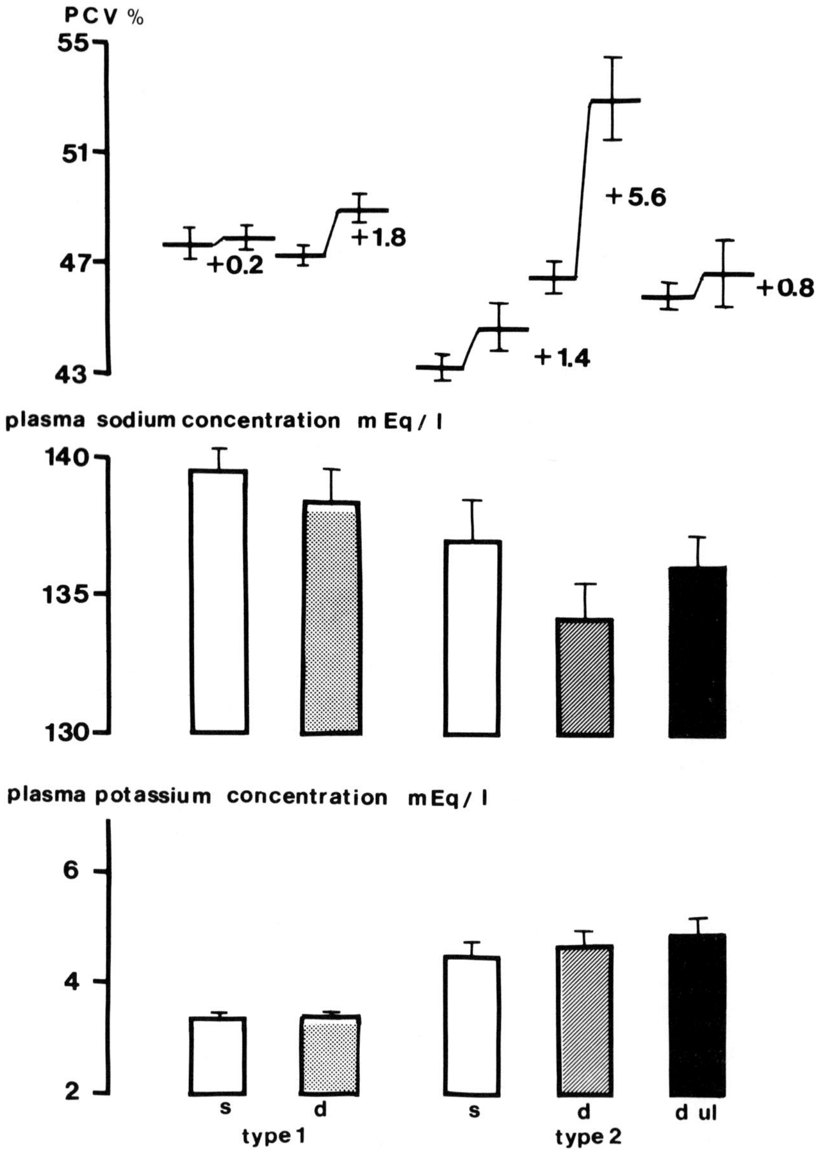

FIG. 6. Packed cell volume (PCV), plasma sodium and potassium concentrations before and after removal of one renal artery stenosis. Groups correspond to those in Figure 3.

within the observation period of six hours. Other investigators reported contradictory results; they observed a close relationship between the fall in blood pressure and the loss of salt and water during a 24-hour period after the removal of the sole clip in unilaterally nephrectomized rats [9].

When, in a hypertensive rat, the clip is removed from one renal artery, the vascular bed is suddenly exposed to a higher pressure, whereby the degree of the pressure increase depends upon the gradient between the pre- and poststenotic pressure. The larger this difference, the more pronounced will be the pressure increase in the renal vascular bed after the removal of the clip. Within 30 minutes after declamping, some vascular damage was demonstrable if either peroxidase or ferritin was injected intravenously as marker. Both the enzyme and the iron-protein compound, which has a much larger molecular weight (about 450.000) than peroxidase (about 40.000), were deposited in the walls of small arteries and arterioles in the declamped kidney. The deposition became more marked during the following hours, and, after 42 hours, severe morphological lesions in the form of fibrinoid necrosis and perivascular infiltrations were seen. Hence, it must be supposed that the sudden exposure of the renal vascular bed to high blood pressure induces severe arteriolar damage, which is not prevented by the subsequent fall in blood pressure. It seems that a relatively short exposure to high blood pressure causes arteriolar lesions, especially if the vascular wall is not gradually but suddenly subjected to the increase in pressure. This observation corresponds to findings after the administration of high doses of pressor agents [1].

After unilateral declamping, the rapid fall is followed by a slow rise in blood pressure, which either will reach the level of the hypertensive controls, which have not been declamped, or will remain on somewhat reduced values, provided the period of observation is extended to about two weeks. The individual response to declamping differs widely, and so does the remounting of pressure during the period afterwards. Some animals may develop an acute malignant phase, with negative sodium balance due to increased excretion by the declamped kidney, whereas others may maintain an equilibrated sodium and water balance, despite the fact that their blood pressure rises to high levels. In a group of rats that had hypertension caused by bilateral clamping of the renal arteries, the declamping of one kidney resulted in the development of an acute malignant phase of hypertension in 11 of 16 rats during an observation period of two weeks. These rats had only water to drink, but if, in addition, a 2% saline solution was offered, only five of 14 rats showed symptoms of an acute malignant phase. Although the offering of saline could not prevent the development of an acute malignant phase, it reduced its frequency, and the general condition of the animals that had the possibility of drinking saline was better than that of the rats that had water only.

Antihypertensive Drugs

In the renin-dependent forms of malignant hypertension, the administration of either saralasin [10] or converting enzyme inhibitors [11], of pepstatin (Lazar, personal communication) or antirenin [12] may lower the blood pressure. However, such an antihypertensive effect is restricted to the period of administration of these substances, which are therefore useful for diagnostic purposes, but hardly as therapeutic agents. Beta-adrenergic blockers have themselves only little or no effect in experimental renal hypertension, but may be more effective if they are administered together with a diuretic. However, such a combined treatment is not a specific measure against malignant hypertension. It must be stressed that it may even be dangerous to administer diuretics during the acute malignant phase caused by negative sodium balance, since more sodium and water will be lost and the renin-angiotensin system will be further stimulated. Although the vasoconstrictor response to angiotensin is reduced in animals with negative sodium balance [13], it has been demonstrated that under these conditions the renin-angiotensin system may contribute to the maintenance of high blood pressure [14].

In renal hypertensive rats, some reduction in blood pressure was obtained when a diuretic (chlorthalidone) was added to propranolol. Either of the drugs, given alone, exerts little or no effect on the high blood pressure (Fig. 7).

In conclusion, we may say that of the various measures that affect malignant hypertension (a) salt supply is indicated only

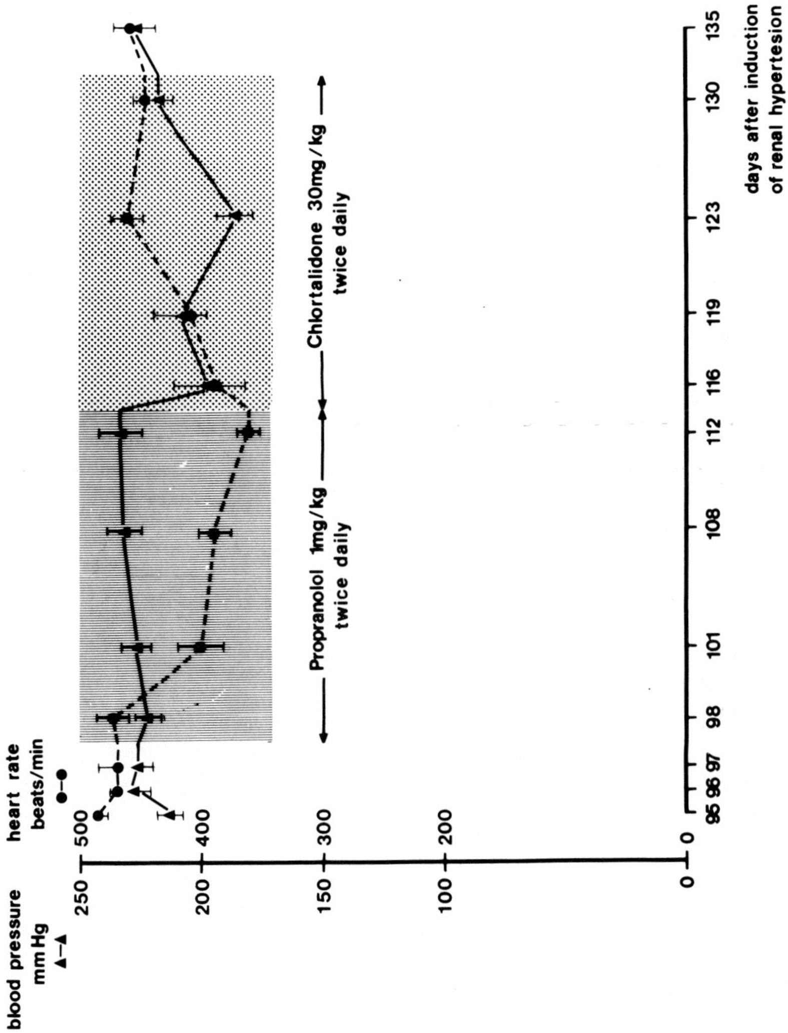

FIG. 7. Effects of propranolol and chlorthalidone on blood pressure and heart rate in rats with renal hypertension due to bilateral renal artery stenosis. n: 9.

in a limited number of cases, in which a negative sodium balance is demonstrable; (b) correction of the renal artery stenosis by removal of the clip has to avoid the sudden exposure of the renal vascular bed to high pressure levels; (c) inhibitors or antagonists interfering with the renin-angiotensin system are useful diagnostic tools in renin-dependent forms of hypertension, but their therapeutic value is very limited; (d) antihypertensive drugs induce a nonspecific fall in high blood pressure; they may control various forms of malignant hypertension, independent of their pathogenesis. Progress of arterial damage may be prevented by an effective reduction of pressure and, in addition, repair of vascular lesions may be favored, at least to a certain degree.

Acknowledgments

The studies were supported in part by the German Research Foundation within the SFB 90, "Cardiovasculäres System."

We are grateful to Mrs. K. König-Garbade and Miss B. Kurzenhäuser for their technical assistance and to Mr. J. Hollatz for drawing the graphs.

References

1. Giese, J.: The Pathogenesis of Hypertensive Vascular Disease, thesis. Munksgaard, Copenhagen, 1966.
2. Byrom, F.B.: The Hypertensive Vascular Crisis. An Experimental Study. London:W. Heinemann Medical Books Limited, 1969.
3. Selye, H., Hall, C.E. and Rowley, E.M.: Malignant hypertension produced by treatment with desoxycorticosterone acetate and sodium chloride. Canad. Med. Ass. J. 49:88-92, 1943.
4. Gavras, H., Brunner, H.R., Laragh, J.H. et al: Malignant hypertension resulting from deoxycorticosterone acetate and salt excess. Role of renin and sodium in vascular changes. Circ. Res. 36:300-309, 1975.
5. Dauda, G., Möhring, J., Hofbauer, K.G. et al: The vicious circle in acute malignant hypertension of rats. Clin. Sci. Molec. Med. 45 (suppl. 1):251-255, 1973.
6. Möhring, J., Möhring, B., Näumann, H.-J. et al: Salt and water balance and renin activity in renal hypertension of rats. Am. J. Physiol. 228:1847-1855, 1975.
7. Dietz, R., Mast, G.J., Möhring, J. et al: Aldosterone and corticosterone production in renal hypertensive rats. Acta Endocrinol. 79:317-328, 1975.

8. Gross, F., Dietz, R., Mast, G.J. et al: Salt loss as a possible mechanism eliciting an acute malignant phase in renal hypertensive rats. Clin. Exp. Pharmacol. Physiol. 2:323-333, 1975.
9. Liard, J.F.: Sodium retention versus renin-angiotensin system in experimental renal hypertension. Canad. J. Physiol. Pharmacol. 51:238-241, 1973.
10. Brunner, H.R., Kirshman, J.D., Sealey, J.E. et al: Hypertension of renal origin: Evidence for two different mechanisms. Science 174:1344-1346, 1971.
11. Gavras, H., Brunner, H.R., Gavras, I. et al: Hypotensive effect of angiotensin-converting-enzyme inhibitor SQ 20,881. Lancet 2:353, 1974.
12. Romero, J.C., Hoobler, S.W., Kozak, T.J. et al: Effect of antirenin on blood pressure of rabbits with experimental renal hypertension. Am. J. Physiol. 225:810-817, 1973.
13. Bock, K.D. and Gross, F.: Abschwächung pressorischer Wirkungen durch Sali-Diuretica. Naunyn Schmiedeberg Arch. Exp. Path. 238:339-347, 1960.
14. Gavras, H., Brunner, H.R., Vaughan, E.D.,Jr. et al: Angiotensin-sodium interaction in blood pressure. Maintenance of renal hypertensive and normotensive rats. Science 180:1369-1372, 1973.

The Effects of Antihypertensive Treatment on the Kidney

Priscilla Kincaid-Smith, M.D., F.R.A.C.P., F.R.C.P., D.C.P.

When antihypertensive drugs first became available 25 years ago, the most dramatic clinical effect was the reduction in mortality of malignant hypertension in treated patients. Uremia was the major cause of death in untreated malignant hypertension and the kidneys suffered the major "target organ" damage in patients with hypertension and papilledema [1]. The arrest of renal vascular lesions, which caused rapid deterioration in renal function, was largely responsible for the significant alteration in survival in patients with treated malignant hypertension [2].

In this paper the contrast between benign and malignant hypertension in terms of end-organ damage in the kidney and the effects of antihypertensive treatment on renal function and renal parenchymal damage are discussed and illustrated.

End-Organ Damage in the Kidney

Benign Nephrosclerosis

Despite the fact that some textbooks of pathology state that "small kidneys due to benign nephrosclerosis are found in three quarters of individuals over the age of 60" [3], this statement is not in keeping with more accurate studies and measurements of the kidney in patients with benign hypertension.

Priscilla Kincaid-Smith, M.D., F.R.A.C.P., F.R.C.P., D.C.P., University of Melbourne Department of Medicine and Department of Nephrology, The Royal Melbourne Hospital, Victoria, Australia.

Despite the fact that hypertension may be present in as many as 21% of people screened in population studies [4], Zollinger was able to identify the shrunken kidney of benign nephrosclerosis in only 13 cases in a series of 10,000 autopsies. The photograph which he published to illustrate this lesion was the kidney of an 82-year-old woman [5]. The kidney size reduces progressively over the age of 40 years [6]; therefore, normotensive persons of 80 to 90 may show considerable reduction in renal size. If benign hypertension causes significant reduction in renal parenchyma, this should be apparent at all ages however Zollinger stresses the rarity of lesions in young hypertensive subjects [5]. Among a consecutive series of 4,968 autopsies carried out at the Royal Postgraduate Medical School, the findings in the retina had been recorded shortly before death in 131 patients in whom a blood pressure above 180/110 mm Hg was recorded on two occasions. Patients with glomerulonephritis, pyelonephritis, renal artery stenosis or other renal causes of hypertension noted at the time of autopsy were excluded. These 131 patients included those with all grades of hypertensive retinopathy short of papilledema. The mean renal weights in these patients are shown in Table 1. The weights of right and left kidneys in these patients, in whom a diagnosis of benign hypertension had been based on accurate records of the blood pressure and retinal findings, were within normal limits.

These findings serve to emphasize the benign nature of hypertension without papilledema as far as target organ damage in the kidney is concerned. Renal function in patients with

Table 1. Renal Weights in Benign Essential Hypertension

4,968 Consecutive Autopsies

131 Patients Classified as Benign Hypertension (20-80 Years of Age)

1. Two records of BP 180/110 or higher.
2. Retinal examination – no hemorrhages or exudates.
3. No underlying renal disease specified in autopsy findings.

Mean Left Renal Weight	Mean Right Renal Weight
162.9 gm ± 46.9	159.7 gm ± 48.2

benign hypertension is normal in terms of the serum urea and creatinine levels, and on follow-up over many years no increase in blood urea or serum creatinine has been noted in patients with benign hypertension without underlying renal disease. Deterioration in renal function in patients presumed to have benign essential hypertension suggests an underlying renal lesion [7].

The most striking example of the relative immunity of the renal vasculature from the effects of benign hypertension was seen in an 86-year-old woman in whom records showed that diastolic blood pressures above 160 mm Hg had been recorded over a 20-year period. The interlobular arteries in this patient had similar lumen to that seen in normotensive patients in this age group (Fig. 1).

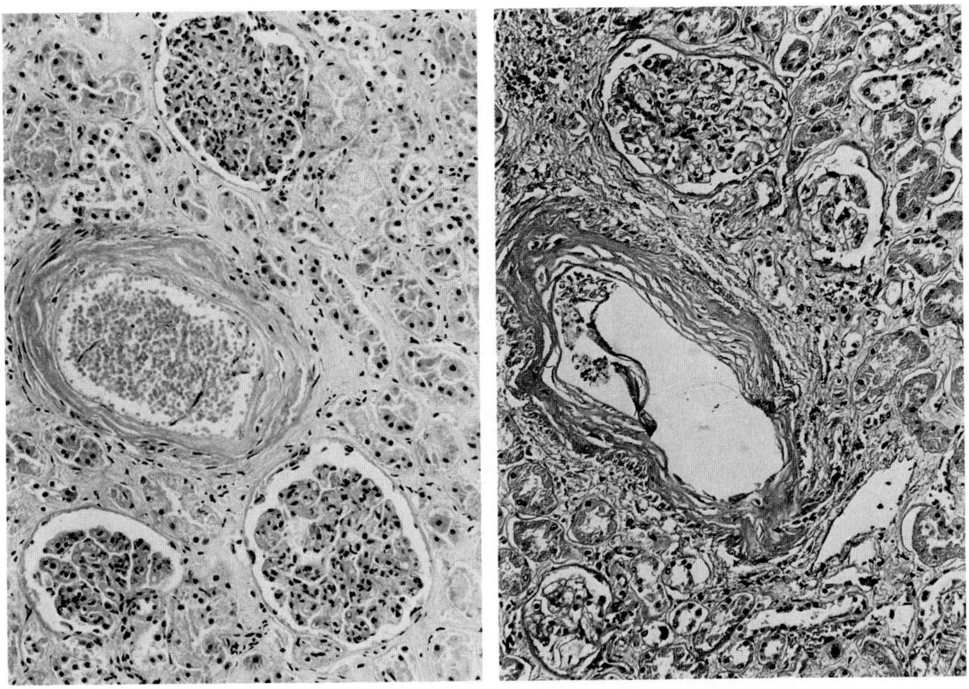

FIG. 1. *Left*, Interlobular artery from kidney of 86-year-old patient with diastolic blood pressure above 160 mm Hg for 20 years (hematoxylin and eosin x 112). *Right*, Interlobular artery from kidney of 92-year-old normotensive woman (Periodic acid Schiff x 112).

Malignant Hypertension

Because the effects of hypertension on the structure and function of the kidney are minimal in benign essential hypertension, the major impact of antihypertensive treatment on the kidney is seen in patients with malignant hypertension.

The fulminating and rapidly fatal course of untreated malignant hypertension was very largely due to uremia [1]. Even with the far from adequate blood pressure control which was possible in the early 1950s treatment of malignant hypertension brought about a dramatic and highly significant reduction in mortality [1].

The major factor which influenced the prognosis in patients with malignant hypertension was the degree of renal damage at the time at which treatment commenced. Patients with an initial blood urea above 60 mg% had a significantly shorter survival than those with a blood urea below 60 mg% [2]. Survival time in treated patients with a blood urea above 60 mg% did not differ significantly from that in untreated malignant hypertension.

A comparison of the above results between 1952 and 1959 and subsequent results in the same hypertension clinic by Breckenridge and his colleagues [8] showed that by 1967 there had been only a slight improvement in the survival of treated patients with malignant hypertension (Fig. 2). The 50% survival at four years is disappointing comparing unfavorably, for example, with the survival of 80% at four years in patients who have received cadaveric renal transplants [9].

Surprisingly, renal failure was still the major cause of death in patients reported by Breckenridge and his colleagues in 1970. Patients with malignant essential hypertension who die of renal failure do so within the first year, 90% dying within six months [1, 2].

Our recent experience suggests that newer methods of treating hypertension have probably altered the survival of patients who present with malignant hypertension and impaired renal function.

Figure 3 shows the serum creatinine levels in 16 patients with malignant essential hypertension who have presented to our clinic with impaired renal function since 1965 (blood urea above 60 mg%), whereas previous experience suggested all these

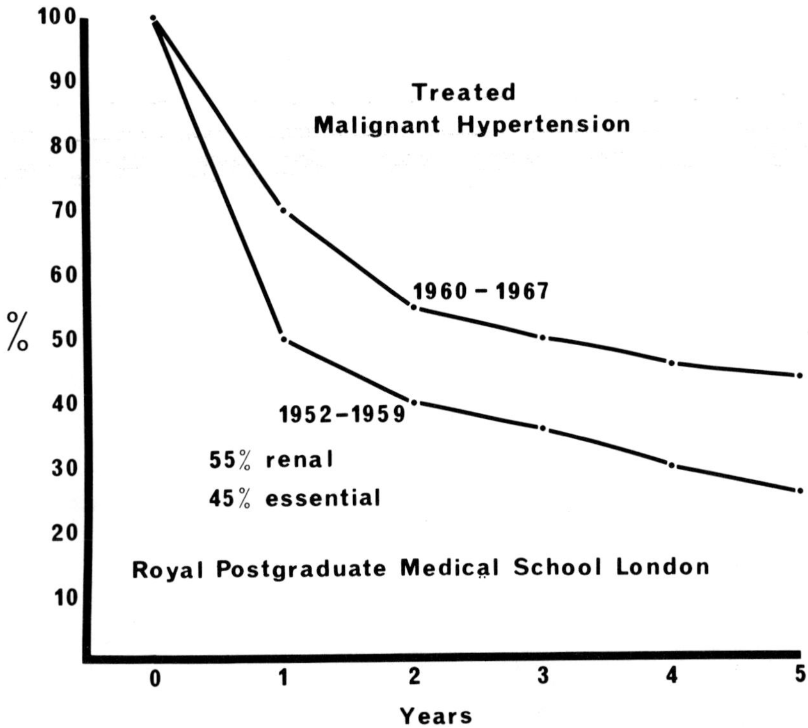

FIG. 2. Survival curves in patients with malignant hypertension treated at the Royal Postgraduate Medical School. (From Breckenridge et al [8].)

patients, even with treatment, should have died of uremia in one year [2], these 16 patients showed a gradual improvement in renal function. Renal function was severely impaired in three patients (serum creatinine levels .65-1.6 mmol/l) and one required initial treatment by dialysis (Fig. 4). Over the same period two patients with impaired renal function and malignant essential hypertension deteriorated to end-stage renal failure. Both had defaulted from the clinic and deterioration occurred during this period when the blood pressure was uncontrolled. Malignant essential hypertension is a rare cause of end-stage renal failure now that effective treatment is available (Table 2).

Care was taken to exclude patients with underlying renal disease such as glomerulonephritis or pyelonephritis and to include only those patients with malignant essential hyper-

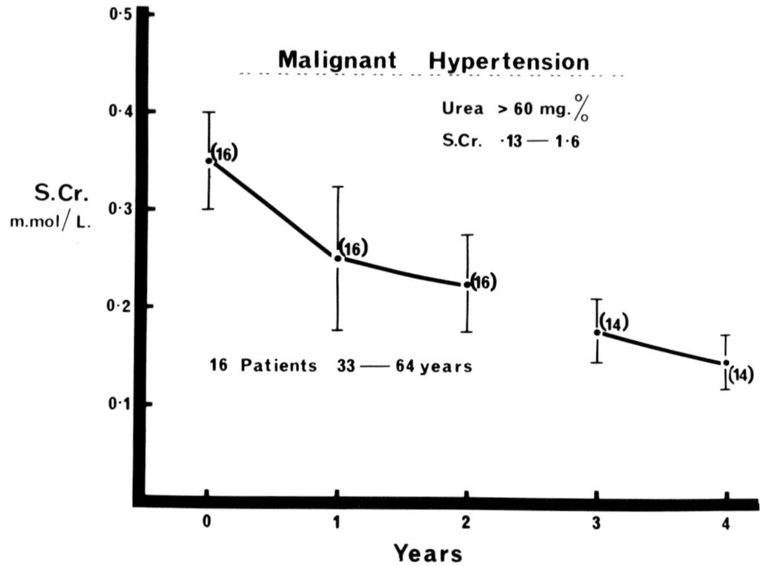

FIG. 3. Mean serum creatinine levels in 16 patients who presented with impaired renal function (serum creatinines 0.13-1.6 mmol/liter). Two of the patients were not followed for the four-year period. One whose course is graphed in Figure 4 died of a C.V.A. after 2½ years. The second is well, having presented with a serum creatinine of 8.6 mmol/liter. This is now .51 mmol/liter two years later (mean and standard deviations charted).

tension. Progression to renal failure was found to be more rapid in patients with malignant essential hypertension than in those with underlying renal disease in the earlier study [2] in which all patients with blood urea levels over 60 mg% and essential hypertension died within a year of diagnosis.

Morphological lesions in malignant hypertension. In contrast to the situation in benign hypertension in which no reduction in size could be demonstrated (Table 1), patients with malignant hypertension show a reduction in renal parenchyma. The mean combined weight of the two kidneys was 260 gm compared with a normal of approximately 320 mg [1].

The lesion in the renal parenchyma in malignant hypertension which causes reduction in size is the "partial infarction" or "ischemic tubular atrophy" which occurs in nephrons distal to severely narrowed interlobular arteries.

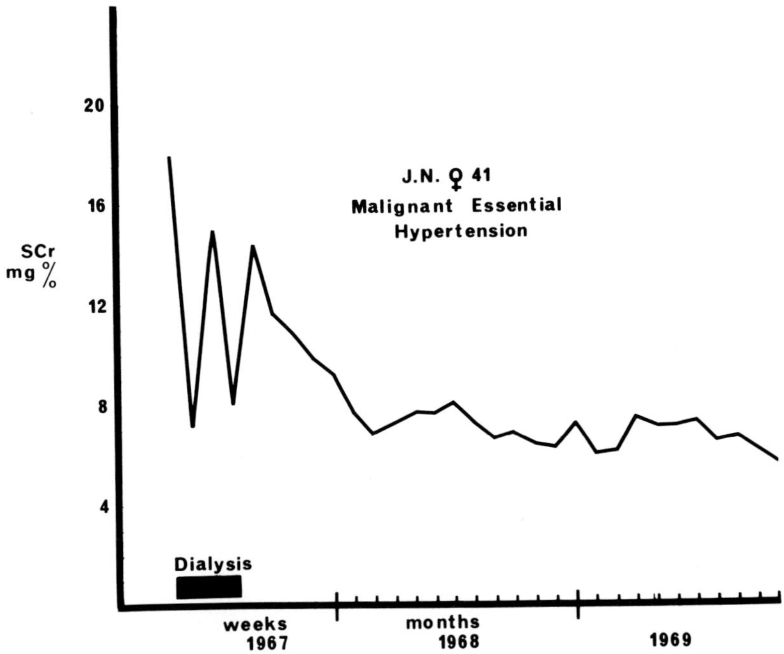

FIG. 4. Course of the patient with the most severe impairment of renal function included in the analysis in Figure 3. She required dialysis on several occasions at the time of presentation but thereafter gradually improved. Renal function was stable at 6 mg/100 ml when she died of a C.V.A. Sections from the kidney are shown in Figures 6 and 7.

Table 2. Cause of Renal Failure in Patients Admitted to Dialysis and Transplantation at Royal Melbourne Hospital, 1963-1972

	Patients	*Percent*
Glomerulonephritis	76	56.3
Atrophic pyelonephritis	25	18.5
Polycystic and medullary cystic	15	11.1
Essential hypertension	2	1.5
Analgesic nephropathy	1	0.7
Other specified	11	8.2
Total	130	

Of 144 cadaveric renal transplants, pathological diagnosis was known in 130 patients.

Interlobular arteries may show lesions ranging from almost total occlusion by the so-called onion layering in the intima to only minor degrees of intimal proliferation. It is the widening of the intimal layer and narrowing of the lumen in interlobular arteries (Fig. 5) which correlates with impairment of renal function. The fibrinoid necrosis in afferent arterioles which may extend into glomeruli is a patchy change and was not found to correlate with impaired renal function [1].

In the acute phase the lumen is narrowed by proliferation of cells within the intima, or by fibrin alone, or by a combination of the two (Fig. 5). In animals lesions ranging from large fibrin thrombi to marked narrowing by cellular intimal proliferation

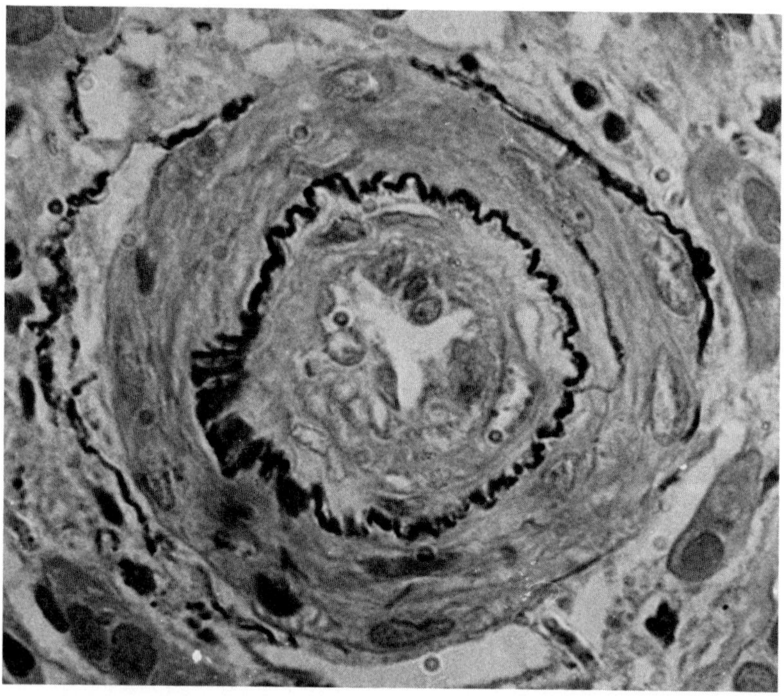

FIG. 5. Interlobular artery from a patient with a recent onset of malignant hypertension. The internal elastic lamina is single and the lumen is narrowed by a newly formed cellular layer which contained fibrinoid material on light microscopy (Weigert's elastic and von Gieson's stain x 900).

appear in interlobular arteries within days of the onset of malignant hypertension [10].

With treatment fibrinoid necrosis disappears in a few days and fibrin within glomeruli and afferent arterioles is replaced by hyaline material [2]. The extent of the narrowing in interlobular arteries determines the degree of impairment of renal function and this change in interlobular arteries does not disappear, it becomes converted from cellular layers which contain no collagen or elastic fibers to acellular fibrous and elastic layers, but the narrowing of the lumen persists [2] (Fig. 6).

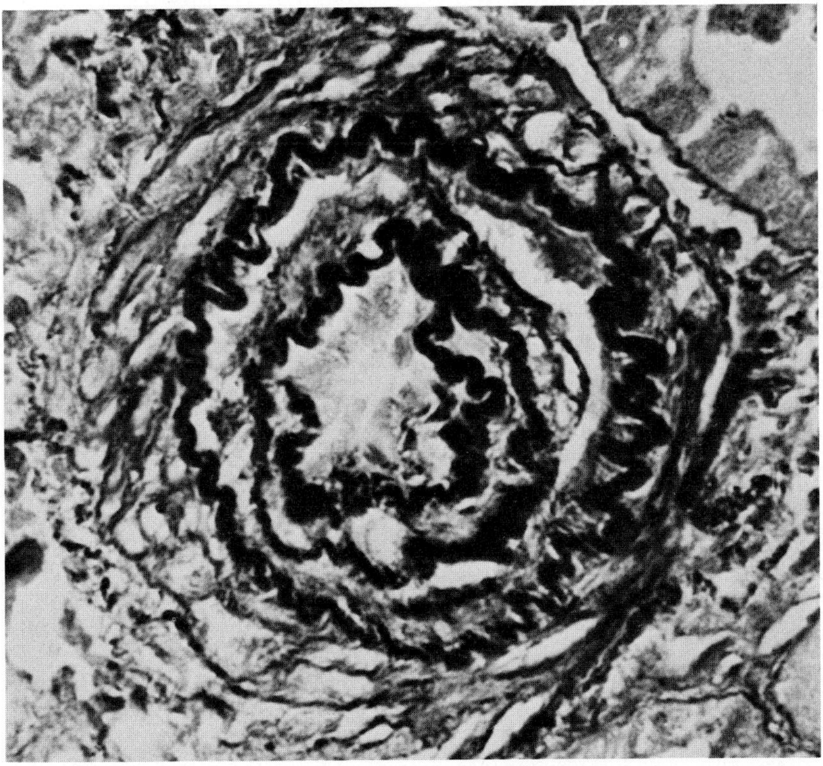

FIG. 6. Interlobular artery from a patient with malignant hypertension for three years. The lumen is now narrow by layers of collagen and elastic tissue (Weigert's elastic and von Gieson's stain x 900).

The gradual improvement in function which occurs over a period of months or years following control of hypertension in patients in whom renal function is impaired (Fig. 3) is due to hypertrophy of those nephrons supplied by interlobular arteries in which the narrowing is less marked.

Figures 7 and 8 show different areas from the kidney of the patient whose course is illustrated in Figure 4. In some areas total occlusion of interlobular arteries and extreme atrophy of related parenchyma were present. In other areas surviving nephrons were supplied by interlobular arteries which showed some narrowing and in other areas marked hypertrophy of nephrons distal to widely patent interlobular arteries was found.

Changes in therapeutic agents which may have contributed to the improved prognosis in patients with malignant hyper-

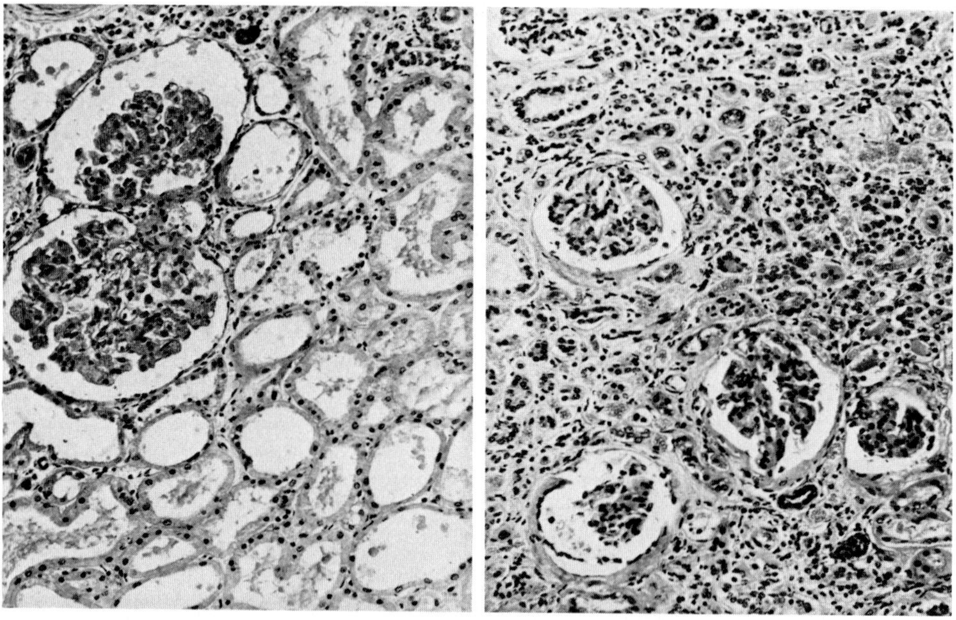

FIG. 7. *Left*, Area of renal cortex from kidney of patient whose course is graphed in Figure 4. This area was supplied by a widely patent interlobular artery (Fig. 8) and has undergone marked hypertrophy. *Right*, Area of renal parenchyma from the same kidney showing marked ischemic atrophy. The interlobular artery supplying this area showed marked narrowing by fibro-elastic layers (Fig. 8) (hematoxylin and eosin x 112).

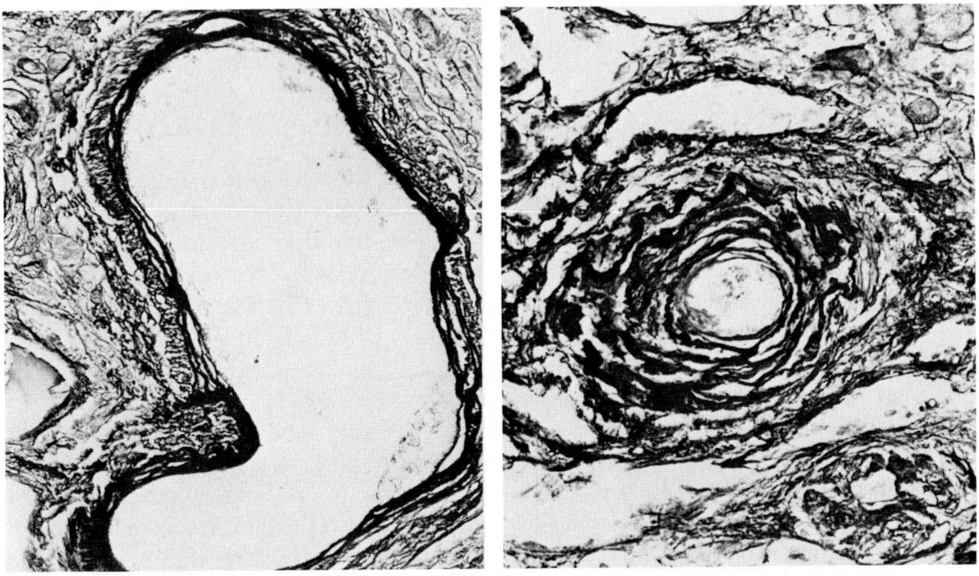

FIG. 8. *Left*, Widely patent interlobular artery supplying the hypertrophied area of cortex in Figure 7. *Right*, Marked narrowing of interlobular artery supplying ischemic area in Figure 7 (Weigert's elastic and von Gieson's stain x 112).

tension and impaired renal function. Between 1952 and 1959 the major agents used to control hypertension had been reserpine and ganglion blocking agents [1, 2]. Chlorothiazide only became available in 1958 and may have been a major factor contributing to the slightly improved results for the period 1960-1967 [8] (Fig. 2).

In the past five years the therapeutic regimes in hypertension have undergone further marked changes [11, 12]. Using a combination of beta-adrenergic blocking agent, a vasodilator such as prazosin or hydralazine and a thiazide, it is now possible to achieve good control of the blood pressure in most patients with little if any difference between the standing and lying blood pressures.

In patients with resistant hypertension in whom the blood pressure cannot be satisfactorily controlled by other means, oral diazoxide will achieve control. One of the striking features of oral diazoxide is its ability to control the lying blood pressure in patients in whom a considerable postural fall on standing had been present using other agents [11].

Conclusion

Hypertensive "target organ" damage in the kidney does not cause impairment of function or loss of renal parenchyma in benign hypertension. The loss of parenchyma in malignant hypertension and the fulminating progression to uremia in untreated malignant hypertension is due to narrowing in interlobular arteries. It is this change in the kidney and not fibrinoid necrosis in arterioles which correlates with impairment of function.

Control of the blood pressure in malignant hypertension arrests the progressive narrowing of interlobular arteries, but the degree of narrowing present when treatment is started persists.

Although the prognosis of patients with malignant essential hypertension and a blood urea over 60 mg% was very poor prior to 1959 this has altered. Whereas all such patients died within a year in the early study [2], renal function now gradually improves when the blood pressure is controlled (Fig. 3). This improvement in function may occur even in patients in whom the renal function shows marked impairment at the time of presentation. Hypertrophy of those areas of renal cortex which are supplied by patent interlobular arteries accompanies improvement in function. Areas supplied by severely narrowed interlobular arteries undergo further ischemic atrophy.

This improved survival in patients with malignant hypertension and impaired renal function has accompanied better blood pressure control achieved in both lying and standing positions with new therapeutic agents.

References

1. Kincaid-Smith, P., McMichael, J. and Murphy, E.A.: The clinical course and pathology of hypertension with papilloedema (malignant hypertension). Quart. J. Med. New Series 27:117, 1958.
2. Harington, M., Kincaid-Smith, P. and McMichael, J.: Results of treatment in malignant hypertension. A seven-year experience in 94 cases. Brit. Med. J. 2:969, 1959.
3. Robbins, S.L: Pathology, ed. 3. Philadelphia:Saunders, 1967, p. 1029.

4. Prineas, R.J., Stephens, W.B. and Lovell, R.R.H.: Blood pressure and its treatment in a community: The Albury blood pressure study. Med. J. Aust. 1:5, 1973.
5. Zollinger, H.: Niere und ableitende Harwege. *In* Doerr, W. and Vehlinger, E. (eds.): Spezielle Pathologische Anatomie Vol. III. Berlin:Springer-Verlag, 1966, p. 578.
6. Hodson, C.J.: Radiology of the kidney. *In* Black, D. (ed.): Renal Disease, ed. 3. Oxford:Blackwell Scientific Publications, 1972, pp. 213-249.
7. Kincaid-Smith, P.: The Kidney. A Clinicopathological Study. Oxford: Blackwell Scientific Publications, 1975, p. 214.
8. Breckenridge, A., Dollery, C.T. and Parry, E.H.O.: Prognosis of treated hypertension. Quart. J. Med. 39:411, 1970.
9. Mathew, T.H., Vikraman, P., Johnson, W. et al: Integrated programme of dialysis and renal transplantation. Results in 155 patients. Lancet 2:137, 1975
10. Kincaid-Smith, P.: The Kidney. A Clinicopathological Study. Oxford: Blackwell Scientific Publications, 1975, p. 258.
11. Kincaid-Smith, P., Fang, P. and Laver, M.C.: A new look at the treatment of severe hypertension. Clin. Sci. Molec. Med. 45 (suppl. 1):75, 1973.
12. Kincaid-Smith, P., Macdonald, I.M., Hua, A. et al: Changing concepts in the management of hypertension. Med. J. Aust. 1:327, 1975.

Discussion

Moderator: Dr. I. H. Page

Dr. Kaplan: I may have had trouble getting through Dr. Gross's maze of rats, but it appears that in the animals with a single clip, when the clip was removed, the other kidney's renin release system was suppressed and would not respond. In the human, even after prolonged suppression as with primary aldosteronism, the suppression of renin is presumably never permanent and with appropriate stimulation can respond.

To Dr. Kincaid-Smith: Perera's data on the natural history of essential hypertension showed that 7% of patients developed malignant hypertension. Why do you find it to be such a rare phenomenon these days; are we able to diagnose secondary causes more accurately or is it a consequence of antihypertensive therapy?

Dr. Gross: After taking away the single clip the renin-angiotensin system did not respond but this is an experiment of only six hours duration. Our aim in this type of experiment was to show that when one takes away a single clip then the renin-angiotensin system is suppressed, measured by plasma angiotensin II levels. When one takes one clip away and leaves the other kidney clipped then the renin-angiotensin system is much stimulated and angiotensin II levels go up, although we have a fall in blood pressure of about 90 mm Hg. In the first case plasma angiotensin level comes down and in the second case it goes up, but the fall in blood pressure is the same. After one day or two the renin-angiotensin system in the contralateral kidney becomes responsive also after removal of the single clip.

Dr. Page: Dr. Kincaid-Smith, do you want to answer the other part of this question?

Dr. Kincaid-Smith: I do not think I can answer the question. We tried to analyze the Hammersmith Hospital data, the population from which our malignant hypertensive patients were derived. They came from a fairly stable and defined area. We estimated that the percentage of patients who developed malignant hypertension was much lower than that estimated by Dr. Perera, namely, between 1% and 2%. There is no way in which I can give an estimate of how many patients in Melbourne with essential hypertension developed malignant hypertension. Our hospital would certainly draw a greater proportion of patients with renal disease because of our active dialysis and transplantation program. Certainly in our hospital 75% of patients with papilledema have underlying renal disease. I think the answer will come from population screening studies and I think that these may prove that malignant hypertension is less frequent now than it used to be.

Dr. Page: Don't you think that a lot depends upon the ethnic background of people? If you have a large black population you will probably get more.

Dr. Thurau: To Dr. Gross's paper: The dependency on sodium chloride raises a question about the intracellular mechanism. It is now becoming clear that many diuretics interfere with chloride transport in the kidney. Chloride transport, however, is linked with bicarbonate transport. Could it be that the dependency on sodium chloride finally reflects changes in intracellular bicarbonate or hydrogen? The second comment is about our recent observation showing that autoregulation is abolished following the removal of a clip from a clipped kidney.

Dr. Page: Does anybody have an answer to either question that Dr. Thurau asked? No.

Dr. Onesti: I would like to support the seemingly paradoxical effect of a high salt diet on severe renal hypertension in the rat. In rats with hypertension produced by ligation of the aorta between renal arteries, 1% NaCl solution as drinking water reduces significantly the blood pressure in the chronic phase (20 and 30 days after aortic constriction). High salt intake, however, has an effect on the onset of this hypertension (five to ten days after aortic constriction).

Dr. Doyle: I would just like to make a few points about Dr. Gross's paper because we have been doing some rather similar studies but using a different technique. The technique that we have been using differs, quite markedly, from his in that while he gives his rats sodium in the diet, we have been using a sodium

22 equilibration technique, a technique for looking at total exchangeable sodium in the rat. This involves giving a sodium-free diet as the solid food. When we do this, and when we clip one kidney, we find contrary to your data, that although the rats lose weight, although they develop polyuria and polydipsia, nevertheless the total body sodium actually increases very sharply. In spite of this, blood pressure becomes highly elevated, the renin levels go up, and we are left with a situation in which these rats lose weight, are sick, but do, in fact, have sharply raised exchangeable sodiums. In the single kidney model we find no change at all. The question I would like to put to you is your data, really, I think, are derived from animals taking a low salt diet because they are not eating and they are drinking water. We find that when we give animals, right from the start, saline to drink their blood pressures go up just the same as yours did. The belief that we have been formulating is that this effect on urinary output might, indeed, be an effect of the renin-angiotensin system. It might be partly the kind of increased sodium and water output that has been so well described by you in the rat and by us in man. I also wonder if it is not possibly a secondary phenomenon with polydipsia because under these circumstances if you have polydipsia the high renin levels increase free water clearance. This explanation might, in fact, account for both of them and it might not, in fact, be a pressure dependent naturesis at all.

Dr. Page: The question all of us who have treated malignant hypertension have is how much time should be allowed to elapse before vigorous treatment is instituted. I have always believed that this syndrome is a true medical emergency and time was of the essence. Renal excretory efficiency in the latter stages is lost very quickly. The longer the blood pressure remains at excessively high levels, the greater the risk of hypertensive encephalopathy. That is why I have preferred sodium nitroprusside because its hypotensive effect is immediate and the pressure can be accurately controlled.

Whether one is justified taking the time to learn whether a patient is salt deficient and needs to have saline administered seems to me doubtful. After the blood pressure has been brought to normal then, I would suggest, might be the time to measure plasma volume and sodium metabolism. The number of patients who might have a sodium deficit would probably be small. It would be interesting to have the opinion of this audience, since this is a symposium on treatment.

Dr. Kincaid-Smith: An opinion on the clinical side. There is a particular group of patients whom we see quite frequently in whom salt depletion is a prominent clinical feature. They may present with malignant hypertension and salt depletion. These are patients with renal papillary necrosis and theoretically there may be something special about their hypertension. Certainly salt depletion is part of it. Prostaglandin depletion may play a part in the acute hypertension. Among these patients a small number benefit from saline administration in terms of reduction of blood pressure.

Dr. Page: But you have administered saline to these people. How many, roughly, have you seen?

Dr. Kincaid-Smith: We have studied three, but Dr. Nanra in Newcastle, Australia, has studied a larger number. He has a manuscript in preparation but I have not actually seen the data.

Dr. Page: We have time for about two questions.

Dr. MacDonald: We have seen a similar situation, a malignant type of hypertension which seems to respond to saline. This, in patients who are undergoing dialysis.

Dr. Page: Wait a minute. I am not clear, these are patients who have malignant hypertension that are being dialyzed?

Dr. MacDonald: No. These are patients who have hypertension and chronic renal failure. During the course of removing extracellular volume, the blood pressure may attain diastolic levels of 120 to 140 mm Hg. These patients frequently develop headaches, confusion and a clinical picture similar to that seen in patients with encephalopathy. It has been our experience that these patients not infrequently will respond to an infusion of 200 or 300 ml of saline. In this syndrome some patients are quite predictable, developing it time after time.

Dr. Denton: I was interested in the experiments of Dr. Gross with DOC. You might recall that we described this phenomenon of natriuresis when one kidney is constricted and the other kept intact some years ago in *Endocrinology*. The chronology was that when you clamp one kidney and leave the other one intact with the rise in blood pressure there was a massive diuresis, negative sodium balance and, as well, a rise in renin and in aldosterone measured in peripheral blood. Aldosterone was very high so perhaps this was an instance when you were superimposing DOC on already maximum endogenously increased aldosterone because of the negative sodium balance. Have you done these experiments in adrenalectomized animals with a clip on the sole kidney and then produced negative sodium balance under those conditions? Second, in relation to your observations on appetite, have you observed in the single clip animal any decrease in hedonic sodium intake analogous to what Landis and colleagues have described from Harvard some 20 odd years ago?

Dr. Page: Did you say hedonic?

Dr. Denton: Yes.

Dr. Gross: It seems that some of the rats, when they get saline, like it and drink more than they really need to compensate the previous sodium loss. This is perhaps a consequence of the long-term deprivation of saline. Regarding your first question, the aldosterone secretion is high in these animals, but interestingly enough, also that of corticosterone is markedly elevated. When we give DOCA we certainly suppress the aldosterone production. The dose of 10 mg DOCA per day per rat may be so high as to favor the manifestation of vascular lesions. As to your second question, we have not worked on adrenalectomized rats.

Dr. Zanchetti: I would like to follow on the question raised by Dr. Page: how to deal with malignant hypertensive patients. I think this is a very important clinical problem. I am convinced that they are to be dealt with as an emergency but, however, that measurement of the hematocrit and possibly of plasma sodium and plasma volume, which can be done very quickly in most hospitals might provide some useful indication on the best way of managing these patients. While diuretic and sympatho-inhibitory agents are common indications, if some patients give signs of being dehydrated, then we should at least delay the use of diuretics in these patients.

Dr. Page: I think we want to keep in mind when we talk about this sort of thing that most of these patients are treated not in University hospitals but in homes or county hospitals. You have to be very careful in recommending measurements which are not readily available unless the patient is in the hands of a competent cardiologist. To me the main effort should be to get the blood pressure under cóntrol in a matter of minutes and then do the other less urgent diagnostic procedures.

Hemodynamic Changes During Acute and Chronic Administration of Thiazide Diuretics

Edward D. Freis, M.D.

The thiazide diuretics have become established as the drugs of first choice in the treatment of hypertension. While not entirely free of side effects, they are usually well tolerated by hypertensive patients. Dosage is fairly uniform from one patient to another because of the relatively flat dose response curve in the therapeutic range, a characteristic of these drugs which simplifies their administration in clinical practice. A further desirable quality of the thiazide diuretics is that they enhance the antihypertensive effects of other blood pressure reducing drugs such as alpha methyldopa, reserpine, clonidine, propranolol, guanethidine and hydralazine.

Mechanism of Action

Three main theories have been advanced to explain the antihypertensive effects of the thiazide diuretics. The first two have to do with the sodium-depleting effect, one that the hypotension results from a reduction in extracellular fluid volume (ECF) and the other that it is caused by a reduction in the salt and water content of the arterioles or in the concentration gradient of intracellular to extracellular sodium in arteriolar smooth muscle. The third theory, and the one most popularly accepted, is that the thiazides maintain their antihypertensive effects on chronic administration through a vasodilator action of the drug.

Edward D. Freis, M.D., Senior Medical Investigator, Veterans Administration Hospital, Professor of Medicine, Georgetown University, Washington, D.C.

A specific vasodilator action of chlorothiazide that was independent from its diuretic action was first proposed by Hollander, Chobanian and Wilkins [1]. They claimed that a fall in blood pressure occurred prior to a significant diuresis. This view was supported by the subsequent discovery by Rubin et al [2] of diazoxide, a vasodilator agent which is related chemically to the benzothiadiazine agents. Bartorelli et al [3] and Rose et al [4] found that diazoxide is a vasodilator antihypertensive agent which causes sodium retention.

The hemodynamic effects of diazoxide, however, and the mechanism by which it reduces blood pressure are quite different from the thiazide diuretics. Following intravenous diazoxide, reduction of blood pressure occurs immediately and is rather transient. By contrast, the thiazide diuretics have a delayed onset of antihypertensive action and a longer duration of effect. According to Rowe et al [4] diazoxide produces a reflex increase in heart rate and cardiac output and a considerable decrease in total peripheral resistance similar to that seen with other vasodilator drugs such as amyl nitrate or sodium nitroprusside. Crosley et al [5], Dustan et al [6] and Frohlich et al [7] found that the hemodynamic effects of the thiazides are quite different. Cardiac output decreases and total peripheral resistance increases.

The observations of Hollander et al [1] have not been confirmed. Freis [8], Dollery et al [9] and Macleod et al [10] found that the reduction of blood pressure occurred only after there had been a significant diuresis. Most investigators now agree that at least the acute antihypertensive effects of the thiazide diuretics are related to diuresis and consequent depletion of salt and water. Further support for this view has been provided by the observation that all drugs which can produce a similar degree of sodium loss will exert comparable antihypertensive effects such as parenteral mercurials as observed by Hollander et al [1] and ethacrynic acid as found by Conway and Leonetti [11]. Also, Murphy [12] and Watkin [13] have indicated that the reduction of blood pressure seen with the low sodium "rice diet" was associated with a significant reduction in ECF.

Following administration of the thiazide diuretics the blood pressure falls in association with a reduction in plasma volume and ECF. This has been demonstrated by a number of investigators including Tapia et al [14], Freis et al [15], Dollery et al [9], Winer [16], McQueen and Morrison [17] and Ronnov-Jessen [18]. Wilson and Freis [19] observed that patients given thiazides continuously lose about 2 liters of extracellular fluid included in which are 300 to 400 cc of plasma volume. The dehydration is mild, therefore, comprising about 10% of the extracellular fluid and about 15% of the plasma volume. Murphy [12] and Watkin [13] observed similar depletions in patients taking the rice diet.

According to Dustan et al [6], Dollery et al [9], McQueen and Morrison [17] and Freis [8], the antihypertensive effects of the thiazides can be reversed in many patients by reexpanding the plasma volume with salt-free dextran solution or, as Freis et al [15] and Winer [16] have shown, by administering large salt loads of 15 to 30 gm orally per day sufficient to cause a return of body weight.

Freis et al [20] demonstrated that patients whose sympathetic reflex responses have been depressed by ganglioplegic or other blocking drugs are extremely sensitive to even small degrees of blood volume reduction. Patients who are not receiving such drugs, while less sensitive than those who are, still will show a reduction of blood pressure with any procedure that reduces extracellular fluid volume including mercurials, thiazides as shown by Dustan et al [6] or salt-free diet. Freis et al [15] indicated that the only situation in which a reduction of blood pressure does not occur is in young normal subjects.

As shown by Wanko and Freis [21], thiazide diuretics, probably by reason of their volume-depleting action, enhance the blood pressure reducing effects of various depressor stimuli, whereas the blood pressure raising effects of pressor influences such as infusion of norepinephrine are depressed. Thus, volume depletion could work at least in part by blunting pressor stimuli and by amplifying the antihypertensive effects of depressor stimuli.

Another possible mechanism by which the relatively small decrement in total ECF may lower blood pressure involves the baroreceptor mechanism. Baroreceptor responsiveness depends upon the compliance of the aorta and carotid artery and these become less distensible with age and hypertension. Therefore, homeostatic adjustments to either depressor or pressor stimuli are not well moderated as was found by Finnerty et al [22] and by Hoobler [23]. In young normal adults given thiazides Freis et al [15] found that the blood pressure did not fall, but the heart rate became rapid indicating baroreceptor-induced compensation for the volume loss. However, Hoobler [23] found that older normotensive subjects fail to show such compensation and their blood pressure declines as in the hypertensive patient. The difference with age is consistent with the hypothesis that baroreceptor activity may play at least a partial role in the antihypertensive effect of the thiazide diuretics insofar as compensation for the volume depletion is not as effective in hypertensive or elderly individuals as it is in young normal subjects with more distensible large arteries.

The third possible way in which volume depletion may reduce blood pressure stems from experimental studies. The subject has been reviewed recently by Guyton [24]. Briefly, the findings have been that with either experimental renovascular hypertension, reduction in renal mass plus salt loading or excess licorice ingestion, the following series of events occur in sequence: (1) expansion of ECF, (2) increased venous pressure and venous return to the heart, (3) increased cardiac output, (4) rise in blood pressure and increase in urine volume with consequent reduction of the expanded ECF, (5) increased total peripheral resistance in response to the inappropriate rise in total blood flow (cardiac output), (6) return of cardiac output to normal, (7) maintenance of a new equilibrium wherein homeostasis of the ECF is maintained at the expense of an increased total peripheral resistance and blood pressure.

According to Guyton, the critical factor is the relationship between urine volume and blood pressure. Urine volume and sodium excretion rise with an increase in blood pressure which is the mechanism that the body uses in many instances where there is a chronic increase in ECF. The height to which the blood pressure rises will depend upon the intrinsic functional capacity of the kidney to handle volume loads which varies from one individual to another and which may also be a function of age. It would also depend upon other supportive mechanisms and their ability to reduce their activity. These other mechanisms include the renin-angiotensin-aldosterone system, the sympathetic nerve supply to the kidney and the ADH mechanism. By reducing ECF, diuretics produce a reversal of the changes seen in experimental hypertension, that is, a fall in cardiac output as was seen by Rowe et al [4], Dustan et al [6] and Frohlich et al [7] after acute administration and a decrease in total peripheral resistance after chronic treatment as was seen by Conway and Lauwers [25] although the latter observation has not been confirmed.

To recapitulate, three possible mechanisms are proposed to explain why the diuretic-induced reduction in extracellular fluid and plasma volumes could lower blood pressure. The mechanisms are (1) decreased responsiveness to pressor stimuli and increased responsiveness to depressor influences; (2) poorly modulated depressor effects of extracellular and plasma volume reduction because of impaired baroreceptor activity in hypertensive patients and (3) effect of volume depletion on hemodynamics including reduced cardiac output. Also, because of the diuresis the blood pressure-urine volume relationship changes permitting the kidney to maintain ECF homeostasis at lower levels of blood pressure.

There has been much discussion concerning the difference between the short-term and long-term effects of thiazides. This has stemmed from the work of Conway and Lauwers [25] who observed plasma and ECF reductions in the first week of treatment with chlorothiazide but not after one month of continuous treatment. They also found an initial fall but then a return to normal of cardiac output after one month of treatment. Strangely, body weight remained reduced during long-term treatment and to explain this they postulated a shift of fluid from the intracellular to the extracellular compartment.

Although their observations have been widely accepted to indicate that the thiazides reduce blood pressure over the long term because of a vasodilator effect, other investigators have failed to corroborate their findings. Wilson and Freis [19] found after six months of continuous treatment with chlorothiazide that ECF remained significantly reduced ($p < 0.01$). Plasma volume also was reduced but not significantly at six months but was reduced significantly ($p < 0.05$) at 12 months. They also found no dichotomy between reductions in body weight and ECF during long-term treatment. Finally, they observed that withdrawal of chlorothiazide after long-term treatment resulted in a prompt and significant rise of plasma volume, ECF, blood pressure and body weight indicating that the treatment still was effective in reducing volume.

More recent studies have fully confirmed the observations of Wilson and Freis on the long-term maintenance of volume depletion with thiazides. Both Tarazi et al [26] and Leth [27] found a continued reduction of plasma volume and ECF during long-term treatment with thiazides, and Tarazi observed a sharp rebound in these volumes when the thiazides were discontinued.

Further evidence for the overriding importance of the ECF in the chronic antihypertensive effect of thiazides is indicated by the studies of Winer [16] who after one month of treatment with hydrochlorothiazide added 10 gm of salt in tablet form daily to the already ad lib salt diet, a total of close to 30 gm/day. This was followed by a return of body weight and blood pressure to approximate control levels despite continued thiazide treatment. Winer's experiment provides strong evidence that the long-term antihypertensive effect of the thiazide diuretics depends upon a reduced ECF rather than any presumed vasodilator effect. Thus, the concept of a dual mechanism of action for the thiazide diuretics has no basis in fact. Rather, the evidence indicates that the antihypertensive action of these agents is the same during both short-term and long-term treatment, namely, it is dependent upon a continued reduction in volume.

The observations of Conway and Lauwers [25] that cardiac output returns to normal during long-term therapy has been confirmed by Lund-Johansen [28]. Preliminary studies in this laboratory by Shah and Freis (unpublished) also have shown that the cardiac output measured in eight patients decreased initially and remained somewhat reduced after eight weeks of treatment with hydrochlorothiazide. Total peripheral resistance was decreased at eight weeks. It has been noted with other types of antihypertensive agents that cardiac output tends to revert toward the pretreatment value during continued treatment. For example, Villarreal et al [29] found that the decrease in cardiac output seen initially with guanethidine rose toward normal with long-term treatment. Also, Reubi [30] observed that hydralazine initially increases cardiac output which later returns toward normal during long-term therapy. Instead of searching for an alteration in fundamental drug action with time it would seem preferable to investigate the nature of the autoregulatory changes which might cause a return of cardiac output toward normal with time regardless of the type of agent used.

Summary

In contrast to prevailing opinion, the evidence available today indicates that there is no essential difference between the mechanisms that initiate and maintain the antihypertensive effect of acute and chronic therapy with thiazide diuretics. There is no valid evidence for a direct vasodilator effect of the thiazide diuretics. The lowering of blood pressure seen during both acute and chronic administration of the thiazide diuretics is associated with a reduction of ECF.

Recent studies in experimental forms of hypertension indicate that it is the expansion of ECF and the resulting increased volume load on the kidney which is the crucial initiating factor in a series of events leading to an elevation of blood pressure. Thus, hypertension seems to be a mechanism in maintaining homeostasis of the ECF. It is suggested that thiazides along with other potent natriuretic agents permit the kidney to excrete the volume load at a lower level of blood pressure. A related antihypertensive treatment is the severely restricted low-salt diet which also results in reduced ECF and a consequent lowering of blood pressure.

References

1. Hollander, W. et al: Studies on the antihypertensive action of chlorothiazide. Clin. Res. 6:21, 1958.
2. Rubin, A.A. et al: Pharmacology of diazoxide, an antihypertensive, nondiuretic benzothiadiazine. J. Pharmacol. Exp. Ther. 136:344, 1962.
3. Bartorelli, C. et al: Hypotensive and renal effects of diazoxide, a sodium-retaining benzothiadiazine compound. Circulation 27:895, 1963.
4. Rowe, G.G. et al: The systemic and coronary hemodynamic effects of diazoxide. Am. Heart J. 66:636, 1963.
5. Crosley, A.P. Jr. et al: The acute effects of carbonic anhydrase inhibition on systemic hemodynamics. J. Clin. Invest. 37:887, 1958.

6. Dustan, H.P. et al: A mechanism of chlorothiazide-enhanced effectiveness of antihypertensive ganglioplegic drugs. Circulation 19:360, 1959.
7. Frohlich, E.D. et al: Hemodynamic alterations in hypertensive patients due to chlorothiazide. N. Engl. J. Med. 262:1261, 1960.
8. Freis, E.D.: The effects of salt and extracellular fluid depletion on vascular responsiveness with particular reference to chlorothiazide. *In* Skelton, F.R. (ed.): Hypertension, Proceedings Council High Blood Pressure Research, November 1958. New York:American Heart Association, 1959.
9. Dollery, C.T., Harrington, M. and Kaufman, G.: The mode of action of chlorothiazide in hypertension: With special reference to potentiation of ganglion-blocking agents. Lancet 1:1215, 1959.
10. Macleod, C. et al: Sequential changes evoked by chlorothiazide in hypertensive patients. Arch. Intern. Med. 106:316, 1960.
11. Conway, J. and Leonetti, G.: Hypotensive effect of ethacrynic acid. Circulation 31:661, 1965.
12. Murphy, R.J.F.: The effect of "rice diet" on plasma volume and extracellular fluid space in hypertensive subjects. J. Clin. Invest. 29:912, 1950.
13. Watkin, D.M. et al: Effects of diet in essential hypertension. II. Results with unmodified Kempner rice diet in fifty hospitalized patients. Am. J. Med. 9:441, 1950.
14. Tapia, F.A. et al: Enhanced effectiveness of ganglion-blocking agents in hypertensive patients during administration of a saluretic agent (chlorothiazide). Lancet 2:831, 1957.
15. Freis, E.D. et al: Chlorothiazide in hypertension and normotensive patients. Ann. N.Y. Acad. Sci. 71:450, 1958.
16. Winer, B.M.: The antihypertensive actions of benzothiadiazines. Circulation 23:211, 1961.
17. McQueen, E.G. and Morrison, R.B.I.: The hypotensive action of diuretic agents. Lancet 1:1209, 1960.
18. Ronnov-Jessen, V.: Variations in blood-volume during treatment of hypertension with ganglion-blocking agents and thiazide-preparations. Acta Med. Scand. 170:263, 1961.
19. Wilson, I.M. and Freis, E.D.: Relationship between plasma and extracellular fluid volume depletion and the antihypertensive effect of chlorothiazide. Circulation 20:1028, 1959.
20. Freis, E.D. et al: The collapse produced by venous congestion of the extremities or by venesection following certain hypotensive agents. J. Clin. Invest, 30:435, 1951.
21. Wanko, A. and Freis, E.D.: Altered vascular responsiveness following chlorothiazide or mercurial diuresis in normotensive subjects. Circulation 18:792, 1958.
22. Finnerty, F.A., Jr. et al: Changes in heart rate during levarterenol infusion: An index of arterial elasticity. Circ. Res. 7:565, 1959.
23. Hoobler, S.: Antihypertensive effects of diuretics. *In* Gross, F. (ed.): Antihypertensive Therapy—Principles and Practice. Heidelberg: Springer-Verlag, 1966, p. 256.

24. Guyton, A.C. et al: A systems analysis approach to understanding long-range arterial blood pressure control and hypertension. Circ. Res. 35:159, 1974.
25. Conway, J. and Lauwers, P.: Hemodynamic and hypotensive effects of long-term therapy with chlorothiazide. Circulation 21:21, 1960.
26 Tarazi, R.C. et al: Long-term thiazide therapy in essential hypertension. Circulation 41:709, 1970.
27. Leth, A.: Changes in plasma and extracellular fluid volumes in patients with essential hypertension during long-term treatment with hydrochlorothiazide. Circulation 42:479, 1970.
28. Lund-Johansen, P.: Hemodynamic changes in long-term diuretic therapy of essential hypertension. Acta Med. Scand. 187:509, 1970.
29. Villarreal, H. et al: Effect of guanethidine and bretylium tosylate on systemic and renal hemodynamics in essential hypertension. Am. J. Cardiol. 14:633, 1964.
30. Reubi, F.C. et al: Quelques aspects du réajustement circulatoire au cours du traitment antihypertensif de longue durée. *In* Milliez, P. and Tcherdakoff, P. (eds.): L'Hypertensión Arterielle. (Club International sur L'hypertension Artérielle. Premiére Réunion. July 5-7th, 1965.) Paris:L'Expansion Scientifique Francaise, 1966.

False Tolerance to Antihypertensive Drugs

Harriet P. Dustan, M.D., Robert C. Tarazi, M.D.
and Emmanuel L. Bravo, M.D.

Introduction

Each antihypertensive drug can evoke a counteraction that limits its ability to reduce arterial pressure. These counteractions occur in systems that participate either directly or indirectly in arterial pressure regulation. They are responsible for the development of false drug tolerance and, in certain circumstances, for drug resistance. Use of other antihypertensive drugs can lessen the counteractions and improve arterial pressure control.

There are three broad groupings of antihypertensive drugs — sympatholytics, diuretics and vasodilators. *Sympatholytics* can cause fluid retention and, with this, arterial pressure rises. Use of a diuretic promptly reestablishes good blood pressure control. *Diuretics* reduce plasma and extracellular fluid volumes and these reductions, in turn, can (1) decrease GFR and enhance renal reabsorption of salt and water and (2) stimulate renin release. The former can prevent maintenance of the necessary degree of negative salt and water balance and blood pressure can rise. The latter introduces a renal pressor factor and the increased renin may lessen the saluretic effect of the diuretic. False tolerance to diuretics can be overcome by increasing diuretic dosage, by use of an adrenergic inhibitor

---

This study supported in part by Grant HL 6835 from the National Heart and Lung Institute, National Institutes of Health, USPHS.

Harriet P. Dustan, M.D., Robert C. Tarazi, M.D. and Emmanuel L. Bravo, M.D., Research Division, The Cleveland Clinic Foundation and The Cleveland Clinic Education Foundation, Ohio.

which will suppress renin release or administration of an aldosterone-blocking agent. *Vasodilators* produce reflex sympathetic stimulation which increases cardiac output and heart rate; they also cause marked fluid retention and stimulate renin release. In contrast to sympatholytics and diuretics, blood pressure control is not adversely affected by increased intravascular volume; neither does the stimulation of the renal pressor system seem to raise arterial pressure. Thus, sympathetic stimulation seems to be the primary factor that lessens the antihypertensive effect of vasodilators. Thus use of central and/or peripheral inhibitors of adrenergic function can improve arterial pressure control.

Polypharmacy is widely used in the treatment of hypertension for the simple reason that better arterial pressure control is achieved for many patients with a combination of drugs rather than with one alone. The reason for this clinical experience is beginning to emerge as it becomes apparent that each type of antihypertensive drug can evoke compensatory responses which can limit the ability of the drug to reduce arterial pressure. In the early 1950s, before oral diuretics were available, it was common experience that the antihypertensive effectiveness of a ganglion-blocking drug lessened during months of therapy. When chlorothiazide first became available, one of its most striking effects was the improvement in blood pressure control that was achieved when it was added to ganglion-blocking therapy. Only much later was it realized that most drugs that suppress neurocirculatory control mechanisms can cause fluid retention and that this, in turn, causes arterial pressure to rise.

It now seems clear that drug therapy does not always eliminate basic pressor mechanisms because arterial pressure responses to drugs are different from those resulting from removal of one of the known causes of hypertension. For example, following surgery for renal arterial stenosis, pressure often falls to normal and remains normal without any apparent stimulation of other pressure control mechanisms to maintain the hypertension. In contrast, each type of antihypertensive drug may influence a variety of control mechanisms with the net result being a reduction in antihypertensive effectiveness. It is the purpose of this paper to examine the various effects of antihypertensive drugs in addition to arterial pressure reduction — effects which in some instances adversely affect their usefulness.

Compensatory Responses to Antihypertensive Drugs

The classification of antihypertensive drugs in three broad groups, sympatholytic, diuretics and vasodilators, has relevance not only in regard to the mechanism of their antihypertensive action but also in regard to similar consequences of their use. These consequences are compensatory responses to either arterial pressure reduction, per se, or some other physiologic effect of the drug.

The known compensatory responses are listed in Table 1. Sympatholytic drugs (with the exception of propranolol) can cause fluid retention. Diuretics initially cause a decrease in extracellular fluid volume and this increases plasma renin activity. However, the oligemia produced can cause antinatriuresis and, therefore, a relative increase in extracellular fluid can result. Vasodilators can produce marked expansion of extracellular fluid, much increase in plasma renin activity and marked stimulation of the sympathetic nervous system. These compensatory responses carry with them the possibility for diminishing the inherent antihypertensive potential of the drugs. In a way, this is not surprising because each compensation involves one or more of the various factors known to

Table 1. Antihypertensive Drugs: Primary Effect and Countereffects

Drug Class	*Primary Effect*	*Countereffects*
Sympatholytics	Decreased sympathetic activity	1) Increased ECF and plasma volume
Diuretics	Decreased ECF	1) Fluid retention 2) Increased PRA with increased aldosterone
Vasodilators	Vasodilation	1) Fluid retention 2) Increased PRA with increased aldosterone 3) Increased sympathetic activity

influence arterial pressure. Since these compensatory responses affect the factors known to influence arterial pressure, our attention was drawn to the possibility that when an antihypertensive regimen became progressively less effective, this might reflect the dominance of the compensatory response over the original depressor effect of the regimen.

Methods

In a number of publications during the past few years we have explored the possibility of compensatory responses to antihypertensive drugs being responsible for the blood pressure control achievable with these medications. The evidence supporting this possibility has come from a variety of studies of hypertensive patients treated with a number of antihypertensive drugs given alone or in combination.

Analytical Methods

To understand whether lessening of responsiveness to sympatholytic drugs was a function of fluid retention, we studied the effects of therapy on arterial pressure and intravascular volume. Brachial arterial pressure was measured at home by the patient twice daily, lying and standing, and in the hospital by the nursing staff four times daily. Plasma volume was estimated from the volume of distribution of 2.5 μCi of I^{125} albumin after at least a 30 minute supine rest [1]; total blood volume was calculated from the plasma volume by using the hematocrit which was measured in triplicate. Both plasma volume (PV) and total blood volume (TBV) were expressed as milliliters per centimeter to lessen differences introduced by differences in amount of body fat. Because these volumes are naturally larger in men than in women, values are often expressed in percent of normal so that data from the two groups can be analyzed together.

To study diuretics, arterial pressure and plasma and total blood volumes were determined as described above and plasma renin activity was estimated by radioimmunoassay of generated angiotensin I [2, 3] from plasma samples obtained at the time of plasma volume measurement. The effect of upright posture on PRA was not studied. It is now widely recognized that the pressor effect of exogenous angiotensin II is directly related to salt and water balance [4], so the possibility arose that the antihypertensive effect of a diuretic in salt- and water-dependent hypertension might represent not only the degree of oligemia achieved (which would favor arterial pressure reduction) but also the degree of stimulation of the renal pressor system that the diuretic produced (this would limit the fall in arterial pressure). To attempt some estimate of this combined effect, we calculated "total circulating renin" by multiplying plasma volume in milliliters per centimeter of height by PRA nanograms per milliliter.

Minoxidil was the vasodilator drug studied. For this, brachial arterial pressure, plasma volume and plasma renin activity were measured, as described above. In addition, cardiac output was performed using indocyanine green [5]. Intra-arterial pressure was recorded continuously using a Statham strain gauge P32db, and total peripheral resistance was calculated from cardiac output and mean arterial pressure. Heart rate was measured from a continuously recorded electrocardiogram. These hemodynamic measurements were made sequentially during minoxidil therapy in 13 patients; in ten of these, pre-minoxidil studies were also made. In four of these patients, extracellular fluid volume (ECF) and total exchangeable sodium (Na_e) were determined. For this purpose, 10-15 μCi of ^{22}Na was injected; ECF was measured as the volume of distribution of the isotope after the three-hour equilibration while Na_e was measured at the end of a 24-hour period of equilibration [6].

Patients and Treatment Regimens

All patients had been thoroughly investigated for known causes of hypertension and were classified by diagnosis accordingly. All measured arterial pressure at home twice daily and returned periodically either for outpatient visits or were admitted to the hospital whenever new therapy (eg, minoxidil) was begun or for readjustment of conventional forms of therapy.

Studies of sympatholytic drugs were carried out in 16 patients, ranging in age from 30-64 years, who had been under treatment for a few months to several years. Four had renal arterial stenosis and 12 were considered to have essential hypertension. Five received methyldopa or guanethidine alone and the remaining 11 were receiving diuretic therapy in addition to the sympatholytic drug — for five it was guanethidine, for four, methyldopa, while for two it was propranolol combined with hydralazine [7].

Responses to diuretic drugs were investigated in three groups of patients. The relationship between intravascular volume and arterial pressure control was determined after months or years of therapy. The influence of hyperreninemia on arterial pressure control during diuretic treatment was studied in three groups — two who received either hydrochlorothiazide or spironolactone [8, 9] and the other, hydrochlorothiazide alone and then in combination with propranolol [10].

The vasodilator drug, minoxidil, was given to 13 patients. Four received it as a single antihypertensive agent to which, later, was added a diuretic and/or one or more sympatholytic drugs. In the remaining nine patients, who were seriously ill with malignant hypertension, minoxidil was added to a regimen that included one or more sympatholytic drugs and a diuretic.

Results

Sympatholytic Drugs

It is now well known that when sympatholytic drugs are used for the treatment of hypertension, salt and water retention may occur with increases in extracellular fluid and plasma volume. This consequence has been reported for reserpine [11], ganglioplegic drugs [12], methyldopa [13] and guanethidine [14]. Sometimes this retention has been so marked that it has caused cardiac failure. In prolonged use these drugs may lose their initial antihypertensive effectiveness, yet the addition of a diuretic usually reestablishes good arterial pressure control. It was this experience that prompted our original study of a possible direct arterial pressure-intravascular volume relationship during sympatholytic drug treatment [7].

As indicated above, this possibility was explored in 16 patients during treatment. Eleven of them had normal, or near normal, arterial pressure, both supine and standing; five were receiving a sympatholytic drug alone and in the other six it was combined with hydrochlorothiazide. In all of these patients plasma volume was reduced; for the group it ranged from 70% to 93% of normal and averaged 84%. In contrast, the remaining five had inadequate blood pressure control as evidenced by supine diastolic pressure averages of 97-114 mm Hg even though they were taking combination therapy with adrenergic-blocking drugs and diuretics; in them plasma volume averaged 109% of normal and ranged from 95% to 135%. To see whether the inadequate pressure control was a function of the absolute or relative hypervolemia, diuretic therapy was intensified. For those who were taking furosemide, the daily dosage was doubled and for the three taking hydrochlorothiazide, that diuretic was discontinued and furosemide substituted. This intensified diuretic therapy caused all patients to lose weight; plasma volume fell to 93% of normal as an average for the group and supine pressure fell promptly toward normal. For the entire group of 16 patients, both systolic and diastolic arterial pressures were found to correlate directly with intravascular volume ($r=+0.666$ and $+0.697$, respectively, $p < 0.01$). Thus, these results supported the possibility that the compensatory fluid retention that may occur during sympatholytic drug treatment could diminish the inherent depressor capability of the drug and they also showed that patients responding to sympatholytic drugs alone did so because the compensatory fluid retention did not occur.

Diuretics

For diuretics to reduce arterial pressure and maintain it at a lower level over a prolonged period of time, they must first produce a negative salt and water balance and then prevent fluid retention during long-term use. However, the chronically depleted plasma and extracellular fluid volumes evoke two compensatory responses each capable of resulting in return of hypertension. One of these mechanisms is fluid retention, which can neutralize the natriuretic effect of the diuretic. This fluid retention comes about because as plasma and ECF volumes are reduced, glomerular filtration rate falls slightly and fractional reabsorption of proximal tubular fluid is increased [15]. Since diuretics act primarily on sodium reabsorption in distal segments of the nephron, their ability to maintain chronic oligemia reflects an interplay between enhanced proximal tubular reabsorption and natriuresis at distal sites.

The other compensatory mechanism that could favor return of hypertension is increased production of renin and angiotensin [16]. Since the pressor potential of exogenous angiotensin is lessened by salt and water depletion and increased by fluid retention, the possibility arose that the ability of this compensatory response to adversely influence the antihypertensive effectiveness of diuretics reflects a balance between oligemia and hyperreninemia. The effects of these two compensatory responses on arterial pressure control were examined in patients during long-term treatment with hydrochlorothiazide and/or spironolactone.

In 11 patients with essential hypertension [17], diastolic arterial pressure during treatment was found to be directly related to intravascular volume ($r=+0.613$, $p < 0.01$). Thus, in these patients with salt- and water-dependent hypertension, the antihypertensive effectiveness of diuretic therapy was a function of the oligemia produced.

The role of hyperreninemia in determining arterial pressure control was investigated by calculating the relationship between decreases in arterial pressure and increases in plasma renin activity and total circulating renin (Table 2) in 46 patients [9, 10]. Although diuretic treatment produced substantial reduction in arterial pressure and increases in both renin activity and circulating renin, the relationship between these functions was not significant. In 24 of these patients propranolol was subsequently added to diuretic therapy. This addition caused

Table 2. Arterial Pressure and Circulating Renin Relationships During Treatment with Diuretic Alone or Combined with Propranolol

	r	*p*
MAP – circulating renin		
diuretic	+0.21	ns
diuretic plus propranolol	+0.19	ns
% Decrease MAP – % increase circulating renin		
diuretic	–0.36	ns
diuretic plus propranolol	+0.16	ns

marked reduction in pressure with varying effects on plasma renin activity and circulating renin [10]. Again, no relationship between pressure and renin was found.

Vasodilators

Although vasodilators seem the most rational therapy for hypertension characterized by increased peripheral resistance, they evoke compensatory responses that can conceivably lessen their ability to decrease arterial pressure. They produce fluid retention, stimulate renin release [17, 18] and cause reflex sympathetic stimulation [19] with resultant increases in cardiac output and heart rate.

To investigate whether any of these compensatory responses influence the pressure level achieved by the drug, studies of the effects of minoxidil were carried out in 13 patients. Four received the drug alone and later a diuretic and/or propranolol was added separately; in nine who were already receiving treatment for severe hypertension with renal insufficiency, minoxidil was added to regimens that included one or more sympatholytics and furosemide as well as, in some, spironolactone. In all patients, fluid retention with increases in plasma volume occurred. Generally speaking, the early weight gain was not so marked in patients already taking a diuretic when minoxidil treatment was begun than it was in those for whom minoxidil was used as a single drug (Tables 3 and 5). It did not seem to influence arterial pressure control adversely, rather the amount of sodium retention was correlated with the antihypertensive effect of the drug ($r=-0.66$, $p<0.05$) in the four patients in whom measurements of extracellular fluid and total exchangeable sodium were made throughout the early weeks of treatment. Also, in these patients, arterial pressure and plasma volume were inversely related ($r=-0.91$, $p<0.001$) indicating that the lower the pressure the greater the tendency for salt and water retention.

Plasma renin activity bore no significant relationship to arterial pressure, intravascular volume or total peripheral resistance (Tables 3 and 5). It varied widely and the changes exhibited no group trends.

Systemic hemodynamic data appear in Tables 3, 4 and 6. Table 3 presents the findings in patients who received minoxidil

Table 3. Effects of Minoxidil Added to Usual Treatment

No.	*Control Rx*	*MAP – mm Hg*		*HR – b/min*		*CI – L/min/M²*		*TPR – U*		*PV – %N*		*PRA – ng/ml*	
		C	*M*	*C*	*M*	*C*	*M*	*C*	*M*	*C*	*M*	*C*	*M*
1	F,P,MD,H,S,G	145	119	62	55	2.2	2.3	65	52	83	95	9	22
3	F,P,MD,S,G	153	99	76	61	3.2	2.4	48	41	87	87	6	5
4	F,MD,H,S,G	152	127	76	86	3.2	2.8	43	46	93	112	14	52
6	F,H,S,G	116	101	81	75	3.1	4.1	37	25	106	132	26	9
10	F,P,MD,R	163	97	66	69	2.1	2.9	77	33	95	118	7	2
13	F,P,G	140	114	60	79	2.6	3.4	54	34	89	107	42	36
	Mean	145	110	70	71	2.7	3.0	54	39	92	109		
	% Change		-25		0		+11		-28		+18		

Abbreviations: MAP – mean arterial pressure, HR – heart rate, CI – cardiac index, TPR – total peripheral resistance, PV – plasma volume, PRA – plasma renin activity

Control Rx: F – furosemide, P – propranolol, MD – methyl dopa, H – hydralazine, S – spironolactone, G – guanethidine, R – reserpine

Table 4. Effects of Minoxidil (M) and Minoxidil Plus Propranolol (M + P)*

No.	MAP – mm Hg			HR – b/min			CI – L/min/M2			TPR – U		
	O	M	M+P	O	M	M+P	O	M	M+P	O	M	M+P
5	200	122	117	65	72	63	3.0	2.9	2.4	66	41	49
7	131	115	128	81	78	66	3.2	3.8	3.0	42	26	42
8	188	159	116	114	112	71	2.9	5.5	4.0	69	28	29
9	168	130	131	69	84	61	2.1	3.3	3.3	81	42	39
Mean	177	132	123	82	87	65	2.8	3.9	3.2	67	35	40
% Change		-25	-30		+6	-20		+39	+14		-48	-40

*Abbreviations as for Table 3 and M – minoxidil

Table 5. Effect of Minoxidil (M) and Minoxidil Plus Propranolol (M+P) on Plasma Volume (PV) and Plasma Renin Activity (PRA)

No.	PV – % Normal			PRA – ng/ml		
	C	M	M+P	C	M	M+P
5	94	101	104	6.7	45	10
7	91	122	107	2.6	2.0	2.7
8	103	143	142	57	27	3.0
9	84	104	95	1.1	1.4	0.5

Table 6. Sequential Hemodynamic Studies During Minoxidil Treatment*

No.	Rx	Duration Minoxidil Rx	MAP	CI	TPR
2	G,MD,F,M,P	2 weeks	123	3.1	40
	MD,P,M,F,S	21 months	121	3.3	37
	MD,M,F,S	30 months	117	4.6	25
	MD,P,M,F,S	31 months	105	3.5	30
11	M,MD	1 week	102	3.5	29
	M,MD,F	1 month	123	3.8	32
	M,MD,F,S	6 weeks	106	3.9	27
12	MD,G,M,R,P	2 months	155	4.3	36
	MD,M,P	9 months	117	3.7	31
	MD,M,P,F	11 months	121	4.3	28

*Abbreviations as for Table 3 and M - minoxidil

in addition to conventional treatment regimens while Table 4 includes pretreatment data, data with minoxidil alone and then with minoxidil plus propranolol. In these two groups of patients (Tables 3 and 4), arterial pressure reduction was similar. In the first group, however, it was associated with less stimulation of cardiac output than in the second group and, therefore, reflected more truly the decrease in peripheral resistance. In contrast, in the second group, cardiac stimulation with minoxidil alone was marked and seemed to limit the antipressor potential of the vasodilator. For example, if blood pressure reduction had resulted from decrease in resistance alone and output had not increased, mean pressure would have fallen from 177 mm Hg to 92 rather than to 130 mm Hg. When propranolol was added, pressure was slightly reduced, cardiac output also fell and total peripheral resistance rose slightly.

Three patients were studied only during treatment with minoxidil (Table 6). These patients were severely azotemic and were, accordingly, anemic. The anemia may well have influenced systemic flow as much as the vasodilation produced by the drug. The data show how variable hemodynamic functions can be during long-term treatment with minoxidil regardless of the other drugs used.

Discussion

These results indicate that compensatory responses to antihypertensive drugs can either lessen the blood pressure lowering effect from the very beginning of treatment or result in return of hypertension after a period of good blood pressure control. Although the mechanisms of these responses seem clear, the reasons why they should occur are not at all clear. Thus, as indicated earlier, the consequences of arterial pressure reduction by medication stand in sharp contrast to those produced either clinically [20] or experimentally [21] when renal artery stenosis is relieved. In such circumstances, peripheral resistance falls but no compensation occurs to block the decrease of arterial pressure. These contrasts indicate that antihypertensive drugs do not always abolish the basic mechanism of a hypertension — no matter how effective they may be. Further, the compensatory responses evoked provide the basis for multiple drug therapy that experience has shown to be so successful.

In most types of hypertension, untreated, there is an inverse relationship between diastolic pressure and intravascular volume [22]. Yet when sympatholytic drugs are given, the relationship becomes a direct one [7]. Although this finding is unexplained, there is substantial experimental evidence that an intact autonomic nervous system is necessary to maintain arterial pressure at normal levels in response to intravascular volume expansion [23-26]. In fact, the suggestion has been made that when autonomic reflexes are deficient, systemic flow is the hemodynamic variable that is controlled in contrast to arterial pressure that is controlled when reflexes are intact [25, 26]. The information is not yet available whether this situation obtains in patients treated with sympatholytic drugs because sequential measurements of cardiac output during long-term therapy are not yet available. Certainly, the rise in arterial pressure that occurs during treatment with adrenergic-blocking drugs, when plasma volume approaches normal levels, is suggestive of the development of vasoconstriction because it seems unlikely that cardiac output would become elevated just because of normovolemia [27, 28].

The finding of a direct arterial pressure-intravascular volume relationship during diuretic therapy, similar to that observed during treatment with sympatholytic drugs [7], suggests that diuretics have an effect on neurocirculatory control mechanisms. Again there is substantial experimental evidence to support this suggestion because diuretics have been shown to diminish the vasoconstriction produced by sympathetic nerve stimulation [29] and to suppress cardioinhibitory reflexes [30]. It is not now known whether these effects reflect salt and water depletion or a direct effect of the drugs on the autonomic nervous system. To answer this question similar studies must be performed during dietary salt restriction.

Diuretics also increase renin release and this is not only transient as an early manifestation of oligemia, but seems to be present on a chronic basis. It seems likely, then, that a renal pressor factor could lessen the antipressor effectiveness of diuretics. However, the results of our two studies [9, 10] do not support this possibility because plasma renin activity both in actual values and percentile changes bore no relationship to the arterial pressure responses. Also, these variables were not consistently affected by propranolol. Since the pressor effectiveness of exogenous angiotensin II is directly related to sodium balance [4], another approach was to assess the relationship of "total circulating renin" to arterial pressure in order to obtain a rough estimate of the combined effect of these two variables. Since no quantitative relationship was found, this could indicate that there is no influence of the renal pressor system on arterial pressure during diuretic therapy. This, however, seems unlikely because we have demonstrated a significant quantitative relationship between plasma renin activity and arterial pressure in patients with renovascular hypertension [31]. The other possibility is that the renal pressor system increased the activity of the sympathetic nervous system and that this overrode the neurosuppressant effects of the diuretics.

Of the three types of drugs, vasodilators — particularly minoxidil — seem to present the most complicated physiologic background for hemodynamic adjustments during treatment because all factors known to influence arterial pressure are affected in a significant degree. With minoxidil, fluid retention is more frequent and of greater magnitude than occurs with any other antihypertensive drug, yet it does not seem to influence arterial pressure control adversely. Rather, the blood pressure reduction itself seems to be the factor determining the degree of sodium reabsorption because both the increase in plasma volume as well as the cumulative sodium balance were significantly related to the degree of blood pressure reduction. Minoxidil can also cause marked increases in plasma renin activity but these did not seem to have an effect on arterial pressure. The facts that volume expansion and increases in the renal pressor component did not seem to restrict the antipressor potential of the drug suggest that its site of action is at some arteriolar site "distal" to that influenced by salt and water, angiotensin and the nervous system.

Minoxidil-induced vasodilation also causes reflex increases in heart rate and cardiac output [22]; these seem likely to reflect increases in sympathetic vasomotor outflow, but this is ineffective because of the direct effect of the drug on vascular smooth muscle. Both increases in cardiac output and heart rate could limit the effectiveness of a vasodilator. It was this possibility that prompted the addition of propranolol [22]. Our data show that without some form of adjunctive sympatholytic therapy, the rise in cardiac output does, in fact, limit the blood pressure fall. This is clearly shown in Table 4 which presents the arterial pressure levels that would have been achieved if the fall in pressure had not increased cardiac output. The fact that propranolol did not completely normalize arterial pressure may well be because cardiac output was not returned to control levels.

References

1. Tarazi, R.C., Dustan, H.P. and Frohlich, E.D.: Plasma volume in men with essential hypertension. N. Engl. J. Med. 278:762, 1968.
2. Haber, E., Koener, T., Page, L.B. et al: Application of radioimmunoassay for angiotensin I to the physiologic measurement of plasma renin activity in normal human subjects. J. Clin. Endocrinol. 29:1349, 1969.
3. Sealey, J.E. and Laragh, J.H.: Limitations of some commonly used methods. Am. J. Med. 55:303, 1973.
4. Laragh, J.H.: Dependence of the vasoactivity of angiotensin in the state of sodium balance. *In* Milliez, P. and Tcherdakoff, P. (eds.): L'Hypertension Arterielle (First Meeting of International Club on Arterial Hypertension, July 5-7, 1965). Paris:Expansion Scientifique Francaise, 1966, pp. 92-103.
5. Frohlich, E.D., Tarazi, R.C., Ulrych, M. et al: Tilt test for investigating a neural component in hypertension. Its correlation with clinical characteristics. Circulation 36:387, 1967.
6. Rovner, D.R. and Cohn, J.W.: A simple and precise method for the simultaneous measurement in man of plasma volume, radiobromide space, exchangeable potassium, and exchangeable sodium. J. Lab. Clin. Med. 62:492, 1963.
7. Dustan, H.P., Tarazi, R.C. and Bravo, E.L.: Dependence of arterial pressure on intravascular volume in treated hypertensive patients. N. Engl. J. Med. 286:861, 1972.
8. Dustan, H.P., Bravo, E.L. and Tarazi, R.C.: Volume-dependent essential and steroid hypertension. Am. J. Cardiol. 31:606, 1973.
9. Acchiardo, S., Dustan, H.P. and Tarazi, R.C.: Similar effects of hydrochlorothiazide and spironolactone on plasma renin activity in essential hypertension. Cleveland Clin. Quart. 39:153, 1973.
10. Bravo, E.L., Tarazi, R.C. and Dustan, H.P.: β-Adrenergic blockade in diuretic-treated patients with essential hypertension. N. Engl. J. Med. 292:66, 1975.

11. Perera, G.A.: Rauwolfia serpentina in hypertensive vascular disease. Proc. Soc. Exp. Biol. Med. 86:453, 1954.
12. Ronnov-Jessen, V.: Blood-volume and tolerance to pentolinium in the treatment of hypertension. Lancet 2:669, 1960.
13. Hansen, J.: Alpha-methyl-dopa (Aldomet®) in the treatment of hypertension: The effects of blood volume, exchangeable sodium, body weight and blood pressure. Acta Med. Scand. 183:323, 1968.
14. Ronnov-Jessen, V. and Hansen, J.: Blood volume and exchangeable sodium during treatment of hypertension with guanethidine and hydrochlorothiazide. Acta Med. Scand. 186:255, 1969.
15. Earley, L.E.: Salt and water transport in the kidney: Mechanism of action of diuretics utilizing the thiazide diuretics as a model. *In* Hoffman, F. (ed.): Diuretics in Clinical Medicine. Amsterdam, The Netherlands:Excerpta Medica Foundation, 1968, pp. 34-52.
16. Maebashi, M. and Yoshinaga, K.: Effect of dehydration on plasma renin activity. Jap. Circ. J. 31:609, 1967.
17. Pettinger, W.A. and Keeton, K.: Altered renin release and propranolol potentiation of vasodilatory drug hypotension. J. Clin. Invest. 55:236, 1975.
18. Ueda, H., Yagi, S. and Kaneko, Y.: Hydralazine and plasma renin activity. Arch. Intern. Med. 122:387, 1968.
19. Gilmore, E., Weil, J. and Chidsey, C.: Treatment of essential hypertension with a new vasodilator in combination with beta-adrenergic blockade. N. Engl. J. Med. 282:521, 1970.
20. Tarazi, R.C., Frohlich, E.D. and Dustan, H.P.: Contribution of cardiac output to renovascular hypertension. Am. J. Cardiol. 31:600, 1973.
21. Ferrario, C.M., Page, I.H. and McCubbin, J.W.: Increased cardiac output as a contributory factor in experimental renal hypertension in dogs. Circ. Res. 27:799, 1970.
22. Tarazi, R.C., Dustan, H.P., Frohlich, E.D. et al: Plasma volume and chronic hypertension. Relationship to arterial pressure levels in different hypertensive diseases. Arch. Intern. Med. 125:835, 1970.
23. Folkow, B.: A study of the factors influencing the tone of denervated blood vessels perfused at various pressures. Acta Physiol. Scand. 27:99, 1953.
24. Levy, M.N., Brind, S.H. and Brandlin, F.R.: The acute effects of elimination of the moderator reflexes upon cardiac output and total peripheral resistance in the anesthetized dog. Circ. Res. 3:415, 1955.
25. Granger, H.J. and Guyton, A.C.: Autoregulation of the total systemic circulation following destruction of the central nervous system in the dog. Circ. Res. 25:379, 1969.
26. Liedtke, A.J., Urschel, C.W. and Kirk, E.S.: Total systemic autoregulation in the dog and its inhibition by baroreceptor reflexes. Circ. Res. 32:673, 1973.
27. Werkö, L., Sannerstedt, E., Varnauskas, E. et al: Experimentally induced hypervolemia during ganglionic blockade: The effects on cardiac function in patients with mitral disease. Scand. J. Clin. Lab. Invest. 14:289, 1962.

28. Frye, R.L. and Braunwald, E.: Studies on Starling's law of the heart. I. The circulatory response to acute hypervolemia and its modification by ganglionic blockade. J. Clin. Invest. 39:1043, 1960.
29. Aoki, V.S. and Brody, M.J.: The effect of thiazide on the sympathetic nervous system of hypertensive rats. Arch. Int. Pharmacodyn. 177:423, 1969.
30. Eckstein, J.W., Wendling, M.G. and Abboud, F.M.: Circulatory responses to norepinephrine after prolonged treatment with chlorothiazide. Circ. Res. 18 & 19 (suppl. 1):48, 1966.
31. Dustan, H.P., Tarazi, R.C. and Frohlich, E.D.: Functional correlates of plasma renin activity in hypertensive patients. Circulation 41:555, 1970.

Discussion

Moderator: Dr. E. D. Freis

Dr. Sambhi: Dr. Dustan, you showed that those patients who responded to therapy maintained the contraction in their plasma volume and others did not. Do you think this will be reflected in their body weight? Did you have the body weights?

Dr. Dustan: Since hypertensives tend to be obese and since their weights often fluctuate with various attempts to reduce, changes in weight are unreliable. Measurements of extracellular fluid and plasma volume should be made for proper assessment.

Dr. Doyle: I just wonder whether the two speakers have not left a factor as to the question of venous capacity. Plasma volume is going to be related not in an absolute sense to plasma volume, but is going to be related to the capacity of the venous system to accommodate it. Some experiments we have done recently may perhaps make this a little easier to interpret. We have been studying, not the effects of drugs, but simply the effects of bed rest on untreated patients in terms of blood pressure. We found that approximately half the patients who are admitted to the hospital are just put to bed for three days, give a substantial fall in blood pressure which seems to be entirely associated with fall in cardiac output which is associated with no change in plasma volume or weight but which is associated with a demonstrable reduction in venous stiffness and venous compliance. These considerations are particularly important in the interpretation of certain acute studies of the effects of diuretics. I would like to ask Dr. Freis whether he thinks, for example, the acute fall in cardiac output simply could be related to the effect of bed rest. The other point I would like to make is that in these patients who do have falls in cardiac output and changes in venous compliance there is evidence of a fall in plasma adrenalin also at the same time.

Dr. Freis: I would agree that the relationship between venous compliance and blood volume are the main determinants of venous return to the heart. One could have, for example, with excessive sympathetic stimulation an increase in venous constriction. One of the effects of bed rest is the same as that of sleep, that is, that there is a general turning off of the sympathetic nervous system outflow. With sleep one sees a marked decrease in cardiac output and heart rate and probably an increase in venous compliance. The other question was the effect of bed rest on the cardiac output changes. Although our initial studies on cardiac output were in hospitalized patients, the last studies that I showed you were done in outpatients.

Dr. Kincaid-Smith: I wonder if you would comment on the controlled trials which have shown that thiazides are more effective than furosemide and ethacrynic acid in the control of blood pressure in spite of a stronger diuretic and natriuretic effect of these agents. I would like to ask Dr. Dustan about minoxidil. I think her slide showed that when she added propranolol to minoxidil there was quite a striking increase in renal blood flow. I wonder if she has comments about that. I also wonder if she has observed long-term tolerance to this combination.

Dr. Freis: I think the reason why furosemide is a poor treatment for patients with chronic, essential hypertension is that the duration of its action is very short. If the drug is given twice daily, it is simply not providing adequate diuretic coverage. However, if you gave 100 mg of furosemide four times a day, you would find a similar antihypertensive effect as with the thiazides, perhaps more. Furosemide does not in any way disprove the diuretic theory for the reduction of blood pressure. Rather, it is simply not a good agent from the point of view of duration of action for the treatment of chronic, essential hypertension.

Dr. Dustan: I agree with Dr. Freis concerning the explanation for the apparent lesser effectiveness of furosemide as an antihypertensive drug. In regard to the effect of propranolol on the renal vascular bed in minoxidil-treated patients, the rise in renal blood flow that occurred has not been explained. We do know that it was not positively correlated with a suppression of PRA. Since minoxidil causes increased sympathetic activity, it may well have blocked a neurally mediated renal vasoconstriction.

Dr. Freis: I would like to comment on the subject of tolerance in general and also as it applies to Dr. Dustan's report. We have seen it and I think it is primarily due to the fact that we are seeing fluid accumulation over a long period of time. Also I would interpret what Dr. Dustan reported a little differently. She said that the reduction blood pressure was dependent upon the increase in plasma volume. I would say that the increase in volume was dependent upon the blood pressure reduction.

Dr. Dustan: If I said that, I did not mean to. My interpretation is that the sodium retention and rise in intravascular volume result from vasodilatation and arterial pressure reduction.

Dr. Freis: Good, then we agree. I think that eventually if we continue treatment long enough without diuretics we will see in patients with renal failure the development of resistance to minoxidil.

Dr. Thurau: I would like to come back to the discussion concerning the importance of peripheral hemodynamics on blood pressure. Under normal conditions peripheral resistance to flow is primarily governed by local, metabolically linked mechanisms. If any centrally originated increase in peripheral resistance is superimposed, one would have to expect that arteriovenous oxygen difference should be increased because the blood flow through the tissue is relatively too low to the state of metabolism. My question then is whether someone has measured a decrease in arteriovenous O_2 difference after the administration of diuretics, which would indicate that the superimposed increase in peripheral resistance was removed or taken away by the treatment. My other comment is concerned with what Dr. Freis said about the origin of volume which is excreted after diuretics. There is no question it is primarily extracellular volume and plasma volume. But if one is talking about the constituent ions, then I think there is a tremendous shift of ions from intracellular compartments to extracellular compartments as a result of diuretic therapy.

Dr. Freis: I agree with what Dr. Thurau has said. Certainly there are many hemodynamic factors which ought to be taken into account. It seems to me we have oversimplified matters by just considering the blood pressure.

Dr. Zanchetti: Of course I am not ready to play ex-officio defendant of the theory that extracellular blood volume comes back to normal in a late period of diuretic treatment. I certainly agree that the picture presented by textbooks is oversimplified, white against black. I do not agree with that. However, I think it is also indisputable that even your old data with Wilson show that some of the patients during the chronic period of treatment had extracellular volume or plasma volume returned toward normal values. In the slides summarizing your recent work on patients followed for eight weeks, which is not a very long observation period, if I read them correctly, extracellular fluid volume certainly was decreased at the eighth week as in the earlier period, but plasma volume seemed to show some trend to come back closer to control values. The change at eight weeks was not significant, whereas the other ones were significant. So I think that probably some of the different and apparently conflicting information could be made to agree if we think that there is a trend toward control values, although this is a very slow one, that may not be complete in all patients but only in a few. Another factor which could be brought into this picture, at least hypothetically, is that when plasma volume comes back, another factor which is the container, that is, the vein stiffness, can be changed. So even what seems apparently a normal plasma volume can work as a smaller plasma volume if there is a change in stiffness. There is no clearcut evidence, on this point, but some vague evidence is suggested by the observation that intravenous furosemide causes a decreased venous stiffness. In your recent series of patients did you measure the right atrial pressure at different weeks of treatment to assess whether it had decreased?

Dr. Freis: No we did not. We were strictly noninvasive in our study. But I think that the evidence is overwhelming if you read all of the papers that volume is reduced during long-term treatment. There was some tendency to return towards control, in certain cases in our study, for example, plasma volume in our early study was reduced but not significant at 6 months, but the reduction was significant at 12 months. It was still greatly reduced at six months, it just missed statistical significance. Also, ECF volume was significantly reduced at six months. However, when you look at Tarazzi and Dustan's paper the reductions in both ECF and plasma volume were significant over the long term. With respect to venous tone I wish I knew how to measure that accurately. Maybe Dr. Doyle would comment. However, one would expect that, with the initial reduction in cardiac output and blood pressure with thiazide, there would be an increase in venous tone due to sympathetic reflex activity via the baroreceptors. With the passage of time this would tend to disappear because the baroreceptors would get tired and would reset. I imagine that is what occurs.

Dr. Sambhi: I have a problem accepting Dr. Freis's explanation that furosemide is a poor antihypertensive agent because of its duration of action. If what we are concerned about is merely the contraction of plasma volume, then I think you can cause an adequate *reduction* in plasma volume and extracellular volumes with good doses of furosemide.

Dr. Freis: As long as we eat salt during the day we do not maintain reduction in ECF and plasma volume and it is very quickly restored. If you give furosemide only in the morning and in the evening in a dose of 40 mg by the time the patient has had his noon and evening meal you have restored your plasma volume. The result is a fluctuating ECF rather than a maintained reduction.

Effect of Long-Term Beta-Blockade on Central Hemodynamics at Rest and During Exercise in Essential Hypertension

A Comparison Between Alprenolol, Atenolol and Timolol

Per Lund-Johansen, M.D.

Introduction

In recent years the beta-blockers have become very popular in the therapy of hypertension. Since the introduction of propranolol as a blood pressure lowering drug about ten years ago [1], several new beta-blockers have appeared on the market and many are under investigation [2, 3]. The beta-blockers seem to have a common acute or short-term hemodynamic effect: reduction in heart rate (HR) and cardiac output (CO) rise in total peripheral resistance (TPR) and little effect upon blood pressure (BP) [4-8]. However, after weeks or months on propranolol therapy the TPR seems to decrease due to readjustment, the CO remains low or increases slightly and the blood pressure remains low or decreases further [6, 7]. Other mechanisms responsible for the pressure drop have also been discussed [9].

Little is known about the hemodynamic long-term effects of the newer compounds. A preliminary study has suggested a different long-term effect of one of the new compounds, timolol [8]. The purpose of this study is to compare the

---

Per Lund-Johansen, M.D., Associate Professor, Medical Department A., University of Bergen, School of Medicine, Bergen, Norway.

hemodynamic long-term effects of three beta-blockers with different pharmacological characteristics: alprenolol (non-cardioselective with intrinsic sympathicomimetic activity), atenolol (cardioselective without intrinsic sympathicomimetic activity) and timolol (non-cardioselective without intrinsic sympathicomimetic activity).

Material

The study includes 39 men, aged 20-56 years, with previously untreated essential hypertension in WHO stage I. Secondary hypertension was excluded by the usual routine procedures [10]. All were without symptoms, the hypertension being discovered by routine control at health offices and established by at least three visits to the outpatient clinic at Medical Department A, Haukeland Hospital.

The subjects were divided in groups according to therapy, but were not matched. The age, weight, body surface area (BSA) and pretreatment BP and HR are seen in Table 1. After one year on therapy the body weight had not changed significantly in any group.

Methods

The subjects were studied hemodynamically during strictly standardized conditions at rest supine and sitting and during bicycling in steady state at 300, 600 and 900 kpm/min. Oxygen consumption, intra-arterial pressure (brachial artery), heart rate (ECG) and cardiac output (Cardiogreen) were measured in duplicate in each situation. The methods have been described previously in detail [10]. The subjects were informed about the

Table 1. Age (Range and Mean) and Mean Values for Weight, Body Surface Area (BSA), Casual Blood Pressure (BP) and Heart Rate (HR) Before Therapy

	n	*Age (years)*	*Weight (kg)*	*BSA (m^2)*	*BP (mm Hg)*	*HR (beats/min)*
Alprenolol	10	30-42 (37.1)	80.6	1.99	171/116	94
Atenolol	13	20-48 (33.8)	75.8	1.93	163/106	86
Timolol	16	32-56 (47.4)	79.8	1.97	171/114	89

nature and the purpose of the study and consent was obtained from all.

All studies were made on an outpatient basis. After a treatment period of 11 to 12 months the hemodynamic study was repeated. The difference between the hemodynamic results at the first and the second study was tested by Student's t-test.

The present study does not include any untreated control group. However, it has been documented in a previous work [11] that in similar untreated subjects the hemodynamic parameters at the restudy after one year were not significantly different from the first.

Treatment

The subjects received one sole drug. The beta-blockers were administered as tablets at 7:00 A.M. and 5:00 P.M. The dosages were alprenolol 200-400 mg bds, atenolol 50-100 mg bds and timolol 5-10 mg bds. No other drugs or diet restrictions were given. On the day of the second hemodynamic study the subjects took their morning dose at 7:00 A.M. The hemodynamic study was performed between 9:00 and 12:00 A.M.

Side Effects

No subjects had to be withdrawn from the study. During the first two to three weeks a few temporary side effects, sometimes necessitating reduction in dose, were seen: alprenolol: none; atenolol: fatigue in legs and thighs during stair-climbing, 3; dizziness after exercise, 1; timolol: fatigue in legs and thighs, 3; dizziness, 1; cold feet, 1. Later, all subjects were without complaints, many enjoying rather vigorous physical exercise like running in the mountains and cross-country skiing.

Results

Casual Blood Pressure and Heart Rate

The casual BP and HR dropped in all subjects during treatment. The mean values before and one year after therapy are seen in Table 2. The reductions in BP obtained by the three drugs are rather similar; the reduction in heart rate most marked with timolol. All subjects in the alprenolol and atenolol groups experienced at least 10 mm Hg reduction in DAP, and all but three in the timolol group.

Table 2. Casual Blood Pressure and Heart Rate (Mean Values) Before = I and During = II Therapy and Number of "Non-responders"

	BP (mm Hg)			*HR (beats/min)*			*"Non-responders"*
	I	*II*	Δ	*I*	*II*	Δ	*(Δ DAP $\leqslant$ 10 mm Hg)*
Alprenolol	171/116	139/97	−32/19	94	70	−24	0
Atenolol	163/106	135/90	−28/16	86	63	−23	0
Timolol	171/114	142/97	−29/17	89	58	−31	3

Hemodynamics

Since details about the alprenolol and atenolol study have been published elsewhere [12, 13], only the major findings will be presented in this comparative survey.

The hemodynamics at rest sitting before therapy is seen in Table 3. It is seen that the groups compare well in spite of some differences with respect to age. The hemodynamics in relation to oxygen consumption at rest and during exercise before and after therapy is seen in Figures 1, 2 and 3.

Oxygen consumption. The VO_2 did not change at rest, but during exercise the values tended to be higher after therapy. In the timolol group the VO_2 was significantly increased at the two highest work levels.

Blood pressure. The changes in SAP, DAP and MAP were rather similar and therefore only the changes in MAP will be presented. Table 4 shows the relative changes in MAP at rest supine and sitting and at the 600 kpm/min work load. The pressure reduction was more pronounced by atenolol and timolol than by alprenolol. At rest sitting only 3 of 10 subjects in the alprenolol group had reduction in MAP greater than 10 mm Hg, in contrast to 12 of 13 and 15 of 16 in the atenolol and

Table 3. Hemodynamics at Rest Sitting Before Therapy (Mean Values ± SD)

	n	*VO_2 ml/min/m^2*	*HR beats/min*	*CI l/min/m^2*	*SI ml/stroke/m^2*	*MAP mm Hg*	*TPRI dyn sec cm^{-5} m^2*
Alprenolol	10	148 ± 13	83 ± 11	3.2 ± 0.5	38.9 ± 5.6	124 ± 15	3136 ± 426
Atenolol	13	150 ± 21	79 ± 15	3.3 ± 0.9	41.1 ± 5.5	122 ± 7	3150 ± 707
Timolol	16	145 ± 14	75 ± 9	3.1 ± 0.5	41.2 ± 5.4	127 ± 10	3368 ± 512

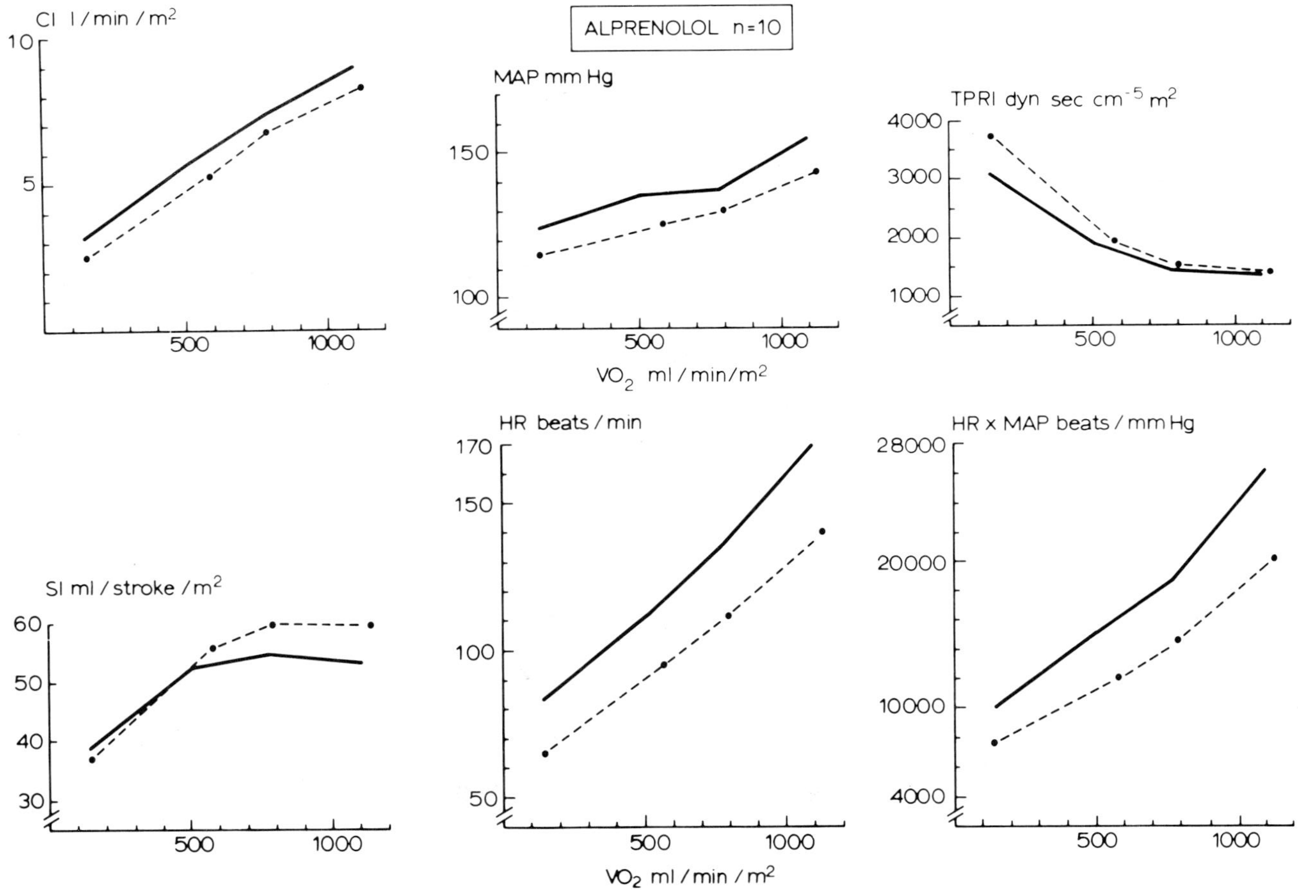

FIG. 1. Cardiac index (CI), mean arterial pressure (MAP), total peripheral resistance index (TPRI), stroke index (SI), heart rate (HR) and heart rate-pressure product (HR × MAP) in relation to oxygen consumption (VO_2) at rest and during exercise before (———) and during (--------) alprenolol therapy, mean values.

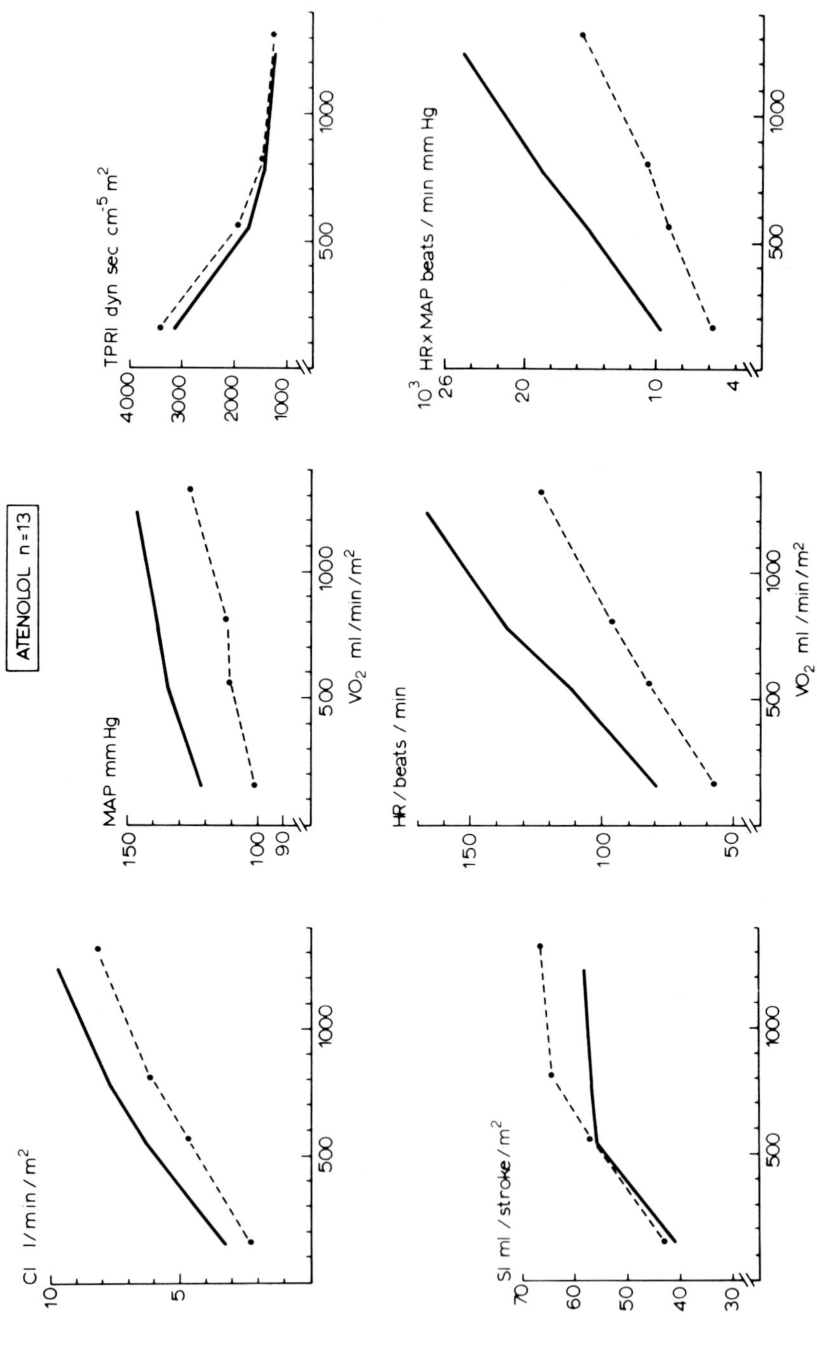

FIG. 2. Central hemodynamics before and during atenolol therapy. Legend and abbreviations as in Figure 1.

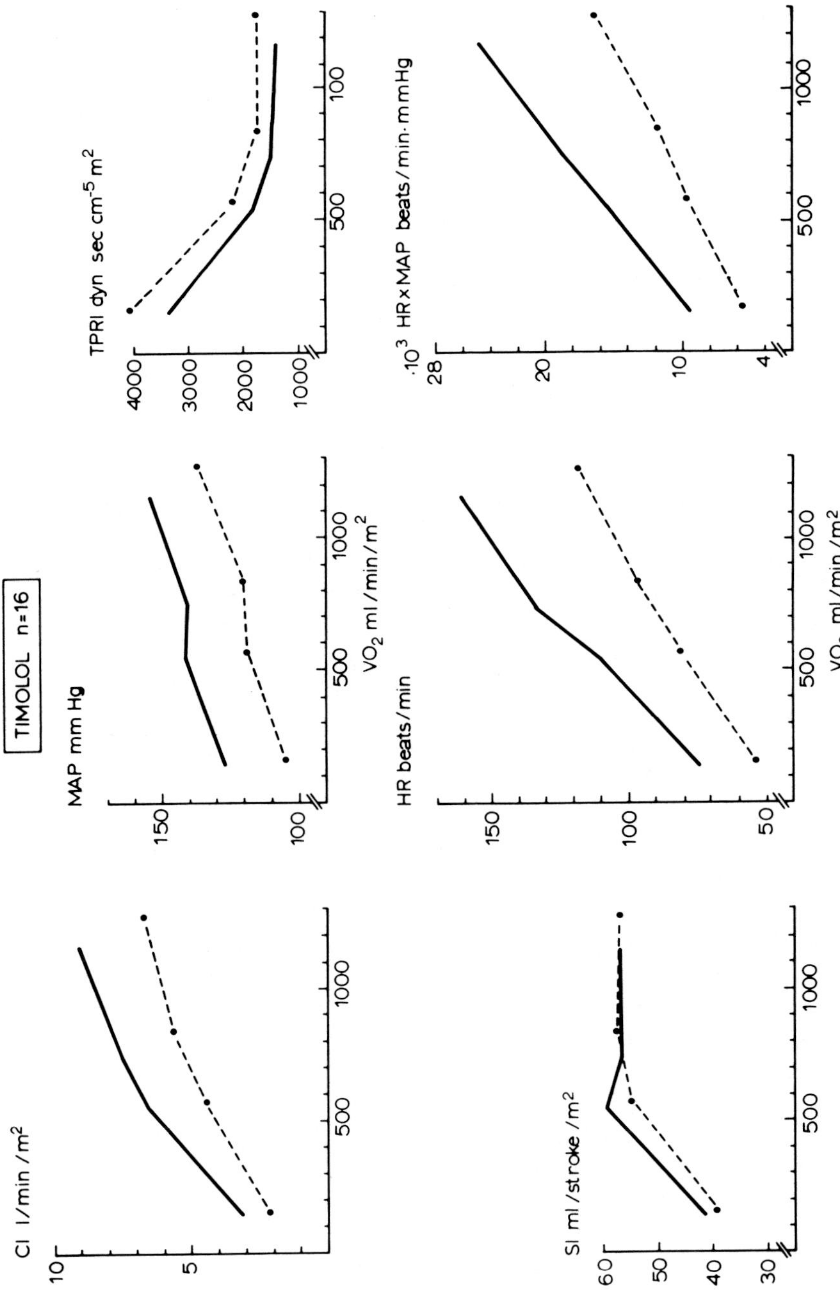

FIG. 3. Central hemodynamics before and during timolol therapy. Legend and abbreviations as in Figure 1.

Table 4. Relative Changes in Mean Arterial Pressure, Cardiac Index and Total Peripheral Resistance Index

	MAP (%)			*CI (%)*			*TPRI (%)*		
	Rest		*Work*	*Rest*		*Work*	*Rest*		*Work*
			600			*600*			*600*
	Supine	*Sitting*	*kpm/min*	*Supine*	*Sitting*	*kpm/min*	*Supine*	*Sitting*	*kpm/min*
Alprenolol	−11	− 7	− 6	−13	−23	−10	+ 2	+21	+ 5
Atenolol	−17	−17	−19	−16	−27	−20	− 3	+ 9	+ 1
Timolol	−18	−17	−14	−28	−32	−25	+12	+21	+15

timolol groups. The pressure reductions in these two groups were very similar (Table 4; Figs. 2 and 3).

The mechanisms behind the pressure drop are seen in Table 4 and Figures 1, 2 and 3.

Cardiac index. With only one exception, the CI was lower after therapy in all subjects at rest as well as during exercise. The greatest decrease was seen at rest sitting: 23%, 27% and 32% in the three groups. This corresponds to a reduction in CO of approximately 1.5, 1.7 and 2.0 l/min. During exercise the absolute reductions in CO were even greater, about 1.5, 3.0 and 4 l/min, respectively. As the VO_2 was increased or unchanged, this implies an increase in the A-V 0_2 difference.

Total peripheral resistance index. All subjects had an increased TPRI before therapy. The TPRI did not decrease significantly in any group compared to the pretreatment levels, but tended to be increased in most situations, and was significantly increased in the sitting position by all drugs. In the alprenolol and atenolol groups the changes were small and insignificant at rest supine and during work. Timolol, however, induced a significant increase in TPRI in all situations. Only two subjects (alprenolol 1 and atenolol 1) demonstrated a 10% decrease in TPRI at rest and during work.

Heart rate. The HR dropped in all subjects in all situations most pronounced (about 28%) by atenolol and timolol (Table 5). Nine subjects on these drugs had HR $\leqslant$ 48 beats/min at rest supine. It should be noted that subjects with low pretreatment values responded with a marked drop in HR. The HR during exercise was much lower than what has been found in normotensive healthy subjects of the same age [10].

Table 5. Relative Changes in Heart Rate and Stroke Index

	HR (%)			*SI (%)*		
	Rest		*Work 600*	*Rest*		*Work 600*
	Supine	*Sitting*	*kpm/min*	*Supine*	*Sitting*	*kpm/min*
Alprenolol	–20	–20	–18	+ 8	–4	+ 8
Atenolol	–24	–28	–29	+10	+3	+13
Timolol	–26	–28	–27	– 2	–5	+ 2

Stroke index. In the alprenolol and atenolol groups the reductions in HR were partly compensated by greater posttreatment SI at rest supine and during exercise. At rest sitting, however, the SI was practically unchanged and consequently the CI reduced similarly to the HR. In the timolol group the posttreatment SI did not show any compensatory increase, but even tended to be decreased; thus, the CI was reduced even more than the HR at rest and during light work.

Pressure-heart rate product. The MAP × HR product was markedly decreased by all drugs, the reduction being about 40% at rest sitting and during work on atenolol and timolol and about 25% on alprenolol.

Discussion

All three beta-blockers reduced BP in the majority of the subjects with mild essential HT who took part in this study. Only three of 39 had reduction in casual DAP less than 10 mm Hg. Based on this criterion almost all were "responders." The pressure reduction was less with alprenolol than with the two other drugs. Whether this is due to the intrinsic sympathicomimetic activity of alprenolol or to the dose being too small, compared to the doses of atenolol and timolol, is not possible to determine since the dose was not increased above 800 mg/day. Others have found the BP reduction by a mean dose of 460 mg alprenolol and 24 mg of timolol similar, but greater reduction in HR by timolol [14]. Also in this study the reduction in HR was less with alprenolol than with timolol (and atenolol).

The reduction in BP and HR obtained by atenolol is in accordance with results reported by Hansson et al [15] in the same type of patients on similar doses, and the BP changes induced by timolol compare well with results in clinical trials by Morgan et al [14].

The study of the hemodynamic mechanisms behind the drop in pressure demonstrated that in all three groups the BP drop was associated with a pronounced decrease in CO at rest as well as during exercise. Reduced CO on "long-term" therapy with propranolol has been reported by others after four weeks [7], after five weeks [8], after nine weeks [16], after 10 months [17] and after 20 months [6]. In the last of these studies, the CI after 20 months was reduced about 17% at rest supine compared to the pretreatment situation.

The present study demonstrates that the long-term use of the newer beta-blockers is also associated with a considerable decrease in CO at rest as well as during exercise, mainly due to the persistent decrease in HR. The changes induced by atenolol resemble those reported in a short-term study by Amery et al [18]. It was not possible to confirm the preliminary observations by Franciosa et al [8] and by Franciosa and Freis [19] suggesting no reduction in CO by long-term use of timolol. On the contrary, timolol induced the greatest decreases in CI. The reason for this discrepancy is not clear. However, their patients had more severe hypertension, the mean arterial pressure being 140 mm Hg in contrast to 113 in our group. The patients in their study must have responded less to timolol because a daily dose of 40 mg did induce only 6% reduction in mean arterial pressure, 5% reduction in CO (n.s.) and 16% reduction in heart rate in contrast to 18% reduction in pressure, 28% reduction in CO and 26% reduction in heart rate in our study. In the long-term study on propranolol by Tarazi and Dustan [6] the HR was decreased 25% at rest supine, very similar to what was seen at rest supine by atenolol and timolol in the present study.

If the CO during beta-blockade is to be less reduced than corresponding to the drop in HR, then the posttreatment SV must be increased. The present study seems to indicate small differences between the three drugs in this respect. At rest supine and during the two highest work levels the posttreatment SI was significantly higher on alprenolol and atenolol, but not on timolol. This SV response is responsible for the particularly low CI at rest supine and during exercise in the timolol group. The mechanism behind this difference in the SV responses is not possible to determine from this study. One might ask whether this difference is of clinical importance. In the type of patients who took part in this study there were no more complaints related to reduced CO, such as muscular fatigue, in the timolol group than in the atenolol group. It was indeed puzzling how well the marked deviations from a normal circulatory pattern were tolerated. After the first few weeks, during which local adjustments in the circulation in the muscles probably took place, no subjects had any unpleasant sensations carrying out daily activities or even vigorous exercise. No subjects found the 900 kpm/min load (duration eight minutes) more strenuous after therapy than before. It is possible that in subjects with a more disturbed heart pump function could the differences between the drugs be of importance and a decrease in cardiac contractility be dangerous. However, all three drugs induced a drastic reduction in the MAP × HR product at rest as well as during exercise. This should lead to a marked reduction in myocardial oxygen need. It has recently been shown that even in subjects with significant coronary disease a decrease in CI from 3.4 to 2.6 $l/min/m^2$ induced by propranolol did not change myocardial contractility [20]. Since the greatest hazard for subjects with mild and moderate HT in the Western societies is to die too early from a myocardial infarction, it is to be hoped that the benefit of the beta-blockers on the heart will be greater than the possible dangers of a reduced CO.

The calculated peripheral resistance did not decrease significantly in any group. Still, one year after the therapy the TPRI was significantly *higher* than the pretreatment values in the timolol group. This is somewhat disappointing, since the increased TPRI is the cardinal hemodynamic disturbance in most forms of established HT [10].

The long-term effects of the beta-blockers in mild essential HT differ from the long-term effects of the thiazide diuretics and peripheral vasodilators. The thiazide diuretics induce a temporary reduction in CO due to decrease in SV. After months on therapy the CO increases back to pretreatment level at rest and during exercise and the decrease in BP is due to significant reduction in TPR. The HR is left undisturbed at rest as well as during exercise [11].

The new vasodilator prazosin induces an even greater reduction in TPR and the posttreatment CO is increased at rest as well as during exercise [21].

A crucial question in the discussion of antihypertensive therapy is whether early interference with blood pressure lowering drugs will prevent the structural changes in the heart and blood vessels resulting from the high BP and also being partly responsible for the maintenance of the high blood pressure. Recent data from animal experiments have demonstrated that many of these changes already appear a few weeks after the increase in BP [22-24]. In the beginning these changes are reversible if the BP is reduced. The ability of the various antihypertensive drugs to reverse or prevent cardiac and vascular changes in different forms of HT in animals is insufficiently explored. However, it should be noted that whereas guanethidine and hydralazine have been shown to lower BP and induce regression of vascular changes in the spontaneous hypertensive rat, with established HT, beta-blockers alone did not have this effect. Only if the beta-blockers were given to the SHR rats in their prehypertensive age and continued through eight months could BP be kept normal and vascular changes be prevented [23]. Hypertension induced by stellate ganglion stimulation may be prevented by phenoxybenzamin, but not with propranolol although it nearly abolishes the increase in CO [25].

Most of the patients in this study were in their forties and fifties. Although the duration of the HT was uncertain in most of them, they had permanent, albeit mild, HT. The beta-blockers reduced pressure in almost all, in contrast to what has been reported in rats, but by changing the "high pressure-almost normokinetic circulation" to an "almost normotensive and markedly hypokinetic" system. Further studies are required to predict the long-term prognoses of these changes in central hemodynamics in man.

Summary

Thirty-nine men with essential hypertension in WHO stage I were treated with a sole drug for one year: alprenolol (10), atenolol (13) or timolol (16). Oxygen consumption, intra-arterial pressure, cardiac output and heart rate were measured at rest and during steady state exercise at 300, 600 and 900 kpm/min before and after one year of therapy. The arterial pressure was significantly decreased in all groups at rest and during exercise, somewhat less in the alprenolol group than in the other two. Cardiac output and heart rate were significantly reduced in all groups at rest and during exercise. The stroke volume increased at rest supine and during exercise in the alprenolol and atenolol group, resulting in less reduction in cardiac output than corresponding to the reduction in heart rate. In the timolol group the stroke volume did not increase, the reduction in cardiac output corresponding to the drop in heart rate. The posttreatment calculated total peripheral resistance tended to be higher than the pretreatment values, particularly in the timolol group where the changes were significant at rest as well as during exercise. The possible clinical significance of these changes is discussed.

References

1. Prichard, B.N.C. and Gillam, P.M.S.: Treatment of hypertension with propranolol. Br. Med. J. 1:7, 1969.
2. Simpson, F.O.: β-Adrenergic receptor blocking drugs in hypertension. Drugs 7:85, 1974.
3. Winchester, J.F.: Drug profile: Trasicor. J. Int. Med. Res. 2:448, 1974.
4. Ulrych, M. and Chrpová, V.: Haemodynamic effects of a new beta-adrenergic blocker (Trasicor®) in man when supine and sitting. Pharmacol. Clin. 1:95, 1968.
5. Johnsson, G., Guzman, DeM., Bergman, H. et al: The haemodynamic effects of alprenolol and propranolol at rest and during exercise in hypertensive patients. Pharmacol. Clin. 2:34, 1969.
6. Tarazi, R.C. and Dustan, H.P.: Beta adrenergic blockade in hypertension. Practical and theoretical implications of long-term hemodynamic variations. Am. J. Cardiol. 29:633, 1972.
7. Hansson, L.: Beta-adrenergic blockade in essential hypertension. Acta Med. Scand. suppl. 550, p. 20, 1973.
8. Franciosa, J.A., Freis, E.D. and Conway, J.: Antihypertensive and hemodynamic properties of the new beta adrenergic blocking agent timolol. Circulation 48:118, 1973.
9. Nies, A.S. and Shand, D.G.: Clinical pharmacology of propranolol. Circulation 52:6, 1975.
10. Lund-Johansen, P.: Hemodynamics in early essential hypertension. Acta Med. Scand. 181 (suppl. 482):18, 1967.

11. Lund-Johansen, P.: Hemodynamic changes in long-term diuretic therapy of essential hypertension. Acta Med. Scand. 187:509, 1970.
12. Lund-Johansen, P.: Hemodynamic changes at rest and during exercise in long-term β-blocker therapy of essential hypertension. Acta Med. Scand. 195:117, 1974.
13. Lund-Johansen, P.: Hemodynamic long-term effects of a new beta-blocker atenolol (ICI 66082) in essential hypertension. Br. J. Clin. Pharmacol. (In press.)
14. Morgan, T.O., Sabio, J., Anavekar, S.N. et al: A comparison of beta adrenergic blocking drugs in the treatment of hypertension. Postgrad. Med. 50:253, 1974.
15. Hansson, L., Åberg, H., Karlberg, B.E. et al: Controlled study of atenolol in treatment of hypertension. Br. Med. J. 2:367, 1975.
16. Lydtin, H., Kusus, T., Daniel, W. et al: Propranolol therapy in essential hypertension. Am. Heart J. 83:589, 1972.
17. Frohlich, E.D., Tarazi, R.C., Dustan, H.P. et al: The paradox of beta-adrenergic blockade in hypertension. Circulation 37:417, 1968.
18. Amery, A., Billiet, L., Joossens, J.W. et al: Preliminary report on the haemodynamic response of hypertensive patients with a beta blocker (ICI 66082). Acta Clin. Belg. 28:358, 1973.
19. Franciosa, J.A. and Freis, E.D.: Normal cardiac output during beta blockade with timolol in hypertensive patients. Clin. Pharmacol. Ther. 18:158, 1975.
20. Shubrooks, S.J., Zir, L.M., Dinsmore, R.E. et al: Left ventricular wall motion response to intravenous. Circulation 52:124, 1975.
21. Lund-Johansen, P.: Hemodynamic changes at rest and during exercise in long-term prazosin therapy of essential hypertension. *In* Cotton, D.W.K. (ed.): Prazosin — Evaluation of a New Antihypertensive Agent. Geneva:Excerpta Medica, 1974, pp. 43-53.
22. Farmer, B.B., Harris, R.A., Jolly, W.W. et al: Studies on the cardiomegaly of the spontaneously hypertensive rat. Circ. Res. 35:102, 1974.
23. Folkow, B., Hallbäck, M., Lundgren, Y. et al: Importance of adaptive changes in vascular design for establishment of primary hypertension, studied in man and in spontaneously hypertensive rats. Circ. Res. 32 (suppl. 1) and 33:1, 1973.
24. Henry, J.P., Stephens, P.M. and Santisteban, G.A.: A model of psychosocial hypertension showing reversibility and progression of cardiovascular complications. Circ. Res. 36:156, 1975.
25. Liard, J.-F., Tarazi, R.C., Ferrario, C.M. et al: Hemodynamic and humoral characteristics of hypertension induced by prolonged stellate ganglion stimulation in conscious dogs. Circ. Res. 36:455, 1975.

Discussion

Moderator: Dr. A. Grollman

Dr. Freis: I wanted to respond to Dr. Lund-Johansen. Dr. Franciosa and I measured the hemodynamics of timolol on two occasions. First was in a double-blind comparison with propranolol and to our great surprise we found that although both agents lowered the cardiac output initially, that after two weeks timolol no longer showed a drop in cardiac output whereas the fall was still maintained with propranolol. Therefore we repeated the cardiac output studies with timolol and found the same thing in another series of hypertensive patients. I do not know why we did not get the same results as yours. I suspect you are correct but I think probably the most significant difference is that we saw very little reduction in blood pressure, almost none. In fact, if you took away the drop in diastolic pressure due to decrease in heart rate we had almost none. It is difficult to make hemodynamic conclusions from such small changes in blood pressure and, therefore, I am not going to dispute your results. With respect to the other comments you made about the long-term effects of prazosin and other drugs on cardiac output, I think what we require is a comparison between the acute effects and the chronic effects rather than control versus chronic effects. The point is, does cardiac output return toward control as compared to the acute effects of the drug.

Dr. Lund-Johansen: Perhaps a short comment to Dr. Freis's statement. It would of course have been very interesting to follow the hemodynamic effects of various antihypertensive drugs by measurements taken before therapy, after some hours then after a few weeks, a few months and so on but, obviously, this is difficult. However, I think if you get experience with the method and you study your subjects exactly in the same way, it should be possible to get a picture of the long-term effects of the various types of drugs. I think the results can ultimately show that there is a real difference in the long-term effects of the various antihypertensive drugs. Maybe I could just add what happens if you do *not* treat. We have a one-year follow-up in an untreated group and over a period of one year very little happens to central hemodynamics. Over a period of eight years, however, in a relatively young person, the main change is an increase in the total peripheral resistance at rest and during exercise. As this is the cardinal hemodynamic disturbance in essential hypertension I think we would all like to see a drug which not only reduces pressure but brings the circulatory system as close to normal as possible.

Dr. Onesti: I would like to comment on prazosin. In contrast with other pharmacologic agents it seemed to exert exactly the same hemodynamic effect acutely and chronically. We studied the acute effect of prazosin in essential hypertension.* The hemodynamic effects of prolonged administration of prazosin have been studied by Lund-Johansen.† Acute and long-term hemodynamic effects are identical.

---

*Fernandes, M., Smith, I.S., Weder, A. et al: Prazosin in the treatment of hypertension. Clin. Sci. Molec. Med. 48:181s, 1975.

†Lund-Johansen, P.: Hemodynamic changes at rest and during exercise in long-term prazosin therapy of essential hypertension. *In* Cotton, D.W.K. (ed.): Prazosin — Evaluation of a New Antihypertensive Agent. Geneva:Excerpta Medica, 1974.

Potential Effects of Antihypertensive Therapy on Intravascular Thrombosis

Arthur Grollman, M.D., Ph.D.

The beneficial effects of treating patients with a consistent elevation in diastolic blood pressure is now so generally accepted that it has become ethically difficult to justify denial of such treatment to any patient. The House of Delegates of the American Medical Association, in 1973, stated that "the benefits of treatment were so significant" that they recommended strongly "the prompt and vigorous treatment of hypertensive patients" [1] and that "measurements of diastolic pressure averaging 105 mm Hg or higher on three separate follow-up visits usually indicate the need for the initiation of drug therapy." Accordingly, it would be ethically difficult to justify perfectly controlled studies to determine the validity of this generally accepted directive. Nevertheless, a number of questions remain which deserve consideration and it is the purpose of this paper to discuss one of these, namely, the potential of the antihypertensive drugs to induce thrombosis of the cerebral and coronary arteries or infarction of the brain and heart.

The antihypertensive drugs are used to lower the diastolic (and incidentally the systolic) blood pressure; accordingly, their use is empiric in the sense that they correct a manifestation of the disease rather than its cause. The available actuarial insurance data indicate that any elevation in blood pressure, regardless of whether it be systolic or diastolic, causes an

---

Arthur Grollman M.D., Ph.D., Professor of Experimental Medicine, Department of Pathology, The University of Texas, Health Science Center at Dallas, Tex.

increased mortality. A decrease in the systolic level of the blood pressure in such conditions as atherosclerosis, arteriovenous fistulae, hyperthyroidism, etc., in which there is no or little increase in diastolic blood pressure is not tolerated, since this is accompanied by a decrease in perfusion of the tissues. The use of antihypertensive drugs is therefore limited to diastolic hypertension induced by an increase in reversible peripheral resistance which most commonly occurs in "essential" hypertension. An increased diastolic pressure may, however, also occur when arteriosclerosis involves the smaller arteries and arterioles. In this case lowering the blood pressure would decrease perfusion of the tissues as it does in other forms of atherosclerosis.

Since diastolic hypertension may differ in the morphologic disturbances which it causes in the blood vessels as well as in its pathogenesis, one would anticipate that the response to lowering the blood pressure might differ and that consideration of the underlying pathophysiology of the disturbance would have to be considered in any rational therapeutic regimen. Decreasing the blood pressure might be harmful depending upon the mechanism of action of the drug used and the nature of the cardiovascular disturbance characteristic of the particular form of hypertension under treatment. Surgical intervention would obviously be the desired treatment in aldosterone-producing tumors and the substitution of other antifertility measures in patients in whom drugs have induced hypertension. The use of antihypertensive drugs is considered by many to be satisfactory in cases of surgically remediable (renovascular) hypertension only because of the failure to diagnose this form of hypertension accurately by the currently used procedures [2].

It would be of great practical importance to differentiate the extent to which atherosclerosis elevates the blood pressure by reducing the elasticity of the blood vessels and essential hypertension which acts by increasing the peripheral resistance. This differentiation, however, is not made easily clinically and is further complicated by the fact that essential hypertension accelerates the production of arteriosclerosis and the latter when involving the kidney may contribute to the elevation of blood pressure by a renal mechanism similar to that believed to be involved in the pathogenesis of essential hypertension. The blood pressure in essential hypertension, particularly in the older patient, reflects in fact the existence of a combination of two basically different pathological processes [3], and lowering the blood pressure may induce distinctly different side effects which must be considered in any therapeutic regimen. This paper will be concerned with only one of these side effects, namely, intravascular thrombosis and infarction, common occurrences in hypertension, and a leading cause of death when they involve the heart or brain.

Thrombosis and Infarction as Complications of Antihypertensive Therapy

Thrombosis most commonly results from slowing with loss of the axial stream and laminar flow-pattern of the bloodstream which leads to the deposition of the formed elements of the blood on the vessel walls. Thrombosis is thus favored by bed rest with its attendant muscular inactivity and congestive heart failure, both of which result in slowing of the circulation. Any drug which concomitantly with its antihypertensive action reduces the cerebral, coronary or peripheral blood flow would also tend to provoke thrombosis, cerebral or myocardial infarction (common complications of hypertension) and thromboembolism of peripheral vessels which is believed to cause the focal manifestations of cerebral ischemia observed in hypertension.

The precipitating factors in thrombosis may also be a consequence of increased coagulability of the blood secondary to the direct effects of drugs, but there is no evidence to indicate that the antihypertensive drugs activate coagulation factors. Common causes of thrombosis are stasis of the circulation secondary to cardiac arrhythmia, congestive heart failure, dehydration, immobilization, myocardial infarction, obesity and varicosities of the veins. Congestive heart failure, the most common complication of hypertension, dehydration induced by the use of diuretics, and hemodynamic changes resulting in a reduction of the perfusion pressure of the tissues must be considered as potential causes of thrombosis and infarction when the blood pressure is lowered. The significance of this complication of antihypertensive therapy has been generally ignored, but a critical examination of the literature indicates that it must be considered as a potential precipitating factor in the death of patients receiving antihypertensive drugs.

That the above-described undesirable complications of antihypertensive therapy are of practical importance is demonstrated by patients, particularly the elderly, who respond adversely to therapy and, therefore, discontinue taking their antihypertensive medications. To exclude such patients from a study, as was done in the investigation sponsored by the Veterans Administration Hospitals [4], is obviously misleading. The exclusion of patients dying within six months of the initiation of therapy [5] would likewise be unjustified since this procedure excludes patients most vulnerable to any potentially harmful effects of therapy. In short-term experiments, cerebral blood flow is maintained constant, despite variations in perfusion pressure, by its intrinsic autoregulatory capacity. In advanced cerebral arteriosclerosis, however, or in the face of a marked reduction in cerebral blood flow one would anticipate thrombosis or circulatory insufficiency to ensue.

Incidence of Cerebral Thrombosis in Patients Receiving Antihypertensive Drugs

Any comparison of the data of the literature on the effects of antihypertensive therapy is rendered difficult by the lack of uniformity in the manner in which the experiments were performed. As already indicated, exclusion of patients who failed to take their medications, or who died within six months of therapy, would fail to reveal adverse effects of therapy. Since arteriosclerosis in the hypertensive patient increases with age, the use of younger patients would yield more favorable results than those obtained with older ones. Studies with different drug regimens would also not be comparable since they may affect differently the hemodynamics of the circulation.

As pointed out by Dickinson [6], examination of the literature reveals considerable variation in the incidence of stroke during treatment with antihypertensive drugs in marked contrast to the effect of lowering the blood pressure on congestive heart failure. His review of the earlier literature indicated that the majority of investigators found that medical treatment of hypertension did not appreciably lessen the incidence of strokes. In fact, in most published series the relative importance of strokes as causes of death was increased as a result of treatment. Thus Beem [7] noted that complications of cerebral origin were twice as frequent in treated as compared to control subjects. Hood et al [8] list cerebrovascular accidents as the most common specific cause of death encountered in the treatment of hypertension. Ueda et al [5] noted an increase in death from cerebrovascular accidents in treated as compared to control patients. Gormsen et al [9] also noted that in 202 patients with acute cerebral infarction, 30 were being treated, in eight of whom the cerebrovascular accident was attributable to treatment.

Contrary to the above findings are those, among others, of Hodge et al [10] who noted 32 out of 82 (40%) strokes in controls as compared to 33% in treated patients; Lee et al [11]; Hamilton [12]; Hood et al [13]; Freis [14]; and the Veterans Administration Cooperative Study Group [4]. Hood et al [13], however, noted no change in the five-year mortality in myocardial infarction; one half of the deaths from this complication occurred when the patient was under good or excellent blood pressure control.

Several explanations may be offered to account for the wide discrepancies of the conclusions drawn from the above-cited studies. As already suggested, the reasonable assumption that patients who failed to take or discontinued their medication did so because of cerebral ischemia induced by lowering of their blood pressure biases the conclusions drawn from data based on studies in which such patients were excluded. The inclusion of younger patients with lesser degrees of atherosclerosis would tend to reduce the susceptibility to thrombosis but not to myocardial infarction which may account for the findings of Hood et al [13].

It might be anticipated that even if lowering the blood pressure might predispose to cerebral thrombosis, it would protect against cerebral hemorrhage. This conclusion, however, is erroneous since hemorrhage may occur as a result of changes in the cerebral tissue rather than from increased intravascular pressure.

Although lowering the blood pressure by hypertensive drugs may be life-saving in many cases of malignant hypertension, patients suffering from this disorder may nevertheless succumb to the effects of cerebral thrombosis and hemorrhage [15] even when the blood pressure has been lowered by effective antihypertensive treatment. This form of hypertension is not simply an exacerbation of chronic essential hypertension, as was once believed, but is accompanied by the presence of a pressor agent (not found in chronic essential hypertension) which is apparently responsible for the vascular necrosis and other unique characteristics of this condition [16].

Conclusion

The ideal treatment of essential hypertension would be to initiate therapy during the early stages of the disease in the hope of avoiding its most serious complication, arteriosclerosis. Even if such treatment were feasible, it would not necessarily avoid all the complications of the disease since other organic and functional disturbances are demonstrable, particularly in the heart and blood vessels [17-22]. Nevertheless, visceral changes are preventable in experimental hypertension [23] and reversible to some extent when the blood pressure is reduced in the human by a salt-free diet [24] or by drug therapy [25]. Once an elevated blood pressure has been attained, the ideal drug should act by reducing the peripheral resistance without decreasing the cardiac output and blood flow through the coronary, cerebral and other vessels. The mere reduction of the blood pressure at the expense of interfering with adequate tissue perfusion will be counterproductive and potentially harmful, since it would favor the development of coronary and cerebrovasular thromboses and myocardial and cerebral infarctions and interfere with normal cardiac, renal and cerebral functions, the chief complications of chronic essential hypertension.

The goal of therapeutics is to overcome the basic defect responsible for a clinical disability or, if this is not possible, to alleviate its symptoms and prevent its complications. The currently available hypotensive drugs reduce the blood pressure without affecting the basic defect responsible for the disease or its progress [1]. Such empirical therapy nevertheless is of established value in ameliorating congestive heart failure and malignant hypertension. Antihypertensive drugs and salt restriction are the best procedures presently available for the treatment of essential hypertension, but studies must continue to determine its pathogenesis and a search made for a therapeutic regimen to correct the basic defect responsible for the disease and its use at an early stage prior to the development of atherosclerosis and other irreversible organic changes.

The extent to which the blood pressure should be lowered is controversial. Dorph et al [25] noted no advantage in lowering the blood pressure to normal in severe hypertension. Toguchi and Freis [26], on the other hand, argue for normal control at an early state of the disease in order to reduce the increased risk of coronary artery disease. In addition to the level of the blood pressure, it is important to consider the clinical evidence of cerebral and myocardial change as a guide to therapy. It is also necessary to avoid precipitous drops in blood pressure when using such potent agents as diazoxide or sodium nitroprusside and the induction of dehydration and azotemia when using diuretics.

References

1. Moyer, J.H.: Hypertension: National significance, general principles of management, and choice of drugs. *In* Russek, H.I. (ed.): New Horizons in Cardiovascular Practice. Baltimore, Md.: University Park Press, 1973, pp. 253-271.
2. McNeil, B.J. and Adelstein, S.J.: Measures of clinical efficacy: The value of case finding in hypertensive renovascular disease. N. Engl. J. Med. 293:221, 1975.
3. Grollman, A.: The pathogenesis and treatment of hypertension. J. Am. Geriatr. Soc. 1:223, 1953.
4. Veterans Administration Cooperative Study Group on Antihypertensive Agents. JAMA 213:1143, 1970.
5. Ueda, H., Nakajima, K., Takeda, T. et al: Effectiveness of prolonged antihypertensive treatment on survival of patients with essential hypertension. Jap. Heart J. 5:399, 1964.
6. Dickinson, C.J.: Neurogenic Hypertension. Oxford:Blackwell Scientific Publications, 1965, pp. 135-140.
7. Beem, J.R.: Causes of death due to hypertension: The effect of therapy. *In* Moyer, J.H. (ed.): Hypertension (1st Hahnemann Symposium). Philadelphia, Pa.:Saunders, 1959, pp. 106-111.

8. Hood, B., Björk, S., Sannerstedt, R. et al: Analysis of mortality and survival in actively treated hypertensive disease. Acta Med. Scand. 174:393, 1963.
9. Gormsen, J., Drybye, M., Eiken, M. et al: Acute cerebral infarct: Extracerebral genesis with particular reference to cardiovascular status. Acta Med. Scand. 169:455, 1961.
10. Hodge, J.V., McQueen, E.G. and Smirk, H.: Results of hypotensive therapy in arterial hypertension. Based on experience with 497 patients treated and 156 controls observed for periods of one to eight years. Br. Med. J. 1:1, 1961.
11. Lee, R.E., Seligmann, A.W., Clark, M.A. et al: Freedom from cerebral vascular accidents during drug-induced blood pressure reduction in benign hypertensive disease. Am. J. Cardiol. 11:738, 1963.
12. Hamilton, M.: Selection of patients for antihypertensive therapy. *In* Gross, F. (ed.): Antihypertensive Therapy. Berlin-Heidelberg-New York:Springer-Verlag, 1966, pp. 196-206.
13. Hood, B., Aurell, M., Falkheden et al: Analysis of mortality and survival in actively treated hypertensive disease. *In* Gross, F. (ed.): Antihypertensive Therapy. Berlin-Heidelberg-New York:Springer-Verlag, 1966, pp. 370-387.
14. Freis, E.D.: Effect of antihypertensive treatment on morbidity. Milbank Mem. Fund Quart. 47:153, 1969.
15. Farmer, R.G., Gifford, R.W., Jr. and Hines, E.A., Jr.: Effect of medical treatment of severe hypertension. A follow-up study of 161 patients with group 3 and group 4 hypertension. Arch. Intern. Med. 112:118, 1963.
16. Grollman, A.: The pathogenesis of malignant hypertension. Int. Res. Commun. Syst. 1:16, 1973.
17. Laramore, D.C. and Grollman, A.: Water and electrolyte content of tissues in normal and hypertensive rats. Am. J. Physiol. 161:278, 1950.
18. Muirhead, E.E., Turner, L.B. and Grollman, A.: Hypertensive cardiovascular disease. Nature and pathogenesis of the arteriolar sclerosis induced by bilateral nephrectomy as revealed by a study of its tinctorial characteristics. Arch. Pathol. 52:266, 1951.
19. Deming, Q.B.: Experimental atherosclerosis and hypertension. *In* Gross, F. (ed.): Antihypertensive Therapy. Berlin-Heidelberg-New York:Springer-Verlag, 1966, pp. 111-124.
20. Hazama, F., Ooshima, A., Tomimoto, K. et al: Vascular changes in the various substrains of spontaneously hypertensive rats, untreated and treated with sodium chloride in diet. Jap. Heart J. 14:174, 1973.
21. Grollman, A. and Krishnamurty, V.S.R.: Contractile response of the aorta of the normotensive and acute and chronic hypertensive rat. Arch. Int. Pharmacodyn. 203:376, 1973.
22. Yamori, Y., Tomimoto, K., Ooshima, A. et al: Developmental course of hypertension in the SHR-substrains susceptible to hypertensive cerebrovascular lesions. Jap. Heart J. 15:209, 1974.

23. Griffith, R. and Hummel, R. Effect of treatment on the development of vascular lesions in the hypertensive rat. Triangle 12:75, 1973.
24. Kempner, W.: Treatment of kidney disease and hypertensive vascular disease with rice diet. N.Carolina Med. J. 5:125, 1944.
25. Dorph, S., Leth, A., Degnbol, B. et al: Visceral changes in severe hypertension and their response to drug therapy. Acta Med. Scand. 187:411, 1970.
26. Toguchi, J. and Freis, E.D.: Partial versus complete control of blood pressure. Circ. Res. 36(suppl. 1): 257, 1975.

Low Renal Papillary Plasma Flow in Both Dahl and Kyoto Spontaneously Hypertensive Rats

Louis Tobian, M.D., Mukul Ganguli, Ph.D. and Lewis Dahl, M.D.

The renal medulla has several possibly important connections to hypertension. For instance, the renal interstitial cells are all located in the inner medulla [1]. These cells appear to be secretory in nature and are known to secrete prostaglandin E_2 [2]. Moreover, when implants of these cells are placed subcutaneously in a hypertensive rat or rabbit, some humoral agent issuing from them lowers the level of arterial pressure [3, 4]. These interstitial cells also contain a distinctly reduced number of cytoplasmic lipid granules in five separate forms of experimental rat hypertension [1, 5-8]. These cells not only secrete prostaglandins but also appear to elaborate Muirhead's antihypertensive neutral lipid [2, 3]. Moreover, in three forms of experimental rat hypertension, the sodium concentration in the papilla was significantly lower than that in normotensive controls [1, 5, 6]. The reduction in sodium concentration in the papilla paralleled the reduction in the number of interstitial cell granules with a fairly strong correlation [1, 5, 6]. Moreover, prostaglandins are very powerful vasoactive agents; in the kidney they are mainly synthesized (90%) in the renal medulla [9], largely by the interstitial cells and the collecting

---

Louis Tobian, M.D., Professor of Internal Medicine and Chief of Hypertension Unit, University of Minnesota Medical School, Minneapolis; Mukul Ganguli, Ph.D., Research Associate, Department of Internal Medicine, University of Minnesota Medical School; Lewis Dahl, M.D., Chief of Hypertension Research Unit, Brookhaven National Laboratory, Upton, N.Y.

duct cells [2, 10]. The renal medulla also contains the collecting ducts, powerful regulators of ultimate sodium excretion [11-13]. Since hypertension is affected profoundly by the sodium balance in the body, the collecting ducts of the medulla could conceivably have an important connection to hypertension.

With this background, we became interested in measuring plasma flow to this important region in hypertensive rats. It has been reported by several investigators that while renal cortical blood flow is well autoregulated, renal medullary blood flow is not. Kramer et al [14] and Miyamoto and Gordon [15] found that during a sudden rise in the perfusion pressure, the blood flow through the renal medulla increased, while the cortical and total renal blood flow remained constant. If this were indeed true under all circumstances, then hypertensive rats could well have very large papillary plasma flows. Ganguli and Tobian [16] noted in rats with "post-salt" hypertension that the renal papilla does indeed chronically "autoregulate" its flow, since they observed a reduced renal papillary plasma flow in rats with "post-salt" hypertension. Since the "post-salt" hypertensive kidneys had a considerable amount of nephrosclerosis which led to the atrophy of some nephron units, we further endeavored to test this hypothesis in Kyoto spontaneously hypertensive rats (SHR) and in Dahl salt-sensitive ("S") rats. Both of these strains have almost no nephrosclerosis at 17 weeks of age if fed a normal salt intake. Furthermore, the SHR and "S" rats are recognized as models resembling human essential hypertension [17-19].

Methods

The renal papillary plasma flow was measured in rats under Inactin (100 mg/kg) anesthesia using a method essentially similar to Lilienfield et al [20] with slight modifications by Ganguli and Tobian [16] and subsequently by Solez et al [21] to make it applicable to the rat. In brief, albumin-^{125}I at the concentration of 4 Mμ Ci/ml in normal saline (0.9%) is steadily infused into the right atrium. Then for about 60 seconds in the dog and for about 36 seconds in the rat, the radioactive counts in the papilla increase approximately linearly with time after the start of the infusion. Because of the small amount of mixing and slow flow and long length of the vessels in the papilla, this represents the time that elapses before plasma entering the papilla actually leaves it. During the precise time interval in which radioactive albumin is entering the kidney, blood in the carotid artery was slowly but continuously sampled for radioactivity at approximately the same rate of withdrawal as fluid containing radioactive albumin entered the right atrium. After a time interval of 24 seconds, the kidney pedicle was instantaneously ligated and the collection of blood from the carotid artery was terminated. Since the time interval for linear accumulation of radioactive albumin in the papilla lasts 36 seconds, an accumulation time of 24 seconds is well within the linear period and should provide an accurate index of plasma flow to the papilla.

At the end of the prescribed time interval, the papilla of the kidney was quickly dissected out and placed in an air-tight pre-weighed weighing bottle to obtain the net weight of the papilla. Then the radioactivity of the papilla was ascertained in a gamma scintillation counter. The samples of blood from the carotid artery were similarly weighed and counted. Tissue radioactivity was expressed as counts per minute per gram of tissue. Blood radioactivity was expressed as counts per minute per milliliter of plasma after making corrections for the hematocrit. When the radioactive counts per gram of papilla were divided by counts per milliliter of plasma, one has an estimate of the volume of plasma accumulating in a gram of papilla during 24 seconds of elapsed time. This should represent papillary plasma flow. Just prior to infusion of radioactive albumin, mean blood pressure was measured directly from the carotid artery with a Hg manometer. Statistical analyses of the data were made using Student's "t" test [22].

Experiment 1

We used the two strains of rats developed by Dahl [19]. One group, the "S" strain, invariably becomes hypertensive when fed a high NaCl intake (8% NaCl in dry chow). The other group, the "R" strain, never becomes hypertensive when fed an 8% high salt intake. The "S" strain is so named because it is sensitive to salt hypertension. The "R" strain is so named because it is resistant to salt hypertension.

A total of 77 female rats of "S" and "R" strains, about 16 weeks of age and weighing between 235 and 285 gm, were used. They were divided into eight categories as follows:

One Week Feeding

	0.3% NaCl	8.0% NaCl
"S"	Group I (n=10)	Group II (n=9)
"R"	Group III (n=13)	Group IV (n=12)

Four Weeks Feeding

	0.3% NaCl	8.0% NaCl
"S"	Group V (n=8)	Group VI (n=7)
"R"	Group VII (n=9)	Group VIII (n=9)

The two levels of dietary NaCl, 0.3% and 8.0%, could be considered as either "normal" or "high salt," respectively [23]. All rats had received 0.3% NaCl chow since weaning. After that, high salt feeding was carried out in both "S" and "R" rats for one- and four-week periods. Concomitant feeding of a diet with 0.3% NaCl was carried out in other "S" and "R" rats. The papillary plasma flow was then measured as described above. This was done in a "round-robin" fashion among groups I through IV, as well as in groups V through VIII.

Experiment 2

Twenty-six male Kyoto spontaneously hypertensive (SHR) rats (BP 170-200) and 24 Kyoto normotensive controls (BP 100-130), weighing between 280 and 360 gm and all about 17 weeks of age, were used. The mean arterial pressure for the Kyoto SHR was 182 mm Hg; the mean pressure for the Kyoto normotensives was 118 mm Hg. All rats had received 0.3% NaCl chow since weaning. The plasma flow to the renal papilla was measured using the method described above. The measurements on Kyoto hypertensive and Kyoto normotensive rats were alternated.

Results

Experiment 1 (Table 1)

When eating a normal Na diet with 0.3% NaCl, 18 hypertension-sensitive ("S") rats and 22 hypertension-resistant ("R") rats (all 20-weeks old) had blood pressures close to the normal range, the two groups averaging 144 and 129 mm Hg, respectively. The "S" rats could be considered to have borderline hypertension, since their average mean blood pressure was about 15 mm Hg above that of the "R" rats. After both groups had been on the normal (0.3%) NaCl intake for several weeks, the borderline hypertensive "S" rats had a mean papillary plasma flow of 19.2 ml/100 gm/min of papilla, which was 25% lower than the 25.6 papillary plasma flow of the normotensive "R" rats. The difference in flow here was highly significant with a p value much less than 0.001.

Table 1.

Group	Type of Rat	No. of Rats	% NaCl in Diet	Blood Pressure* (mm Hg)		Papillary Plasma Flow* (ml/100 gm/min)	
				One Week			
I	S	10	0.3	145 ± 4.2		20.4 ± 1.30	[p ≤ 0.05]
II	S	9	8.0	152 ± 3.1		24.8 ± 1.56	
III	R	13	0.3	130 ± 2.4		25.6 ± 0.81	[p ≤ 0.001]
IV	R	12	8.0	128 ± 1.8		33.8 ± 1.84	
				Four Weeks			
V	S	8	0.3	142 ± 3.3	[p ≤ 0.001]	17.7 ± 1.13	
VI	S	7	8.0	162 ± 3.3		20.0 ± 1.74	
VII	R	9	0.3	127 ± 2.9		25.7 ± 0.72	[p ≤ 0.025]
VIII	R	9	8.0	127 ± 2.5		29.5 ± 1.41	

*Mean ± SEM.

[p ≤] = Whenever p values are written between two means, they indicate a significant difference between those two means. When p values are not listed, it indicates that the difference between means was not statistically significant.

When the "R" rats are challenged with a high (8%) NaCl diet for seven days, the papillary plasma flow rose to 33.8 ml/100 gm/min, while it was only 25.6 in comparable "R" rats that remained on the normal (0.3%) NaCl intake. Thus, exposure to the high salt intake led to a 32% increase in papillary flow in the "R" rats. The "p" value of the difference was less than 0.001.

The same 8% high salt feeding was carried out for one week in "S" rats. After the one-week challenge with a high salt intake, the "S" rats had an average papillary flow of 24.8, compared to a flow of 20.4 in "S" rats on a normal salt intake. The high salt intake increased papillary flow 22% in these "S" rats, with a p value less than 0.05.

We next studied the effect of a four-week challenge with the high salt feeding. In "R" rats on the high salt intake, the flow was 29.5, compared to 25.7 in "R" rats on a normal salt intake. Thus, even after four weeks of high salt feeding, there is a 15% increase in papillary flow above control, with a p value of 0.025. This is a considerably smaller rise than the 32% increase seen after one week on the high salt intake. Evidently, some degree of adaptation to the high salt intake had taken place.

When the four-week salt challenge was tested on "S" rats, we found only a small rise in flow compared to the control group. The difference was not statistically significant. Thus, the "S" rats appear to undergo little increase of papillary flow after four weeks of high salt feeding, a much smaller response than was present after one week of high salt feeding.

A contrast in blood pressure and papillary flow was found in the two strains of rats after one week of high salt feeding. The "R" rats show no increase in blood pressure. It is still 128. The "S" rats have risen up to 152 after only one week of salt feeding. The "R" rats have a papillary flow of 33.8, while the "S" rats have a flow of only 24.8. This is a 27% difference in papillary flow, with a p value less than 0.005.

The same comparison was made after four weeks of high salt feeding. The blood pressure of the "R" rats still remains low at 127. The blood pressure of the "S" rats has risen to 162. The papillary flow of the "R" rats is 29.5 while that of the "S" rats is only 20.0. This is quite a large difference, with the "S" rats having a flow 32% lower than that of the "R" rats. The p value of this difference was less than 0.001.

Experiment 2

On a normal salt intake, the papillary flow of 26 Kyoto spontaneously hypertensive rats (age 17 weeks — BP 182) was compared with that of 24 Kyoto normotensive rats (age 17 weeks — BP 118). The Kyoto hypertensives had an average papillary flow of 29.5 ml/100 gm/min, while the Kyoto normotensives averaged 33.2. Thus, the Kyoto hypertensives had an 11% lower papillary flow than the Kyoto normotensives ($p < .001$).

Discussion

In previous studies of "S" and "R" rats on either 0.3% NaCl or 8.0% NaCl by Ben-Ishay and Dahl [24], the PAH clearance was virtually the same in either strain on either high or normal salt diets. Thus, the total renal blood flow in the "S" rat is not reduced, compared to the "R" rat. The elevation of total renal vascular resistance just matches the rise in arterial pressure so that the total renal blood flow in the "S" rat remains normal. This is in striking contrast to our finding of a markedly lower papillary plasma flow in the "S" rat. The vascular resistance of vessels supplying the papilla in the "S" rat must be disproportionally much greater than the vascular resistance in the "S" kidney as a whole.

This disproportionate vasoconstriction in vessels supplying the "S" papilla, when the "S" rat has only borderline hypertension, may well be related to this rat's susceptibility to NaCl hypertension. Our findings indicate that papillary plasma flow increases significantly in normotensive "R" rats when they are challenged with a high salt intake. This increase in papillary flow may be a physiologic aid in the expeditious excretion of the large NaCl load. It is well demonstrated by Stein et al [11], Sonnenberg [12] and Diezi et al [13] that the collecting duct participates very importantly in the excretion of a large Na load. The increase in papillary plasma flow during a high sodium intake may be related to this collecting duct action. The "S" rat has an abnormally low papillary flow while on a normal sodium intake. However, as long as the sodium intake is fairly low, the reduced papillary flow of the "S" rat may be of little importance in sodium homeostasis, and the rat's blood pressure does not rise above the borderline hypertensive range. However, when the "S" rat begins to eat the high salt intake, he has only a limited rise in papillary flow, which remains a striking 32% below the papillary flow of the "R" rat after four weeks on the same high salt intake. One might theorize that the limited papillary flow in the "S" rat somehow brings about a limited capacity of the kidney to excrete sodium rapidly. If this were indeed the case, other, alternative natriuretic forces might then be needed to expedite a brisk Na excretion. It is well established that an increase in renal arterial pressure will bring about a natriuresis in an isolated kidney [25]. Thus, one can further theorize that the low papillary flow of the "S" rat limits the usual rapid excretion of Na, thereby necessitating a rise in arterial pressure to bring about Na excretion through the mechanism of a "pressure natriuresis." We hasten to add that this formulation is at present only a working hypothesis, and further information on several key points is needed before it can be accepted or rejected with any confidence.

If indeed low papillary flow retards the rate of sodium excretion and higher papillary flow facilitates it after a sodium load, this could very well be related to the development of hypertension. In a previous study [26] ordinary rats were fed a diet containing 8% NaCl, and 40% of them became hypertensive. Another group of similar rats were fed the same high salt diet and at the same time were given a thiazide diuretic in their drinking water. None of the rats in this group became hypertensive. Both groups came into sodium balance on the high salt intake, but one group had a high prevalence of hypertension and the other group had no hypertension. The group on the straight high salt diet had a 5% increase of ECF volume above control after one week on the diet. The group on the high salt diet plus thiazide had an ECF volume very close to control levels. Even though rats in both groups excreted the ingested NaCl, the thiazide facilitated this excretion in one group, thereby achieving Na balance with a normal ECF volume. In the other group without thiazide, Na balance was achieved in association with an expanded ECF volume. Hypertension was frequently present in the group with the expanded ECF volume but was absent in the group with the normal ECF volume. When the ECF volume is expanded for a considerable period of time, as in mineralocorticoid or renal parenchymal hypertension, hypertension often supervenes. It is conceivable that the marked difference in papillary plasma flows in the "S" and "R" rats may have had a differential effect on sodium excretion just as the presence or absence of thiazide did.

The low plasma flow to the renal papilla in "S" rats and Kyoto hypertensive rats may have another implication. The low flow indicates an unusual degree of increase in vascular resistance, more than is found in other vascular beds in hypertension. The hypertensive state, in general, is associated with narrow vascular lumens and increased vascular resistance. It could be that the vessels supplying the papilla are especially sensitive to this "hypertensive" effect, more sensitive than any other set of vessels in the body. They could be so sensitive that they produced a 25% reduction of papillary plasma flow even in "S" rats with borderline hypertension eating a normal salt intake. The vessels supplying the papilla in these rats could be narrowed quite a bit while other vessels are scarcely narrowed at all. The supersensitivity of papillary vessels in "S" rats could also affect and retard sodium excretion during a high sodium load, which in turn would have the effect of increasing the severity of the hypertension. If this hypothesis were correct, during a large sodium load the key elements would exist for a mildly vicious cycle.

If the vessels to the papilla are especially narrowed in "S" rats, one might suspect excess or deficits of vasoactive humoral agents which are elaborated in close proximity to these vessels. Substances secreted by the interstitial cells could very well be causing the exaggerated narrowing of vessels supplying the papilla of the "S" rat. These would include prostaglandins as well as Muirhead's "neutral lipid" as well as other unrecognized secretory materials put out by the interstitial cells. Moreover, the collecting duct cells also synthesize prostaglandins which could be acting on these blood vessels.

In regard to the increased papillary plasma flow after a high salt intake, one is reminded that volume expansion causes the elaboration in the rat of a humoral agent of nonrenal, nonadrenal origin which dilates renal blood vessels and heightens natriuresis [27]. It would be of interest to know if this factor were stimulated by a high NaCl diet and whether it affects the caliber of blood vessels supplying the renal papilla.

The Kyoto spontaneously hypertensive rats also had an 11% lower papillary flow than the Kyoto normotensive controls. This is of particular interest considering that Nishiyama and Frohlich [28] found the blood flow to the Kyoto hypertensive kidney as a whole to be the same as that of the Kyoto normotensive kidney as a whole. Thus, here again the resistance in vessels supplying the papilla is disproportionally higher than the vascular resistance to the kidney as a whole. The vessels supplying the papilla appear to be especially sensitive to the narrowing associated with the hypertensive process. The flow to the papilla in Kyoto hypertensives is only 11% below Kyoto controls. This is a smaller difference than was seen between Dahl "S" and "R" rats and is consistent with the observation that the Kyoto hypertensive strain shows a much more modest rise in blood pressure in response to a high salt intake than that of the Dahl "S" rat.

In a previous study it was noted that the papillary flow in rats with "post-salt" hypertension is 15% lower than that of normotensive controls [16]. Thus, we have studied three distinct types of experimental rat hypertension, all of which have significantly reduced papillary plasma flow. It is possible that this low papillary flow is a genuine repeating hallmark for all types of experimental rat hypertension. More studies will definitely be needed to get a firm answer to this question.

References

1. Tobian, L., Ishii, M. and Duke, M.: Relationship of cytoplasmic granules in renal papillary interstitial cells to "post-salt" hypertension. J. Lab. Clin. Med. 73:309-319, 1969.
2. Muirhead, E.E., Germain, G., Leach, B.E. et al: Production of renomedullary prostaglandins by renomedullary interstitial cells grown in tissue culture. Circ. Res. 31 (suppl 2):161-172, 1972.
3. Muirhead, E.E., Brown, G.B., Germain, G.S. et al: The renal medulla as an antihypertensive organ. J. Lab. Clin. Med. 76:641-651, 1970.
4. Tobian, L. and Azar, S.: Antihypertensive and other functions of the renal papilla. Trans. Ass. Am. Physicians 84:281-288, 1971.

5. Ishii, M. and Tobian, L.: Interstitial cell granules in renal papilla and the solute composition of renal tissue in rats with Goldblatt hypertension. J. Lab. Clin. Med. 74:47-52, 1969.
6. Tobian, L. and Ishii, M.: Interstitial cell granules and solutes in renal papilla in "post-Goldblatt" hypertension. Am. J. Physiol. 217:1699-1702, 1969.
7. Muehrcke, R.C., Mandal, A.K., Epstein, M. et al: Cytoplasmic granularity of the renal medullary interstitial cells in experimental hypertension. J. Lab. Clin. Med. 73:299-308, 1969.
8. Mandal, A.K., Frohlich, E.D., Chrysant, K. et al: Renal interstitial cells in spontaneously hypertensive rats. Circulation 48:IV-46, 1973
9. Van Dorp, D.: Recent developments in the biosynthesis and the analyses of prostaglandin. Ann. N.Y. Acad. Sci. 180:181-199, 1971.
10. Janszen, F.H.A. and Nugteren, D.H.: Histochemical localization of prostaglandin synthetase. Histochemie 27:159-164, 1971.
11. Stein, J.H., Kirshenbaum, M.A., Bay, W.H. et al: Role of the collecting duct in the regulation of sodium balance. Circ. Res. 36 and 37 (suppl. 1):I-119-124, 1975.
12. Sonnenberg, H.: Medullary collecting-duct function in antidiuretic and in salt or water-diuretic rats. Am. J. Physiol. 226:501-506, 1974.
13. Diezi, J., Michoud, P., Aceves, J. et al: Micropuncture study of electrolyte transport across papillary collecting duct of the rat. Am. J. Physiol. 224:623-634, 1973.
14. Kramer, K., Thurau, D. and Deetjen, P.: Hämodynamik des Nierenmarks. Capilläre Passagezeit, Blutvolumen, Durchblutung, Gewebshemätokrit und O_2-Verbrauch des Nierenmarks in situ. Arch. Ges. Physiol. 270:251-269, 1960.
15. Miyamoto, J. and Gordon, S.: The cortical and medullary blood flows of the isolated dog's kidney. Jap. J. Physiol. 20:584-597, 1970.
16. Ganguli, M. and Tobian, L.: Does the kidney autoregulate papillary plasma flow in chronic "post-salt" hypertension. Am. J. Physiol. 226:330-333, 1974.
17. Folkow, B., Hallbäck, M., Lundgren, Y. et al: Structurally based increase of flow resistance in spontaneously hypertensive rats. Acta Physiol. Scand. 79:373-378, 1970.
18. Undenfriend, S. and Spector, S.: Spontaneously hypertensive rat. Science 176:1155-1156, 1972.
19. Dahl, L.K., Heine, M. and Tassinari, L.: Effects of chronic salt ingestion. Evidence that genetic factors play an important role in susceptibility to experimental hypertension. J. Exp. Med. 115:1173-1190, 1962.
20. Lilienfield, L.S., Maganzini, H.G. and Bauer, M.H.: Blood flow in the renal medulla. Circ. Res. 9:614-617, 1961.
21. Solez, K., Kramer, E.C., Fox, J.A. et al: Medullary plasma flow and intravascular leukocyte accumulation in acute renal failure. Kidney Int. 6:24-37, 1974.
22. Snedecor, G.D. and Cochran, W.G.: Statistical Methods. Ames, Iowa:Iowa State University Press, 1967.

23. National Research Council, 1972: Nutrient requirements of domestic animals — Nutrient requirements of laboratory animals. Nat. Acad. Sci. Nat. Res. Council Publ. 990.
24. Ben-Ishay, D., Knudsen, K.D. and Dahl, L.K.: Renal function studies in the early stage of salt hypertension in rats. Proc. Soc. Exp. Biol. Med. 125:515-518, 1967.
25. Selkurt, E.E.: Effect of pulse pressure and mean arterial pressure modification on renal hemodynamics and electrolyte and water excretion. Circulation 4:541-551, 1951.
26. Tobian, L., Lange, J., Magraw, S. et al: Body sodium and hypertension, sodium retention by "hypertensive" kidneys. Trans. Ass. Am. Physicians 87:225-232, 1974.
27. Tobian, L., Coffee, K. and McCrea, P.: Evidence for a humoral factor of non-renal and non-adrenal origin which influences renal sodium excretion. Trans. Ass. Am. Physicians 80:200-206, 1967.
28. Nishiyama, K., Nishiyama, A. and Frohlich, E.D.: Regional blood flow in spontaneously hypertensive rats (SHR). Circulation 50:III-10, 1974.

Discussion

Moderator: Dr. E. D. Freis

Dr. Schepers: Since we have reached the stage of speculation I think I would be capable of contributing some facts and some thoughts. During the past day and this morning an enormous amount of technical detail was presented concerning the kidneys, the adrenals and other organs. I do not clearly recall the lungs having been mentioned. Figure 1 shows how one can produce hypertension by irritating the lung. So far everybody has talked about sodium as a hypertensiogenic agent. In this case we produced systemic hypertension without sodium. Instead, silica (SiO_2) was used. This was one of a series of 24 experiments which I performed about 15 years ago, as yet unpublished. The steeply ascending curve with the markers XYA shows what happened to the left ventricular pressures of rabbits when they had been continuously exposed to submicron amorphous silica dust by inhalation at a concentration of 10.2 mg/cu ft of air. The solid line which represents the inhalation phase rises steeply until the animals reach a state of malignant hypertension. Their pressures now were enormously high and the rabbits had all the symptoms of malignant hypertension. Indeed, some start dying from congestive cardiac failure and other hypertension related conditions.

But note what happens when we stopped the exposure. The pressure still went up for about a month, then it dropped sharply in the direction of normal. Does this mean that one can cure hypertension by exposing the animals to normal air instead of to thiazides?

Now look at curve C which is the exposure of another group of animals to a much lesser concentration of silica (0.8 mg/cu ft of air). Now the blood pressure rose more slowly but steadily. It reached after 24 months what would be, in man, category II or category III level of systemic hypertension. If we now look at the dotted line Y it will be noted that the animals that were

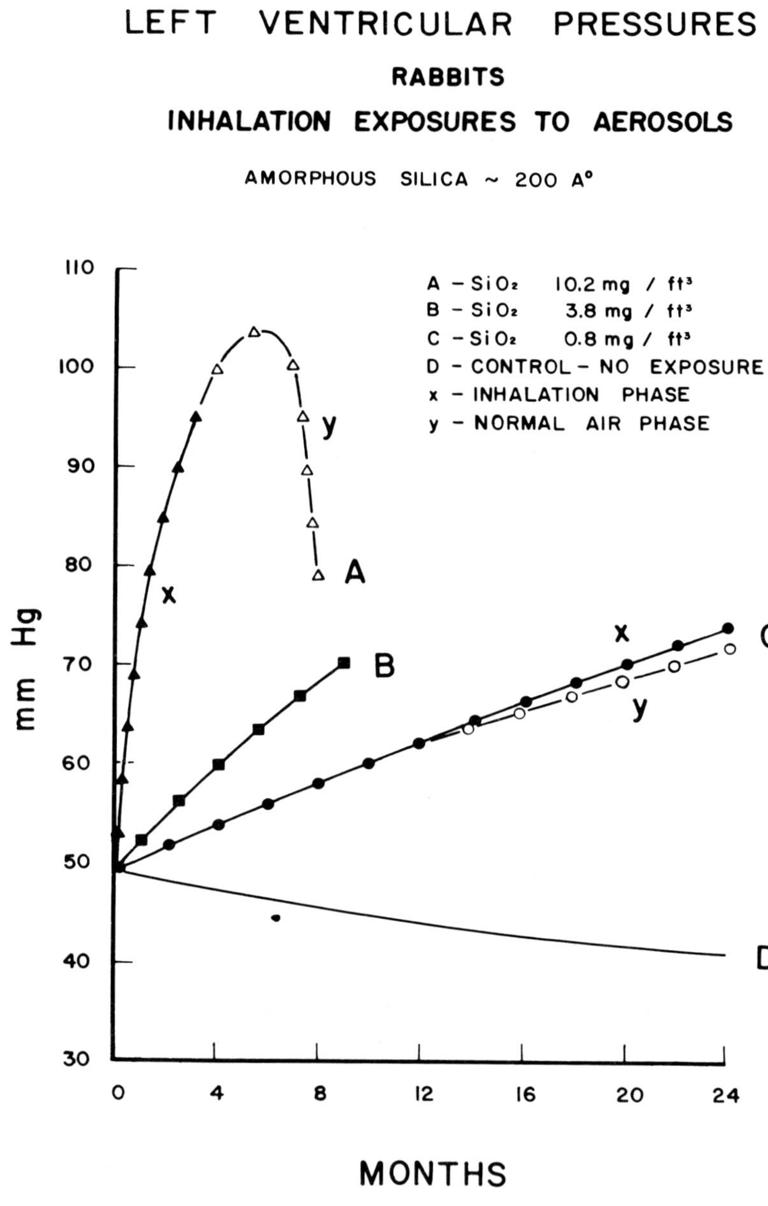
LEFT VENTRICULAR PRESSURES
RABBITS
INHALATION EXPOSURES TO AEROSOLS
AMORPHOUS SILICA ~ 200 A°
A - SiO2 10.2 mg / ft³
B - SiO2 3.8 mg / ft³
C - SiO2 0.8 mg / ft³
D - CONTROL - NO EXPOSURE
x - INHALATION PHASE
y - NORMAL AIR PHASE
mm Hg
MONTHS
110
100
90
80
70
60
50
40
30
0
4
8
12
16
20
24
A
B
C
D
x
y

FIGURE 1.

returned to normal air after 12 months of dust exposure did not lose their hypertension. In other experiments with similar substances the pressure even went higher in the animals exposed to the lesser level of the toxic substance. This phenomenon I long speculated about and I hope that you will all speculate about it. You will notice the curve D is the normal pressure of the control rabbits as they got older. When they were 24 months in the experiments, their blood pressures were much lower than when they started. So we are not dealing with something intrinsic to that particular group of rabbits.

These particles are extremely small and are strictly invisible to the naked eye. I offer you these data to think about. You scientists of the new generation I hope you will do something with this knowledge derived from inhalation studies with submicron amorphous silica.

Dr. Puschett: Dr. Tobian, I wonder if I can ask you about your blood flow studies in view of the fact that several years ago Dr. Buckalew and I participated in a study in hypertensive man in which we compared their response to saline infusion to that of normal patients. They demonstrated an exaggerated natriuresis which we explained on the basis of defective sodium reabsorption in Henle's loop. I wonder if you would consider it compatible with your data to conclude that rather than the collecting duct being the bad actor here that perhaps inappropriate loop function might be producing the exaggerated natriuresis, perhaps resulting from an increase in papillary blood flow.

Dr. Tobian: I think it is a distinct possibility. The way my thinking is going along these lines presumes that this basic defect is there; and, as a result of it, hypertension supervenes in an attempt to correct the physiologic abnormality. So now that this individual is hypertensive, you get a different, exaggerated response to a salt load. In other words, the fact that that individual has become hypertensive may completely overcome the initial effect of the low flow in the papilla and permit exaggerated natriuresis. I am not going to be very positive about either one of these possibilities and I would say the ball game is still quite open.

Dr. Kincaid-Smith: Did you measure the papillary flow when giving thiazides?

Dr. Tobian: No. I hope to have that done within the next three or four months.

Dr. Genest: How did you measure this papillary plasma flow and what factors govern it, and what is your interpretation about the decreased papillary flow in salt-sensitive hypertensive rats and spontaneously hypertensive rats?

Dr. Tobian: This is basically the method thought up by Dr. Lilienfield of Georgetown. He did it in the dog and we did not do anything very original. We just adapted it to the rat and validated it in the rat. One has to change the original method somewhat. The principle involves the slow flow and the long vessels in the papilla. When an albumin molecule enters the papilla, it takes quite a while for it to emerge. So for a certain length of time, every albumin molecule that arrives there stays there. It will stay there for 60 seconds in the dog and 35 seconds in a rat. In other words, the rate of accumulation is linear for 36 seconds and then it begins to tail off. So if one picks a time such as 24 seconds and then quickly clamps off the kidney, every bit of plasma that entered the papilla is still there. It is all still there for 24 seconds. In our system you have to be collecting blood slowly out of an artery at the same time as the blood is entering and accumulating in the kidney. So if you know the amount of radioactive albumin per microliter of blood plasma and if you have the total amount of radioactive albumin accumulated in the papilla during that time and if you divide one into the other, you will have papillary plasma flow. Then dividing by papilla weight can give plasma flow per gram of papilla. That is the basic principle of it. Now in terms of what it means, there are two thoughts about it. One possibility is that hypertension in general increases with resistance of all organs, roughly to an equivalent degree. Some people say that maybe the splanchnic resistance increases a little bit more than that of the other organs. The reason I say that resistance is roughly equivalent in most beds is the flow in most organs in hypertensive subjects remains about the same. So the arterial pressure is up and the resistance increase just about matches it and the flow comes out to be just about what it normally is. There are some claims though that the splanchnic bed is an exception, and this may well be true. Even when Dahl's "S" rats have borderline hypertension, they had a markedly diminished papillary flow. One possibility is that the papilla is by far the most sensitive bed in hypertension and it gets more than its share of vasoconstriction. This could be the result of the hypertensive process. That is one possibility. The other possibility is that for some reason not understood, a genetic factor tends to produce an increased resistance in the papilla and this could have an effect on the excretion of salt. Anything which tends to retard the excretion of salt would have a prohypertensive effect. One could have a combination of these things. You could have a slight, genetic tendency to hypertension which gave you this tendency to extra vasoconstriction in the papilla and this tended to cause salt retention which resulted in even more hypertension. It could be that this particular circulation is particularly sensitive to the hypertensive vasoconstriction. It might be the part of the body that gets the greatest share of the hypertensive vasoconstriction. The implications of this are at present just purely speculative.

Dr. Weinberger: I wonder, Dr. Tobian, if you might speculate on the possible role of thiazides in influencing vascular reactivity? A few years ago we reported some studies* in normotensive rats where we could demonstrate those animals taking a high sodium diet had a much greater rise in blood pressure when given angiotensin II intravenously compared to animals maintained on a normal or low sodium diet. Then we treated a third group with thiazide diuretics and permitted them free access to saline. The amount of sodium repletion, as judged by measurements of renin activity and aldosterone, was comparable to that of the animals receiving saline but without thiazide diuretics. Yet their vascular or blood pressure response to the same dose of angiotensin II was markedly diminished.

Dr. Tobian: There are different ways of looking at this. The way I look at it is that in the one animal you tended to have expansion, and in the other animal, even though he was getting a lot of salt, you tended to have less expansion. The varying degrees of expansion would have a varying effect on the kidneys. The varying degrees of expansion have vascular consequences. In other words, the blood vessels, over a period of time, become aware of varying degrees of expansion. The

*Weinberger, M.H. et al: Effect of chlorothiazide and sodium on vascular responsiveness to angiotensin II. Am. J. Physiol. 223:1049-1052, 1972.

principle that with expansion animals become more sensitive to various kinds of pressor substances is well known. So the way I interpret it is that it is not so much the direct effect of the thiazide on the blood vessel, but it is the effect of expansion versus no expansion on the vascular tree. After a period of expansion one gets extra sensitivity to the various pressor substances like angiotensin, etc.

Thiazide Diuretics and Salt Consumption in the Treatment of Hypertension

Walter M. Kirkendall, M.D. and Merrill L. Overturf, Ph.D.

Our experiences have suggested that a modest reduction of sodium chloride intake to the level of 4 to 6 gm/day is desirable in that it enhances the hypotensive effect of the thiazide diuretics even in hypertensives without azotemia. Others believe that salt restriction is an unnecessary imposition. Currently, a controversy has developed over whether salt should be restricted in the diet of patients being treated for hypertension with diuretics [1, 2]. The purpose of this paper is to review the evidence pro and con and bring the controversy into perspective.

It has been shown that large quantities of dietary salt will produce hypertension in susceptible rats, rabbits and man. Nevertheless, in short-term studies using up to 400 mEq of sodium per day hypertension was not produced in normotensive men despite changes in forearm blood flow, creatinine clearance, plasma renin activity, or aldosterone excretion [3]. On the other hand, when borderline hypertensive individuals were fed similar salt diets for similar intervals, there was an increase in blood pressure and an increase in forearm vascular resistance [4].

There is no question that a 10 mEq sodium diet will cause a sharp reduction of blood pressure in patients with essential

---

Supported in part by the National Institutes of Health Grant HL-15171 from the National Heart and Lung Institute, Bethesda, Md.

Walter M. Kirkendall, M.D., Professor and Chairman, Department of Internal Medicine and Merrill L. Overturf, Ph.D., Assistant Professor of Internal Medicine, The University of Texas Medical School at Houston.

hypertension [5]. This reduction of blood pressure is sodium related and when salt is increased in the diet, blood pressure becomes elevated. Dahl [6] has separated the effects of weight reduction and salt reduction in the diet as causes for blood pressure lowering in obese hypertensives.

Despite this information, few clinicians and patients believe that the 10 mEq sodium diet is a practical one for most hypertensives. Even when it represented a major therapeutic effort few patients were able to follow this program for long intervals. Since the advent of the thiazide diuretics, much of the interest in the use of very low sodium diets for the treatment of hypertension has waned. Indeed, considerable sentiment has now developed for the position that there should be no restriction of sodium intake in hypertensive patients with normal renal function. A typical statement recently appeared in *Lancet*: "The doctor who tells his hypertensive patient with normal renal function to avoid salt is wrong" [1].

Our interpretation of the literature and experiences indicate that even a modest reduction of sodium chloride intake enhances the hypotensive effect of the thiazide diuretics. Thus, reduction of salt intake appears to be good advice.

Mechanism of Action of Diuretics

If sodium depletion has nothing to do with the action of thiazide diuretics, the restriction of sodium under any circumstances would be unnecessary to achieve an antihypertensive effect. The evidence, however, suggests that both initially and in the long term some measure of salt and water depletion is necessary for the full expression of the thiazide hypotensive action [7, 8].

In chronic treatment with thiazide diuretics other non-volume related effects are seen. Peripheral vascular resistance falls in long-term studies and blood pressure stays reduced even when cardiac output has returned to normal or near normal levels [9-11]. It is not known whether this is the result of (a) removal of sodium from vascular smooth muscle cells [12], (b) a change in response to sympathetic nerve stimulation [11, 13, 14], or (c) a change in the capacity of nerve terminals to take up or release norepinephrine [15]. The thiazide diuretics increase the urinary excretion of magnesium, potassium and aldosterone and usually decrease calcium in the urine. It is possible that these changes, involving materials which have profound effects on biologic tissue, are important in the reduction of peripheral vascular resistance.

Thus, the action of thiazide diuretics on blood pressure represents a combination of sodium and water depletion and a reduction in peripheral vascular resistance caused most likely by either an alteration of autonomic function or local cellular electrolyte changes.

It is obvious from the physiological responses that the NaCl depletion which results from dietary restriction is different from that which results from the action of thiazides. The plasma potassium level rises slightly or remains unchanged with dietary restriction [16] and falls with thiazides [17]. Furthermore, the sodium content of the arterial wall may be diminished with reduced dietary salt intake [18] but is unaffected by thiazide therapy [13]. Urinary magnesium and potassium are not increased with salt depletion, although the excretion of both is increased with thiazide diuretic use. Hyperglycemia is not seen with salt restriction as it is with the administration of thiazide diuretics. In addition, thiazides variably have a carbonic anhydrase inhibiting effect, which alkalizes the urine and causes an increase in bicarbonate excretion, and reduce free-water clearance [19].

There are conflicting data concerning the effect of volume replacement by Dextran and saline on the response of the blood pressure after thiazide diuretics, but there is a consensus that a major portion of the hypotensive action associated with thiazide administration is lost if sodium is replaced equal to the quantities eliminated [9, 20, 21].

Thus, though there are other components in the action of the thiazides it is generally agreed that a major factor in their effectiveness is their ability to produce chronic salt and water depletion.

Potency of the Thiazide Diuretics

The thiazide diuretics and agents related to them work primarily on the distal nephron where an active sodium chloride pump is located [22]. However, only relatively small amounts of filtered sodium can be reabsorbed at this locus — perhaps no more than 5% under optimal circumstances. Therefore, rejection of sodium at this site is small and finite. The dose-response curve of thiazide dose to sodium load is a relatively flat one. This means that the mechanism for sodium reabsorption effected by thiazides is quickly eliminated and increased doses of the drug do not promote additional release of sodium. Chlorothiazide in a dose of 1 to 2 gm/day produces maximal salt excretion. Several authors have quantified the amount of salt which taken in the diet can overwhelm the ability of the thiazide diuretics to create volume and sodium depletion [9, 20, 21]. These figures have ranged from 12 to 20 gm of salt added to the diet per day. Above this value additional weight loss is not seen and the hypotensive effect of thiazide diuretics is impaired or completely lost.

What Is the Salt Consumption of Hypertensives?

Habits concerning salt ingestion are known to vary widely over the world and within the United States. Dahl estimated that the salt consumption in the country varied from 4 to 24 gm of salt (69-413 mEq of sodium) per day with an average of 10 gm of salt (172 mEq of sodium) per day [6].

At the University of Iowa in 1970, 24 white unselected hypertensives coming to the clinic taking only a thiazide diuretic had the sodium chloride content in their 24-hour urine measured. Six of these patients were excreting over 18 gm of sodium chloride daily; one excreted 25 gm of sodium chloride per day. None were excreting less than 10 gm of salt per day. At the Hypertension Clinic of the University of Texas Medical School at Houston, the population is predominantly black. Here the sodium chloride intake as measured by the 24-hour urine sodium appears generally greater, with the majority excreting over 200 mEq/day. Many patients, particularly those quite obese, excrete over 300 mEq/day, and one 18-year-old hypertensive man excreted 540 mEq (31 gm) for 24 hours.

There is evidence from animal studies that a diuretic (furosemide) induces salt-craving [23]. The evidence on this point in man is still limited but if such salt-craving develops, it may be a factor in the relatively large consumption of sodium chloride seen in our hypertensive population. Langford et al [24] found, for example, that hypertensive women on antihypertensive medication excreted 170 mEq of sodium per day; hypertensives not treated excreted significantly less (126 mEq of sodium per day). Parijs et al [25] also observed an increase in salt excretion of those hypertensives on diuretics. Whether salt substitutes would be effective in counteracting such apparent craving is unstudied.

Can One Lower Blood Pressure if Dietary Salt Content Is Moderately Lowered?

We observed six hypertensive patients in a metabolic ward while they were taking chlorothiazide, 500 mg, twice a day. During an initial period in the metabolic ward the patients were given a general diet containing approximately 12 gm of salt. Their blood pressure was monitored in the supine and upright position four times a day and the averages of the blood pressures were used for calculations. They were then given a formula diet designed to maintain their body weight but containing only 4 gm of sodium chloride. After 12 days, while taking the same formula, the sodium chloride was increased to 12 gm. After an additional ten-day period, the formula was once more changed to 4 gm of sodium chloride daily. After ten more days the studies were discontinued. In four of the six subjects the lowest values for systolic and diastolic blood pressure, both supine and upright, were observed at the end of the second 4 gm sodium chloride diet interval. The blood pressure reductions in these four patients averaged 9 mm Hg for the systolic pressure and 6 mm Hg for the diastolic pressure, compared to the pressures found during the 12 gm sodium chloride interval. Data from a representative patient who had a reduction in blood pressure with the lower salt diets are shown in Figure 1. There was no consistent change in body weight. In two subjects there was no reduction in blood pressure during the 4 gm sodium chloride intervals. Perhaps this disparity identifies salt-resistant individuals [26].

A second study which indicates that salt reduction with diuretic therapy can lower blood pressure was done by Parijs et

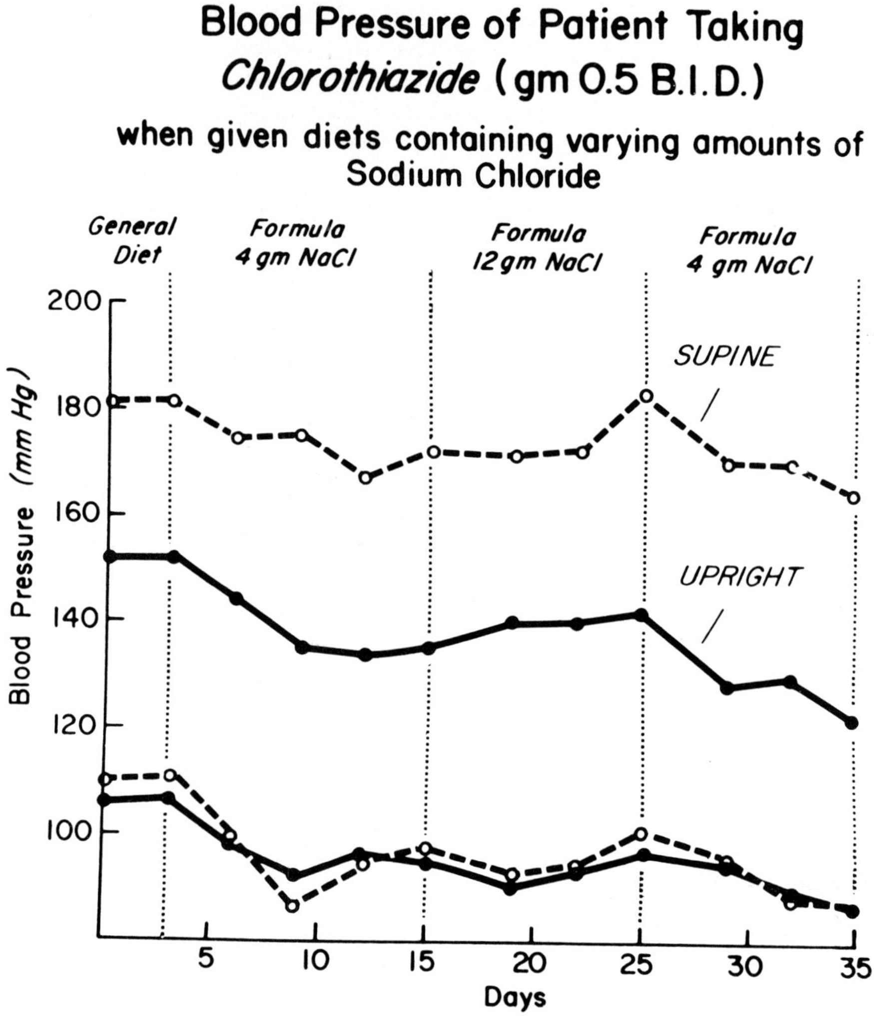

FIG. 1. Data from representative patient showing blood pressure responses to varying amounts of sodium chloride in diet.

al [25]. They did a crossover study of 22 patients comparing, among other things, the effect of a usual salt intake against a low salt intake (5 gm sodium chloride) while the patients were taking 100 mg of spironolactone and 100 mg of hydrochlorothiazide daily. With the sodium chloride restriction before drug therapy the patients reduced their sodium excretion by approximately 50%, that is, from 93 to 42 mEq/24 hrs. This resulted in a small but statistically significant decrease of blood pressure averaging 9.1 mm Hg systolic and 5.8 mm Hg diastolic. The reduction of sodium excretion between the regular diet drug period and the low salt diet drug period was from 200 to 139 mEq/day. In terms of sodium chloride this represents a reduction from 11.6 to 8.1 gm/day. This resulted in a reduction of 5.6 mm Hg systolic and 1.6 mm Hg diastolic supine and 8 mm Hg systolic and 5 mm Hg diastolic upright. Since there was a positive correlation between the height of the systolic and diastolic blood pressure and the excretion of sodium, it is quite possible that additional blood pressure reductions might have been realized had the subjects consumed only the recommended 5 gm of salt daily.

Fallis and Ford [20] have observed that the antihypertensive effect of 50 mg of hydrochlorothiazide could be virtually negated by changing the sodium intake from 50 to 100 mEq/day. Freis et al [27] have observed that raising the salt intake from 4.25 to 11.25 gm/day abolished the antihypertensive effect of 1.5 gm of chlorothiazide in one patient and greatly attenuated the blood pressure reduction in a second study.

Winer [28] has observed that a thiazide-induced reduction of systolic pressure of 26 mm Hg and a diastolic blood pressure reduction of 10 mm Hg in ten patients with essential hypertension could be abolished by the ingestion of 20 gm of sodium chloride. Furthermore, the addition of salt obliterated the effects of hydrochlorothiazide on the responses of systolic and diastolic pressures from intravenous trimethyphan, erythrol tetranitrate and protoveratrine B. The diastolic blood pressure response to norepinephrine remained slightly reduced as compared to the control response before the addition of salt.

Patients with azotemia, indicated by creatinine clearances below 10 ml/min, are acutely sensitive to a large sodium chloride intake and tend to gain weight and develop hypertension [29]. Some of such patients have an obligate sodium chloride loss which renders severe sodium restriction hazardous. Since patients with end stage renal disease have a relatively low finite limit to the sodium chloride they can excrete, the question has been raised as to whether patients with lesser degrees of renal function impairment have a similar reduction in their capacity to excrete large loads of sodium. If this is so, it is likely that patients with hypertension and minor degrees of renal function impairment, short of azotemia, may have their blood pressure elevated by amounts of salt which have no effect on persons with normal kidney function.

Why the Controversy?

The evidence presented indicates that the antihypertensive effect of thiazide diuretics may be either abolished or attenuated by from 10 to 28 gm of salt per day. It is also evident that in at least two locations in the United States and most likely in many others, hypertensive patients consume diets containing sodium chloride in these amounts.

Despite the evidence, many physicians do not believe it is necessary to recommend a 4-6 gm sodium chloride diet. They believe that their patients will not follow such a salt-restricted diet and do not recommend it for this reason. However, if maximal or useful antihypertensive effect from the thiazide diuretic only occurs with this lower level of sodium chloride ingestion, this argument is irrelevant. Even less acceptable is the practice of ignoring salt consumption and resorting to larger doses of thiazide diuretics and more potent loop diuretics to remove the sodium chloride consumed.

Some physicians object to the limitation of dietary sodium to 4-6 gm/day because they believe that certain hypertensives may actually be salt depleted when first seen. Hypertensives who fall into this group may be those who have certain forms of "two-kidney" renal artery stenosis with salt losing from the contralateral kidney [30], certain patients with salt losing nephropathy [31] and perhaps other patients with high renin essential hypertension who respond to thiazide diuretics with tachycardia, weakness and little reduction of blood pressure. This argument has no relevance for the majority of hypertensive patients who do not have these characteristics. Furthermore, careful monitoring of patients and their serum electrolytes will quickly identify such individuals. Indeed, if a patient cannot tolerate salt restriction to 4-6 gm/day, he probably should not be treated with a thiazide diuretic.

Conclusions

Thiazide diuretics have their major action on blood pressure by causing a contraction of plasma volume and mild sodium chloride depletion.

Dietary salt in amounts of 12 to 28 gm/day will abolish much of the blood pressure reduction of a thiazide diuretic in patients with benign essential hypertension. Many hypertensives in the United States consume more than this amount of salt per day. There is evidence that the reduction of salt consumption to less than 7 gm will enhance the effect of thiazide diuretics in the majority of this group.

Thiazide diuretics may produce salt-craving and thus contribute to loss of their effectiveness in patients on an unrestricted diet.

There is a need to better define the degree and extent to which sodium chloride should be restricted in hypertensive patients on diuretic agents, particularly with regard to the patient's renal functional status.

A major medical problem is the need to make such mild sodium chloride restricted diets attractive to patients. Perhaps more palatable salt substitutes would provide a simple answer to the salt-restriction controversy, because lack of patient compliance appears to be the major contraindication to a 4-6 gm salt diet.

Acknowledgment

The authors wish to gratefully acknowledge Ms. Gail Russell for aiding in the preparation of the manuscript.

References

1. Editorial: Salt and Hypertension. Lancet 1:1325, 1975.
2. Morgan, T.: Editorial. Med. J. Aust. 1:603, 1975.
3. Kirkendall, W.M., Connor, W.E., Abboud, F. et al: The effect of dietary sodium chloride on blood pressure, body fluids, electrolytes, and renal function of normotensive man. J. Lab. Clin. Med. (In press.)

4. Mark, A.L., Lawton, W.J., Abboud, F.M. et al: Effects of high and low sodium intake on arterial pressure and forearm vascular resistance in borderline hypertension. Circ. Res. 36 and 37 (suppl. 1):1-194, 1975.
5. Corcoran, A.C., Taylor, R.D. and Page, I.H.: Controlled observations on the effect of low sodium diet therapy in essential hypertension. Circulation 3:1, 1951.
6. Dahl, L.K.: Salt and hypertension. Am. J. Clin. Nutr. 25:231, 1972.
7. Leth, A.: Changes in plasma and extracellular fluid volumes in patients with essential hypertension during long-term treatment with hydrochlorothiazide. Circulation 42:479, 1970.
8. Tarazi, R.C., Duston, H.P. and Frohlich, E.D.: Long-term thiazide therapy in essential hypertension. Evidence for persistent alteration in plasma volume and renin activity. Circulation 41:709, 1970.
9. Winer, B.M.: The antihypertensive actions of benzothiadiazines. Circulation 23:211, 1961.
10. Gifford, R.W., Mattox, V.R., Orvis, A.L. et al: Effect of thiazide diuretics on plasma volume, body electrolytes, and excretion of aldosterone in hypertension. Circulation 24:1197, 1961.
11. Villarreal, H., Exaire, J.E., Revollo, A. et al: Effects of chlorothiazide on systemic hemodynamics in essential hypertension. Circulation 26:405, 1962.
12. Daniel, E.E.: On the mechanism of antihypertensive action of hydrochlorothiazide in rats. Circ. Res. 11:941, 1962.
13. Tobian, L.: Why do thiazide diuretics lower blood pressure in essential hypertension?Ann. Rev. Pharmacol. 7:399, 1967.
14. Aoki, V.S. and Brody, J.: The effect of thiazide on the sympathetic nervous system of hypertensive rats. Arch. Int. Pharmacodyn. 177:423, 1969.
15. Beeler, G.W. and Suenson, M.: Voltage clamp measurements on myocardial tissue under the influence of isoproterenol. Fed. Proc. 32:432, 1973.
16. Jose, A., Crout, J.R. and Kaplan, N.M.: Suppressed plasma renin activity in essential hypertension. Roles of plasma volume, blood pressure, and sympathetic nervous system. Ann. Intern. Med. 72:10, 1970.
17. Fichman, M.P., Vorherr, H., Kleeman, C.R. et al: Diuretic-induced hyponatremia. Ann. Intern. Med. 75:853, 1971.
18. Tobian, L.: Effect of a low sodium diet on electrolyte composition of arterial wall. Am. J. Physiol. 181:599, 1955.
19. Goldberg, M.: The renal physiology of diuretics. *In* Handbook of Physiology, Section 8, Renal Physiology, American Physiological Society, Washington, D. C., 1973, p. 1003.
20. Fallis, N. and Ford, R.V.: Electrolyte excretion and hypotensive response. JAMA 176:99, 1961.
21. Johnson, O.D., Ruchelman, H. and Ford, R.V.: Diuretics and hypertension. Effect of sodium balance. New Engl. J. Med. 267:336, 1962.

22. Kunau, R.T., Weller, D.R. and Webb, H.L.: Clarification of the site of action of chlorothiazide in the rat nephron. J. Clin. Invest. 56:401, 1975.
23. Jalowiec, J.E.: Sodium appetite elicited by furosemide: Effects of differential dietary maintenance. Behav. Biol. 10:313, 1974.
24. Langford, H.G., Watson, R.L. and Gouras, J.: Increased salt appetite in the treated hypertensive. Clin. Res. 23:55A, 1975.
25. Parijs, J., Joossens, J.V., Van der Linden, L. et al: Moderate sodium restriction and diuretics in the treatment of hypertension. Am. Heart J. 85:22, 1973.
26. Knudsen, K.D., Iwai, J. and Dahl, L.K.: Salt, heredity, and hypertension. *In* Onesti, G., Kim, K.E. and Moyer, J.H. (eds.): Hypertension: Mechanisms and Management. New York:Grune & Stratton, 1973, p. 111.
27. Freis, E.D., Wanko, A., Wilson, I.M. et al: Treatment of essential hypertension with chlorothiazide (Diuril). Its use and combined with other antihypertensive agents. JAMA 166:139, 1958.
28. Winer, B.M. : The antihypertensive mechanisms of salt depletion induced by hydrochlorothiazide. Circulation 24:788, 1961.
29. Weidmann, P., Maxwell, M.H., Lupu, A.N. et al: Plasma renin activity and blood pressure in terminal renal failure. New Engl. J. Med. 285:757, 1971.
30. Dauda, G., Mohring, J., Hofbauer, K.G. et al: The vicious circle in acute malignant hypertension of rats. Clin. Sci. Molec. Sci. 45:251s, 1973.
31. Kincaid-Smith, P., MacDonald, I.M., Hua, A. et al: Changing concepts in the management of hypertension. Med. J. Aust. 1:327, 1975.

Some Biochemical Consequences of Diuretic Therapy of Low Renin Essential Hypertension

John W. Hollifield, M.D., Paul E. Slaton, Jr., M.D. and Grant W. Liddle, M.D.

Introduction

Diuretics are well recognized as the cornerstone of contemporary antihypertensive therapy. The National High Blood Pressure Education Program guidelines for the standard therapy of the uncomplicated hypertensive patient call for the use of a thiazide-type diuretic as the primary antihypertensive agent. Certain hypertensive patients generally considered to have milder forms of hypertension normalize their blood pressure during thiazide therapy alone. However, diuretic therapy is not confined to mild hypertension and is well established as adjunctive therapy to the use of other antihypertensives. Indeed, the antihypertensive activity of any adrenergic blocking agent is potentiated by the use of diuretics. In 1971, Beevers et al [1] presented a series of 227 moderate to severe hypertensive patients chronically treated with thiazide diuretics as their sole antihypertensive therapy with "adequate blood pressure control." Subsequently, a number of investigators have suggested that there does exist a sizable group of hypertensive patients (mild, moderate and severe), recognized by their peripheral plasma renin activity, who have volume related, hence diuretic-responsive hypertension [2-6].

This investigation was supported in part by the following grants-in-aid from the National Institutes of Health, United States Public Health Service: 5-TO1-AM-05092, 5-P17-HL-14192, and 5-MO1-RR-95.

John W. Hollifield, M.D., Paul E. Slaton, Jr., M.D. and Grant W. Liddle, M.D., Department of Medicine and Endocrinology, School of Medicine, Vanderbilt University, Nashville, Tenn.

Methods

The Vanderbilt University Hospital studies with diuretics as primary antihypertensive agents began during our investigations of low-renin essential hypertension. Through these studies a carefully categorized, dependable hypertensive population has been developed whose responses to various medication regimens can be studied on a well-controlled outpatient basis. Low-renin essential hypertension (LREHT) is defined as low plasma renin activity (PRA) which resists acute furosemide stimulation in the essential hypertensive patient. Normal renin essential hypertension is defined as essential hypertension in a patient whose peripheral PRA responds to orally administered furosemide. The therapeutic implication of the stimulated renin method of renin categorization of the hypertensive patient is best seen in the blood pressure responses to spironolactone. Favorable blood pressure response to spironolactone is predicted by the failure of PRA to exceed 1.67 ng/ml/hr following oral ingestion of 120 mg furosemide given in three divided doses at 6 P.M., 12 mn., 6 A.M. and assumption of upright posture for three hours. Patients whose PRA exceeds 1.67 ng/ml/hr are relatively unresponsive to spironolactone [3]. Spironolactone-responsive (low renin) essential hypertensives have also been shown to respond to other diuretic agents such as hydrochlorothiazide [5], chlorthalidone [4] and hydrochlorothiazide-triamterene combination [6]. In our experience, 75%-80% of LREHTs respond favorably to these diuretic agents [6]. However, many patients in this group require the use of higher than traditionally recommended doses of diuretics to normalize their blood pressure. Only 25% of patients categorized as normal renin hypertensives generally with milder disease and lower stimulated PRA respond with normalization of blood pressure during diuretic therapy [4] (unpublished observations) and only rarely is favorable blood pressure response to spironolactone observed [3]. In this paper we will present only data from studies in low-renin essential hypertensives with serum creatinine, on no therapy, of 1.7 mg%, or less, and address ourselves to the controversy [7] if newer diuretic agents offer the clinician rational pharmacologic alternatives to the thiazides.

Antihypertension therapy with the thiazide diuretics although well tolerated relative to more potent antihypertensive drugs, however, may cause a number of well-known undesirable biochemical alterations. It behooves us, therefore, to ask if some of the newer diuretic agents are capable of avoiding these biochemical consequences of thiazide therapy.

The various diuretic agents which have been investigated by the Vanderbilt University Hospital Endocrine Hypertension Group are listed in Table 1. Hydrochlorothiazide (HCTZ), the most widely used thiazide diuretic in the United States, is used in our studies as a standard against which other diuretic agents are compared in terms of their effects on serum potassium, uric acid, calcium and PRA.

Chlorthalidone is a sulfonamide diuretic which differs structurally from the thiazides. Its diuretic effect may continue for 48 to 72 hours following a single dose [4]. Furosemide is a potent diuretic which inhibits sodium reabsorption in the proximal tubule as well as in the ascending limb of the loop of Henle. Its potency as a natriuretic causes increased delivery of sodium to the distal tubule where excess potassium secretion can occur [7]. Metolazone is a quinazolinesulfonamide with potent diuretic properties and prolonged serum and biologic

Table 1.

Sulfonamide diuretics
Hydrochlorothiazide (HCTZ)
Chlorthalidone
Metolazone
SKF 62,698
Loop diuretics
Furosemide
Potassium sparing diuretics
Triamterene
Spironolactone
Win 24,540
Aminoglutethimide
Combination diuretics
Hydrochlorothiazide-triamterene
Hydrochlorothiazide-spironolactone
Furosemide-triamterene
Furosemide-spironolactone

half-life [8]. SKF 62,698 is a uricosuric diuretic which effectively lowers uric acid while promoting natriuresis [9]. Win 24,540 is a 19-carbon steroid analog which inhibits an early step in aldosterone biosynthesis [10]. Aminoglutethimide is another inhibitor of aldosterone biosynthesis which inhibits the conversion of cholesterol to pregnenolone [11]. The diuretic combinations HCTZ-triamterene and HCTZ-spironolactone are both currently marketed as fixed combinations of a potassium-sparing agent plus HCTZ.

All studies were conducted at the Clinical Research Center Outpatient Facility of Vanderbilt University Hospital. Informed consent was obtained prior to initiation of the studies. For the sake of analysis, blood pressure is represented as the physiological mean pressure (1/3 pulse pressure added to the diastolic pressure). Mean blood pressures were then used to calculate percentage blood pressure response by the following formula:

$$\% \text{ response} = \frac{\text{Control BP mm Hg} - \text{treatment BP mm Hg} \times 100}{\text{Control BP mm Hg} - 107 \text{ mm Hg}}$$

Our target response was to obtain a reduction in blood pressure to 140/90 or less; 107 mm Hg is the physiological mean of 140/90. Control blood pressure is plotted as zero percent and a reduction of pressure to 107 mm Hg or less is represented by 100%.

Results and Discussion

Studies using HCTZ were accomplished in an open-label fashion with each patient receiving 50 mg HCTZ daily for four weeks. Only one of 13 patients studied normalized his pressure at this dose. The remaining 12 patients then received 100 mg HCTZ daily for an additional four-week period. At this dose four additional patients normalized their blood pressure. The remaining eight patients then received 150 mg HCTZ daily for four weeks with all but one normalizing their pressure. The results of this study are depicted in Figure 1. The remaining diuretic studies were performed using a double-blind protocol previously described [3, 6]. Blood pressure responses and the plasma or serum levels of the biochemical parameters followed are reported as the average of the last two weeks of a control or treatment period.

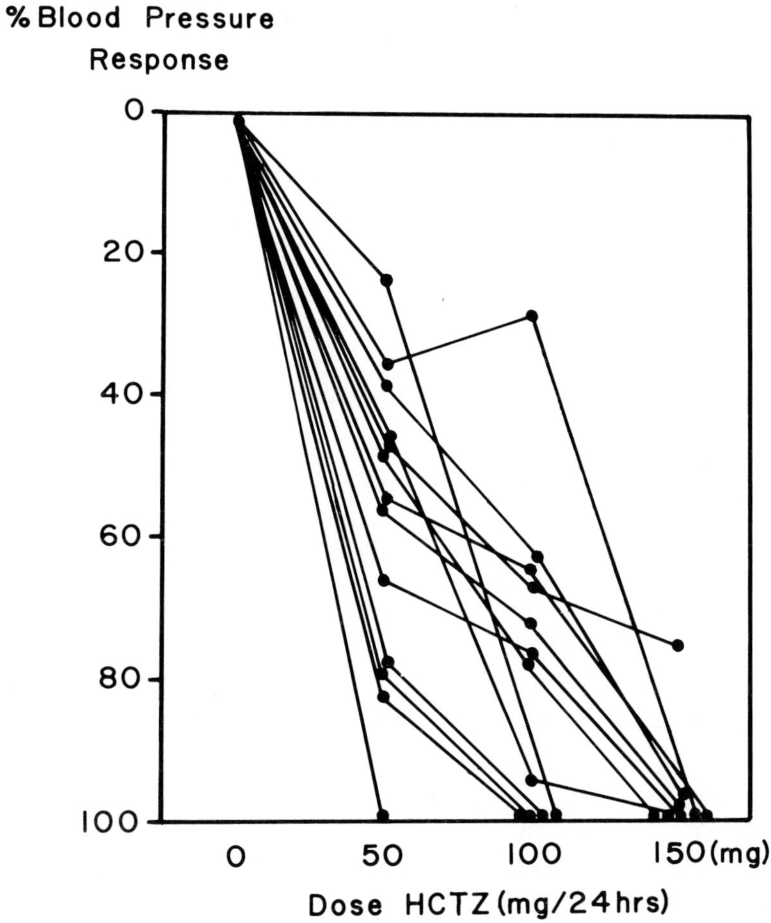

FIG. 1. The effect of graded doses of hydrochlorothiazide (HCTZ) in the blood pressure of 13 patients with low renin essential hypertension.

Blood Pressure

The mean change in blood pressure of a group of LREHT patients during therapy with one of the diuretics listed in column A is shown in column B (Table 2). Column C contains the mean change in blood pressure during HCTZ therapy in the same patients whose mean blood pressure is listed in column B. Column D indicates the number of patients receiving both diuretic agents. Significance analysis (column E) of data was performed by paired t-test.

Table 2. Comparison of BP-Lowering Effects of Various Diuretics (A) with HCTZ. Decrease in BP During Non-HCTZ Therapy (B) Is Compared with Change During HCTZ Therapy in Same Patients (C)

A	*B*	*C*	*D*	*E*
	Mean Δ *BP*	*Mean* Δ *BP With HCTZ*	*N*	*P*
Chlorthalidone 150 mg QD	28.8 ± 1.9	29.8 ± 3.1	4	NS
Furosemide 20 mg QID or 40 mg TID	21.2 ± 3.9	20.4 ± 2.1	5	NS
Metolazone 20 mg QD	24.8 ± 3.4	25.8 ± 2.0	4	NS
SKF 62,698 250 mg BID	22.8 ± 2.7	25.0 ± 3.9	5	NS
Spironolactone 400 mg QD or 100 mg QID	27.1 ± 1.7	23.1 ± 2.1	14	< .05
HCTZ 100 mg – Triamterene 200 mg QD	26.4 ± 2.0	22.8 ± 2.4	12	< .05
HCTZ 100 mg – Spironolactone 100 mg QD	30.0 ± 1.8	22.8 ± 2.6	11	< .001
Triamterene 200 mg BID	6.9 ± 0.74	25.3 ± 3.0	8	< .001

HCTZ compares favorably with comparable doses of metolazone, furosemide, chlorthalidone and SKF 62,698 in its antihypertensive activity in the small number of patients (Table 2). The data indicate more clearly that spironolactone and the diuretic combinations HCTZ-spironolactone, or HCTZ-triamterene, are more effective than HCTZ alone; while triamterene alone is less effective.

Hypokalemia

Studies with HCTZ (50-150 mg/day) in 13 patients with LREHT are shown in Figure 2. On smaller doses of HCTZ (50-100 mg daily), the changes in serum potassium were not so impressive as with 150 mg daily therapy. Figure 3 depicts the changes in serum and total body potassium (measured by K-40 technique) [13] in four LREHT patients. Other recent reports indicate that total body potassium is not altered despite decreases in serum potassium during thiazide administration [12]. All the same, in the case of HCTZ, hypokalemia, defined as serum potassium less than 3.5 mEq/L, appears to be a predictable consequence of normalization of the blood pressure (Fig. 2). Similar findings are encountered in the treatment of LREHT with other sulfonamide diuretics. Table 3 compares the hypokalemia seen with HCTZ with that observed for other diuretic agents. One patient receiving furosemide developed serum K of 2.7 mEq/L and premature ventricular

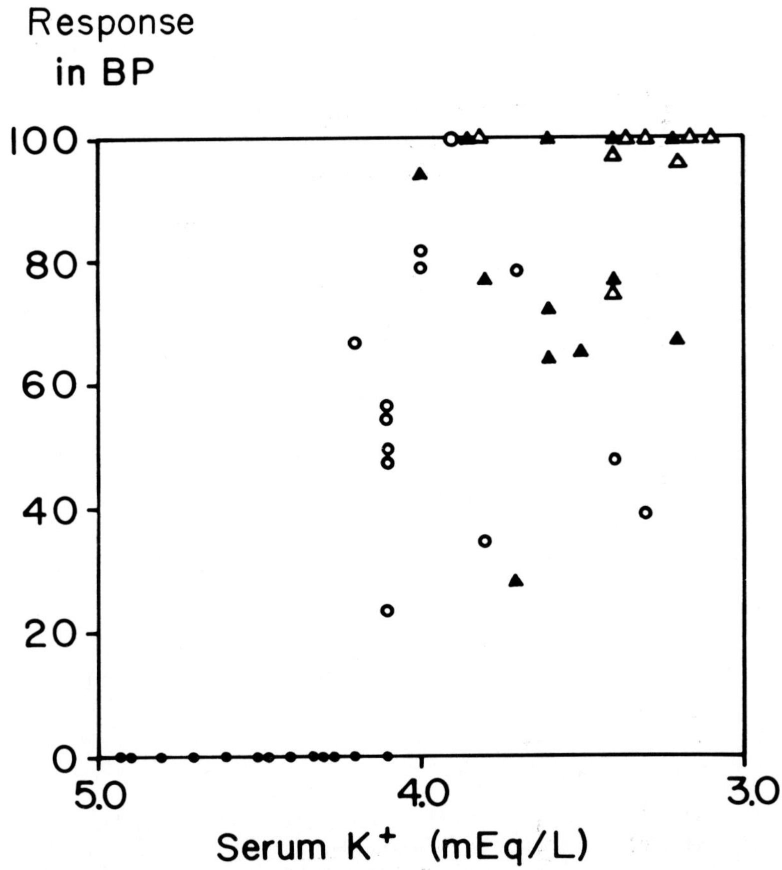

FIG. 2. Effect of increasing doses of HCTZ on blood pressure response and serum K. Closed circles indicate serum K^+ on no therapy, open circles 50 mg HCTZ daily, closed triangles 100 mg daily and open triangles 150 mg daily.

contractions. Paired data analysis of serum K^+ during chlorthalidone or furosemide versus HCTZ therapy in the same patients (Table 3) indicates significantly lower serum K^+ during therapy with furosemide or chlorthalidone. Metolazone and SKF 62,698 are also capable of inducing hypokalemia, but hypokalemia is less marked than with HCTZ (Table 3), as are the changes in whole body potassium with these agents depicted in Figure 4.

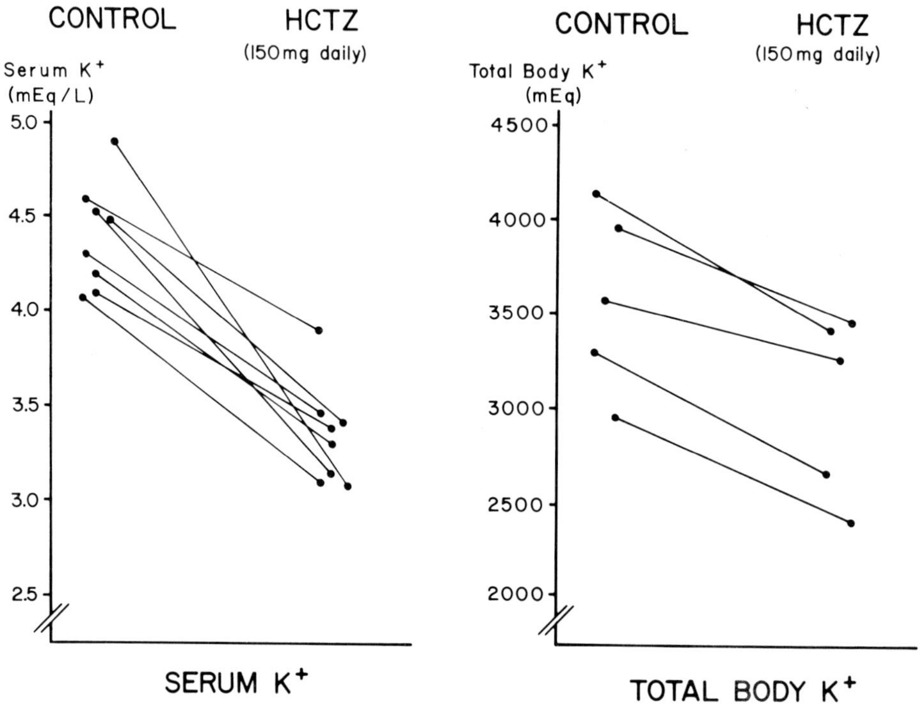

FIG. 3. Serum K^+ and whole body (K-40) after 12 weeks of HCTZ therapy in four patients with LREHT.

Table 3. Comparison of Effect of Various Diuretics (A) on Serum K^+ (B). Column C Indicates Serum K^+ in Same Patients During HCTZ Therapy

A	*B* Mean Serum K	*C* Mean Serum K With HCTZ	*D* N	*E* P
Chlorthalidone 150 mg QD	3.10 ± .09	3.6 ± .12	4	< .05
Furosemide 20 mg QID or 40 mg TID	3.00 ± .09	3.4 ± .13	5	< .05
Metolazone 20 mg QD	3.50 ± .13	3.4 ± .08	4	NS
SKF 62,698 250 mg BID	3.90 ± .12	3.3 ± .06	5	< .01
Spironolactone 400 mg QD or 100 mg QID	4.90 ± .08	3.5 ± .08	13	< .001
Triamterene 200 mg BID	5.00 ± .09	3.4 ± .09	8	< .001
Win 24,540 30 mg QID	4.60 ± .06	3.2 ± .09	3	< .002
Aminoglutethimide 250 mg QID	4.80 ± .15	3.2 ± .88	3	< .002
HCTZ 100 mg – Triamterene 200 mg QD	4.10 ± .11	3.47 ± .09	12	< .001
HCTZ 100 mg – Spironolactone 100 mg QD	4.20 ± .06	3.4 ± .09	11	< .001

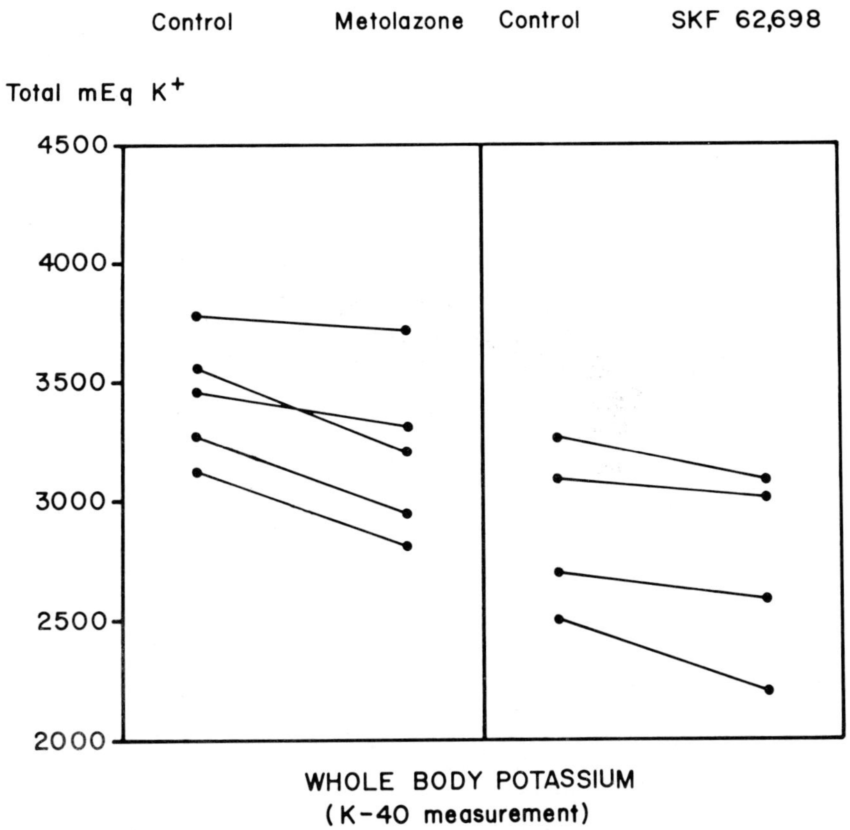

FIG. 4. Total body K^+ (K-40) determinations performed in LREHT patients during 6 weeks of therapy with metolazone and SKF 62,698.

The potassium-sparing effect of diuretic agents such as triamterene, spironolactone [3, 6], Win 24,540 and aminoglutethimide [10] have also been evaluated. Serum potassium rose during therapy with each agent (Table 3). Diuretic therapy involving the combination of a thiazide plus a potassium-sparing diuretic has been reported to improve diuretic effect without the development of hypokalemia [14, 15]. We have evaluated the currently marketed combination agents, triamterene-hydrochlorothiazide and spironolactone-hydrochlorothiazide. The incidence of hypokalemia in these studies is considerably less than with other agents, with only 3/17 developing hypokalemia during HCTZ (100 mg)-triamterene (200 mg daily) therapy (mean decrease 0.6 mEq/L); and 0/20 developing hypokalemia during HCTZ (100 mg)-spironolactone (100 mg) therapy (mean decrease 0.5 mEq/L). In addition, blood pressure control seemed considerably improved when compared to HCTZ 150 mg daily.

Stote et al [16] found triamterene (50-100 mg) capable of blocking the kaliuretic effect of a single 40 mg dose of furosemide in normal control subjects. We have performed similar studies in patients with LREHT using furosemide and metolazone. The effect of 100 mg triamterene or 100 mg spironolactone on the 24-hour kaliuresis, induced by either 40 mg furosemide or 10 mg metolazone administered as a single 8 P.M. dose, is shown in Figure 5. Both potassium-sparing agents potentiate the natriuresis and block the kaliuresis induced by furosemide and metolazone.

Thus, it appears that combination therapy with thiazide or loop diuretic plus a potassium-sparing agent such as triamterene or spironolactone offers considerable advantage over thiazide alone in the prevention of hypokalemia. The fact that spironolactone, a mineralocorticoid antagonist, abolishes the excess kaliuresis induced by metolazone and furosemide suggests the important role of aldosterone in the development of diuretic-induced potassium loss. The inhibitors of aldosterone biosynthesis such as Win 24,540 or aminoglutethimide should be investigated as potassium-sparing adjunctive therapy for the thiazides and loop diuretics.

Uric Acid

The thiazide diuretics are well known to cause elevation of serum uric acid and may precipitate acute gout in the susceptible individual. There appears to be a dual mechanism for this phenomenon. The sulfonamide and loop diuretics are weak acids which compete for uric acid at secretion sites in the distal renal tubule. Furthermore, Suki et al have argued that any substance which results in contraction of extracellular fluid volume will result in increased proximal tubular reabsorption of uric acid and hence hyperuricemia [17]. Figure 6 indicates the effect of HCTZ (50, 100, 150 mg daily) on serum uric acid. With increased dosage there is an incremental increase in uric acid as well as an incremental decrease in blood pressure (Fig. 1).

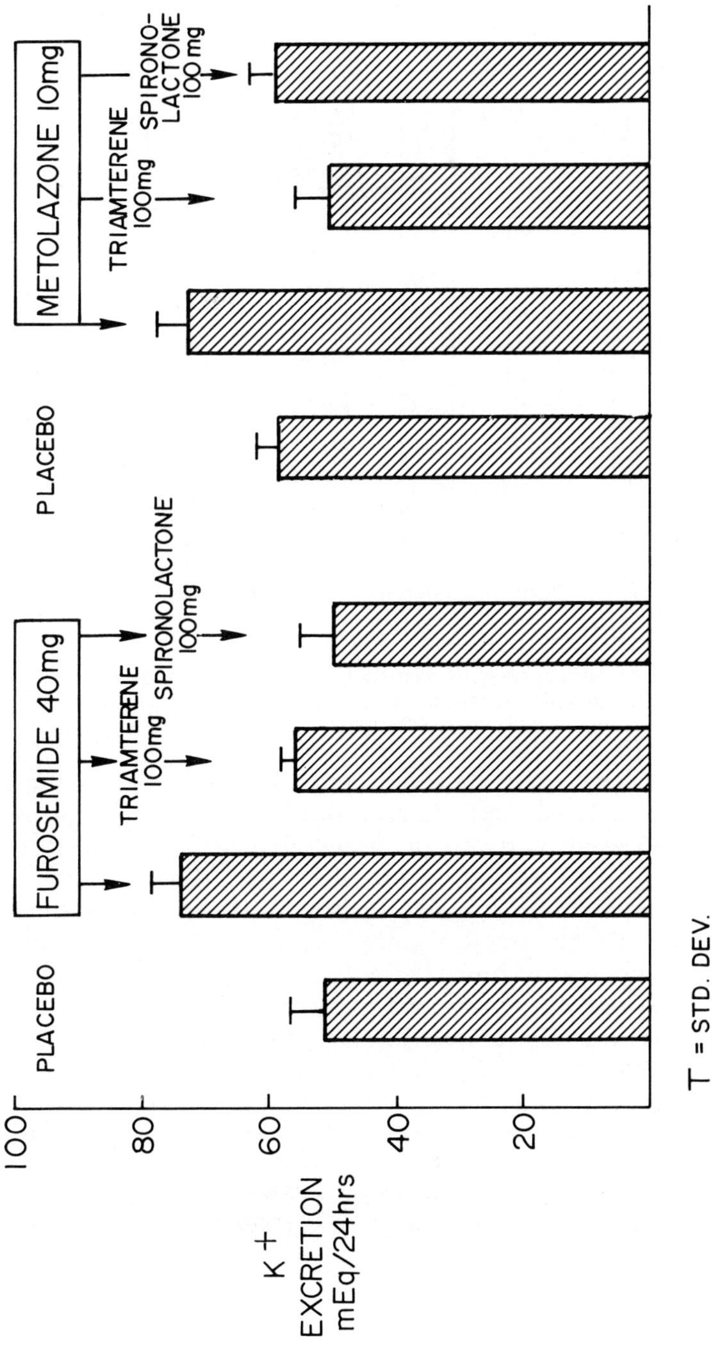

FIG. 5. The effect of triamterene and spironolactone on the kaliuresis following ingetion of 40 mg furosemide or 10 mg metolazone.

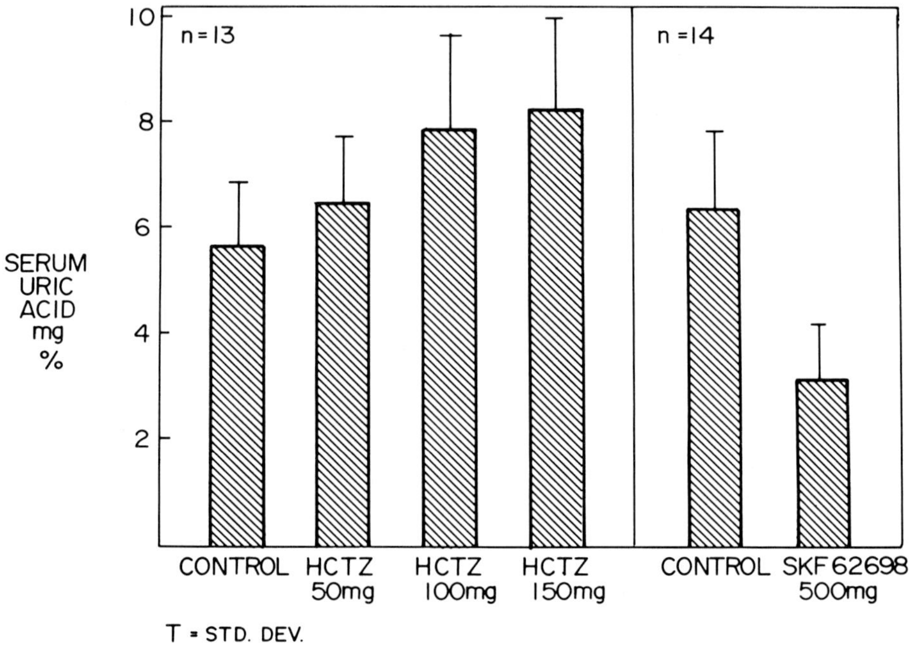

FIG. 6. Effect of HCTZ (N=13) and SKF 62,698 (N=14) on serum uric acid at the conclusion of four weeks of therapy.

The effects of other diuretic agents on serum uric acid are shown in Table 4. All patients receiving chlorthalidone, furosemide, metolazone and, to a lesser degree, spironolactone demonstrated elevation of serum uric acid. The changes in serum uric acid were not significantly different from those observed for HCTZ by the paired t-test for chlorthalidone, furosemide and metolazone. Patients receiving SKF 62,698, a uricosuric diuretic agent, realized consistent drops in their uric acid. Five to seven days after initiation of therapy with 250-500 mg SKF 62,698 daily, the serum uric acid plateaus and reaches levels approximately 50% of pretreatment values (Fig. 6). As with other uricosuric agents, there is the theoretical possibility of precipitating clinical gout.

Thus, SKF 62,698 or spironolactone may provide a satisfactory alternative to thiazide diuretic therapy in the gout-prone, hypertensive patient.

Table 4. Comparison of Changes in Serum Uric Acid During HCTZ or Other Diuretic Therapy. Only During SKF 62,698 Therapy Was There Consistent Fall in Serum Uric Acid

A	*B*	*C*	*D*	*E*
	Δ *Uric Acid*	Δ *Uric Acid With HCTZ*	*N*	*P*
Chlorthalidone 150 mg QD	+2.70 ± .35	+2.88 ± .51	4	NS
Furosemide 20 mg QID or 40 mg TID	+1.18 ± .41	+1.92 ± .69	5	NS
Metolazone 20 mg QD	+1.80 ± .51	+2.43 ± .75	4	NS
SKF 62,698 250 mg BID	−2.76 ± .54	+3.06 ± .38	5	< .002
Spironolactone 400 mg QD or 100 mg QID	+1.05 ± .20	+2.98 ± .39	6	< .002

Hypercalcemia

The effects of the thiazide diuretics on calcium metabolism with a resultant drop in urinary calcium excretion and elevation of serum calcium are well documented [18-20]. The mechanisms through which thiazides produce hypercalcemia are poorly understood. Studies in uremic and anephric man indicate that hypercalcemia can occur without functional renal tissue [21]. Other investigators have suggested that parathyroid hormone is required for this phenomenon [20], while still another hypothesis contends that thiazides themselves stimulate release of calcium from bone particularly in states which are characterized by rapid bone turnover [19]. The hypercalcemia associated with thiazide therapy is generally mild and aside from the necessity of considering other etiologies of the hypercalcemia, there is no clinical significance to thiazide-induced hypercalcemia. Stote et al [18] noted that seven of nine normal subjects treated with HCTZ, 50 mg twice daily, developed hypercalcemia. In our studies using HCTZ in LREHT patients, seven of 13 patients treated with sufficient HCTZ to result in normalization of blood pressure developed pathologic serum calcium elevations (Fig. 7). None of these patients, however, developed complications which could be related to their hypercalcemia. The rise in serum calcium appears to be a dose-dependent phenomenon with each incremental increase in HCTZ dose from 50 mg daily to 150 mg daily resulting in significant increases in serum calcium.

Table 5 indicates the effect of other diuretics or diuretic combinations on serum calcium during six-week studies. Use of

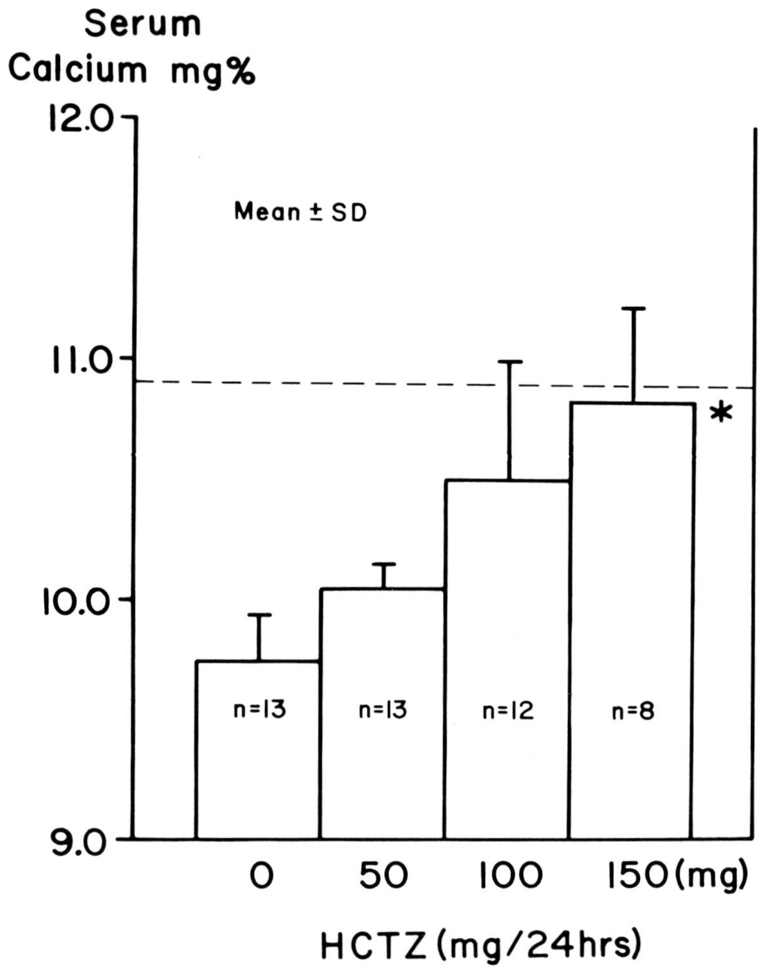

FIG. 7. Effect of HCTZ on serum calcium during dose escalation. Serum calcium levels are expressed as the average of determinations obtained during the third and fourth week of HCTZ therapy, hence, do not represent the maximal values obtained earlier in therapy.

any of the sulfonamide diuretics results in significant increases in serum calcium. However, the loop diuretic furosemide (80 mg daily) showed no significant elevation in serum calcium level. With thiazides the elevation of serum calcium is maximal one to two weeks following initiation of therapy and then

Table 5. Changes in Serum Calcium Developing During Diuretic Treatment

	Control Serum Calcium	*Treatment Serum Calcium*	*Patients Developing Hypercalcemia*
Chlorthalidone 150 mg QD	9.6 ± .23	10.30 ± .21	2/4
Furosemide 20 mg QID or 40 mg TID	9.7 ± .14	9.60 ± .28	0/5
Metolazone 20 mg QD	9.6 ± .10	9.95 ± .19	1/5
SKF 62,698 250 mg BID	9.8 ± .17	9.90 ± .23	2/14
Spironolactone 400 mg QD or 100 mg QID	9.6 ± .24	9.70 ± .18	0/7

returns toward, but not to control values. This initial rise in serum calcium is not noted with furosemide. Consistent increases in serum calcium were observed during spironolactone therapy; however, the values did not exceed the upper limits of normal. It can be hypothesized that this increase results from enhancement of proximal tubular reabsorption of calcium in the face of extracellular fluid volume depletion. Hence, furosemide and spironolactone can be used as an alternative to thiazide therapy in the hypercalcemic hypertensive patient.

Renin System

Elevation of PRA follows chronic use of diuretics. Although low renin hypertensives are relatively nonresponsive to the acute effects of diuretic agents, on prolonged therapy they regain renin responsiveness. Figure 8 depicts the correlation between percent fall in blood pressure and random upright PRA drawn between 9 a.m. and 10 a.m. The data points clustered about the origin (solid circles) reflect pretreatment PRA (hence 0% fall in BP). The percentage fall in blood pressure and peripheral PRA during treatment with 50 mg HCTZ daily is indicated by open circles, 100 mg HCTZ daily by closed triangles and 150 mg HCTZ daily by open triangles. There is an apparent correlation between the fall in blood pressure and rise in PRA. The effect of other diuretic regimens on PRA is depicted in Table 6. All of the diuretics which result in normalization of BP also result in an elevation of PRA.

The vasculotoxicity of renin has been discussed in animal models by Giese [22]. Concern has been expressed that the elevation of renin which accompanies diuresis may cause an increase in morbidity and mortality associated with hyper-

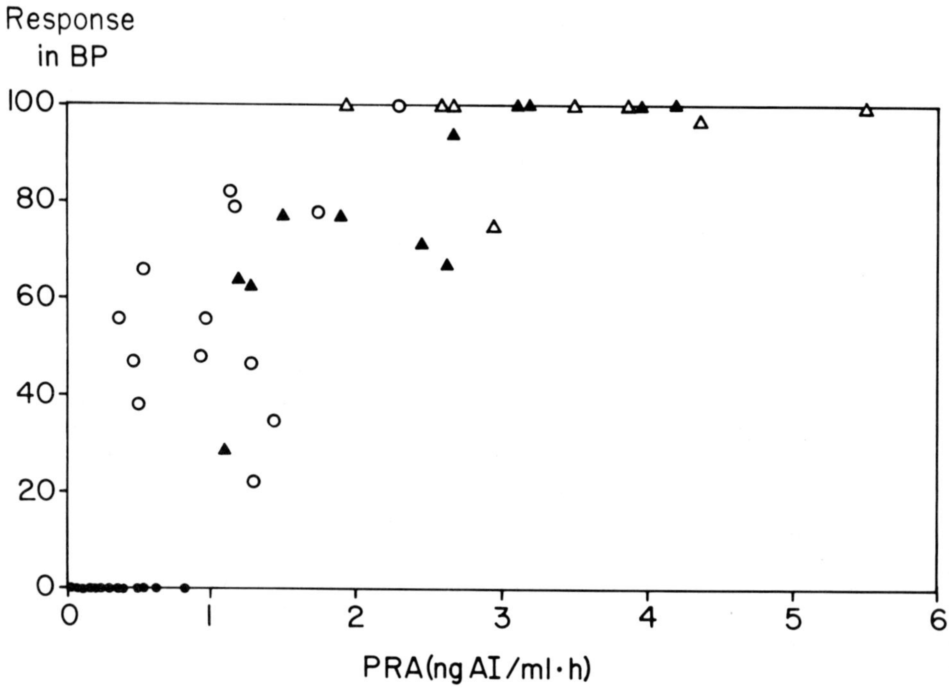

FIG. 8. The effect of diuretic-induced blood pressure control on PRA in LREHT patients. The percentage blood pressure response is calculated as fall in blood pressure from control values (0%) divided by fall necessary to normalize the blood pressure (100%). Solid circles (●) are control values, open circles (○) 50 mg HCTZ daily, closed triangles (▲) 100 mg HCTZ daily and open triangles (△) 150 mg HCTZ daily.

Table 6. Comparison of PRA During Therapy With Various Diuretic Regimens

	PRA	*PRA with HCTZ*	*N*	*P*
Chlorthalidone 150 mg QD	3.26 ± 0.81	3.60 ± .62	4	NS
Furosemide 20 mg QID or 40 mg TID	3.63 ± 0.51	3.49 ± .70	5	NS
Metolazone 20 mg QD	4.11 ± 0.31	3.90 ± .54	4	NS
SKF 62,698 250 mg BID	2.86 ± 0.51	3.16 ± .41	5	NS
HCTZ 100 mg – Triamterene 200 mg QD	4.82 ± 1.30	3.19 ± .44	11	$< .01$
HCTZ 100 – Spironolactone 100 mg QD	5.10 ± 1.20	3.44 ± .20	11	$< .01$

tension rather than reducing it. For this reason, the effects of diuretics on PRA have been investigated for a variety of diuretic regimens. Table 6 illustrates a comparison of PRA obtained during four to six week studies with chlorthalidone, furosemide, metolazone, SKF 62,698, HCTZ-spironolactone combination and HCTZ-triamterene combination as compared with HCTZ. Only with the combination agents (which also demonstrated improved blood pressure control) was there a significant elevation of PRA over HCTZ. Furosemide has been suggested as having a short-lived effect on PRA [23]. To investigate this contention, we obtained PRA at frequent intervals throughout the day in patients whose blood pressure was normalized during therapy with metolazone, HCTZ-spironolactone combination and furosemide (Table 7). Metolazone and the combination were administered once daily and furosemide was administered on a twice daily schedule. The PRA demonstrates a diurnal variation with all three agents, but furosemide does not evidence a pattern appreciably different from the combination or metolazone.

Conclusions

The data suggest that hypokalemia, hyperuricemia, hypercalcemia and hyperreninemia are commonly associated with thiazide therapy sufficient to normalize blood pressure. Chlorthalidone, furosemide, metolazone, SKF 62,698 are effective antihypertensive agents in LREHT. The combination agents HCTZ-triamterene, HCTZ-spironolactone and spironolactone alone are more effective in controlling the blood pressure of

Table 7. PRA Values Obtained at 9 A.M., 12 Noon, 4 P.M., 8 P.M. During Therapy With Metolazone, HCTZ-Spironolactone Combination and Furosemide

	N	*9 A.M.*	*12 N*	*4 P.M.*	*8 P.M.*
Metolazone 20 mg QD	3	4.26 ± 0.40	4.03 ± 0.56	3.74 ± 1.00	2.10 ± .50
HCTZ 100 mg – Spironolactone 100 mg QD	5	5.68 ± 1.50	6.22 ± 1.50	4.62 ± 1.10	3.62 ± .67
Furosemide 20 mg QID or 40 mg TID	3	3.67 ± 0.60	3.96 ± 1.00	3.19 ± 0.58	2.04 ± .11

LREHT than HCTZ and prevent the hypokalemia seen with thiazide use. Chlorthalidone and furosemide cause significantly greater hypokalemia than HCTZ alone. SKF 62,698 should be considered for the gout-prone hypertensive patient and furosemide may be substituted for HCTZ in the hypercalcemic hypertensive. All of the diuretics used to treat LREHT cause an elevation of the circulating renin. The rise in PRA during therapy is closely associated with a fall in blood pressure.

The newer antihypertensive agents do offer rational alternatives to the thiazide diuretics. The knowledge of the pharmacology of these agents can permit individualization of a patient's diuretic program to avoid or correct certain side effects of the thiazides. We suggest that the combination diuretics using a thiazide cogener plus a potassium-sparing agent should be considered as the standard primary therapy for the uncomplicated hypertensive patient rather than thiazide alone.

Acknowledgments

The authors wish to thank Mrs. Nancy Schultz for preparation of the manuscript, Ms. Carolyn Bayless for specimen collection and Mrs. Glenda Rye and Jackie Goodman for the PRA determinations.

References

1. Beevers, D.G., Hamilton, M. and Harpin, J.E.: The long-term treatment of hypertension with thiazide diuretics. Postgrad. Med. J. 47:639, 1971.
2. Tarazi, R.C., Frohlich, E.D. and Dustan, H.: Plasma volume and chronic hypertension. Arch. Intern. Med. 125:835, 1970.
3. Carey, R.M., Douglas, J.G., Liddle, G.W. et al: The syndrome of essential hypertension and suppressed plasma renin activity. Arch. Intern. Med. 130:849, 1972.
4. Vaughn, E.D., Laragh, J.H., Gavras, I. et al: Volume factor in low and normal renin essential hypertension. Am. J. Cardiol. 32:523, 1973.
5. Adlin, E.V., Marks, A.D. and Channick, B.J.: Spironolactone and hydrochlorothiazide in essential hypertension. Arch. Intern. Med. 130:855, 1972.
6. Douglas, J.G., Hollifield, J.W. and Liddle, G.W.: Treatment of low-renin essential hypertension. JAMA 227:518, 1974.
7. Frohlich, E.D.: Use and abuse of diuretics. Am. Heart J. 89:1, 1975.
8. Steinmuller, S.R. and Puschett, J.B.: Effects of metolazone in man: Comparison with chlorothiazide. Kidney Int. 1:169, 1972.

9. Stote, R.N., Cherrill, D.A., Maass, A.R. et al: SKF 62,698, a diuretic with significant uricosuric activity. Abstract presented at 6th International Congress of Nephrology, Florence, Italy, 1975.
10. Hollifield, J.W., McKenna, T.J., Wolff, J. McD. et al: Inhibition of adrenal biosynthesis in the treatment of steroid excess states. Abstract presented at The Endocrine Society, New York, 1975.
11. Dexter, R.N., Fishman, L.M., Ney, R.L., et al: Inhibition of adrenal corticosteroid synthesis by aminoglutethimide. J. Clin. Endocrinol. Metab. 27:473, 1967.
12. Wilkinson, P.R., Hesp, R., Issler, H. et al: Total body and serum potassium during prolonged thiazide therapy for essential hypertension. Lancet 1:759, 1975.
13. Lorimer, A.R., Sinclair-Smith, B.C., Constantinides, C. et al: Clinical applications of whole body potassium determination. *In* Radioactivity in Man. Meneely, G.R. and Linde, S.M. (eds.). Springfield, Ill.:Charles C Thomas, 1966, p. 248.
14. Hansen, K.B. and Bender, A.D.: Changes in serum potassium levels occurring in patients treated with triamterene and a triamterene-hydrochlorothiazide combination. Clin. Pharmacol. Ther. 8:392, 1966.
15. Ogilvie, R.I. and Ruedy, J.: Treatment of hypertension with hydrochlorothiazide and spironolactone. Canad. Med. Ass. J. 101:591, 1969.
16. Stote, R.M., Alexander, F. amd Familiar, R.G.: Effect of triamterene on furosemide-induced kaliuresis in normal volunteers. J. Int. Med. Res. 2:379, 1974.
17. Suki, W.N., Hull, A.R., Rector, F.C., Jr. et al: Mechanism of the effect of thiazide diuretics on calcium and uric acid. Am. Soc. Clin. Invest. 46:1121, 1967.
18. Stote, R.M., Smith, L.H., Wilson, D.M. et al: Hydrochlorothiazide effects on serum calcium and immunoreactive parathyroid hormone concentrations. Ann. Intern. Med. 77:587, 1972.
19. Brickman, A.S., Massry, S.G. and Coburn, J.W.: Changes in serum and urinary calcium during treatment with hydrochlorothiazide: Studies on mechanisms. J. Clin. Invest. 51:945, 1972.
20. Popouitzer, M.M., Subryan, V.L., Alfrey, A.C. et al: Acute effects of chlorothiazide on serum ionized calcium. J. Clin. Invest. 55:1295, 1975.
21. Koppel, M.H., Massry, S.G., Shinaberger, J.R. et al: Thiazide-induced rise in serum calcium and magnesium in patients on maintenance hemodialysis. Ann. Intern. Med. 72:895, 1970.
22. Giese, J.: Renin, angiotensin and hypertensive vascular damage: A review. Am. J. Med. 55:315, 1973.
23. Gordon, R.D., Pawsey, C.G.K., O'Halloran, M.W. et al: Use of home blood pressure measurement to compare the efficacy of two diuretics. Med. J. Aust. 2:565, 1971.

Discussion

Moderator: Dr. A. E. Doyle

Dr. Genest: I would like to report on some experiments that were done by Drs. Kusumoto and Constantopoulos in our laboratories on the effect of hydrochlorothiazide on the content of water, cations (Na, K, Ca, Mg) and norepinephrine in cardiovascular tissues. These experiments were part of a large study of the effects of various antihypertensive drugs on the same parameters.

Hydrochlorothiazide was studied in normotensive mongrel dogs and in dogs made hypertensive with one clipped kidney and the contralateral kidney removed. It was given at 3.75 mg/kg/day for 45 days. Hydrochlorothiazide given to normotensive mongrel dogs resulted in a 9% (not statistically significant) decrease in plasma volume, in a significant decrease in plasma potassium and magnesium concentrations without any change in blood pressure. As shown in Figure 1, there is a significant decrease in water and potassium content of the cardiovascular tissues studied in normotensive dogs receiving hydrochlorothiazide. Another finding of interest is the significant increase in myocardial content of calcium which was also seen in renal hypertensive dogs receiving hydrochlorothiazide. Norepinephrine content was also decreased in all cardiovascular tissues, but significantly only in mesenteric and carotid arteries.

These studies were repeated in dogs made hypertensive by clipping one renal artery and with contralateral nephrectomy (Fig. 2). Only dogs which showed a significant increase in mean blood pressure of more than 30 mm Hg above control levels were used. They were divided into three groups: (1) receiving hydrochlorothiazide alone, (2) receiving hydrochlorothiazide plus a potassium supplement of 45 mg/kg/day and (3) hypertensive dogs which served as controls and did not receive any drug.

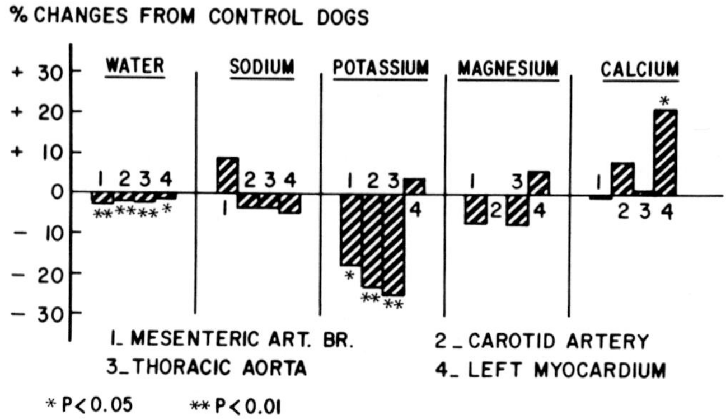

FIG. 1. Changes in water and cations (Na, K, Mg, Ca) contents of various cardiovascular tissues in dogs receiving hydrochlorothiazide (3.75 mg/kg/day for 45 days) in comparison to control normotensive dogs.

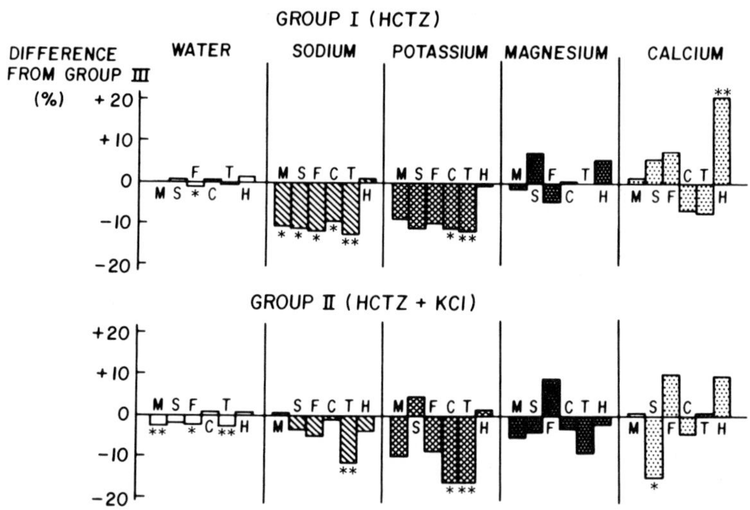

FIG. 2. Changes in water and content of cations (Na, K, Mg, Ca) in various arteries and myocardium of renal experimental hypertensive dogs treated with hydrochlorothiazide alone (group 1) with hydrochlorothiazide plus KCl (group 2) for 42 days. The results are compared to a third group of renal hypertensive dogs which did not receive any drug. M = branches of mesenteric arteries; S = saphenous artery; F = femoral artery; C = carotid artery; T = thoracic aorta; H = left myocardium.

$*p < 0.05$; $**p < 0.01$

The same dosage was used in these dogs as in the first experiment.

In the first group of dogs receiving hydrochlorothiazide alone, there was a significant decrease of 19% in plasma volume and in plasma potassium concentration. When this group was compared to the hypertensive dogs not receiving any drug, there was a significant decrease in cardiovascular tissue contents of sodium and in general also of potassium. Again, myocardial content of calcium was significantly increased. No change was seen in the norepinephrine content in the cardiovascular tissue studied. On the other hand, in the second group of dogs receiving hydrochlorothiazide and a potassium supplement, the plasma volume decreased only by 4% which was not significant. Plasma potassium concentration decreased significantly. There was again a significant decrease in potassium content in both carotid and thoracic arteries and a significant decrease in sodium content in the latter with a decrease in water content in most of the tissues studied. Again in this group there was no significant change in norepinephrine content.

So, in conclusion, it seems that the antihypertensive action of hydrochlorothiazide may be through a decrease in plasma volume and total body potassium reflected in part by the significant decrease in potassium content of cardiovascular tissues. This is not accompanied by changes in norepinephrine content which were striking when hydrochlorothiazide was given to normotensive dogs.

Question: I just had one question with relationship to your next to the last slide which showed the relationship between renin fall or renin stimulation of the diuretics and blood pressure fall. I wonder if the reason why the combination diuretics work better is because they are better dosewise or for some other reason they are better volume depleters since they also have the highest renin response. If you looked at your chlorothalidone or any of the other groups so that you had comparable renin responses, was there any difference in the blood pressure response, regardless of which therapy you used?

Dr. Hollifield: The statisticians say that the numbers are too small to say that yet. I think that is probably true, though.

Dr. Zanchetti: You did not mention serum urea and serum creatinine levels during administration of these diuretics. Have you observed by any chance if the combination diuretics cause a greater increase in serum urea or serum creatinine than do single diuretics?

Dr. Hollifield: Yes. While you have raised that point, I might mention that there is one unique property that we see with respect to metolazone, that is, it has been the only effective diuretic that we have used to date which does not cause an elevation in creatinine. It does in fact cause an elevation of urea. I guess that probably means that there is enough proximal reabsorption of urea to cause the elevation. But we are really not seeing the elevations of creatinines that we would anticipate, with the degree of elevation of PRA and the degree of fall in blood pressure. We hope to do some studies with GFR and renal plasma flow in this group of patients.

Dr. Weinberger: For those of you who may recall the data that we presented yesterday, even though I did not provide a detailed analysis of the changes in blood pressure and plasma renin activity in the various hypertensives and in the various treatment regimens utilized, we made extensive analysis of that data, both with regard to absolute and relative changes in both plasma renin activity and blood pressure. We observed no discernible correlation, however. Thus, I think our data are somewhat different from the data which you have just examined. Having said that, I would like to propose a potential explanation and ask you to comment upon it. As you recall, our patients were a broad spectrum of mild hypertensive patients. Your patients, by definition, were a very homogeneous group of patients who not only had low plasma renin activity but had a beneficial response to spironolactone, implying that they were homogeneous with respect to a volume or a mineralocorticoid etiology for hypertension. Could this then not be the explanation for the difference in response? I reiterate, though, what I said yesterday: that 75%-83% of our total population achieved a normal blood pressure with the use of any of the diuretic agents, yet we could not demonstrate any relationship between change in blood pressure and change in plasma renin activity.

Dr. Hollifield: I guess that might be one of the reasons why we see this. I will comment that our hypertensive population is an extremely select one. They have been studied on a weekly basis for three years. They have drug compliance assays every week. They are more or less "mothered" and smothered to "death" with their hypertensive care. Most of them would not dare to miss a dose of medicine or fail to keep a doctor's appointment. I wonder whether compliance is not one of the reasons why patients do not have a good correlation. Some patients do not have a good correlation between PRA and change in BP. That might be the other reason. Did you measure compliance assays in your study?

Dr. Weinberger: Our assessment of compliance was made by pill count. We did not include markers which could be measured to indicate the compliance. One point that I would offer, even though it is not necessarily direct proof of compliance, is that those patients under treatment, if you recall the mean plasma renin response of the 4, 8 and 12 week period of treatment, were very consistent, which surprised us for two reasons. First, it should imply that the patient was complying and consistently so during the duration of the treatment period. Second, many patients can overcome hypotensive therapy by an increase in their sodium intake. Had this been the case, I would anticipate that over a three-month treatment period we would see a decline in plasma renin levels. But we did not see that.

Renal Transport and Blood Flow Effects of Certain Antihypertensive/Diuretic Agents

Jules B. Puschett, M.D. and Martin Kuhrman, B.S.

For a number of years, my colleagues and I have been interested in evaluating the site or sites of action within the nephron of certain diuretic agents, many of which also possess antihypertensive effects. In particular, we have directed our attention to the investigation of those drugs which can be demonstrated to have a proximal tubular effect, either as their primary site of action, or as a secondary finding, in addition to a more major sodium transport inhibitory effect in another tubular segment. In these investigations, we have utilized both classical clearance methodology and the recollection micropuncture technique in the dog. Before discussing the experimental observations, let us first review the major functional nephron transport sites as depicted in Figure 1.

In the proximal convoluted tubule, two separate forms of sodium reabsorption can be said to occur: that in which sodium transport is accompanied by anionic reabsorption (labeled site 1) and that which represents the variety of sodium transport involving the secretion of hydrogen ion, leading to the regeneration of bicarbonate within the renal tubular cell (site 2). About 70%-80% of filtered sodium is reabsorbed in the proximal convoluted tubule. The next quantitatively important

---

This work was supported (in part) by grants from the US Public Health Service (AM-17575, 5S01RR05709), The Western Pennsylvania Heart Association and the Pennwalt Corporation.

Jules B. Puschett, M.D. and Martin Kuhrman, B.S., Renal-Electrolyte Section, Departments of Medicine, Allegheny General Hospital and the University of Pittsburgh School of Medicine, Pa.

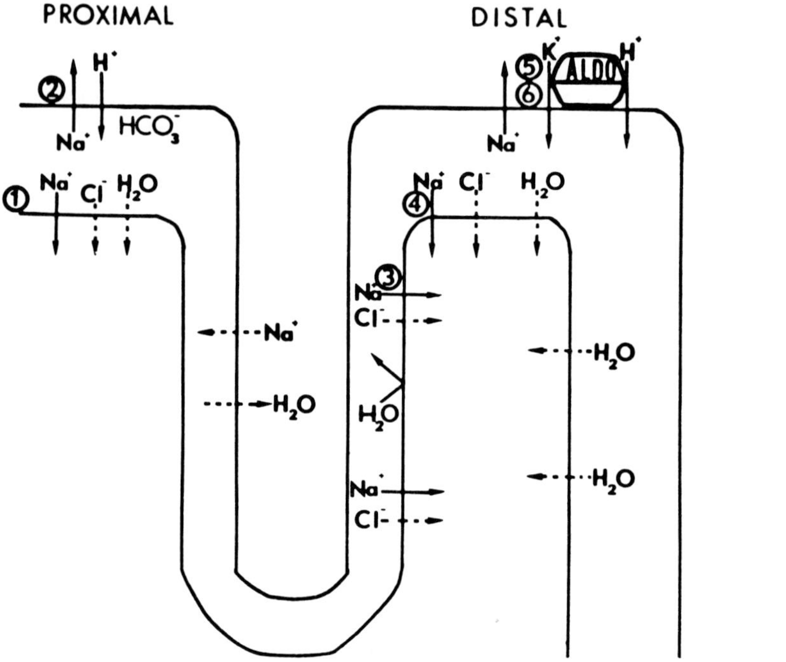

FIG. 1. Diagram of the major sites of sodium chloride and bicarbonate reabsorption in the renal tubular system. (Reproduced with permission from McCurdy, D. and Goldberg, M.: *In* Conn, H.L. and Horwitz, O. (eds.): Cardiac & Vascular Diseases. Philadelphia, Pa.:Lea & Febiger, 1971.)

sodium transport site is located in the thick portion of the medullary ascending limb of the loop of Henle (site 3, Fig. 1). There is current evidence which suggests that active transport at this locus in fact involves chloride reabsorption, with sodium presumably following passively, down an electrochemical gradient [1]. However transport is accomplished at this site, the net effect is the same, namely, the efflux of sodium chloride from the tubular contents. At site 3 the reabsorption of approximately 15%-20% of filtered sodium is accomplished. At site 4, also called the cortical diluting site and functionally located in the early distal convolution, another 5%-8% of filtered sodium is reabsorbed. The sites labeled 5 and 6 represent those at which sodium reabsorption occurs in exchange for hydrogen and/or potassium secretion and are of qualitative rather than quantitative importance, since only an additional 1%-3% of sodium transport appears to occur here. Before leaving the subject of the localization of ionic transport within the nephron, we need to make two other important observations: The first of these concerns phosphate reabsorption and the second the influence of parathyroid hormone on tubular transport. Data from my laboratory, as well as others, indicate that in the animal with intact parathyroid glands, the great bulk of phosphate reabsorption occurs proximally, with only minor distal transport. Additionally, the experimental observations suggest that agents or maneuvers which interfere with the proximal tubular reabsorption of sodium also impair the transport of phosphate in this tubular segment [2-4].

In Figure 2 are depicted the alterations in the tubular handling of sodium and phosphate in the proximal tubule and for the entire micropunctured kidney in recollection experiments performed in the intact dog. These studies were performed in collaboration with Drs. Agus and Goldberg [2]. Notice that the administration of parathyroid hormone resulted in a reduction in both sodium and phosphate reabsorption proximally, and that while a substantial phosphaturia then developed, only a minimal natriuresis ensued. We interpreted these findings as indicating that, since in the intact animal the majority of phosphate reabsorption is accomplished proximally, the bulk of the phosphate escaping proximal reabsorption thereupon appeared in the final urine. On the other hand, sodium transport occurs throughout the nephron, so that the major portion of the proximally rejected sodium must have been reabsorbed in the *distal* nephron, that is, in the loop of Henle and the distal convoluted tubule. Notice, also, that the administration of cyclic 3′, 5′ adenosine monophosphate (or cyclic AMP) produced essentially the same results as did parathyroid hormone, providing strong support for the view that the renal tubular effects of the hormone are mediated by the cyclic nucleotide. That this phenomenon did not represent a nonspecific effect of the infusion of this material is indicated by the fact that 5′ cyclic AMP had no such effect on tubular function. The stability of this dog preparation is verified by the

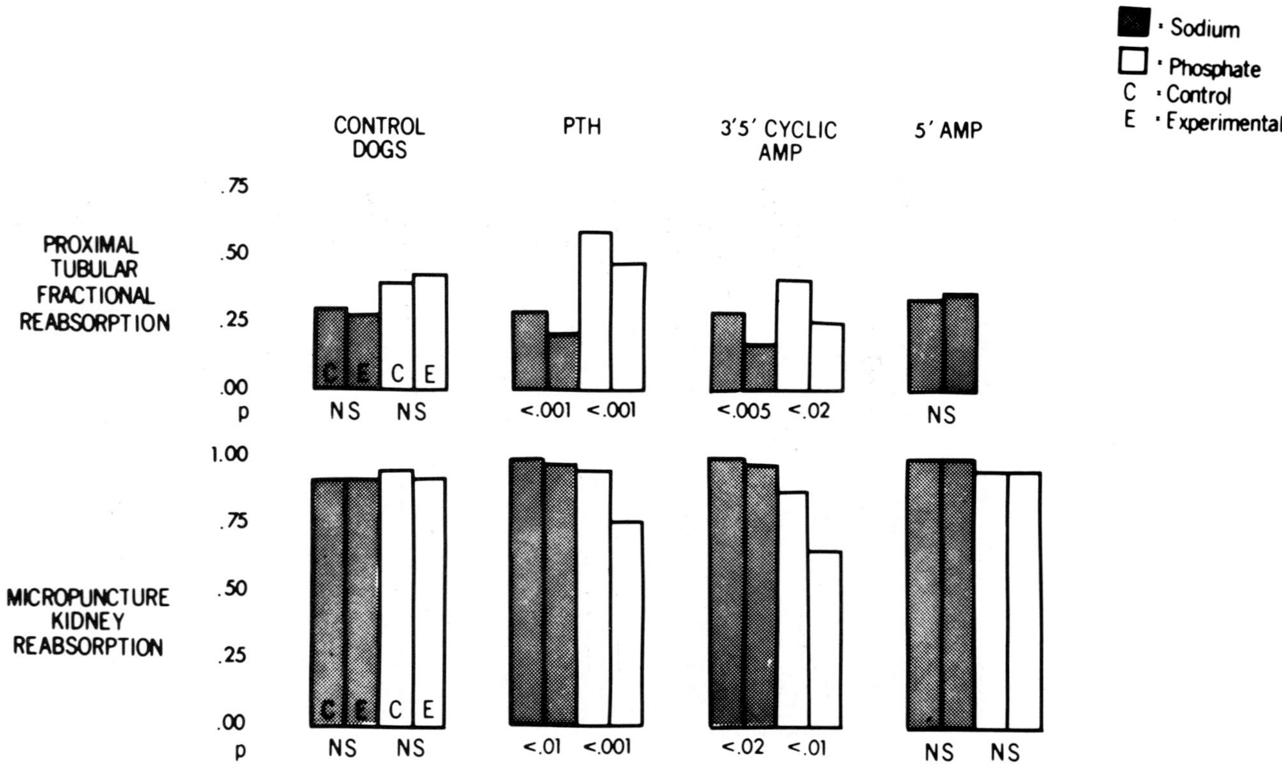

FIG. 2. Effects of parathyroid hormone (PTH) adenosine 3′, 5′ cyclic monophosphate (3′, 5′ cyclic AMP) and 5′ adenosine monophosphate (5′ AMP) on proximal tubular and whole kidney fractional reabsorption of sodium and phosphate in intact dogs. The results are compared to the data obtained in animals utilized as timed controls (panels on the left).

absence of any changes in transport in the timed control animals (Fig. 2). Furthermore, the data suggest that inhibition of sodium transport in the proximal nephron in the *intact* organism may regularly be accompanied by proximal phosphate rejection and, thus, a resultant phosphaturia. Stated in another way, it seemed entirely possible that alterations in urinary phosphate excretion could be utilized as an indicator of proximal tubular function.

Shown in Figure 3 are the changes induced in the percentage of filtered phosphate excreted into the urine as a function of the natriuresis resulting from the administration of several currently employed diuretic agents. On the abscissa is plotted the simultaneously determined increment in percentage

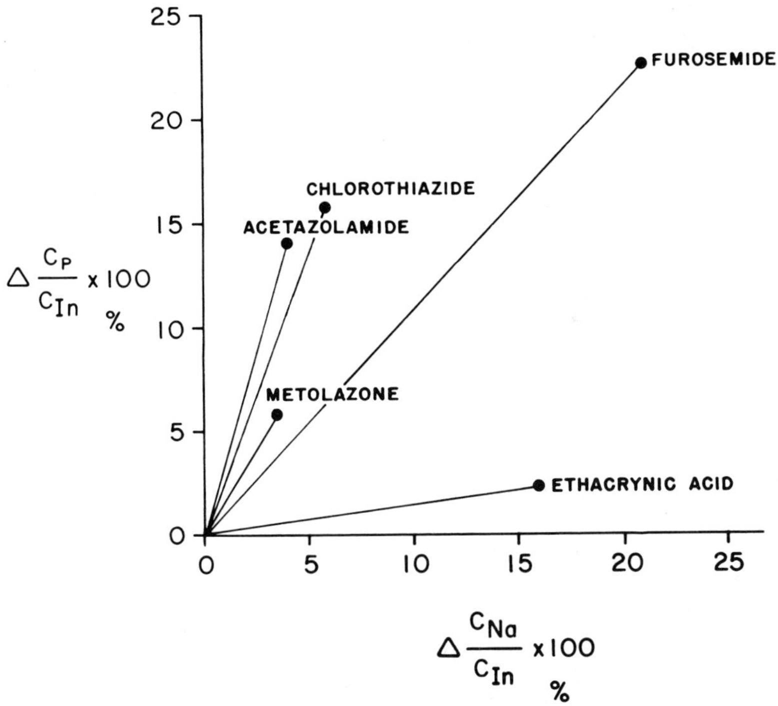

FIG. 3. Changes in the percentage of filtered sodium excreted from control levels (ordinate) produced by each of five diuretic agents, plotted as a function of their respective natriuretic potencies (expressed as the increment in the percentage of filtered sodium excreted, abscissa).

sodium excretion. These experiments were performed in normal man. Acetazolamide, furosemide and chlorothiazide all induced substantial increments in phosphate excretion. Metolazone produced a smaller, but consistent phosphaturia. Ethacrynic acid, on the other hand, demonstrated only minimal and inconsistent effects on phosphate excretion.

Thus far, we have been discussing experimental observations obtained in animals and man in which parathyroid function was intact. However, when the parathyroid glands are removed, the pattern of phosphate reabsorption within the nephron is changed. In Figure 4 are shown fractional reabsorption data for

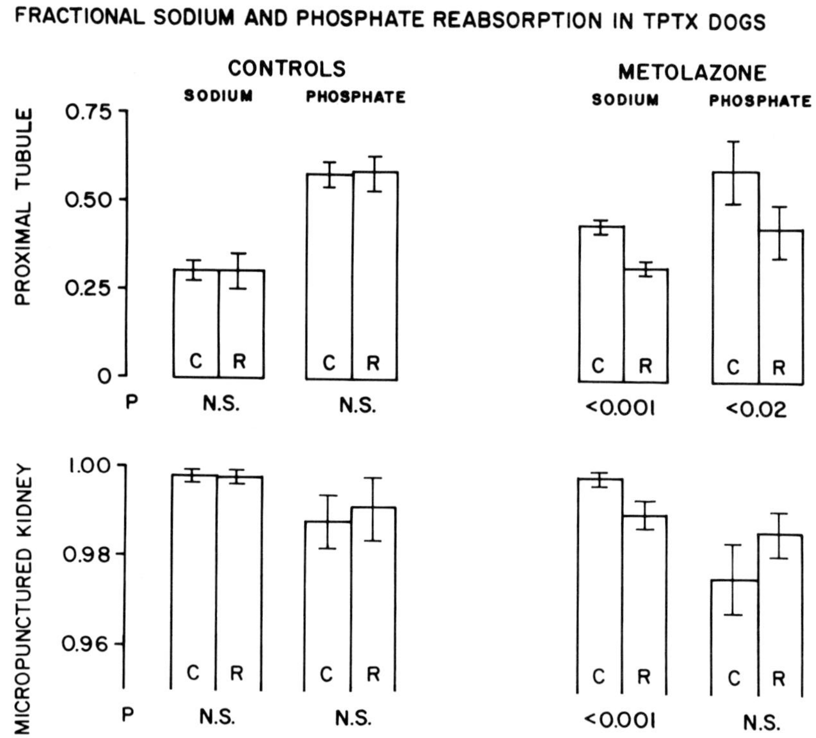

FIG. 4. Effects of metolazone on the fractional reabsorption of sodium and phosphate by the proximal tubule and micropunctured kidney in TPTX animals. The data are compared to those obtained in control animals. C, R = control and recollection phases of the experiments, respectively.

the proximal tubule and for the micropunctured kidney in thyroparathyroidectomized (TPTX) dogs. As demonstrated for the studies in intact animals (Fig. 2), no changes in transport phenomena occurred in the animals utilized as timed controls. The administration of metolazone was followed by a reduction in both phosphate and sodium reabsorption proximally. However, while a natriuresis developed *no phosphaturia occurred.* This means that the phosphate ions rejected proximally were reabsorbed downstream. Thus, in contrast to the situation in the intact animal, there must be substantial *distal* nephron transport of phosphate when parathyroid hormone is absent. This observation, first obtained in our own laboratory [4, 5], has since been confirmed by others [6]. The influence of parathyroid hormone on the pattern of phosphate excretion due to diuretics can be readily appreciated in the studies summarized in Figure 5, in which are presented the mean data for the percentage of filtered sodium and phosphate excreted into the urine following the administration of similar doses of metolazone to both TPTX animals and to dogs with intact parathyroid glands. Whereas the drug caused an equivalent degree of natriuresis in the two groups, *no* phosphaturia occurred in the TPTX animals, but a significant increment in phosphate excretion was observed in the intact dogs. The possibility exists that the differences noted here could have been related to a stimulation of parathyroid hormone secretion brought about by metolazone. However, no changes in serum ultrafilterable calcium concentration occurred. Therefore, we currently favor the thesis that the differences observed in phosphate excretion between the two groups represent an influence of the hormone on the distribution of phosphate reabsorption within the nephron. This question is now under active investigation in our laboratory.

Let us return now to a consideration of the loci of action of the diuretic agents within the tubular system, as well as the possible mechanisms of their transport inhibitory effects. Acetazolamide, the most potent carbonic anhydrase inhibitor in current usage, presumably impairs sodium reabsorption by virtue of its ability to interfere with bicarbonate reabsorption. Since most of the filtered bicarbonate is transported proximally, this drug has as its most important locus of action the

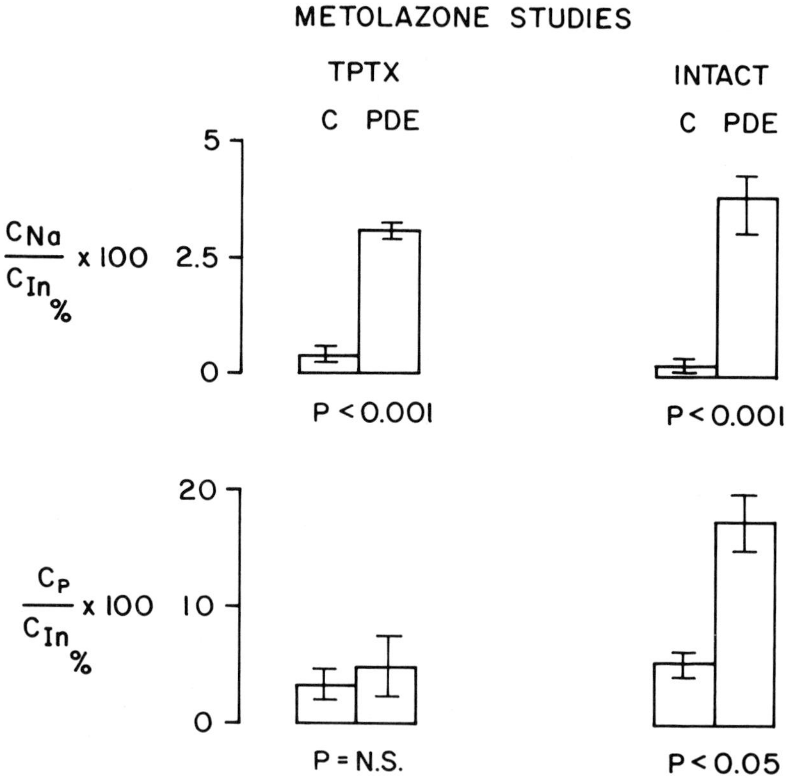

FIG. 5. A comparison of the effects of equivalent doses of metolazone on the percentages of filtered sodium ($C_{Na}/C_{In} \times 100$) and phosphate ($C_p/C_{In} \times 100$) excreted in TPTX and intact animals.

proximal tubular site labeled #2 (Fig. 1). Furosemide has its main effect in the medullary ascending limb of the loop of Henle (site 3), but has an additional action in the proximal tubule, presumably because of a less potent but nevertheless significant ability to inhibit the enzyme carbonic anhydrase [7]. Chlorothiazide owes its diuretic properties to a capacity for impairing sodium transport at site 4 but, like acetazolamide and furosemide, is also a carbonic anhydrase inhibitor with a potency in vitro somewhat less than acetazolamide but greater than that of furosemide [7]. Like chlorothiazide, metolazone acts chiefly at site 4, but its proximal tubular effect is not related to carbonic anhydrase inhibition [8].

As we have demonstrated (Fig. 2), parathyroid hormone, the phosphaturic agent par excellence, has a major effect on proximal tubular transport. Because of the phosphaturia induced by all four of the diuretic agents (Fig. 3), we postulated that they might all share with parathyroid hormone an ability to alter proximal reabsorption by an induction of the adenylate cyclase system. The results of some representative preliminary studies in which we explored this concept are shown in Figure 6. To obviate any problems of data interpretation which might have been introduced by random or induced alterations in circulating levels of parathyroid hormone, all of these studies were performed in thyroparathyroidectomized dogs. Acetazolamide increased phosphate excretion without any concomitant change in urinary cyclic AMP excretion. These results differ, therefore, from those of Klahr and his co-workers, who noted an abrupt increase in urinary cyclic AMP which preceded the phosphaturia in both TPTX and intact rats [9]. Furosemide produced a mild sustained rise in the excretion of the nucleotide which paralleled the increment in phosphate excretion. In confirmation of our earlier studies (Fig. 5), metolazone produced no phosphaturia in the TPTX animal. However, the drug did cause an acute rise in cyclic AMP which was unsustained. We are currently investigating whether this effect of metolazone is the result of variations in glomerular or tubular function, or represents a change in the activity of the adenylate cyclase system within the renal tubular cell. Finally, chlorothiazide, like metolazone, caused no consistent increase in phosphate excretion in the TPTX dog, but unlike metolazone, also did not increase cyclic AMP excretion, suggesting that its proximal effect is not mediated by adenylate cyclase.

One final hypothesis to explain the proximal tubular activity of diuretic agents is suggested by the studies of those workers who have been investigating the possibility that natriuresis may result from alterations in intrarenal blood flow distribution [10]. According to this line of reasoning, a redistribution of blood flow, and hence, glomerular filtrate, from high capacity nephrons located in the juxtamedullary region to low transport capacity nephrons present in the superficial cortex, could account for the increased excretion of sodium. Utilizing the radioactive microsphere technique, we

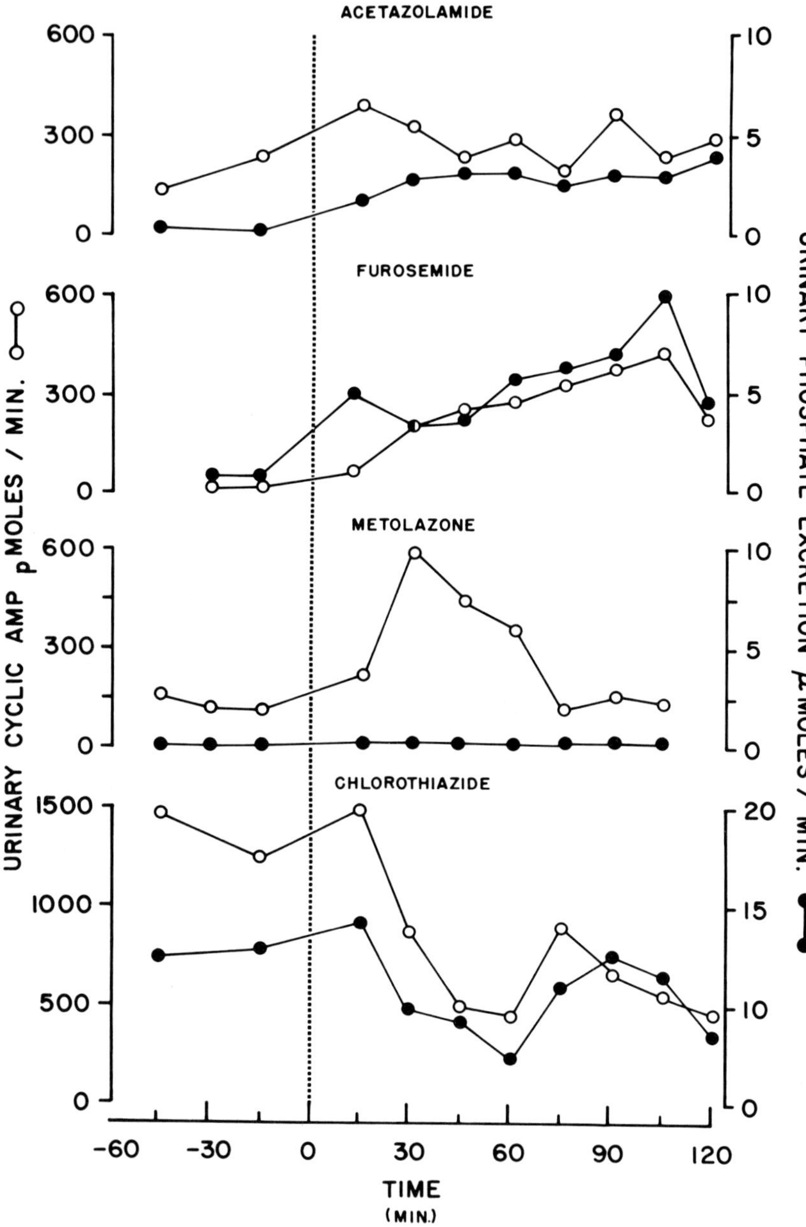

FIG. 6. Representative studies of the effects of four diuretic agents on urinary excretion of cyclic AMP (open circles) and phosphate (closed circles) in TPTX animals. Data points to the left of the dashed vertical line represent the control observations.

have investigated intrarenal blood flow patterns in dogs, with regard to the effects of metolazone. In our studies, the administration of metolazone resulted in no significant alterations in the distribution of blood flow from the control situation. Indeed, the data look quite similar to those obtained in animals utilized as timed controls. Studies with the other diuretic agents are currently in progress; preliminary results of these experiments suggest that no consistent pattern of intrarenal blood flow distribution can be demonstrated for all of the drugs.

In summary, the studies presented here and the available supporting data from the literature suggest the following conclusions: (1) When the parathyroid glands are intact, the transport of phosphate is largely accomplished proximally, so that alterations in phosphate excretion probably reliably indicate changes in proximal tubular function. (2) However, in the absence of parathyroid hormone, significant amounts of phosphate are transported distally. Under these circumstances, therefore, the ability of a proximally active agent to effect a phosphaturia will depend upon its ability to overcome or to inhibit the distal transport mechanisms. (3) With the possible exception of furosemide, none of the diuretic agents studied would appear to exert its proximal action by inducing the adenylate cyclase system. (4) Metolazone does not act proximally by virtue of alterations induced in intrarenal blood flow distribution.

References

1. Burg, M., Stoner, L., Cardinal, J. et al: Furosemide effect on isolated perfused tubules. Amer. J. Physiol. 225:119, 1973.
2. Agus, Z.S., Puschett, J.B., Senesky, D. et al: Mode of action of parathyroid hormone and cyclic adenosine 3′, 5′ monophosphate on renal tubular phosphate reabsorption in the dog. J. Clin. Invest. 50:617, 1971.
3. Puschett, J.B., Agus, Z.S., Senesky, D.J. et al: Effects of saline loading and aortic obstruction on proximal phosphate. Amer. J. Physiol. 223:851, 1972.
4. Fernandez, P.C. and Puschett, J.B.: Proximal tubular actions of metolazone and chlorothiazide. Amer. J. Physiol. 225:954, 1973.
5. Fernandez, P.C. and Puschett, J.B.: Proximal tubular effects of metolazone (M). Clin. Res. 20:891, 1972.

6. Beck, L.H. and Goldberg, M.: Effects of acetazolamide and parathyroidectomy on renal transport of sodium, calcium and phosphate. Amer. J. Physiol. 224:1136, 1973.
7. Puschett, J.B. and Goldberg, M.: The acute effects of furosemide on acid and electrolyte excretion in man. J. Lab. Clin. Med. 71:666, 1968.
8. Puschett, J.B., Steinmuller, S.R., Rastegar, A. et al: Metolazone: Mechanism and sites of action. *In* Modern Diuretic Therapy in the Treatment of Cardiovascular and Renal Disease. Proceedings of a Symposium, held in London, May 1972. Amsterdam:Excerpta Medica Foundation, 1973, pp. 168-175.
9. Rodriguez, H.J., Walls, J., Yates, J. et al: Effects of acetazolamide on the urinary excretion of cyclic AMP and on the activity of renal adenyl cyclase. J. Clin. Invest. 53:122, 1974.
10. Stein, J.H., Boonjarern, S., Wilson, C.B. et al: Alterations in intrarenal blood flow distribution. Circ. Res. 32 & 33 (suppl. 1):1-61, 1973.

Discussion

Moderator: Dr. E. D. Freis

Dr. Kaplan: Dr. Puschett, is metolazone a drug which can be used to increase calcium excretion as other thiazide diuretics?

Dr. Puschett: I can only comment, Dr. Kaplan, on acute studies since we have not performed chronic studies. But, acutely in normal man you get small increases in calcium excretion. I would think that the optimal way to utilize it as a calciuric agent would be to combine it with one of the loop blockers since, perhaps, some of its calciuric effects relate to its ability to act proximally.

Audience: This is for Dr. Puschett. I am trying to figure out the relationship of cyclic AMP in here and I wonder if we were to consider what would a phosphodiesterase inhibitor do and I am thinking of the one that is a diuretic, the xanthines. How do they fit in with this, will they increase the output of cyclic AMP?

Dr. Puschett: I do not know the answer to that question. That is a good question. In view of the fact that most of these agents were not effective in altering urinary cyclic AMP excretion, we have not looked at whether any of them are acting as phosphodiesterase. I think it is certainly a possibility with regard, for example, to furosemide. We are not as yet convinced that the effects of the latter drug are related to any induction of the adenylate cyclase system and our work now is involving us in in vitro methods to test this.

Influence of Metolazone, Hydrochlorothiazide and Spironolactone on Potassium Balance in Hypertensive Patients

Vincent Lanzoni, M.D., Ph.D., Gordon Smith, M.D. and Aram V. Chobanian, M.D.

Introduction

Metolazone is a recently approved diuretic agent whose antihypertensive effect is well documented [1-3]. The drug is a quinethazone derivative with its diuretic action exerted on the cortical diluting segment of the nephron and on the proximal tubule [4]. In patients with mild or moderate hypertension, the reduction of blood pressure with metolazone has been reported to be similar to that of hydrochlorothiazide and chlorthalidone. It has a prolonged duration of action and may therefore have a potential practical advantage over most other diuretics in that it needs to be administered only once daily.

Hypokalemia has been the most troublesome side effect of long-term therapy with metolazone as with most other diuretics. Approximately one fifth of patients with uncomplicated essential hypertension have reductions in serum potassium to abnormal levels with benzothiadiazine derivatives [5]. Although acute studies have suggested that metolazone has less kaliuretic effect than hydrochlorothiazide or furosemide [6], it is uncertain whether differences exist in potassium balance with chronic administration of the drugs.

Supported in part by a grant from the Pennwalt Corporation and by NIH Grant RR 533.

Vincent Lanzoni, M.D., Ph.D., Gordon Smith, M.D. and Aram V. Chobanian, M.D., Boston University School of Medicine, Mass.

Only 2%-3% of total potassium in the body is extracellular in location, and changes in serum potassium may not always reflect the variations occurring in body content. Previous studies have examined the influence of diuretic drugs on exchangeable potassium and total body potassium, but the results have been variable. Substantial reductions in body potassium with benzothiadiazine derivatives have been reported [7, 8], although other investigations have not demonstrated a significant effect [9, 10]. A variety of factors, including the dietary intake of potassium, severity of hypertension, presence of renal disease and duration of therapy, could influence potassium balance and would need to be considered in such investigations.

The current study was carried out to examine the influence of long-term diuretic therapy on blood pressure and serum and body potassium in patients with uncomplicated essential hypertension. Comparisons were made between metolazone, hydrochlorothiazide and spironolactone, as well as the combination of metolazone and spironolactone. In addition, the influence of metolazone and hydrochlorothiazide on sodium and potassium balance, plasma volume, and renin and aldosterone activity was studied under carefully controlled metabolic balance conditions.

Methods

Twelve patients with essential hypertension in the age range of 36 to 66 were included in the study. Seven were black and five white. Secondary causes of hypertension were ruled out by routine diagnostic procedures including intravenous pyelography, urinary VMA or metanephrine levels and, in some cases, by renal angiography and/or renal vein renin assays. All diuretic medications were discontinued for at least one month prior to entry into the study. Pregnant individuals and patients with accelerated hypertension, congestive heart failure, severe renal disease, or severe liver disease were excluded. Informed written consent was obtained from each patient, and the protocol was approved by the Human Studies Committee. All patients were on an unrestricted diet, and no supplementary potassium was administered.

In ten of the patients, following a four-week period of placebo therapy, treatment was instituted with either metolazone 5.0 mg once daily or spironolactone 25 mg four times daily. Treatment was administered for six weeks at which time the other drug was added. The combination was continued for at least six more weeks. In addition, in seven patients, treatment was maintained with one or both drugs for further periods of up to 38 weeks. The daily doses of metolazone in the long-term studies ranged from 1 to 5 mg and of spironolactone from 25 to 100 mg. Six to eight weeks after discontinuation of metolazone and spironolactone, the patients were started on hydrochlorothiazide 100 mg daily and the treatment was continued for six additional weeks. Serum electrolytes, creatinine, uric acid, blood urea nitrogen and blood sugar were measured at one to three week intervals during the study.

Total body potassium content was determined during the control period and following six weeks of therapy with each diuretic and with the combined diuretics. In those patients continued on therapy for longer periods, serial determinations were made over periods of as long as one year. The body potassium measurements were performed by the method of Tyson et al [11] in which the ^{40}K content is assayed directly. Two sodium iodide crystals with matched detector output were used. The subjects lay supine and prone under the detectors, which scanned in a head-to-foot direction. The observed counting error was ± 1%.

In addition, in two patients, comparative studies were carried out between metolazone and hydrochlorothiazide with respect to their acute effects on electrolyte and fluid balance. Two patients with essential hypertension who had been off antihypertensive medications for at least six weeks were studied at the Clinical Research Center under metabolic balance conditions. Dietary sodium intake was maintained at 120 mEq/day and potassium intake at 80 mEq/day. Following a five-day control period, metolazone was administered for eight days at a dosage of 5.0 mg once daily. Measurements of body weight, serum and urinary electrolytes and creatinine clearance were performed on a daily basis. Plasma volume was measured during the control and treatment periods utilizing Evans Blue dye. Plasma renin activity was measured by radioimmunoassay [12] following three hours of ambulation. Aldosterone secretory rate was determined by the method of Melby et al [13]. The same studies were repeated six to eight weeks later utilizing hydrochlorothiazide 50 mg twice daily rather than metolazone.

Results

Significant reductions in blood pressure were observed with each of the diuretics (Table 1). The decreases with metolazone and hydrochlorothiazide were comparable and somewhat greater than those with spironolactone. The combination of metolazone and spironolactone had a greater effect than did either drug alone. The drugs were well tolerated although four of the patients developed hypokalemia (serum potassium < 3.5 mEq/L) with metolazone and three with hydrochlorothiazide. None of these individuals demonstrated any of the signs or symptoms which may be associated with hypokalemia [14].

Mild decreases in total body potassium were present with both metolazone and hydrochlorothiazide (Table 1). The decreases after six weeks of therapy averaged 126 mEq for metolazone (range -60 to -239 mEq) and 104 mEq for hydrochlorothiazide (range -36 to -280 mEq). The largest percentage reductions for total body potassium were 11% for metolazone and 10% for hydrochlorothiazide. The changes in body potassium did not correlate closely with those in the serum. Even in patients who developed hypokalemia to levels as low as 2.9 mEq/L, only minimal reductions in total body content were present.

Spironolactone produced no significant change in body potassium either when used alone or in combination with

Table 1. Influence of Diuretics on Blood Pressure and Serum and Total Body Potassium in Patients with Essential Hypertension

	Blood Pressure (mm Hg)	*Serum K (mEq/L)*	*Total Body K (mEq)*
Metolazone (5 mg/day)	–20/13 ± 5/3	–0.72 ± 0.15	–126 ± 52
Hydrochlorothiazide (100 mg/day)	20/11 ± 6/4	–0.53 ± 0.10	–104 ± 52
Spironolactone (100 mg/day)	–18/ 6 ± 8/3	+0.25 ± 0.06	+ 45 ± 104
Metolazone (5 mg/day) + spironolactone (100 mg/day)	–29/16 ± 13/9	–0.18 ± 0.08	– 94 ± 78

Values represent the mean ± S.E. for the changes observed after six weeks of treatment in 12 patients.

changes following four weeks of hydrochlorothiazide administration although some reduction was present at the end of one week. Anderson et al [10] also did not find any significant decrease in body potassium with hydrochlorothiazide or with furosemide. On the other hand, Healy and associates [7] observed decreases in exchangeable potassium averaging 236 and 250 mEq for three to six weeks of respective treatments with chlorthalidone and furosemide. In addition, Edmonds and Jasani [8] have reported significant reductions in potassium-40 content with bendrofluazide. The differences in results between these investigations may be related to the nature of the patient population studied. Untreated patients with uncomplicated essential hypertension appear to have normal levels of body potassium [15], but significant reductions may be observed in individuals with aldosterone excess such as patients with accelerated hypertension, heart failure, or primary aldosteronism [16]. The latter patients may have very severe degrees of body potassium deficiency and may be very sensitive to the potassium-depleting effects of the kaliuretic drugs. In addition to the type of hypertension present, the dietary intake could also explain differences between the above investigations. Our own patients have been instructed routinely to ingest relatively generous amounts of potassium-containing foods which could serve to minimize the degree of potassium deficiency. It has been observed recently that the addition of 60 mEq of potassium chloride to an unrestricted diet will prevent thiazide-induced hypokalemia in most individuals [17].

It remains uncertain as to whether hypokalemia or total body potassium deficiency is more important in inducing the complications associated with potassium deficiency. However, on the basis of the available evidence, it would appear that the cardiac arrhythmias depend primarily upon the changes in serum potassium. The transmembrane potential of myocardial cells, which is an important determinant of cardiac excitability, appears to depend primarily upon the ratio of extracellular to intracellular potassium. The intracellular potassium reflects total body potassium content and therefore does not generally change rapidly. Any marked variation in serum potassium, however, could have an important influence on membrane polarization. On the other hand, the intracellular concentration of potassium appears to be important for the metabolic functions of the cell. With severe potassium depletion, various harmful tissue effects including muscle atrophy, muscle weakness and renal damage may result [18, 19]. It is of interest that both the myopathy and nephropathy associated with potassium deficiency are rare consequences of diuretic therapy, reflecting probably the lack of severe intracellular potassium depletion. It has been estimated that as much as 30% reduction in body potassium content may be required before these problems develop [20].

The metabolic studies indicated that the effects of metolazone on sodium and potassium balance as well as on PRA, aldosterone secretory rate and plasma volume were essentially similar to that of hydrochlorothiazide. The findings relating to potassium balance contrast with the prior results of Puschett and Rastegar [6] who observed much less of a kaliuretic effect of metolazone than of chlorothiazide and furosemide in water-loaded subjects studied on an acute basis.

Metolazone proved to be an effective and well-tolerated agent for the treatment of hypertension. In collateral studies, we have observed that its antihypertensive potency appears to be similar to that of hydrochlorothiazide when compared on the basis of either 2.5 or 5 mg metolazone and 100 mg hydrochlorothiazide. The 1 mg daily dose of metolazone also lowered blood pressure but to a lesser extent than either the 2.5 or 5.0 mg dosages. In the current work, the combination of spironolactone and metolazone was particularly effective and lowered blood pressure to 150/95 or less in eight of the ten patients studied. Spironolactone also had a beneficial effect in counteracting the hypokalemia induced by metolazone.

Summary

The influence of metolazone, hydrochlorothiazide and spironolactone on potassium balance was examined over prolonged periods of time in ambulatory patients with essential hypertension. Both metolazone and hydrochlorothiazide produced mild reductions in total body potassium as determined by the direct assay of ^{40}K content. The reductions averaged 4%-5% below control levels and did not exceed 11%, even in the patients who developed hypokalemia with the drugs. Spironolactone therapy had little effect on body potassium levels although it produced an increase in serum potassium in all of the patients.

The metabolic effects of metolazone on sodium and potassium balance and on the renin-angiotensin-aldosterone system were comparable to hydrochlorothiazide over an eight-day period of therapy. No differences in kaliuretic or saliuretic activity were apparent at daily doses of 5 mg metolazone and 100 mg hydrochlorothiazide.

Metolazone was well tolerated and produced an antihypertensive effect which was generally of comparable degree to that of hydrochlorothiazide. When used in combination with spironolactone, an increase in antihypertensive activity was observed and the problem of hypokalemia was minimized.

References

1. Pilewski, R.M., Scheib, E.T., Misage, J.R. et al: Technique of controlled drug assay in hypertension. V. Comparison of hydrochlorothiazide with a new quinethazone diuretic, metolazone. Clin. Pharmacol. Ther. 12:843, 1971.
2. Fotiu, S., Finnerty, F.A. and Mroczek, W.J.: Metolazone and chlorthalidone in hypertension — a double-blind evaluation. Int. Res. Commun. Sys. 10:1, 1973.
3. Materson, B.J., Oster, J.R. and Perez-Stable, E.C.: Antihypertensive effects of metolazone (Zaroxolyn). Curr. Ther. Res. 16:890, 1974.
4. Steinmuller, S.R. and Puschett, J.B.: Effects of metolazone in man: Comparison with chlorothiazide. Kidney Int. 1:169, 1972.
5. Hollander, W., Chobanian, A.V. and Wilkins, R.W.: Diuretics in arterial hypertension. *In* Moyer, J.H. (ed.): First Hahnemann Symposium on Hypertensive Disease. New York:W. B. Saunders Company, 1959, pp. 570-580.
6. Puschett, J.B. and Rastegar, A.: Comparative study of the effects of metolazone and other diuretics on potassium excretion. Clin. Pharmacol. Ther. 15:397, 1972.
7. Healy, J.J., McKenna, T.J., Canning, B. St.J. et al: Body composition changes in hypertensive subjects with long-term oral diuretic therapy. Br. Med. J. 1:716, 1971.
8. Edmonds, C.J. and Jasani, B.: Total-body potassium in hypertensive patients during prolonged therapy. Lancet 1:8, 1972.
9. Talso, P. and Carballo, A.J.: Effects of benzothiadiazines on serum and total body electrolytes. Ann. N.Y. Acad. Sci. 88:222, 1960.
10. Anderson, J., Godfrey, B.E., Hill, D.M. et al: Comparison of effects of hydrochlorothiazide and furosemide in treatment of hypertensive patients. Quart. J. Med. 40:541, 1971.
11. Tyson, I., Genna, S., Jones, R.L. et al: Studies of potassium depletion

using direct measurements of total-body potassium. J. Nucl. Med. 11:426, 1970.
12. Sealy, J.E., Gerten-Banes, J. and Laragh, J.H.: The renin system: Variations in man measured by radioimmunoassay or bioassay. Kidney Int. 1:240, 1972.
13. Melby, J.C., Dale, S.L., Grekin, R.J. et al: 18-hydroxy-11-deoxycorticosterone (18-OH-DOC) secretion in experimental and human hypertension. Recent Prog. Hormone Res. 28:287, 1972.
14. Weiner, M. and Epstein, F.H.: Signs and symptoms of electrolyte disorders. Yale J. Biol. Med. 43:76, 1970.
15. Hollander, W., Chobanian, A.V. and Burrows, B.S.: Body fluid and electrolyte composition in arterial hypertension. I. Studies in essential, renal, and malignant hypertension. J. Clin. Invest. 40:408, 1961.
16. Chobanian, A.V., Burrows, B.A. and Hollander, W.: Body fluid and electrolyte composition in arterial hypertension. II. Studies in mineralocorticoid hypertension. J. Clin. Invest. 40:416, 1961.
17. Schwartz, A.B. and Swartz, C.D.: Dosage of potassium chloride elixir to correct thiazide-induced hypokalemia. JAMA 230:702, 1974.
18. Relman, A.S. and Schwartz, W.B.: The kidney in potassium depletion. Am. J. Med. 24:764, 1958.
19. Gross, E.G., Dexter, J.D. and Roth, R.G.: Hypokalemic myopathy and myoglobinuria associated with liquorice ingestion. N. Engl. J. Med. 274:602, 1966.
20. Oliver, J., MacDowell, M., Welt, L.G. et al: The renal lesions of electrolyte imbalance. I. The structural alterations in potassium-depleted rats. J. Exp. Med. 106:563, 1957.

Discussion

Moderator: Dr. A. E. Doyle

Dr. Kincaid-Smith: I have a question for Dr. Chobanian. Your results on potassium appear to be rather different from Dr. Sambhi's results yesterday. I wonder if you have any comments on that. Correct me if I am wrong, but Dr. Sambhi did not show any fall in serum potassium on a very similar trial design.

Dr. Doyle: Dr. Sambhi, would you like to clarify what you said?

Dr. Sambhi: I am afraid I misguided you. There was a fall in serum potassium in our patients also. We however did not quantitate the amount of fall in serum potassium. In general the fall in serum potassium with both drugs — hydrochlorothiazide or metolazone — was comparable. But they both showed this fall in serum potassium.

II

Effects on Renin-Angiotensin System

Antihypertensive Drug Treatment and Plasma Renin

A. E. Doyle, M.D., S. N. Anavekar, M.B.B.S.,
W. J. Louis, M.D. and T. O. Morgan, M.B.B.S.

The fact that renin secreting tumors of the juxtaglomerular cells cause persistent hypertension [1-3] constitutes the best available evidence that renin released from the kidney ever causes high blood pressure. Whether the increased renin release in this syndrome causes hypertension by leading to increased levels of circulating angiotensin II or by local formation of angiotensin within blood vessels is less certain, but there is enough evidence in favor of the latter possibility [4] to cast some doubt on the significance of circulating renin levels in essential hypertension. Nevertheless, it is possible that levels of plasma renin within the rather wide range of normal values could under some circumstances lead to increased local vascular concentrations of angiotensin II.

Although some hypertensive patients have high levels of plasma renin, the majority have levels within the normal range and a significant proportion, on the average about 25%, have low levels. The question remains whether in the latter two groups renin release is significant as a cause of the high blood pressure. An alternative approach to the evaluation of the role of plasma renin in the maintenance of hypertension is the use of means of either reducing renin release, or blocking its action in inducing angiotensin formation, or blocking the action of angiotensin itself. The studies of Haber et al [5], using a

A. E. Doyle, M.D. (Lond.), F.R.C.P., F.R.A.C.P., S. N. Anavekar, M.B.B.S. (Karnatak), F.R.A.C.P., W. J. Louis, M.D. (Melb.), F.R.A.C.P. and T. O. Morgan, M.B.B.S. (Syd.), F.R.A.C.P., Department of Medicine, Austin Hospital Clinical School, University of Melbourne, Heidelberg, Victoria, Australia.

converting enzyme inhibitor, indicate that in sodium-depleted normotensive man, the renin-angiotensin system may have a significant role in the maintenance of blood pressure. Thurston and Swales [4] have reported that angiotensin antagonists reduce blood pressure to the same extent as removal of the ischemic kidney in two kidney hypertensive rats.

In man, renin release from the kidney is controlled to an important extent by the autonomic nervous system. Since most drugs which effectively reduce blood pressure do so *via* an action on the nervous system, it remains possible that their mechanism of action is in part at least related to inhibition of renin release. This paper describes studies of the responses of blood pressure and plasma renin levels in hypertensive patients to a variety of drugs which reduce blood pressure.

Methods

For acute studies, patients were studied in hospital, after three days bed rest, during which time they received a full diet plus 100 mmol of sodium daily as a dietary supplement. When more than one drug was given, one clear day between drug administration was allowed. The effects of chronic administration were studied in outpatients.

Plasma renin activity and concentration were measured by a competitive binding radioimmunoassay [6] and plasma adrenalin and noradrenalin by a double isotope derivative method [7, 8]. Pindolol levels in plasma were measured by a fluorometric technique [9].

Results

Alpha Adrenoceptor Blockade

Acute studies. Nine patients were given phentolamine 5 mg intravenously. Blood pressure did not alter significantly in any patient. There was likewise no change in PRA or PRC. Plasma noradrenalin levels rose significantly from a mean level of 0.153 before the administration of phentolamine to 0.313 (Table 1).

Chronic studies. Eight of the nine patients took phenoxybenzamine in an oral dose of 20 mg twice daily for 14 days. Blood pressures were again unaltered, but there were significant

Table 1. Effect of 5 mg Phentolamine and of 20 mg bid of Phenoxybenzamine on Blood Pressure, Plasma Catecholamine, PRA and PRC in Nine Untreated Hypertensive Patients

		Control	*30 Min. After Phentolamine*	*Two Weeks After Phenoxybenzamine*
Blood pressure				
(9) (mm Hg)		Systolic 150	141	150
		Diastolic 102	99	105
Plasma catecholamines (6) (ng/ml)		.153 ± .046	.313 ± .036	.906 ± .19
PRA	(9)	.177 ± .043	.194 ± .038	0.330 ± 0.33
PRC	(9)	2.34 ± 0.40	2.77 ± 0.44	3.61 ± 0.55

rises in both PRA, PRC and plasma noradrenalin (Table 1). It seems probable that the increases in plasma noradrenalin following alpha-adrenoceptor blockade reflect a disturbance of the re-uptake mechanism at the adrenergic neurone, so that a greater proportion of released noradrenalin enters the circulation. Possibly, the increased levels of circulating noradrenalin stimulated renin release via beta-adrenoceptors in the juxtaglomerular apparatus. It is of interest that the considerable elevation of plasma renin was not associated with a rise in blood pressure.

Ganglion Blockade

Acute studies. Eighteen patients were given an intravenous dose of 5 mg of pentolinium bitartrate. As has been previously reported, ganglion blockade induced a fall in both blood pressure and in plasma noradrenalin levels and the magnitude of change of both parameters correlates closely [10]. By contrast, there was no significant change in either PRA or PRC following pentolinium (Table 2).

Central Sympathetic Blockade

Acute studies. Nine patients were studied. Each was given 150μg of clonidine over a period of five minutes by intravenous injection. Blood pressure and plasma noradrenalin levels both fell sharply, and there was a close correlation between the two. There was no significant fall in either PRA or PRC (Table 3).

Table 2. Effect of Pentolinium Bitartrate, 5 mg IV, on Blood Pressure, PRA, PRC and Plasma Noradrenalin in 18 Hypertensive Patients

		Control	*30 Minutes After Pentolinium*
Blood Pressure:	Systolic	158	135.0
	Diastolic	103	93.3
PRC		2.601 ± 0.4	2.368 ± 0.32
PRA		0.256 ± .04	0.227 ± .034
Plasma Noradrenalin		0.365 ± 0.05	0.257 ± 0.04*

*$p < 0.01$

Beta-adrenoreceptor Blockade

Acute studies. Two studies were performed. In the first, a comparison of the effects of two beta-adrenoreceptor blocking drugs on plasma renin and blood pressure was made. Eleven patients were studied on three occasions at intervals of two days, being given on different days either propranolol, 160 mg, pindolol, 20 mg or four placebo tablets in a random order on a double-blind basis. After control observations of blood pressure and pulse rate, a venous blood sample was drawn for estimations of PRA.

The placebo induced no significant changes in blood pressure, pulse rate or PRA. Propranolol induced a fall of diastolic blood pressure of 10 mm Hg in one patient, and there was no significant fall in the group mean two hours or four hours after the drug was taken. However, mean pulse rate fell

Table 3. Effect of Clonidine 150μg IV in Nine Hypertensive Patients

		Control	*30 Minutes After N*
Blood Pressure:	Systolic	159	134
	Diastolic	101	86
PRC		3.141 ± 1.1	3.66 ± 1.05
PRA		0.387 ± 0.09	0.339 ± 0.021
Plasma NA		0.45 ± 0.06	0.27 ± 0.04

*$p < 0.01$

from 74 to 62 beats per minute at two hours and the mean PRA fell from a control level of 0.60 to 0.33μg/ml/hr.

By contrast, pindolol induced a fall of diastolic blood pressure of 10 mm Hg or more in five of the 11 patients and the group mean fell from 112 mm Hg to 99 mm Hg. The mean pulse rate fell from 75 to 65 beats per minute, and the PRA, although varying a little in individual patients, showed no significant fall in the group mean. These data are summarized in Table 4.

In a second study [11], 15 patients were given 20 mg of pindolol orally, and the effects on blood pressure, PRA and plasma noradrenalin levels measured at intervals over eight hours. These changes were correlated with levels of pindolol in plasma over the same period.

Table 4. Mean Changes in Diastolic Blood Pressure Two Hours After Oral Dose of Propranolol or Pindolol Together With Corresponding Change in PRA

	Diastolic BP mm Hg		*PRA p mol A_1 $ml^{-1}hr^{-1}$*	
	Control	*Two Hours*	*Control*	*Two Hours*
Placebo	112 ± 4.3	111 ± 3.8	0.57 ± 0.11	0.52 ± 0.10
Propranolol	115 ± 4.9	113 ± 5.7	0.60 ± 0.15	0.33 ± 0.09**
Pindolol	112 ± 4.5	99 ± 4.7*	0.61 ± 0.14	0.52 ± 0.14

Mean and S.E. n = 11.
*$p < 0.005$.
**$p < 0.001$ compared with control. Paired "t" test.

The relationship between the mean changes in blood pressure and the mean changes in plasma pindolol is shown in Figure 1. Peak levels of pindolol were reached between two and three hours after administration of the drug, and the trough of the blood pressure fall occurred between three and six hours. There were considerable differences between individuals in the peak concentration in plasma of the drug. The highest concentration achieved was 210 ng/ml; three patients had no detectable drug levels in plasma. There was a close correlation between peak plasma levels and maximal fall in diastolic blood pressure ($r = 0.648$, $p < 0.01$) (Fig. 2). Nine patients had peak

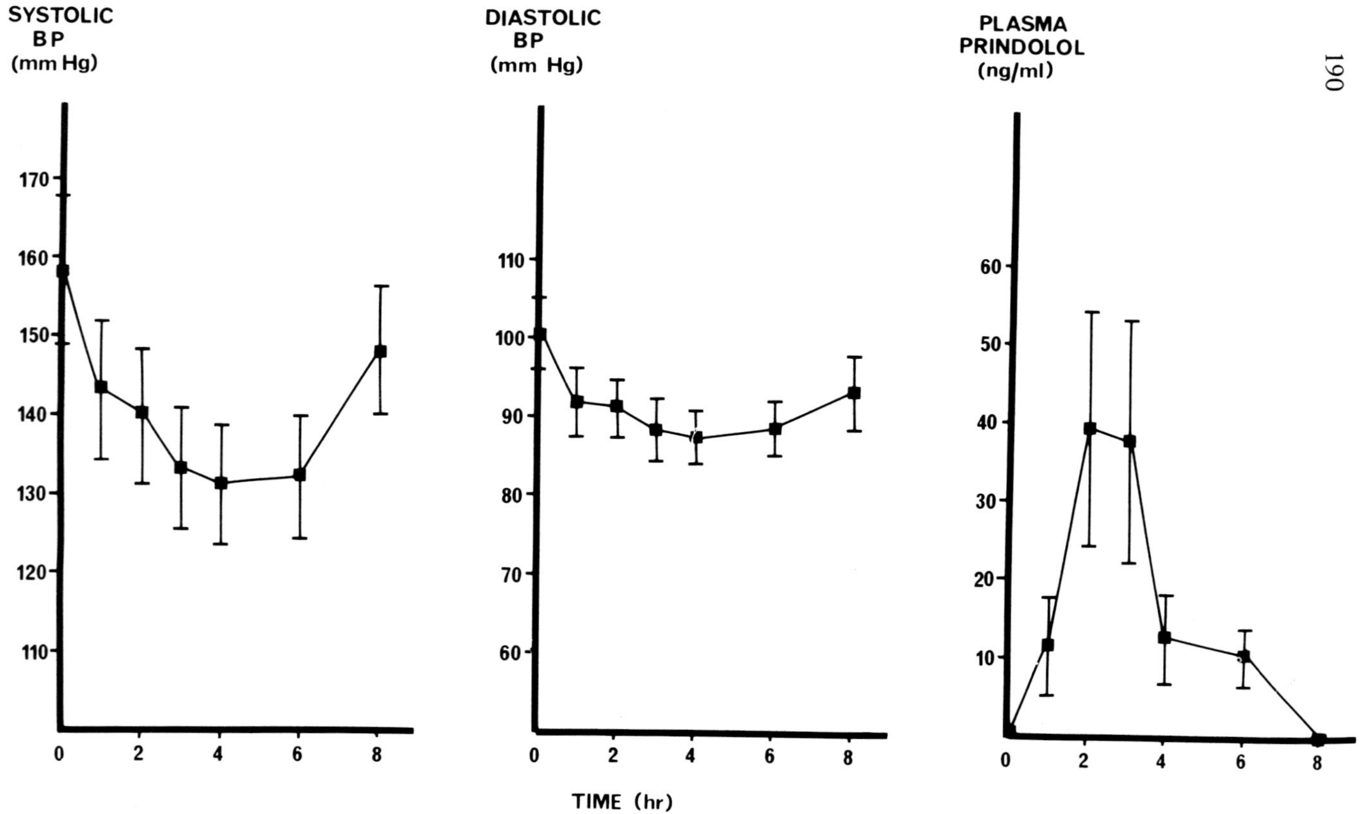

FIG. 1. The effects of 20 mg of pindolol taken by mouth at Ohr on systolic and diastolic blood pressures and plasma drug levels. Points represent means of 15 patients. Bars are S.E.M.

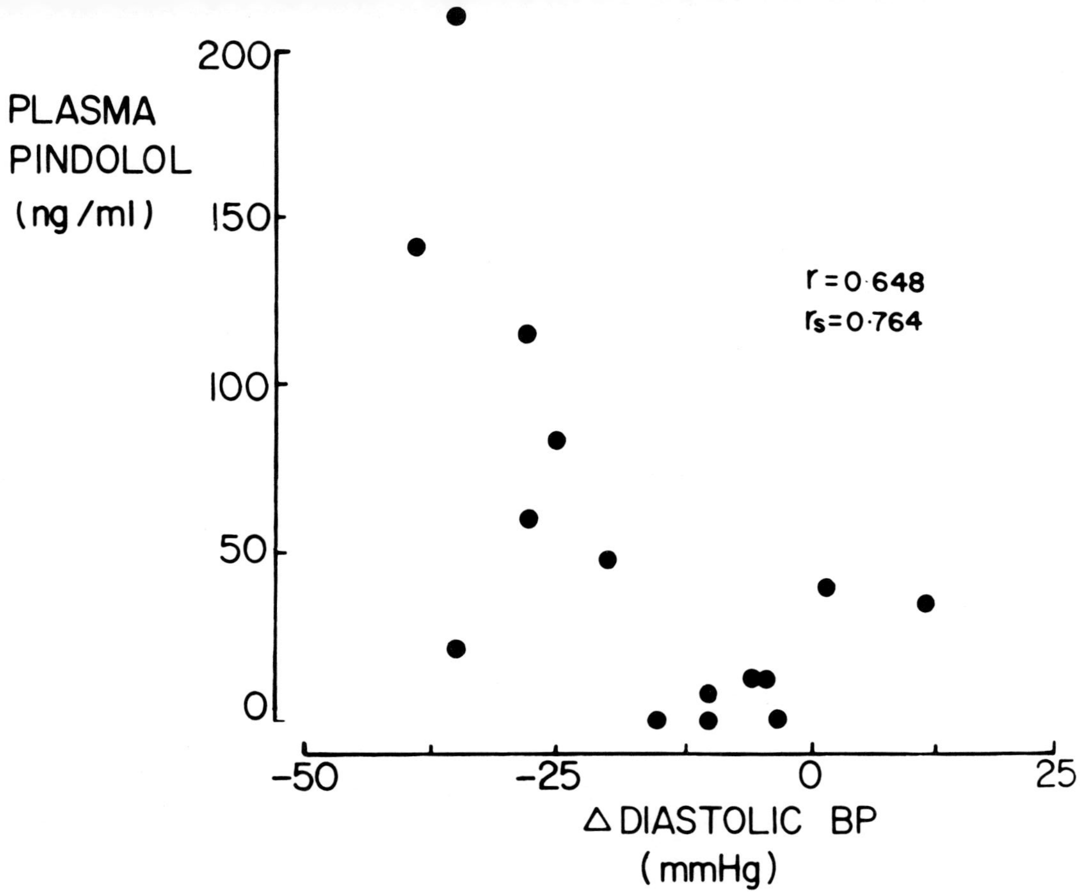

FIG. 2. The relationship between peak plasma levels of pindolol and maximal fall in diastolic pressure following a single dose of 20 mg of pindolol.

levels higher than 15 ng/ml (twice the blank value) and six patients values lower than this. The nine patients who had peak values higher than 15 ng/ml had falls of blood pressure of 41/22 mm Hg, significantly greater than the fall of 16/8 mm Hg in the six with lower levels. In neither group did significant changes occur in either PRA or in plasma noradrenalin levels (Table 5).

Chronic administration. Two studies were carried out. In the first, 76 male patients aged 36-68 (mean 54 years) were studied. All had normal serum creatinine values and none had retinal hemorrhages, exudates or papilledema. All patients were admitted to the hospital and given a diet containing more than 100 mmol of sodium daily. Urinary sodium excretion was measured daily. On the fifth day, patients remained in bed and a venous blood sample drawn for measurement of plasma renin activity to allow classification of patients into high, normal or low renin categories. Patients were discharged from the hospital and given no antihypertensive treatment for three weeks. At this time, PRA and urinary sodium excretion were again measured, as were blood pressure and pulse rate.

Thirty-nine patients then began treatment with propranolol and 37 began treatment with pindolol. The initial dose of propranolol was 80 mg daily and that of pindolol was 10 mg daily. Patients were seen at intervals of two weeks, and if the recumbent diastolic pressure exceeded 95 mm Hg, the dose was

Table 5. Mean Maximal Changes in Systolic and Diastolic BP, PRA, PRC and Plasma NA in Patients With Plasma Pindolol Concentrations Greater or Less Than 15 ng/ml

	Plasma Pindolol > 15 ng/ml (n = 8)		*Plasma Pindolol < 15 ng/ml (n = 6)*		*Significance of Difference Between Mean (t-test)*
Changes in	Mean	S.E.M.	Mean	S.E.M.	
Systolic blood pressure (mm Hg)	-41	9.47	-16.2	3.7	$p < 0.05$
Diastolic blood pressure (mm Hg)	-21	5.7	- 8.0	1.8	$p < 0.05$
PRA*	-0.132	0.14	- 0.174	0.16	$p > 0.4$
PRC*	-1.219	0.86	- 0.73	0.74	$p > 0.3$
Plasma NA (ng/ml)	0.045	0.18	- 0.08	0.06	$p > 0.3$

*ng angiotensin 1/ml/hr.

doubled until an arbitrary maximum dose of 640 mg of propranolol or 80 ng of pindolol had been attained. PRA was measured when recumbent diastolic pressure had fallen below 95 mm Hg for 14 days, or after the maximum dose of each drug had been taken for 14 days. The changes in systolic and diastolic blood pressures and changes in PRA were similar with both drugs (Table 6). Both induced falls in blood pressure of about 12/16 mm Hg, and falls in PRA of 0.20. However, in individual patients there was no correlation between change in plasma renin and change in blood pressure with either drug. The fall in blood pressure did not appear to be related to the fall in the level of PRA (Fig. 3).

The relationship between PRA and daily urinary sodium excretion was also studied. Using our own mean values from normal patients on a high, medium or low sodium diet, patients could be arbitrarily classified into "high," "medium" or "low" renin groups. The "low" renin group had a mean fall in diastolic blood pressure of 20 mm Hg and 13 of the 17 patients in this group had falls of 10 mm Hg or more. The "high" renin group had a mean fall of 15.0 mm Hg, and 14/20 in this group had a fall of 10 mm Hg or more (Table 7).

In a second study, the relationship between response to the chronic administration of pindolol and plasma levels of the drug was studied. Ninety-nine patients, attending as outpatients, were studied. Most were taking other antihypertensive drugs. Pindolol was added to the treatment regime in an initial dose of

Table 6. Change in Blood Pressure and Plasma Renin Activity After Beta-blocking Drugs

	No. of Patients	*Fall in BP (Lying)* *Systolic mm Hg*	*Diastolic mm Hg*	*Fall in PRA* *p mol* A_1 $ml^{-1} hr^{-1}$
Propranolol	39	27.4 ± 2.8*	17.3 ± 2.2*	0.20 ± 0.05**
Pindolol	37	22.5 ± 2.2*	14.4 ± 1.6*	0.20 ± 0.05**
Total	76	24.9 ± 2.0*	15.9 ± 1.4*	0.20 ± 0.04**

Mean and S.E.

*$p < 0.001$ from values before treatment.

**$p < 0.01$ from values before treatment.

No significant difference between effect of propranolol or pindolol on blood pressure or plasma activity $p > 0.05$.

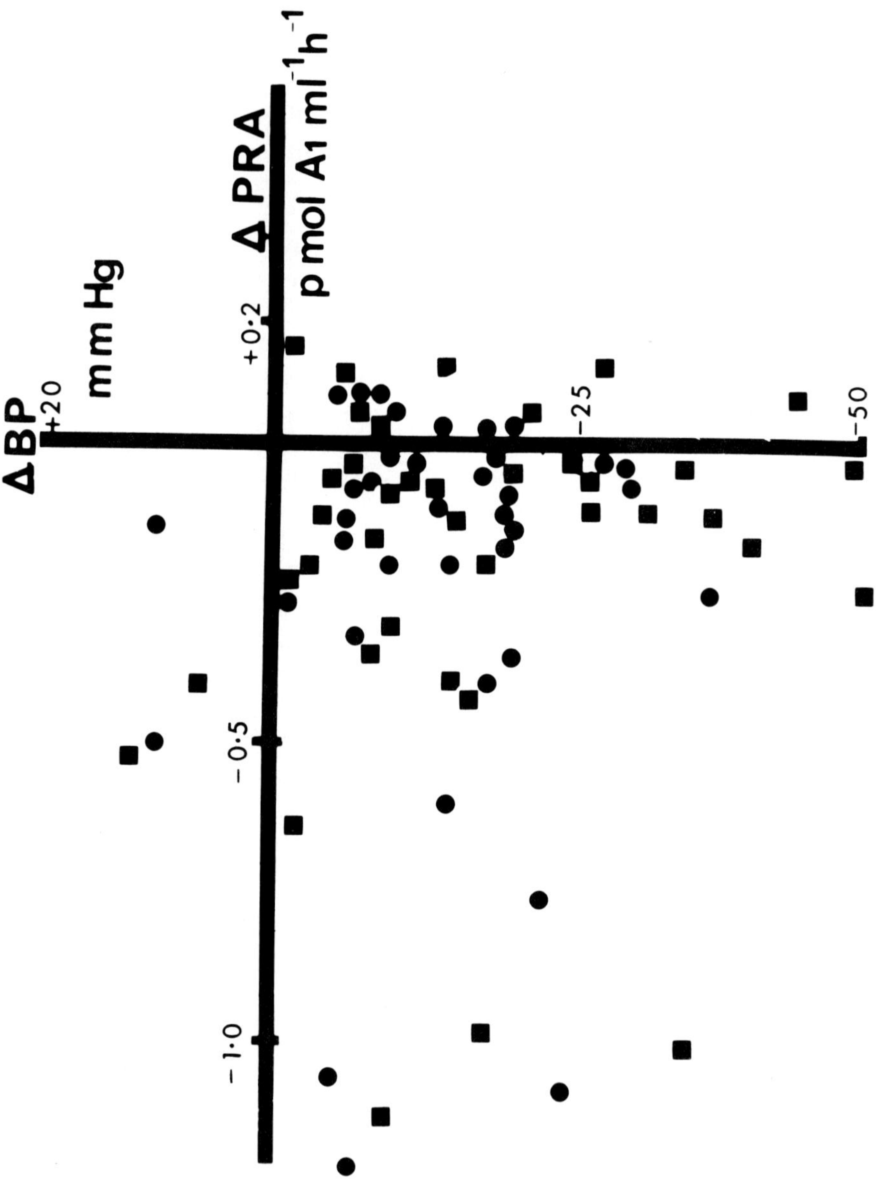

FIG. 3. The relationship between change in PRA and the change in diastolic blood pressure in 39 patients treated clinically with propranolol and 37 patients treated clinically with pindolol.

Table 7. Response of Blood Pressure Related to Plasma Renin Group

Renin Subgroup	*No. of Patients*	*Mean Fall in Diastolic BP mm Hg*	*No. of Patients With > 10 mm Hg Fall*
Low	17	20.0 ± 3.3*	13
Normal	39	15.8 ± 2.1*	24
High	20	15.0 ± 4.6*	14

Mean and S.E.
*$p < 0.001$ from values before treatment.

20 mg daily, increasing to an arbitrary maximum of 80 mg daily. A few patients were unable to take 80 mg daily because of side effects. Patients were classified as having a good response if the recumbent diastolic pressure fell by 15 mm Hg or more and if the diastolic pressure fell below 100 mm Hg, a fair response was a fall of 15 mm Hg, and a final diastolic pressure below 110 mm Hg; patients whose diastolic pressure fell by less than 15 mm Hg, and whose final diastolic pressures exceeded 110 mm Hg, were classified as nonresponders. After a classification of response had been made, plasma pindolol levels were measured two to three hours after the patient had taken his usual dose under supervision. Fifty-nine patients were classified as good responders. In these, the mean plasma pindolol level was 75 ng/ml, at an average daily dose of 24 mg. In the 28 nonresponders the mean pindolol level was 22 ng/ml at an average daily dose of 36.5 mg. In 20 of the 28 patients pindolol levels were absent or nearly so, but in the remaining 8 mean levels were 70 ng/ml with an average daily dose of 44 mg.

Discussion

The results presented here cast considerable doubt on the contribution which plasma renin levels make to the maintenance of the elevated blood pressure in human essential hypertension, for it seems possible to alter plasma renin levels either upward or downward without affecting blood pressure levels. Conversely, it is clear that reduction of blood pressure can be induced in the absence of changes in plasma renin.

Drugs which lower blood pressure by interrupting sympathetic innervation of blood vessels either centrally or peripherally seem to reduce plasma noradrenalin levels by an amount which correlates closely with the magnitude of the fall in blood pressure, but have no apparent action on plasma renin levels. While it remains possible that there is an interaction at local vascular level between locally released angiotensin and locally released neurotransmitter, it seems clear that plasma renin levels offer no help in evaluating this possibility.

It is evident from these data also that there is no simple relationship between the effects of beta-adrenoceptor blockade on blood pressure and plasma renin levels as has been suggested by Buhler et al [12]. It is evident that although the chronic administration of propranolol often reduces both plasma renin levels and blood pressure, changes in the two parameters do not correlate closely in individual patients. Moreover, initial levels of plasma renin do not seem to offer any guide as to the likely response to beta-adrenoceptor blockade in terms of the antihypertensive effect. These findings are reinforced by the fact that single doses of propranolol, although producing a large fall in pulse rate and plasma renin levels, do not affect blood pressure significantly.

Pindolol is a beta-adrenoceptor antagonist which is eight to ten times more potent than propranolol and which also possesses intrinsic sympathomimetic activity [13]. It is likely that the latter property leads to it having a smaller effect than propranolol on pulse rate and may also account for its relatively weak effect on plasma renin levels when given acutely. Nevertheless, it has the capacity to reduce blood pressure acutely in the absence of significant effects on plasma renin activity in man. Similar results have been obtained in the rabbit [14]. The fact that differing beta-adrenoreceptor antagonists have much the same action on blood pressure, but differing effects on plasma renin levels, makes it even less likely that the antihypertensive action of these drugs is mediated via interference with renin release. The pharmacodynamic data presented here suggest that kinetic factors leading to differences in plasma levels are the main determinant of response to these drugs and that the variability of response has usually little to do with the pathogenesis of hypertension.

The mode of action of beta-antagonists remains unclear. Several workers [15-18] have suggested that the mechanism may involve inhibition of sympathetic drive within the central nervous system. If this is so, it is surprising that this is not associated with a fall in plasma noradrenalin levels such as occurs with peripheral ganglion blockade and central inhibition with clonidine. The mechanism of action seems likely to be related to the beta-antagonist properties of the drugs, since their relative potencies in hypertension are related to their relative potencies in blocking isoprenaline-induced tachycardia [16]. The very high doses often needed suggest that their effect may be at a site particularly inaccessible to this group of agents.

It has to be questioned whether measurement of plasma renin levels necessarily gives an indication of the significance of the renin-angiotensin system. In particular, the possibility exists that the pharmacological actions of drugs, which depress both renin levels and blood pressure, may set in train homeostatic mechanisms which may lead by a different mechanism to reversal of one or other component. If this did occur, the information to be derived from studies of plasma renin and blood pressure would be of limited value.

References

1. Robertson, P.W., Klidjian, A., Hardin, L.K. et al: Hypertension due to a renin secreting tumour. Amer. J. Med. 43:963, 1967.
2. Bonnin, J.M., Hodge, R.L. and Lumbers, E.R.: A renin secreting renal tumour associated with hypertension. Aust. N.Z. J. Med. 2:178, 1972.
3. Brown, J.J., Lever, A.F. and Robertson, J.I.S. et al: Hypertension and secondary aldosteronism associated with a renin secreting renal juxtaglomerular cell tumour. Lancet 2:1228, 1973.
4. Thurston, H. and Swales, J.D.: Action of angiotensin antagonists and antiserum upon the pressor response to renin: Further evidence for the local general of angiotensin II. Clin. Sci. Mol. Med. 46:273, 1974.
5. Haber, E., Sancho, J. Re. R. and Barger, A.C.: Third meeting of International Society of Hypertension, Milan, 1974. Clin. Sci. Mol. Med. 1975. (In press.)
6. Johnston, C.I., Mendelsohn, F. and Casley, D.: Plasma renin determination employing a radioimmunoassay of angiotensin I. Proc. Aust. Soc. Med. Res. 2:272, 1969.
7. Engelman, K. and Portnay, B.: Sensitive double isotope derivative assay for norepinephrine and epinephrinic. Circ. Res. 26:53, 1970.
8. Louis, W.J. and Doyle, A.E.: The use of a double-isotope derivative plasma assay for noradrenaline and adrenaline in the diagnosis and

localization of pheaochromocytoma. Aust. New Zeal. Med. 3:212, 1971.

9. Pacha, W.L.: A method for the fluorimetric determination of 4-(2-hydroxy-3-isopropylaminopropoxy)-indole (LB46), a B-blocking agent, in plasma and urine. Experientia 25:802, 1969.
10. Louis, W.J., Doyle, A.E., Anavekar, S.N. et al: Plasma catecholamine dopamine-beta-hydroxylase, and renin levels in essential hypertension. Circ. Res. 34 and 35 (suppl):157, 1974.
11. Anavekar, S.N., Louis, W.J. and Morgan, T.O. et al: The relationship of plasma levels of pindolol in hypertensive patients to effects on blood pressure, plasma renin and plasma noradrenaline levels. Clin. Exp. Pharmacol. Physiol. 1975. (In Press.)
12. Buhler, F.R., Laragh, J.H., Baer, L. et al: Propranolol inhibition of renin secretion. N. Engl. J. Med. 287:1209, 1972.
13. Lubawski, I. and Wale, J.: Studies with LB46, a new B-receptor blocking drug. Europ. J. Pharmacol. 6:345, 1969.
14. Weber, M.A., Stokes, G.S. and Gain, J.M.: Comparison of the effects of renin release of beta adrenergic antagonists with differing properties. J. Clin. Invest. 54:1413, 1974.
15. Laverty, R. and Taylor, K.M.: Propranolol uptake into the central nervous system and the effect on rat behaviour and amine metabolism. J. Pharm. Pharmacol. 20:605, 1968.
16. Morgan, T.O., Louis, W.J. Dawborn, J.K. et al: The use of pindolol in the treatment of hypertension. Med. J. Aust. 2:309, 1972.
17. Morgan, T.O., Sabto, J., Anavekar, S.N. et al: A comparison of beta adrenergic blocking drugs in the treatment of hypertension. Postgrad. Med. J. 50:253, 1974.
18. Dollery, C.T., Lewis, P.J., Myers, M.G. et al: Central hypotensive action of propranolol in the rabbit. Br. J. Pharmacol. 48:343, 1973.

Discussion

Moderator: Dr. A. Grollman

Dr. Zanchetti: I will certainly agree with Dr. Doyle and his position that in mild and moderate hypertensive patients the hypotensive effect of beta-blockade (my experience refers to propranolol) can be completely independent of renin suppression. In the recent paper we published in *Clinical Science* we have been able to calculate dose-response curves and have shown that the dose-response curve for the renin suppression is shifted quite to the left in respect to the dose-response curve for the hypotensive effect of propranolol. So the two effects can be very clearly dissociated. However, I am not against the possibility that in selected groups of patients, the so-called high renin hypertensive patients, renin suppression by beta-blocking agents may have a hypotensive effect. Probably the best way of finding these patients with beta-blockade would be to use small doses of beta-blockers. One hundred sixty milligrams of propranolol a day is a dose which can often have a hypotensive effect independent of the renin-suppressive one. But with smaller doses between the 40 and 80 mg per day then we can have generally a pure renin-suppressive effect, and it is not unlikely that in high renin patients these small doses show that part of their hypertension is renin-dependent.

Dr. Doyle: In general I think that I would suspect that a single dose of propranolol produces a low enough blood level to produce renin block. The point I made was that I think under those circumstances, if one has renin-dependent hypertension one should expect to see an acute fall in blood pressure. I do not think this often occurs. I think the difficulty about long-term administration, even in small doses, is that you get increases in blood levels as the first pass effect is abolished.

Dr. Zanchetti: The dose I mentioned, between 40 and 80 mg a day, were just doses given chronically (chronically meaning one week). In this case you get plasma concentration higher than you can obtain by a single oral dose or by an intravenous dose. I think this is the right way of designing an experiment because just testing the hypotensive effect and the renin-suppressive effect with a single dose, particularly by the intravenous route, can rather confuse the matter because of the acute fall in cardiac output.

Dr. Johnston: The plasma levels are dependent upon the absorption as well as metabolism. Is the variability that you observe in the plasma levels in individual patients due to differences in absorption or metabolism in the liver? Have you given the drug intravenously and studied plasma levels?

Dr. Doyle: Yes, I think that the answer is that it is due to metabolism predominantly. I do not think I would like to leave you with the idea that the only determinant of response is the plasma level because, although on chronic administration it is certainly true that the majority of patients who respond well are those who have detectable blood levels, there are a substantial number of patients who fail to respond to this particular beta-blocking drug or to others in whom it is possible to measure quite high plasma levels so that there are other components which relate to response.

Dr. Winburg: I heard two speakers mention prazosin as being a peripheral vasodilator. We should clarify that since prazosin is a special type of alpha-adrenergic blocker we do not wish to confuse the proceedings. The other point is that of Dr. Doyle, in regard to a central mechanism of action. I do not think that because there were no changes in plasma norepinephrine so we can dismiss this as a possible mechanism of action. Would you agree?

Dr. Doyle: Yes, by inference one would expect that if the beta-blockers were doing something of the same sort as clonidine that they would have had the same effect on plasma noradrenalin. But I think one of the difficulties, of course, is that it may just be a cardiac output effect. However, it still may be acting in an isolated area where it does not produce much in the way of general change. It may, in fact, be selectively on the cardiovascular system in which case noradrenalin output may be hardly modified at all.

Dr. Hollifield: Dr. David Shand and I have also looked at propranolol and renin relationships in low, normal and high renin hypertensives (Fig. 1) as categorized by the Laragh technique of Renin-Sodium index as determined from normotensive middle Tennesseans. We see no response in low renin patients though adequate plasma propranolol levels are achieved on doses of 160 mg daily. We do have favorable blood pressure responses in high and normal renin patients though these responses are less than those noted by Bühler. The high and normal renin patients both responded quantitatively the same. However, it was interesting to us that the majority of blood pressure responses in the high-renin, hypertensive patients occurred during the first increment of dosing, 40 mg daily (not shown). This suggested that we should extend our studies to higher doses of propranolol. Figure 2 shows the effect of high dose propranolol with high plasma levels in low renin hypertensive patients. There was no response of blood pressure on daily doses of up to 160 mg but at each dose level we had incremental decreases in blood pressure though the numbers we

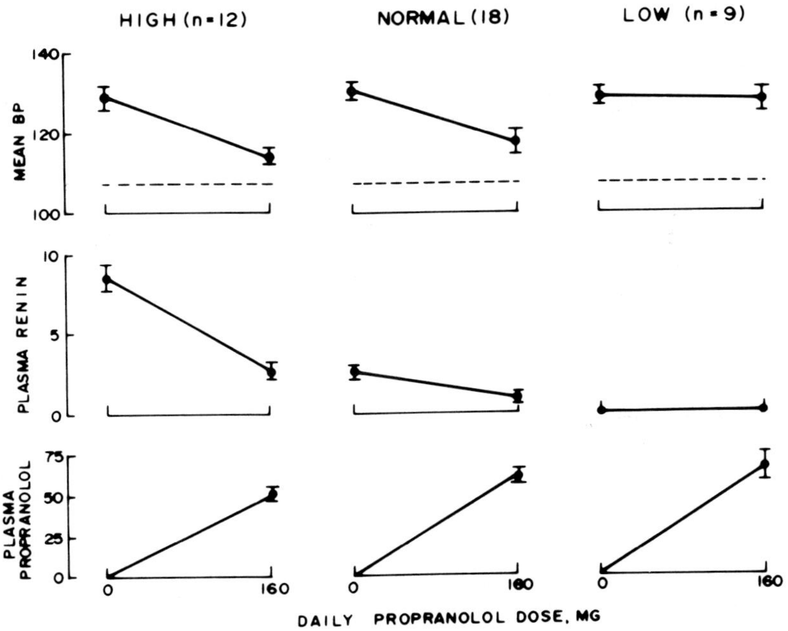

FIGURE 1.

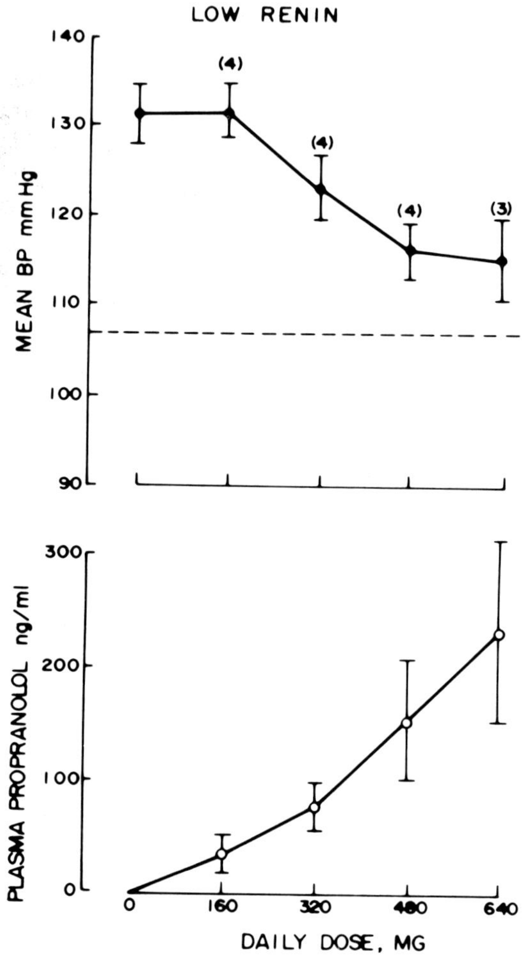

FIGURE 2.

have studied are small. Plasma total propranolol levels demonstrated that we obtained adequate absorption.

Figure 3 shows the same study performed in high renin hypertensive patients. As you can see we have a plateau of plasma renin activity occurring at about the 160 mg dose range but we continue to see a favorable blood pressure response as we escalate the dose as high as 640 mg daily. There was no

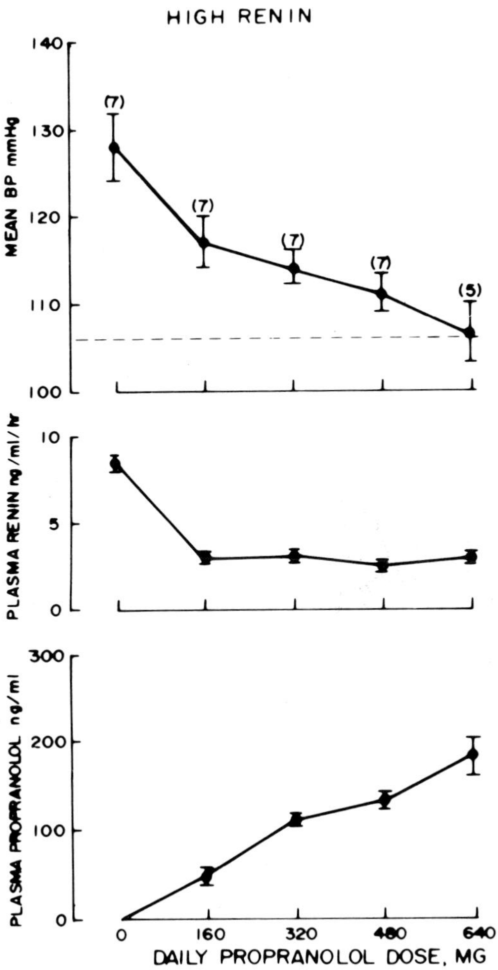

FIGURE 3.

further fall in plasma renin activity at doses of propranolol greater than 160 mg daily. This suggests to us that there are probably two mechanisms of propranolol's antihypertensive activity: one, a low dose effect, seen at plasma levels of about 50 mg/ml Ng which is related to a fall in plasma renin activity and the other, a higher dose effect that is associated with higher plasma propranolol levels and this fall in pressure seems to be renin independent and perhaps might be related to propranolol's effects on the central nervous system.

Dr. Doyle: Clearly I think that if you do get an effect which is on renin, if you do have high blood pressure which is renin independent, or at least a small section of it, as appeared in your slide, you will get a fall of blood pressure, small fall of blood pressure. I suppose you can say that is renin dependent. But maybe people with high renin have a little bit that is renin dependent and a lot more that is something else.

Dr. Hollifield: I think that is very true and we have additional data to suggest this with some P113 studies obtained in these high renin hypertensive patients. We were able to demonstrate that they responded briskly to P113 without propranolol, but during propranolol therapy their blood pressure response to P113 is abolished.

Dr. Onesti: There is a difference between the acute and the long-term effects of some hypertensive agents on renin. Acute administration of pentolinium lowers the blood pressure and has minor effects on renin. However prolonged administration of ganglionic blockers may result in definite renin suppression. It is also interesting to see that after prolonged administration of the ganglionic blockers there is frequently an increase in blood pressure, an increase in blood volume and suppression of renin. This shows an additional example of dissociation between renin effect and blood pressure effect.

Dr. Doyle: One of the problems is that if you keep the blood pressure down for any length of time by any mechanism, it appears that the renin falls. I think in the acute experiment it is very difficult to say this is or is not. I think your point is perfectly valid.

Dr. Freis: I think we are confusing a falling renin as the antihypertensive action of the drug because any of us that have measured renin in hypertension for a long period of time find that in any hypertensive, particularly a hypertensive with high renin, if you treat them for several months with any antihypertensive agents their renins will come down and no one postulates that all the drugs work by renin. I think there is a great danger that we are extrapolating the falling renin as the cause of the antihypertensive action.

Dr. Streeten: I would like to support the view of Dr. Zanchetti and Dr. Hollifield that propranolol probably acts by two distinct mechanisms in these patients. In the data presented by Dr. Doyle, the renin-lowering mechanisms might have been obscured by the fact that, as Dr. Doyle has said, there were very few renin-dependent hypertensives among his patients. It seems to me it is quite unreasonable to expect that propranolol would lower the blood pressure by reducing renin when in fact renin was not the cause of the hypertension. On the contrary, when renin is elevated and is causing the hypertension then it is very difficult to disprove the view that propranolol might be lowering the blood pressure by lowering the renin. And like Dr. Hollifield we have evidence from the use of saralasin in such patients that the blood pressure will come down to normal with this angiotensin II antagonist and will fall equally well during treatment with propranolol with a very high degree of correlation between the responses to the two drugs. Our experience similarly has suggested that with propranolol the effects on the blood pressure last only as long as the renin is reduced. So I think it is very important in this discussion to differentiate between those patients in whom high renin is causing the hypertension — perhaps the best way of finding this is with saralasin — and those patients in whom renin has no relationship to the hypertension where clearly propranolol cannot be acting on blood pressure by lowering renin.

Dr. Doyle: I agree really. I think the only area that we are in any danger of getting into conflict is the frequency with which high blood pressure is renin dependent. If you have a drug which acts in more than one way, and if you accept that reducing the blood pressure often reduces renin, it seems to me devilishly difficult to say that you can prove that it is renin dependent. On the other hand, what has emerged is that many patients apparently with high renins do not seem to have renin-dependent hypertension. I think it is complex. Clearly there must be some patients who are. But how often that is the case I think is really quite obscure and it cannot be determined on a simple estimation of plasma renin.

Dr. Mulrow: I just want to add something to that. Many renin-dependent hypertensives that come into a clinic are markedly volume depleted. Any normal subject who is really volume depleted may have a substantial drop in blood pressure if the renin system is blocked. So sometimes renin-dependent hypertension just may mean a markedly volume depleted subject who depends upon all of his regulatory mechanisms to maintain the blood pressure.

Dr. Stokes: Just to complicate the matter a little further, I think it should be pointed out that there are good grounds to believe that vascular sensitivity to angiotensin varies widely between subjects. I point to the paper recently published by Pinto and others in *Kidney International* suggesting that there may be a factor possibly which governs the degree of binding of angiotensin to vascular receptors from patient to patient within the gamut of essential hypertension. Of course, this is quite apart from the familiar factors such as sodium.

Effects of Antihypertensive Therapy on Plasma Renin Activity

Norman M. Kaplan, M.D., O. Bryan Holland, M.D.
and Celso Gomez-Sanchez, M.D.

Drugs used in the treatment of hypertension may change the level of plasma renin activity (PRA) [1]. There are three broad classes of antihypertensive agents and each class tends to affect PRA levels in a similar direction:

1. Diuretics raise PRA levels.
2. Peripheral vasodilators raise PRA levels.
3. Adrenergic neuronal blockers lower PRA levels.

Brunner et al have claimed repeatedly that higher PRA levels are associated with and are likely causal of cardiovascular damage and death [2, 3]. Though there is increasingly strong evidence against the vasculotoxic potential of normal levels of PRA [4], most would agree that low levels are preferable to very high levels. Though normal levels of renin-angiotensin may not damage blood vessels, high levels may produce enough vasoconstriction to dampen the effectiveness of regimens used to lower blood pressure. The reactive rise in renin following either diuretic-induced volume depletion or vasodilator-induced falls in renal perfusion pressure may blunt the effectiveness of such drugs. On the other hand, the decrease in PRA levels accompanying the use of adrenergic-blocking drugs may explain some of their antihypertensive effectiveness.

Supported by NIH grant NHLI-5-RO1-HL14863.

Norman M. Kaplan, M.D., Deputy Vice President for Research Programs, The American Heart Association and Clinical Professor; O. Bryan Holland, M.D., Assistant Professor; and Celso Gomez-Sanchez, M.D., Assistant Professor, Department of Internal Medicine, The University of Texas Health Science Center, Dallas.

Diuretics are almost always used as initial therapy for hypertension. If the diuretic-induced rise in PRA limits the antihypertensive effectiveness of the agent or serves as a potential vasculotoxic hazard, a drug which lowers renin seems a logical choice if additional antihypertensive action is needed.

We have examined the effects of two adrenergic neuronal blocking drugs, alpha-methyldopa and the beta-blocker, oxprenolol, upon PRA levels and blood pressure in hypertensive patients already on diuretics. The studies were of relatively short duration but should be applicable to the long-term management of hypertension.

Methods

Patients

Twenty patients were used in the study on methyldopa; 15 others were used in the study on oxprenolol. All were between the ages of 30 and 65 and had the diagnosis of essential hypertension based on the absence of clinical features and laboratory data suggestive of secondary causes of hypertension. Their hypertension was considered moderately severe with diastolic pressures above 105 mm Hg at the end of a three-week period on placebo. None had hemorrhagic retinopathy, plasma creatinine levels above 1.5 mg/100 ml or evidences of coronary, cerebral or peripheral vascular disease. Women with childbearing potential were excluded and all patients gave their informed, voluntary consent.

Protocols

The details of the methyldopa study have been published [5]. In brief, patients were given either 250 mg of chlorothiazide or 25 mg of hydrochlorothiazide three times a day or a single tablet of methyldopa, 250 mg, with the same amount of thiazide three times a day. Three weeks later, the medications were switched. Blood for PRA was obtained after the patient had been supine for one hour and measured by a bioassay [6].

For the oxprenolol study, patients were put on 25 mg of hydrochlorothiazide twice a day for four weeks along with a placebo tablet resembling the oxprenolol. At the end of week 4, oxprenolol was started at a dose of 20 mg three times a day. The dose was raised weekly to 40 mg and then to 80 mg three times a day if the patients' standing diastolic blood pressure remained above 90 mm Hg. The medication was continued for four weeks.

Blood pressures were measured with a mercury manometer in the right arm after the patients were supine for five minutes and after two minutes upright posture. Blood for PRA was obtained after the patient was upright for 60 minutes and measured by a radioimmunoassay [7].

Results

Methyldopa

The addition of 250 mg of methyldopa to the thiazide diuretic significantly reduced the blood pressure (Fig. 1) and the PRA (Fig. 2). In those patients first given methyldopa plus diuretic (labeled as A + D in the figures), there was no change in blood pressure when methyldopa was stopped but the diuretic continued (labeled as D). However the PRA level, which had not risen with methyldopa plus diuretic (A + D), rose significantly when the diuretic alone was continued. Thus there is dissociation between the effects of these drugs on blood pressure and PRA.

Oxprenolol

The design of this study provided a more direct approach to the question of whether the renin-lowering effect of the drug was related to its antihypertensive action.

As shown in Table 1 and Figures 3 and 4, there was no relationship between the two effects. The drug significantly ($p < 0.02$) lowered the standing diastolic blood pressure from 104.0 mm Hg to 90.4 mm Hg, with ten of the 15 patients reaching a level of 90 mm Hg or lower. However, the mean PRA levels fell only insignificantly ($p > 0.1$) from 3.38 to 2.87 ng/ml/hr. The fall in blood pressure with the addition of oxprenolol was related neither to the initial pre-oxprenolol, post-diuretic PRA level (Fig. 3) nor to the change in PRA level after four weeks of oxprenolol therapy (Fig. 4).

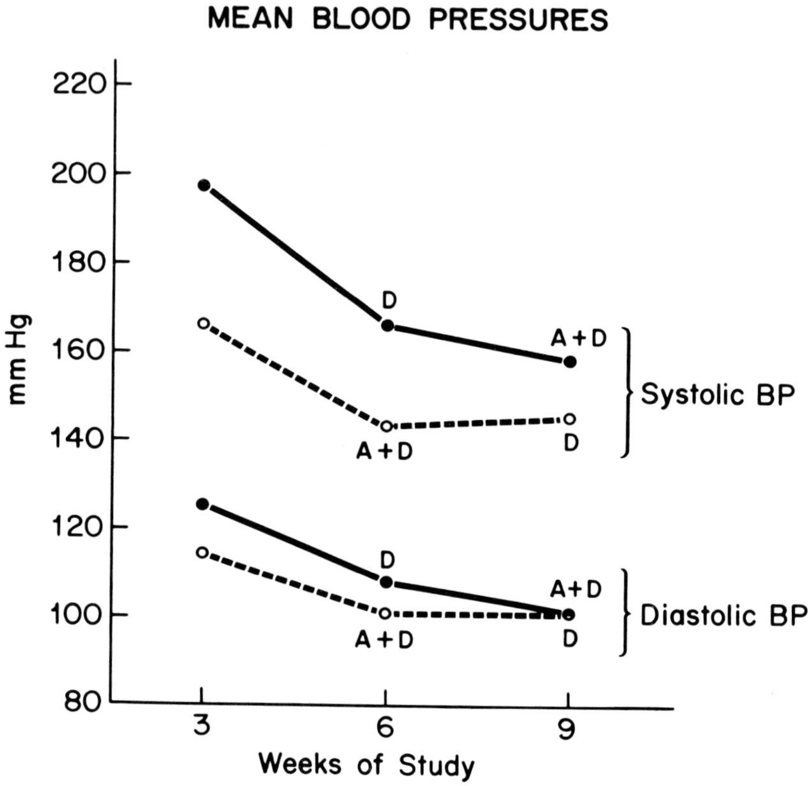

FIG. 1. The mean blood pressures of two groups of hypertensives at end of placebo period (week 3) and two periods of drug therapy (weeks 6 and 9). One group first received thiazide diuretic alone (D), the other first received alpha-methyldopa plus diuretic (A + D). After three weeks the medications were switched. (Reprinted with permission from Archives of Internal Medicine 135:660, 1975. Copyright 1975, American Medical Association.)

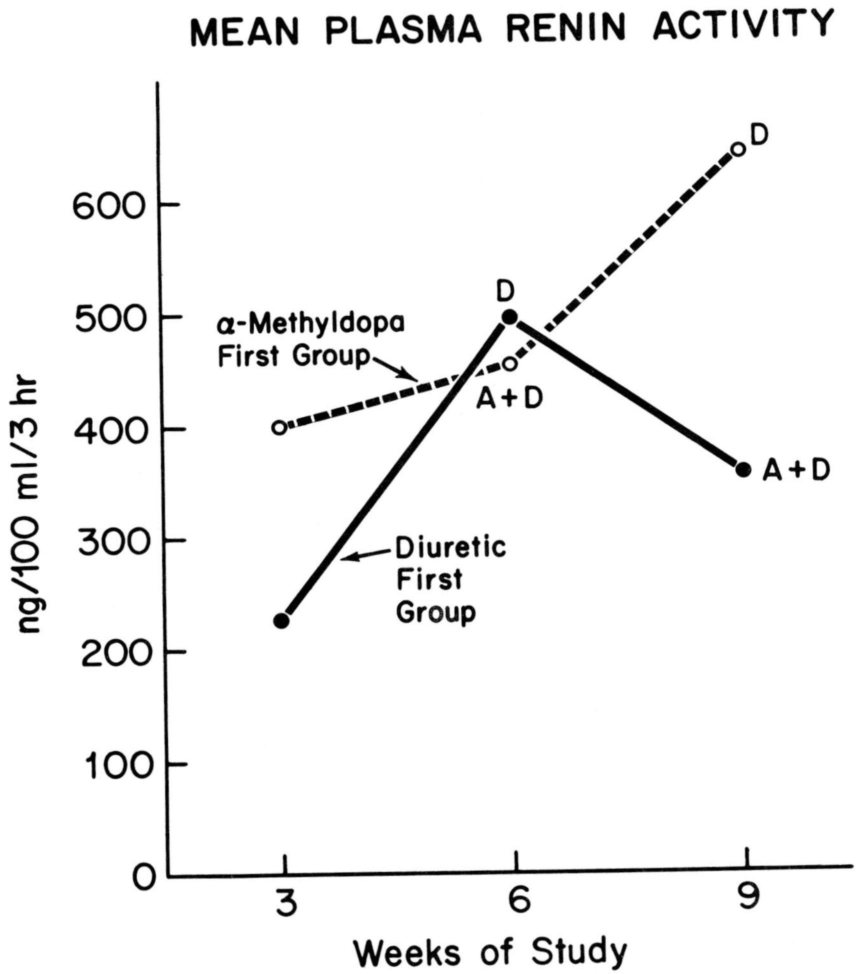

FIG. 2. The mean plasma renin activity (PRA) of the two groups of hypertensives shown in Figure 1 at end of placebo period (week 3) and two periods of drug therapy (weeks 6 and 9). (Reprinted with permission from Archives of Internal Medicine 135:660, 1975. Copyright 1975, American Medical Association.)

Table 1. Changes in Blood Pressure and PRA

Patient	Diastolic Blood Pressure (mm Hg) Diuretic Alone	Trasicor Plus Diuretic	60′ Upright PRA (ng/ml/hr) Diuretic Alone	Trasicor Plus Diuretic	Dose of Trasicor (mg)
1	111	85	2.9	1.9	120
2	101	88	0.5	0.8	60
3	108	83	1.8	2.2	120
4	102	91	1.3	1.9	240
5	101	87	1.6	1.6	240
6	102	94	3.4	4.0	240
7	118	119	0.2	0.1	240
8	102	90	6.3	6.1	60
9	100	84	5.3	5.7	120
10	103	88	1.1	0.5	120
11	97	74	6.0	5.8	60
12	103	104	5.3	2.9	240
13	101	84	1.0	1.1	60
14	111	107	0.9	0.5	240
15	100	78	13.1	7.9	60
Mean:	104.0	90.4	3.38	2.87	

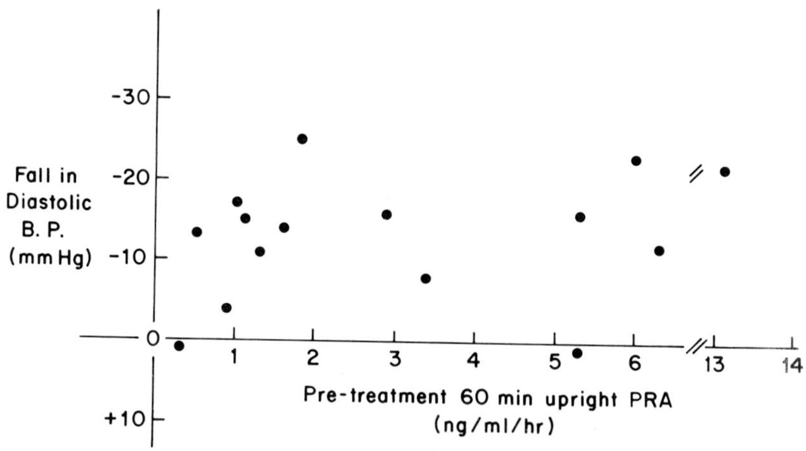

FIG. 3. The individual changes in diastolic blood pressure after four weeks of therapy with oxprenolol plus thiazide diuretic is plotted against the 60 minute upright plasma renin activity obtained prior to the addition of oxprenolol. There is no significant relationship between these variables.

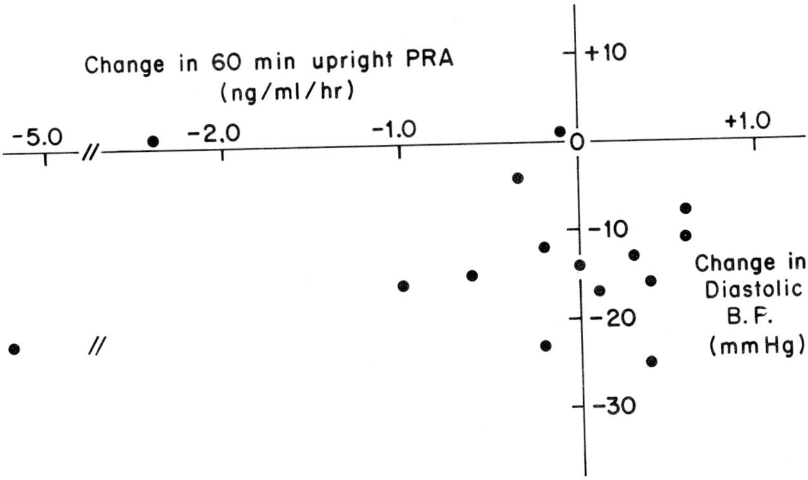

FIG. 4. The individual changes in diastolic blood pressure and 60 minute upright plasma renin activity in patients at the end of four weeks therapy with oxprenolol plus diuretic. There is no significant relationship between these variables.

Discussion

A relationship between the blood pressure-lowering effect of propranolol and its ability to lower PRA was found by Bühler et al [8]. A similar relationship for methyldopa was described by Weidmann et al [9]. These studies suggested that renin-lowering drugs would be effective only in patients with PRA levels that are high either naturally or induced by diuretic therapy. Further, they supported the concept that the choice of antihypertensive therapy should be based, at least in part, upon the patient's renin status.

Attractive as this concept is, the weight of published evidence and our own results suggest that it is wrong. The evidence against a relationship between renin-lowering and blood pressure-lowering effects includes the following:

1. Studies with methyldopa [10], clonidine [11], propranolol [12-17] and practolol [18] showing no relationship between the two effects. Generally, lowering of both renin and blood pressure has been observed but has not been related in degree or by time.

2. The finding that different beta-blockers have variable effects on blood pressure and PRA in experimental animals [19]. Some such as prindolol lower the blood pressure but raise the PRA.

3. The finding that in man, as well, prindolol lowers blood pressure but does not lower PRA [20].

4. Some have found that propranolol may reduce renin but not the blood pressure [21, 22].

5. Propranolol and other drugs which lower PRA are effective in lowering the blood pressure of many more hypertensives than the 15% to 20% who have high levels of PRA [23].

6. Numerous studies, not the least of which is the VA Cooperative Study [24], confirm the long-term effectiveness of drugs which raise PRA in controlling hypertension and preventing cardiovascular damage and death.

We conclude that the addition of a "renin-lowering" drug in the treatment of patients whose blood pressure is not adequately controlled by a diuretic alone is rational and usually effective. However, the second drug may be effective without lowering the renin. Therefore, the choice of antihypertensive drugs remains largely empiric. Clinicians need not be concerned about their patients' renin status in making the choice.

Summary

Two groups of patients with essential hypertension were first given a thiazide diuretic for three to four weeks. One group was then given methyldopa, the other oxprenolol. In both, the blood pressure fell further. With methyldopa the PRA level fell concomitantly but with oxprenolol it did not. We conclude that the blood pressure-lowering effect of antihypertensive drugs is not related to nor dependent upon their ability to lower plasma renin levels.

References

1. Kaplan N.M.: Therapy of hypertension. *In* Clinical Hypertension. Baltimore:Williams and Wilkins Press, 1973, pp. 97-157.
2. Brunner, H.R., Laragh, J.H., Baer, L. et al: Essential hypertension: Renin and aldosterone, heart attack and stroke. N. Engl. J. Med. 286:441-449, 1972.

3. Laragh, J.H., Baer, L., Brunner, H.R. et al: Renin, angiotensin and aldosterone system in pathogenesis and management of hypertensive vascular disease. Am. J. Med. 52:633-652, 1972.
4. Kaplan, N.M.: The prognostic implication of plasma renin in essential hypertension. JAMA 231:167-170, 1975.
5. Kaplan, N.M.: Antihypertensive drugs in combination. Arch. Intern. Med. 135:660-663, 1975.
6. Pickens, P.T., Bumpus, F.M., Lloyd, A.M. et al: Measurement of renin activity in human plasma. Circ. Res. 17:438-448, 1965.
7. Haber, E., Koerner, T., Page, L.B. et al: Application of a radioimmunoassay for angiotensin I to the physiologic measurements of plasma renin activity in normal human subjects. J. Clin. Endocrinol. Metab. 29:1349-1355, 1969.
8. Bühler, F.R., Laragh, J.H., Baer, L. et al: Propranolol inhibition of renin secretion: A specific approach to diagnosis and treatment of renin-dependent hypertensive diseases. N. Engl. J. Med. 287:1209-1214, 1972.
9. Weidmann, P., Hirsch, D., Maxwell, M.H. et al: Plasma renin and blood pressure during treatment with methyldopa. Am. J. Cardiol. 34:671-676, 1974.
10. Solheim, S.B., Sundsfjord, J.A. and Giezendanner, L.: The effect of spironolactone (Aldactone®) and methyldopa in low and normal renin hypertension. Acta. Med. Scand. 197:451-456, 1975.
11. Fyhrquist, F., Kurppa, K. and Huuskonen, M.: Plasma renin activity, blood pressure and sodium excretion during treatment with clonidine. Acta Med. Scand. 197:457-461, 1975.
12. Hansson, L.: Beta-adrenergic blockade in essential hypertension. Acta Med. Scand. 550:1-40, 1973.
13. Hansson, L. and Zweifler, A.J.: The effect of propranolol on plasma renin activity and blood pressure in mild essential hypertension. Acta Med. Scand. 195:397-401, 1974.
14. Bravo, E.L., Tarazi, R.C. and Dustan, H.P.: β-adrenergic blockade in diuretic-treated patients with essential hypertension. N. Engl. J. Med. 292:66-70, 1975.
15. Morgan, T.O., Roberts, R., Carney, S.L. et al: β-adrenergic receptor blocking drugs, hypertension and plasma renin. Br. J. Clin. Pharmacol. 2:159-164, 1975.
16. Geyskes, G.G., Boer, P., Vos, J. et al: Effect of salt depletion and propranolol on blood pressure and plasma renin activity in various forms of hypertension. Circ. Res. 23 (suppl 1):248-256, 1975.
17. Dorhout Mees, E.J., Geyskes, G.G., Vos, J. et al: Observations of the role of body fluid volumes and plasma renin activity in the management of hypertension. Arch. Int. Pharmacodyn. 214:335-346, 1975.
18. Esler, M.D.: Effect of practolol on blood pressure and renin release in man. Clin. Pharm. 15:484-489, 1974.
19. Weber, M.A., Stokes, G.S. and Gain, J.M.: Comparison of the effects on renin release of beta adrenergic antagonists with differing properties. J. Clin. Invest. 54:1413-1419, 1974.

20. Stokes, G.S., Weber, M.A. and Thornell, I.R.: β-blockers and plasma renin activity in hypertension. Br. Med. J. 1:60-62, 1974.
21. Michelakis, A.M. and McAllister, R.G.: The effect of chronic adrenergic receptor blockade on plasma renin activity in man. J. Clin. Endocrinol. Metab. 34:386-394, 1972.
22. Leonetti, G., Mayer, G., Morganti, A. et al: Hypotensive and renin-suppressing activities of propranolol in hypertensive patients. Clin. Sci. Molec. Med. 48:491-499, 1975.
23. Zacharias, J.F., Cowen, K.J., Prestt, J. et al: Propranolol in hypertension. A study of long-term therapy, 1964-1970. Am. Heart J. 83:755-761, 1972.
24. Veterans Administration Cooperative Study Group on Antihypertensive Agents: Effects of treatment on morbidity in hypertension. II. Results in patients with diastolic blood pressure averaging 90 through 114 mm Hg. JAMA 213:1143-1152, 1970.

Discussion

Moderator: Dr. J. Genest

Dr. Genest: Are there either any questions or comments for Dr. Kaplan? Dr. Kaplan, may I ask you a question? I think you have rehabilitated the furosemide test because a number of us who have done the furosemide test at the three or four hour interval, using either 40 or 60 mg IV, have some paradoxical responses. In our own series, which Dr. Guthrie has revised, 15 out of 60 patients have a decrease in PRA instead of the expected increase. Other people have found exactly the same thing. So your results with PRA measured 30 minutes after injection of furosemide may be the answer because of the rapid action of the furosemide. Would you comment on that?

Dr. Kaplan: The procedure we have used initially involved a more prolonged period after IV furosemide. The PRA levels after 60 minutes were slightly higher than at 30 minutes, but the 30 minute data provided just as good separation. In a few we continued drawing blood beyond one hour. The PRA generally fell beyond 60 minutes.

Dr. Zanchetti: We also have experience with the furosemide test and the upright test, both experimentally and clinically, and we certainly agree that the greatest stimulation to intravenous furosemide occurs very early and certainly at three hours it is already in the declining phase or exhausted. I also agree with Dr. Kaplan, that there is a rationale for combining furosemide and upright posture. Indeed, our experiments on cats have shown that both stimuli act by way of the renal innervation. So both are neural stimuli and combined together they are likely to give a stronger neural stimulus to the juxtaglomerular cells.

Dr. Stokes: Further to the same point, I would like to ask Dr. Kaplan this question: What is the within patient replication of this furosemide test? Using the original procedure described by Carey in Liddell's laboratory, we found the test impractical on an outpatient basis because of severe side effects. We subsequently lowered the dose to 80 mg orally and then found poor replication. We did our tests in duplicate on a series of patients and the overall replication was far worse than our assay reproducibility.

Dr. Kaplan: I shall let Dr. Hollifield comment on Dr. Carey's test. How much do you give?

Dr. Hollifield: We give 120 mg.

Dr. Kaplan: In our procedure using 40 mg of furosemide IV we have yet to see postural hypotension or other bothersome side effects. The reproducibility of the procedure is quite good with about a 10% variation in repeat tests.

Dr. Hollifield: Dr. Kaplan, everyone in this room defines low renin hypertension. The problem facing us is that everyone in this room defines it in a different way. I think that you should be able to tell us what the clinical implication is of your method of defining low renin essential hypertension, be it therapeutic or prognostic or whatever. That is my first question.

If I may make a comment about the Carey method of defining low renin essential hypertension, we have done some 400-500 *outpatient* stimulated renins. They have been done by a variety of investigators. Dr. Robert Carey, Dr. Janice Douglas, Dr. Steven Lowder, Dr. Paul Slaton and myself. We have yet to have a serious significant side effect from using 120 mg oral furosemide on an outpatient basis in otherwise healthy hypertensives who have not restricted salt or been on diuretics. We are very careful to use the test only in patients whom we know can tolerate it. We would not give a little old frail lady 120 mg of furosemide because you might predict that she would not make it. Similarly, if a patient has been volume depleted, by previous tests or by low salt diet, then you might also anticipate that they would have difficulty in tolerating the test. We have actually had myocardial infarctions, syncopy, transient cerebral ischemia occurring in patients who have been dehydrated by preparation for radiographic procedures or low salt diet.

That is my comment. Now can I ask you to answer my question?

Dr. Kaplan: We, of course, have no way of proving the validity of this procedure other than comparing it to other, more traditional techniques such as upright posture alone or following a period of salt deprivation. In a small group of patients with the classic low renin state, primary aldosteronism, the test has correctly shown the PRA to be suppressed.

Dr. Weinberger: I would like to speak to Dr. Hollifield's question about the utility of stimulatory maneuvers and assessment of renin status. A few months ago we presented data regarding an approach that we use for the evaluation of hypertensive patients referred to our Hypertension Center. This includes a saline infusion to evaluate suppressibility of the renin-aldosterone system, a stimulatory procedure for measurement of renin activity which utilizes 120 mg of furosemide orally in three divided doses in association with equivalent sodium intake and two hour upright posture the following day. In addition, the patients have renal arteriography. We have currently studied about 350 hypertensive patients using this approach. We have excluded from this population patients who were referred by their primary physician because of known or strongly suspected renal artery stenosis or primary aldosteronism. Thus, these patients are from all evidence from the referring physician and our initial outpatient evaluation essential hypertensives. Using this procedure, we have uncovered roughly 5% (about 18 cases) of unsuspected primary aldosteronism and about 15% of such patients have been found to have unsuspected renal artery stenosis. This is a lengthy roundabout way of responding to Dr. Hollifield's question. I think such a standardized procedure does have a great deal of validity in detecting potentially curable forms of hypertension.

A Crossover Comparison of the Effects of Metolazone and Hydrochlorothiazide Therapy on Blood Pressure and Renin Angiotensin System in Patients With Essential Hypertension

Mohinder P. Sambhi, M.D., Ph.D., Peter Eggena, Ph.D., Jack D. Barrett, Ph.D., Chalemphol Thananopavarn, M.D., Michael Tuck, M.D. and Charles Wiedeman, B.A.

Introduction

Metolazone* is a potent diuretic acting on both the proximal tubule and the cortical diluting segment of the nephron [1-3]. This quinethazone derivative (1,2,3,4-tetrahydro-4-quinazolinone) has been introduced recently as an antihypertensive agent administered once daily. Its antihypertensive potency has been reported to be equal to [4] or somewhat superior [5] to that of benzothiadiazine compounds with which it shares many of the common side effects. It has been suggested that the hyperglycemic effect of metolazone in experimental animals [6] and its kaluretic action in man [7] may be less marked than that of thiazides. The present study

---

Supported by Veterans Administration Research Grant 7697 and National Institutes of Health Grant 15039, and Research Grant from Pennwalt Corporation.

*Trade name Zaroxolyn ®; a trademark of Pennwalt Corporation, Pharmaceutical Division, Rochester, New York.

Mohinder P. Sambhi, M.D., Ph.D., Peter Eggena, Ph.D., Jack D. Barrett, Ph.D., Chalemphol Thananopavarn, M.D., Michael Tuck, M.D. and Charles Wiedeman, B.A., Hypertension Division, Department of Medicine, Veterans Administration Hospital, Sepulveda, Calif., and the Department of Medicine, University of California (Los Angeles) School of Medicine.

was designed with the following objectives: (1) To compare the antihypertensive potency of metolazone used as the sole agent administered once daily with that of hydrochlorothiazide given twice daily in selected patients with benign essential hypertension. (2) To study the alterations of the renin angiotensin system in response to acute and chronic administration of the two diuretic agents and relate these changes, if possible, to the antihypertensive response.

Methods

Clinical Methods

Thirty-three male subjects with a diagnosis of essential hypertension, ranging in age from 25 to 80 years, were selected from the outpatient clinics and the wards of Sepulveda Veterans Administration Hospital. Secondary causes for hypertension were systematically excluded by urinalysis, urine culture, serum creatinine, rapid sequence intravenous pyelography, serum and urinary electrolytes, plasma cortisol, chest x-ray, urinary metanephrines and a clinical history and physical examination. Patients with a previous history or existing evidence of target organ damage, except minor degrees of cardiomegaly and fundoscopic changes (less than grade 2), were excluded from the study. The patients had either not been previously treated for hypertension or discontinued medication for at least four weeks before entering the study. The patients were followed in a special outpatient clinic and were on an unselected diet. During each visit, the patients were weighed and blood pressure was recorded in sitting, standing and recumbent positions. Twenty-four-hour urinary samples were analyzed for total volume, electrolytes and creatinine. Blood samples were taken for measurements of the parameters of the renin angiotensin system as outlined below. Oral potassium supplements were prescribed routinely.

Protocol of Study

The patients were studied following a four-week period of no medication (control period). Diuretics were started at this time (metolazone 5 mg qd or hydrochlorothiazide 50 mg bid) and the patients returned at one week for acute studies and subsequently at one, two and three months for chronic studies. Following three to four months of therapy, the initial diuretic was discontinued and one month was allowed as a washout period. Patients were then crossed over to the other diuretic and studied at the same time periods for another three to four months.

Nineteen patients (group I) completed the first crossover study starting first with hydrochlorothiazide (HCT) and later crossing over to metolazone (MET). Group II included 14 patients that started with MET first and were later crossed over to HCT.

Laboratory Methods

Plasma renin activity (PRA ng/ml/hr) and plasma renin substrate (PRS ng/ml) were measured by radioimmunoassay of generated angiotensin I [8]. Circulating levels of angiotensin I and II in blood were measured simultaneously by a method using saline extraction of whole blood followed by radioimmunoassay [9]. Plasma renin reactivity (PRS_R) was studied according to previously described methods [10]. A short-term incubation (20 minutes) of plasma with added renin (PRS_R 20) is used as an estimation of angiotensin generation rate. Longer incubation (180 minutes) under the same conditions is a measure of total consumable renin substrate (PRS). Plasma renin-substrate reactivity is defined as a ratio of PRS_R 20 to PRS and expressed as a percent index. In group II patients, all parameters of the renin angiotensin system were measured in all patients. In group I patients, circulating levels of angiotensin peptides and the indices of renin reactivity were not measured in all patients. Statistical treatment on all data was done by paired analysis of all parameters using the t test.

Results

Control blood pressures in the two groups of patients are listed in Table 1. The fall in systolic and diastolic blood pressure in group I and group II patients during the crossover treatment periods with the two diuretics is shown in Figures 1 and 2. The

Table 1. Control Blood Pressures* After a Four-Week Period of No Medication

		Sitting	*Standing*	*Recumbent*
Group I	Systolic	157 ± 13.8	164 ± 10.9	160 ± 17.3
	Diastolic	104 ± 11.4	111 ± 8.6	103 ± 10.6
Group II	Systolic	152 ± 13.7	160 ± 15.8	153 ± 14.0
	Diastolic	97 ± 5.4	106 ± 12.8	100 ± 9.5

*Blood pressures mm Hg ± S.D. Group I (HCT → MET) Group II (MET → HCT)

drop in both systolic and diastolic blood pressures is less marked with HCT, especially in group II patients. Differences in the blood pressure lowering effects of the two agents become more apparent when changes in diastolic blood pressure are compared (Fig. 2). Metolazone therapy during both crossover periods resulted in a significant drop (indicated by asterisks) during all time periods in diastolic blood pressure recorded in all positions: sitting, standing and recumbent (Fig. 2). In contrast, the drop in diastolic blood pressure was sporadic during hydrochlorothiazide treatment. In group I patients on HCT, the drop in diastolic blood pressure at 14 weeks did not achieve statistical significance in sitting, standing or recumbent positions. In group II patients, recumbent diastolic pressures did not change significantly during the entire period of treatment with HCT.

Significant drops in body weight were observed at one week of diuretic therapy in all patients except in group II patients on HCT treatment (Fig. 3). During chronic treatment, body weight returned toward control values in all patients except in the group II patients at 14 weeks of HCT treatment, at which time a significant decline in body weight was observed. Serum creatinine did not change in both groups of patients during the entire treatment period with either of the two diuretics except at 14 weeks in group II patients on hydrochlorothiazide. The rise in serum creatinine in this group was very mild albeit highly significant (1.07 ± 0.2 during control period to 1.18 ± 0.27 mg% at 14 weeks, $n = 12$, $p < 0.01$). This rise in serum creatinine coupled with a significant drop in body weight (Fig.

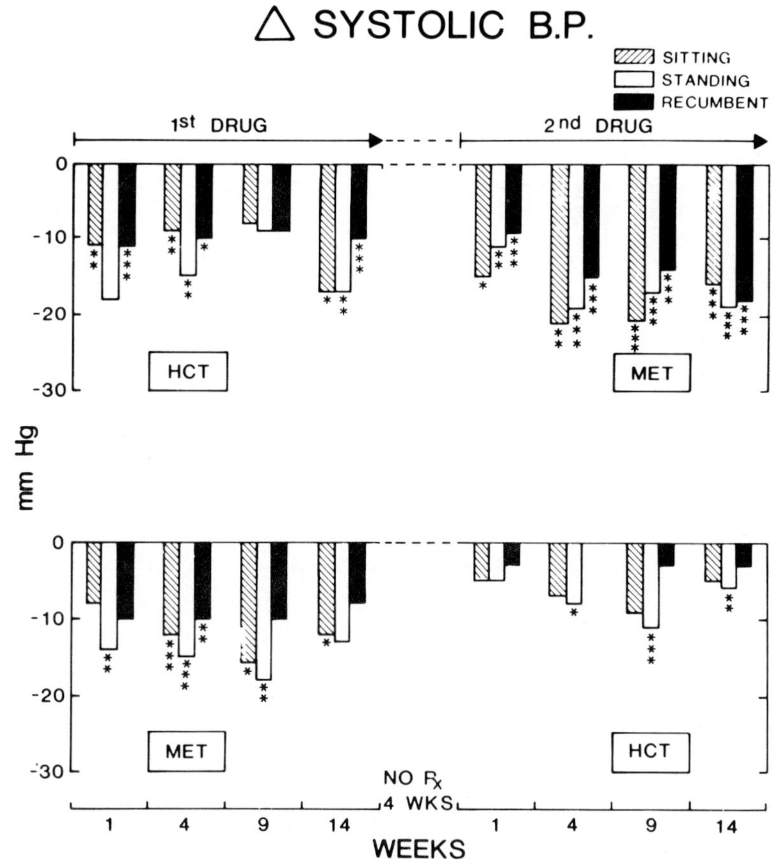

FIG. 1. Change in systolic blood pressure from control value (mm Hg) vs. treatment in the sitting, standing and recumbent position. HCT→MET (n = 14-17), MET→HCT (n = 10-12); * $p < 0.05$, ** $0.025 < p < 0.01$, *** $0.005 < p < 0.001$.

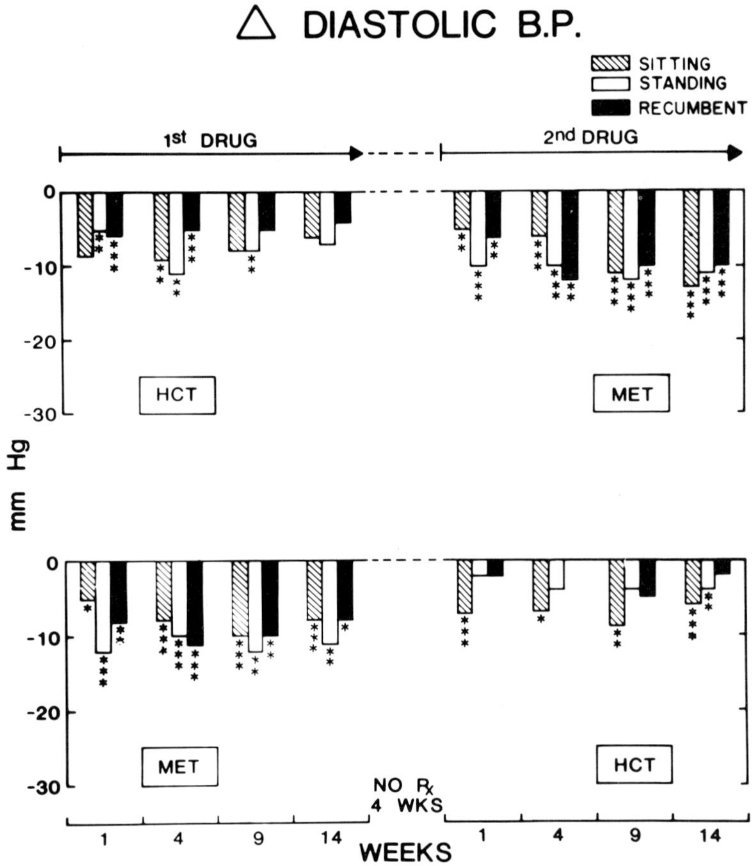

FIG. 2. Change in diastolic blood pressure from control values (mm Hg) vs. duration of treatment (weeks) in the sitting, standing and recumbent position. HCT→MET (n = 14-17), MET→HCT (n = 10-12); *p < 0.05, ** 0.025 < p < 0.01, *** 0.005 < p < 0.001.

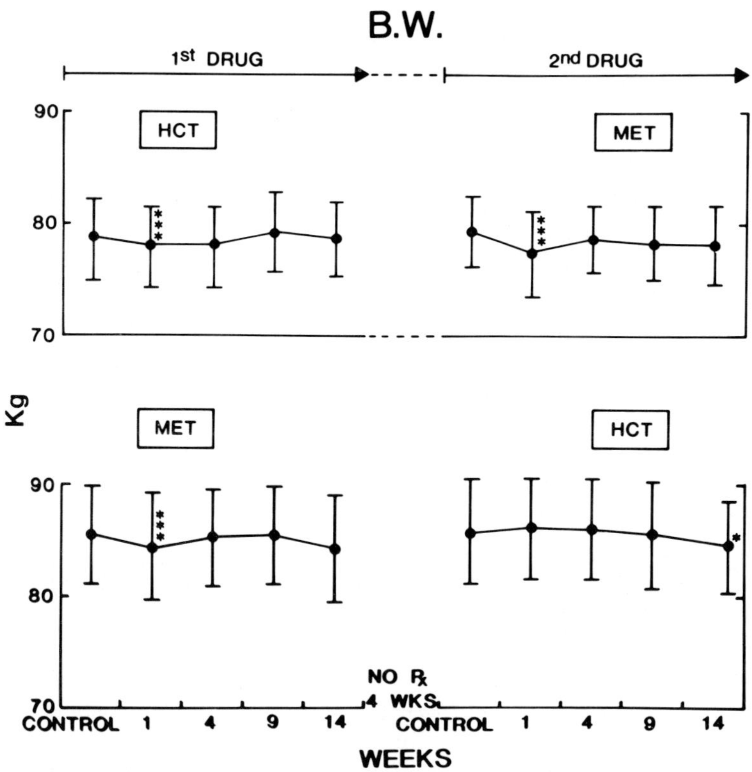

FIG. 3. Body weight in Kg ± S. E. vs. duration of diuretic therapy. HCT→MET (n = 9) MET→HCT (n = 14); * $p < 0.05$, *** $0.005 < p < 0.001$. Significant reductions in body weight are obtained with both diuretics only during the first week of therapy with the exception of thiazide given as the second drug. In that case a significant reduction is obtained after 14 weeks.

3) in the same patients supports the possibility that a chronic contraction of intravascular volume was maintained in these subjects. Blood glucose showed insignificant changes except at 14 weeks on metolazone in group II patients where the elevation of blood glucose was significant (114.5 ± 30.7 vs. 147.8 ± 60.8 mg% – $p < 0.05$ – $n = 12$).

Changes in urinary sodium and potassium and serum potassium during the treatment periods with the two diuretics in the two groups are shown in Tables 2 and 3. Serum potassium showed a significant decline during metolazone therapy in both groups of patients at all time periods except at nine weeks (Table 2). During hydrochlorothiazide treatment, changes in serum potassium were not significant except at four weeks in group II patients (Table 3). Changes in urinary potassium were similar with the two diuretic agents, but differed in the two crossover groups. Enhanced kaluresis of a significant degree was maintained through the entire period of study in group I patients during metolazone therapy. In group II patients, urinary excretion of potassium increased initially but had returned toward control values at 9 and 14 weeks of treatment with both drugs. Urinary sodium did not differ significantly from control levels in any group at any time period.

PRA values during control and treatment periods with both diuretics in group I and II patients are shown in Figure 4. Metolazone treatment in both groups caused a relatively greater rise in PRA that remained significantly elevated above control values at 14 weeks. In contrast during thiazide treatment, significant elevations of PRA were observed only at nine weeks in group I patients. At 14 weeks of HCT treatment, PRA in both groups declined and did not differ from control values.

Plasma renin substrate showed small and inconsistent increases during treatment with both diuretics that achieved significance only in group I patients at 14 weeks of HCT therapy (Fig. 5). PRS_R index showed a significant decline in group I patients only at 14 weeks of metolazone therapy (Fig. 6). Changes in circulating levels of angiotensin I (A I) and angiotensin II (A II) in patients of group I and II are listed in Tables 4 and 5. A I did not increase significantly during the acute administration of either diuretic in either group of

Table 2. Serum Potassium and Urinary Electrolytes During Metolazone Therapy

		Group I (HCT → MET)				*Group II (MET → HCT)*			
		Cont.	*(n)*	*MET*	*p*	*Cont.*	*(n)*	*MET*	*p*
Serum K	1 wk.	4.2 ± 0.3	(8)	3.4 ± 0.6	< 0.001	4.4 ± 0.3	(13)	3.7 ± 0.7	< 0.001
	4 wk.	4.1 ± 0.4	(7)	3.4 ± 0.3	< 0.001	4.4 ± 0.3	(12)	3.7 ± 0.9	< 0.05
	9 wk.	4.1 ± 0.3	(9)	3.7 ± 0.7	< 0.1	4.4 ± 0.2	(11)	3.9 ± 0.7	< 0.1
	14 wk.	4.1 ± 0.3	(9)	3.6 ± 0.5	< 0.005	4.4 ± 0.3	(13)	3.7 ± 0.7	< 0.005
Uk meq/V	1 wk.	49.8 ± 25.2	(8)	96.4 ± 54.2	< 0.025	67.9 ± 25.2	(13)	91.6 ± 25.7	< 0.005
	4 wk.	53.6 ± 27.2	(7)	88.4 ± 55.8	< 0.05	73.0 ± 23.8	(11)	80.9 ± 18.3	< 0.4
	9 wk.	52.7 ± 25.2	(9)	78.0 ± 34.8	< 0.025	68.1 ± 27.5	(11)	76.5 ± 28.8	< 0.5
	14 wk.	52.7 ± 25.2	(9)	91.2 ± 37.5	< 0.01	67.9 ± 25.2	(13)	73.4 ± 24.6	< 0.5
Una Meq/V	1 wk.	136.0 ± 20.0	(7)	145.0 ± 19.0	> 0.5	181.0 ± 20.0	(11)	198.0 ± 18.0	< 0.4
	4 wk.	153.0 ± 18.0	(8)	172.0 ± 21.0	> 0.1	166.0 ± 20.0	(12)	194.0 ± 18.0	< 0.4
	9 wk.	153.0 ± 18.0	(8)	189.0 ± 28.0	> 0.2	164.0 ± 18.0	(14)	167.0 ± 21.0	< 0.5
	14 wk.	153.0 ± 18.0	(8)	174.0 ± 15.0	> 0.1	166.0 ± 19.0	(13)	182.0 ± 34.0	< 0.5

Table 3. Serum Potassium and Urinary Electrolytes During Hydrochlorothiazide Therapy

		Group I (HCT → MET)				Group II (MET → HCT)			
		Cont.	*(n)*	*HCT*	*p*	*Cont.*	*(n)*	*HCT*	*p*
Serum K	1 wk.	3.9 ± 0.5	(9)	3.6 ± 0.4	< 0.1	4.1 ± 0.6	(11)	3.8 ± 0.6	< 0.4
	4 wk.	3.9 ± 0.5	(9)	3.6 ± 0.4	> 0.5	4.1 ± 0.5	(12)	3.7 ± 0.7	< 0.05
	9 wk.	3.9 ± 0.5	(9)	3.7 ± 0.4	< 0.2	4.1 ± 0.5	(12)	3.9 ± 0.6	< 0.04
	14 wk.	3.9 ± 0.5	(9)	3.7 ± 0.4	< 0.2	4.1 ± 0.5	(13)	4.0 ± 0.5	> 0.5
Uk	1 wk.	58.7 ± 33.2	(9)	88.1 ± 34.9	< 0.005	51.7 ± 22.5	(11)	83.9 ± 34.0	< 0.005
	4 wk.	58.7 ± 33.2	(9)	80.7 ± 31.4	< 0.05	52.9 ± 21.4	(12)	75.0 ± 31.1	< 0.05
	9 wk.	58.7 ± 33.2	(9)	82.1 ± 45.0	< 0.025	52.9 ± 21.4	(12)	66.4 ± 26.2	< 0.1
	14 wk.	58.7 ± 33.2	(9)	75.7 ± 31.3	< 0.1	52.2 ± 20.6	(13)	59.3 ± 32.1	< 0.5
Una	1 wk.	135.0 ± 30.0	(7)	143.0 ± 36.0	> 0.5	180.0 ± 29.0	(11)	201.0 ± 35.0	< 0.4
	4 wk.	153.0 ± 32.0	(8)	141.0 ± 16.0	> 0.5	177.0 ± 26.0	(12)	184.0 ± 28.0	> 0.5
	9 wk.	153.0 ± 32.0	(8)	174.0 ± 29.0	< 0.4	171.0 ± 24.0	(14)	222.0 ± 24.0	> 0.1
	14 wk.	153.0 ± 32.0	(8)	208.0 ± 28.0	< 0.2	171.0 ± 28.0	(13)	183.0 ± 28.0	< 0.5

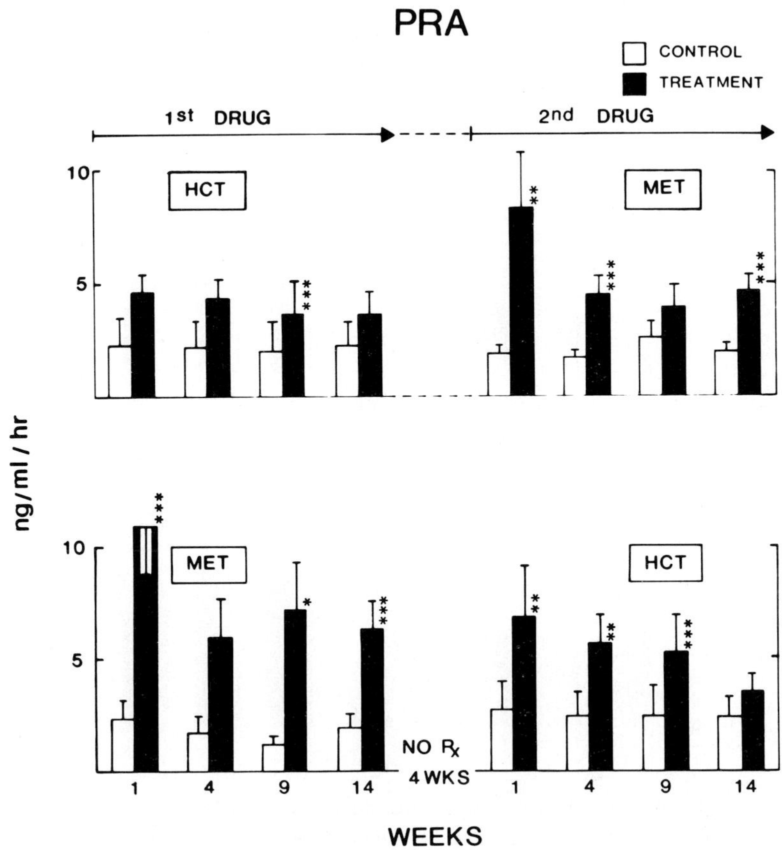

FIG. 4. Plasma renin activity (ng/ml/hr) vs. duration of treatment (weeks). HCT→MET (n = 12-14) MET→HCT (n = 8-12); * $p < 0.05$, ** $0.025 < p < 0.01$, *** $0.005 < p < 0.001$. Both diuretics increase PRA, but the increase on metolazone is much more pronounced, especially after the first week of therapy.

patients. Changes in A I were also insignificant during the chronic period of diuretic administration except at 14 weeks of hydrochlorothiazide administration in group I patients (Table 4). A II, on the other hand, was significantly elevated in group II patients during the acute period of diuretic administration (Table 5). After 14 weeks of treatment with both drugs, however, the circulating levels of A II were not significantly

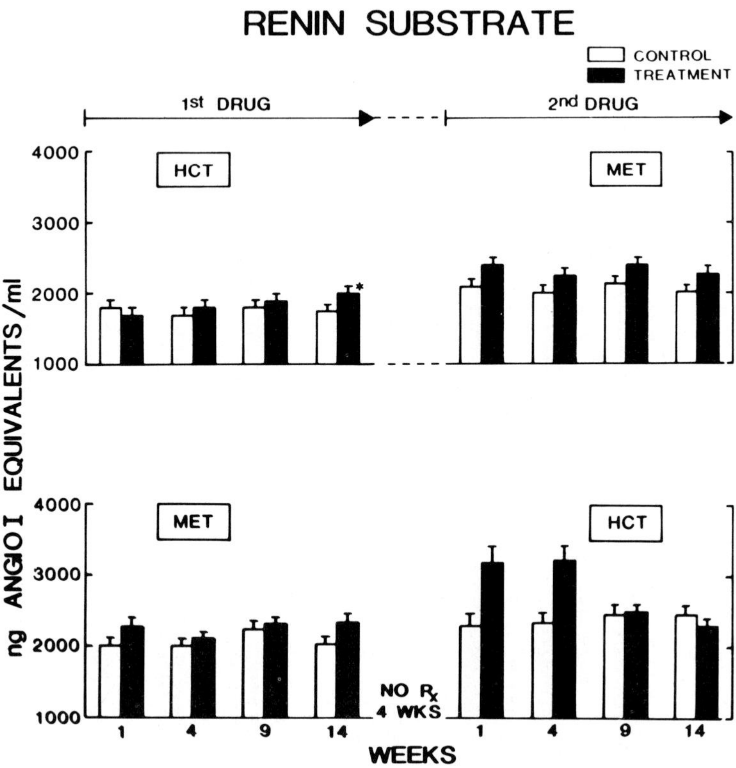

FIG. 5. Renin substrate levels (ng angiotensin I equivalents/ml) vs. duration of diuretic therapy (weeks) HCT→MET (n = 10-15); MET→HCT (n = 7-10); * $p < 0.05$. There is no significant change in renin substrate on either drug with the exception of thiazide treatment (14 weeks) where a small but significant rise in renin substrate levels is observed.

different from control values (Tables 4 and 5). A close scrutiny of the data on the circulating levels of angiotensin further indicates that the stimulation resulting from chronic administration of the two diuretic agents is dependent more upon whether it was the first drug in the crossover than the particular diuretic metolazone or hydrochlorothiazide. Figure 7 compares the circulating levels of angiotensin I and II during the control period with the average of chronic periods (4, 9 and 14 weeks) of diuretic administration. It appears that the first diuretic agent of each crossover segment leads to a greater degree of

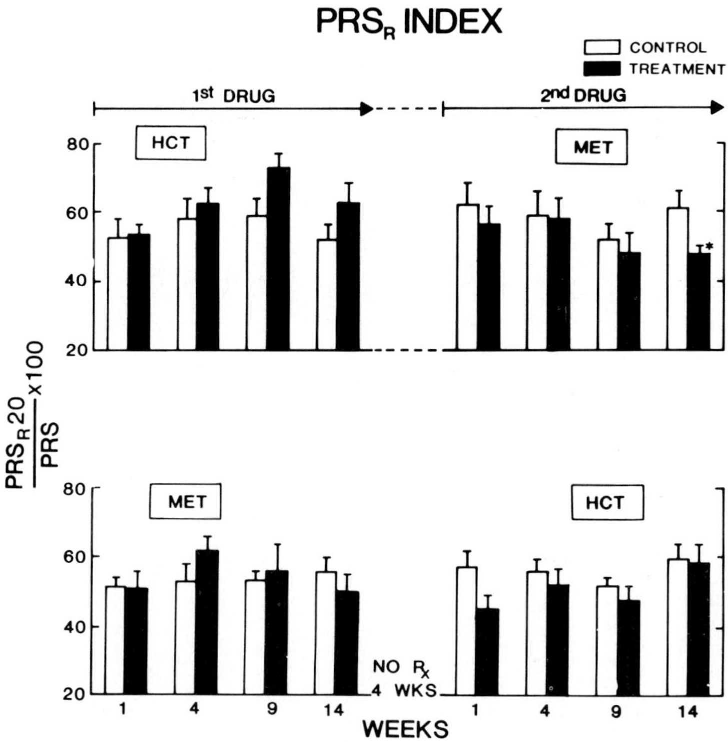

FIG. 6. Plasma renin substrate reactivity (PRS$_R$) index (PRS$_R$ 20/PRS x 100) vs. duration of therapy (weeks). In the top panel the first drug is thiazide, in the lower panel metolazone. HCT→MET (n = 8-13); MET→HCT (n = 6-9); * $p < 0.05$. PRS$_R$ index is not influenced by drug therapy except on metolazone at 14 weeks, where a significant decrease in PRS$_R$ index is observed.

stimulation of circulating angiotensin. At 14 weeks and during the washout period, angiotensin levels statistically do not differ from the control values. The administration of the second diuretic agent in each crossover, on the other hand, does not result in chronic elevations of circulating levels. On the contrary, a tendency toward decline is observed (Fig. 7).

Figure 8 summarizes the changes from control in diastolic blood pressure and in the measured parameters of renin angiotensin system at 14 weeks of treatment with the two diuretics.

Table 4. Circulating Levels of Angiotensin (A I and A II) in Group I Patients (HCT → MET)

	Control	*HCT Rx Weeks*				*Control*	*MET Rx Weeks*			
		1	*4*	*9*	*14*		*1*	*4*	*9*	*14*
AI pg/ml ± S.D.	72 ± 48	93 ± 48	89 ± 42	105 ± 48	113 ± 50	336 ± 375	117 ± 46	107 ± 67	100 ± 49	87 ± 61
(n)		7*	8	8	8		7**	8	8	8
p		> 0.5	< 0.4	< 0.2	< 0.05		< 0.2	< 0.1	< 0.2	< 0.2
	(Control value for * was 79 ± 47)					(Control for ** 370 ± 391)				
AII pg/ml ± S.D.	4 ± 7	20 ± 29	42 ± 73	43 ± 49	10 ± 8	72 ± 135	116 ± 46	12 ± 8	6 ± 3	8 ± 5
(n)		7*	8	8	8		7**	8	8	8
p		< 0.1	< 0.2	< 0.05	< 0.2		> 0.5	< 0.4	< 0.4	< 0.4
	(Controls for * 5 ± 7)					(Control for ** 78 ± 145)				

Table 5. Circulating Levels of Angiotensin (A I and A II) in Group II Patients (MET → HCT)

	Control	*MET Rx Weeks*				*Control*	*HCT Rx Weeks*			
		1	*4*	*9*	*14*		*1*	*4*	*9*	*14*
AI pg/ml ±S.D.	90 ± 157	188 ± 184	130 ± 103	98 ± 104	89 ± 63	153 ± 197	90 ± 77	88 ± 55	84 ± 55	72 ± 60
(n)		10	10	9*	12**		10	10	9*	12**
p		< 0.4	> 0.5	< 0.4	> 0.5		< 0.4	< 0.4	< 0.4	< 0.4
	Control for	* 52 ± 47 ** 86 ± 145				Control for	* 166 ± 205 ** 143 ± 180			
AII pg/ml ± S.D.	7 ± 9	39 ± 53	34 ± 22	6 ± 5	19 ± 19	14 ± 21	23 ± 32	5 ± 5	8 ± 7	6 ± 4
(n)		10	10	9*	11**		10	10	9*	11**
p		< 0.05	< 0.005	< 0.2	< 0.1		> .05	< 0.4	< 0.4	< 0.4
	Control for	* 4 ± 6 ** 6 ± 8				Control for	* 13 ± 22 **13 ± 20			

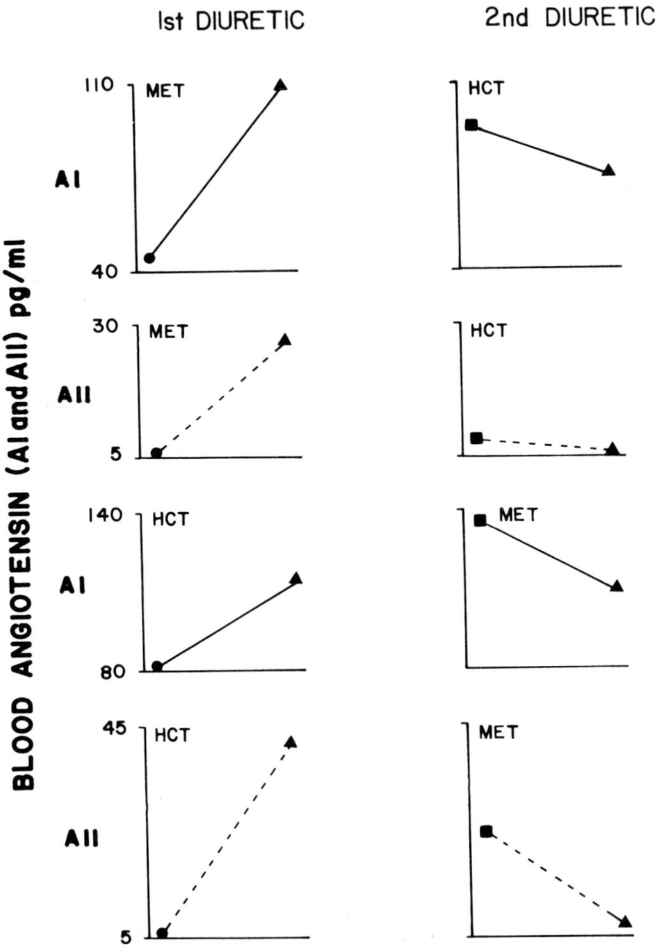

FIG. 7. Comparison of changes in circulating levels of blood angiotensin I (A I) and angiotensin II (A II) in response to chronic therapy with either metolazone or hydrochlorothiazide considered as the first or the second diuretic to be used in the sequence of crossover study design. Blood levels of the two angiotensin peptides are shown: during the initial no medication control period (●), during the control period before the administration of the second diuretic following a four-week washout period (■) and during the chronic period of diuretic therapy, as an average figure of values measured at 4, 9 and 14 weeks of treatment (▲).

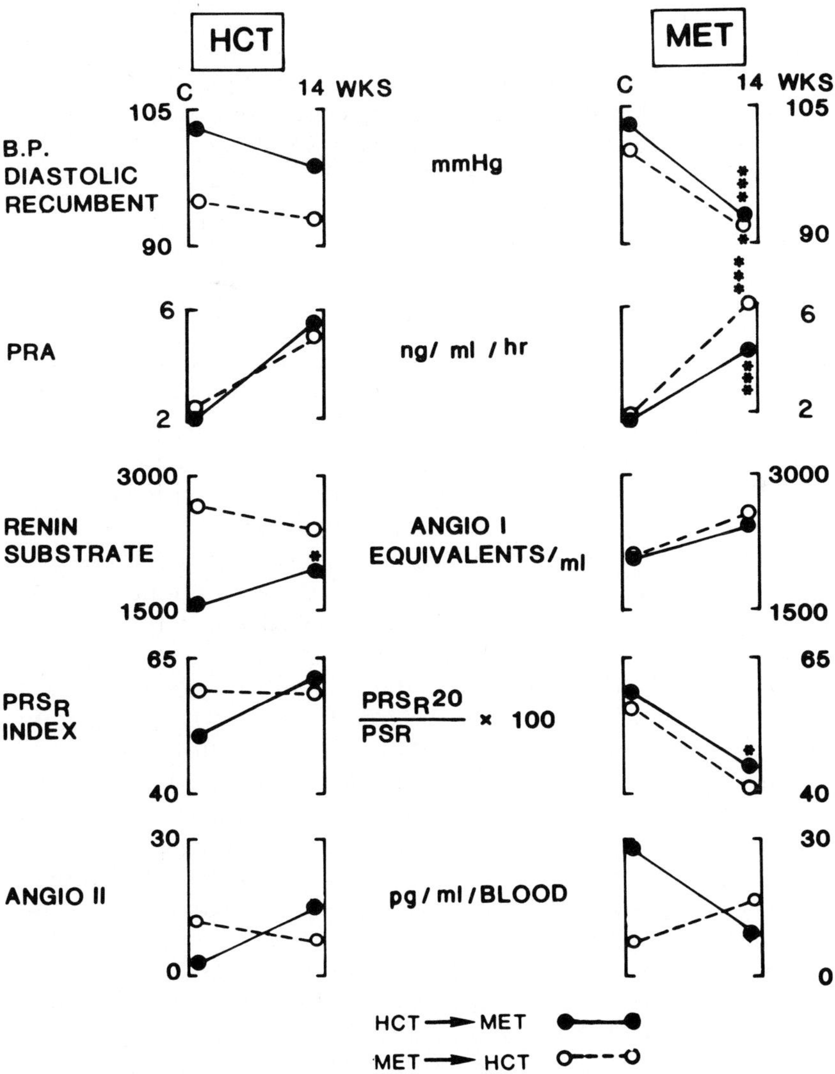

FIG. 8. Comparison of mean changes in recumbent diastolic blood pressure and the measured parameters of the renin angiotensin system at 14 weeks of therapy with hydrochlorothiazide (HCT) and metolazone (MET) in the two crossover groups. The asterisks indicate the level of the statistical significance of the difference from the control values, same as Figure 4.

Discussion

The results of this crossover study indicate clearly that metolazone 5 mg once daily is a significantly more effective antihypertensive agent than hydrochlorothiazide 50 mg twice a day. Reasons for the greater potency of antihypertensive action are entirely obscure and are not elucidated by the present study. Certain observations from these data, however, are noteworthy. A greater fall in body weight or a greater degree of sustained natriuresis was not the basis for the more potent antihypertensive action of metolazone as compared with hydrochlorothiazide. Urinary sodium excretion did not differ significantly from control values during treatment with the two diuretic agents. The significant fall in body weight and a mild albeit significant elevation of serum creatinine were observed in one group of patients only during treatment with hydrochlorothiazide. These observations support the probable existence of a continued contraction of intravascular volume that has been implicated as one of the major mechanisms of long-term antihypertensive action of benzothiadiazine compounds [11]. It is probable, therefore, that additional mechanisms are utilized by metolazone for its antihypertensive action.

The results of this study did not support the suggestions that the hyperglycemic and kaluretic actions of metolazone used as an antihypertensive agent in man are less marked as compared with those of hydrochlorothiazide; lowering of serum K of significant degree, on the other hand, was observed only with metolazone. The lowering of serum potassium, however, did not correlate either with the fall in blood pressure or in the rise in PRA secondary to the administration of metolazone.

It has been suggested that the diuretic-induced stimulation of PRA limits the full antihypertensive potential of diuretic agents and contributes toward the development of partial tolerance of their long-term antihypertensive action [12]. This hypothesis, however, does not derive support from the results of the present crossover study on blood pressure and PRA, since the higher and more significant elevation of PRA along with a greater and more significant fall in blood pressure was maintained during metolazone therapy as compared with hydrochlorothiazide. The reported failure of propranolol to suppress the diuretic-stimulated PRA in patients with essential hypertension and yet cause a further lowering of blood pressure in these subjects further mitigates the importance of stimulated PRA in opposing the antihypertensive action of diuretic agents [13, 14].

Elevations of circulating angiotensin levels during the initial treatment periods and their return toward control in the chronic period of therapy is consistent with previous findings, our own [14] and of others [15]. The results of the present study do not bring out any differences in the circulating levels of angiotensin in response to the two diuretic agents. However, more data are required to be decisive. The observation that the effects on circulating angiotensin I and II, of the first diuretic of either crossover study, are different from the second diuretic agent requires confirmation. It is possible that complete normalization is not achieved during the four-week washout period. Longer washout periods, however, are impractical in this type of study design.

The possible significance of changes in renin reactivity following metolazone therapy has been discussed previously and supports our earlier findings [10]. A decline in renin reactivity, coupled with a decline of blood angiotensin levels, may indicate an overall reduction of the activity of the renin angiotensin system and certainly does not support the notion that the renin angiotensin system is overactive during chronic metolazone therapy despite significant and sustained elevations of PRA. The question, however, of whether alterations in renin angiotensin system caused by long-term diuretic administration, particularly metolazone, are related to and contribute to the mechanisms of its antihypertensive action must remain unanswered until more data are available.

In order to explore the possible identifiable reasons for differences in blood pressure response to the two diuretics, changes in the recumbent diastolic blood pressure were examined in the individual patients as shown in Figure 9. The lack of antihypertensive response is indicated by interrupted lines and it is apparent that approximately 50% of the patients on hydrochlorothiazides in both groups did not achieve an antihypertensive response and the overall change in blood pressure in both groups was insignificant ($p > 0.4$). In contrast, the

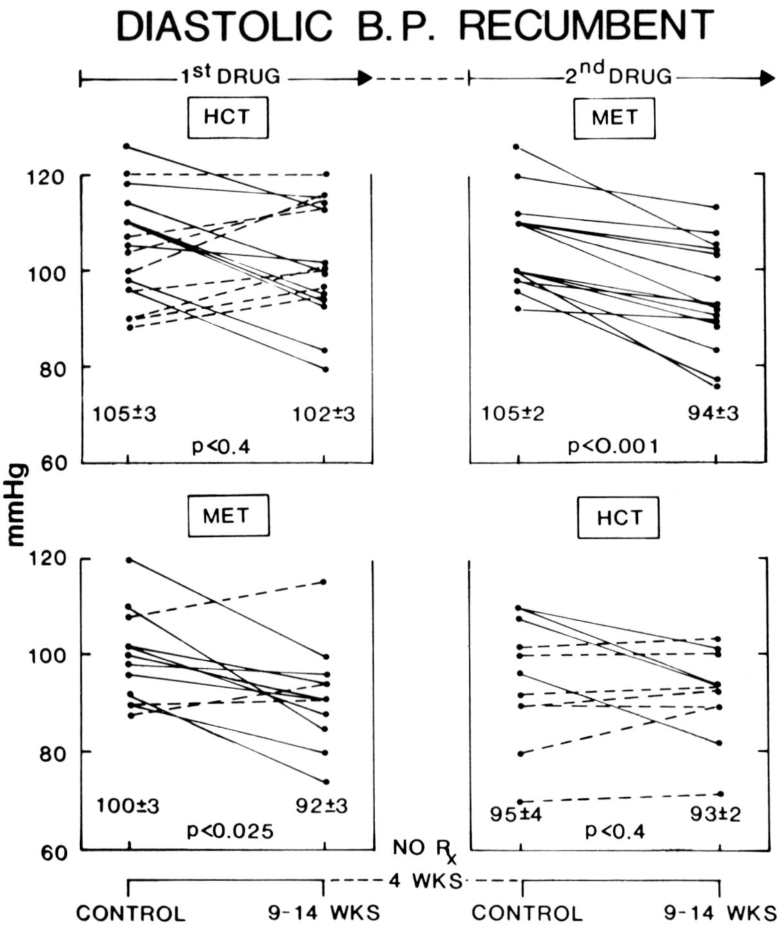

FIG. 9. Diastolic blood pressure in the recumbent position (mm Hg) during control period and following treatment (average of 9 and 14 week data). HCT → MET (n = 15 to 17), MET → HCT (n = 9 to 12). Solid line —— indicates patients who responded but interrupted line — — — represents patients who did not respond to therapy on either diuretic. The data demonstrate that metolazone either as a first or second drug is more effective than hydrochlorothiazide in lowering the diastolic recumbent blood pressure.

majority of the same patients receiving metolazone in both groups respond with a significant drop in blood pressure (group I, $p < 0.001$ and group II, $p < 0.025$).

All patients who did not respond to hydrochlorothiazide in both group I and II were classified as "thiazide nonresponders" (Fig. 10). In these subjects at one and nine weeks of therapy, there was actually a significant increase in recumbent diastolic

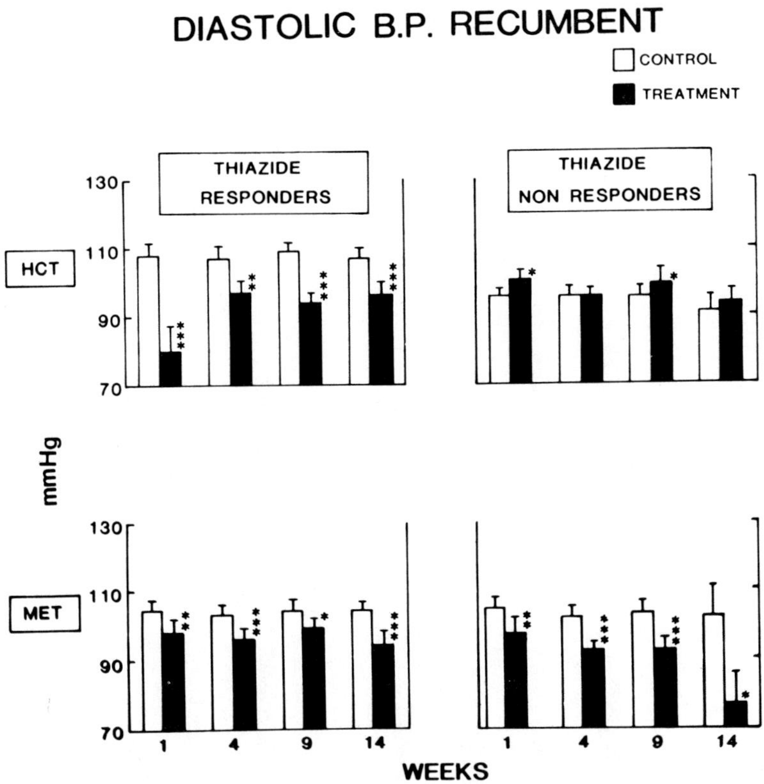

FIG. 10. Recumbent diastolic BP (mm Hg) vs. duration of drug treatment. Patients were divided into two groups, those responding to thiazide treatment (n = 11-13) and those who do not (n = 11-15). For comparison, the same patients on metolazone are also given; * $p < 0.005$, ** $0.025 < p < 0.01$, *** $0.005 < p < 0.001$. The data indicate that only about 50% of the patients respond to thiazide therapy; diastolic blood pressure is lowered in all patients given comparable doses of metolazone.

blood pressure (Fig. 10). On the other hand, patients showing a good antihypertensive response to hydrochlorothiazide in both groups were accordingly classified as "thiazide responders." For comparison, Figure 10 also shows that the highly significant antihypertensive response to metolazone is equally distributed among the thiazide responders as well as nonresponders. No differences were identified in the thiazide nonresponders compared to the responders with respect to changes in body weight, serum potassium, or urinary sodium and potassium. Changes in PRA and plasma renin substrate are shown in these patients in Figures 11 and 12. Thiazide responders had

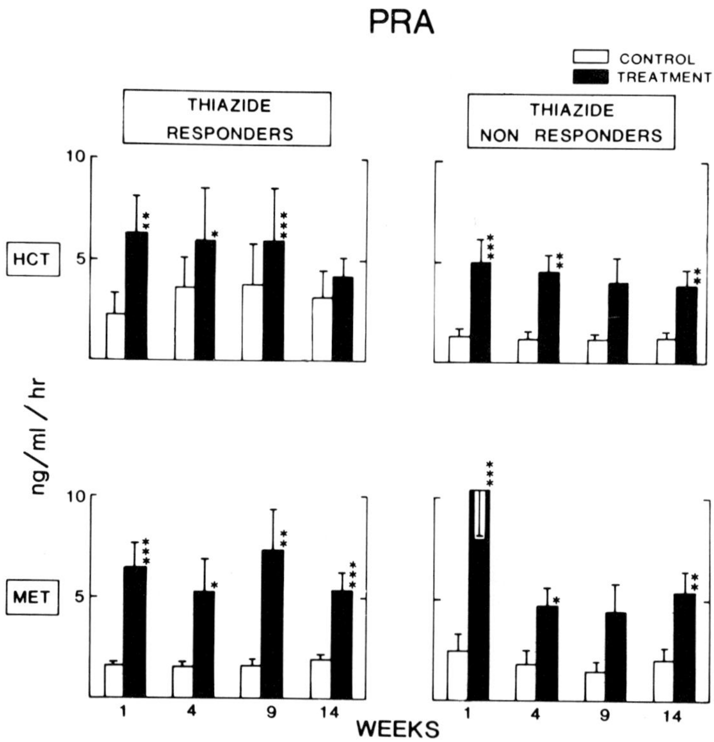

FIG. 11. PRA (ng/ml/hr) vs. duration of treatment (weeks). Thiazide responders (n = 9-14), nonresponders (n = 9-13). The same patients on metolazone treatment are shown in lower panel; * $p < 0.05$, ** $0.025 < p < 0.01$, *** $0.005 < p < 0.001$. Stimulation of PRA at one week of metolazone therapy in nonresponders (thiazide) appears more marked than in the group of responding thiazide patients.

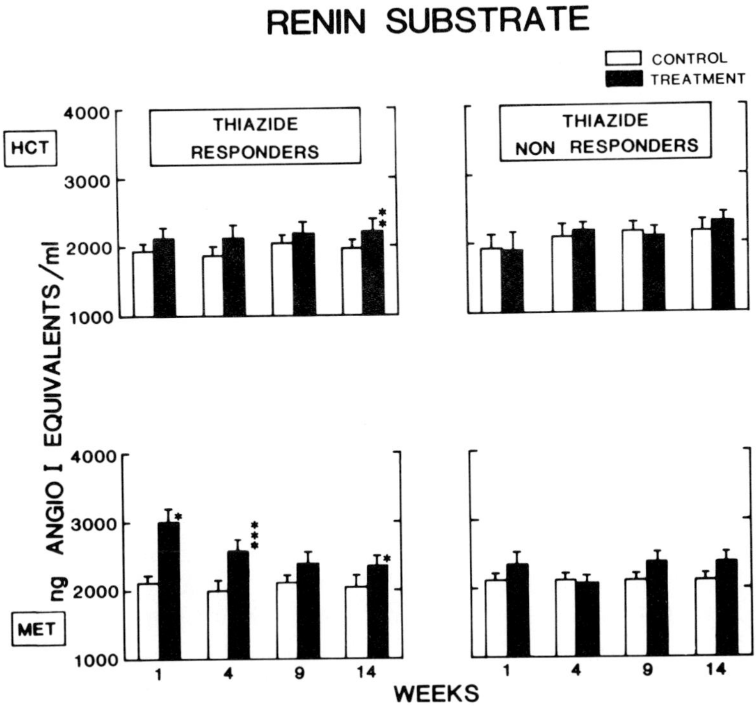

FIG. 12. Renin substrate (ng equivalents angiotensin I/ml plasma) vs. duration of treatment (weeks). Thiazide responders (n = 7-13) and nonresponders (n = 8-14) are shown with their respective controls. The data indicate that nonresponders show no elevation in renin substrate levels whereas those patients which respond demonstrate elevations in substrate levels when placed on metolazone.

somewhat higher values for control PRA but the treatment PRA at 14 weeks did not differ from control. In the thiazide nonresponders the control PRA values were comparatively lower, but PRA at 14 weeks of hydrochlorothiazide treatment was significantly elevated above control (Fig. 11). This pattern does not lend itself for classification of these subjects into the so-called low versus normal renin hypertension. Plasma renin substrate was significantly elevated above control at 14 weeks of hydrochlorothiazide treatment, and at most periods of metolazone treatment, only in the "thiazide responders." The "thiazide nonresponders" showed no significant changes in plasma renin substrate during treatment with either diuretic.

The present study does not allow any basis for implicating the renin substrate elevation to the mechanisms of antihypertensive response. Renin substrate elevations occurred and were confined to the "thiazide responders" during metolazone therapy although comparable antihypertensive response to metolazone was observed both in thiazide responders and nonresponders. Further observations are required to elucidate the possible significance of these findings.

Summary

Metolazone (qd) under conditions of this study proved to be a significantly superior antihypertensive agent than hydrochlorothiazide (bid) in patients with benign essential hypertension. This superiority of antihypertensive action of metolazone, as compared with hydrochlorothiazide, was not related to a greater weight loss or sodium excretion. Kaluresis was comparable with the two diuretics; hypokalemia was more marked with metolazone. PRA showed initial elevations in response to both diuretics but returned toward normal at three months of hydrochlorothiazide therapy. In contrast, PRA remained significantly elevated above control during metolazone therapy. Concomitant with sustained elevations of plasma renin however, renin reactivity and blood angiotensin levels declined toward control values during chronic therapy with metolazone. It was concluded that elevated plasma renin was not accompanied by an overall increase in the activity of the renin angiotensin system during metolazone therapy. Hydrochlorothiazide therapy was effective in lowering diastolic blood pressure only in half of the patients. The thiazide responders showed a relative lack of plasma renin stimulation and an exclusive propensity for stimulation of plasma renin substrate at three months of hydrochlorothiazide therapy.

References

1. Suki, W.N., Dawoud F., Eknoyan, F. et al: Effects of metolazone on renal function in normal man. J. Pharmacol. Exp. Ther. 180:6-12, 1972.
2. Smiley, J.W., Onesti, G., and Swartz, C.: The acute effects of metolazone on electrolyte and acid excretion in man. Clin. Pharmacol. Ther. 13:336-342, 1972.

3. Steinmuller, S.R. and Puschett, J.B.: Effects of metolazone in man: Comparison with chlorothiazide. Kidney Int. 1:169-181, 1972.
4. Pilewski, R.M., Scheib, E.T., Misage, J.R. et al: Technique of controlled drug assay in hypertension. V. Comparison of hydrochlorothiazide with a new quinethazone diuretic, metolazone. Clin. Pharmacol. Ther. 12:843-848, 1971.
5. Cangiano, J.L., Campos, J.A., Trevino, A. et al: The effects of metolazone in the long-term treatment of essential hypertension. Curr. Ther. Res. 16:778-785, 1974.
6. Shetty, B.V., Campanella, L.A., Thomas, T.L. et al: Synthesis and activity of some 3-aryl- and 3-aralkyl-1,2,3,4-tetrahydro-4-oxo-6-quinazolinesulfonamides. J. Med. Chem. 13:886-895, 1970.
7. Puschett, J.B. and Rastegar, A.: Comparative study of the effects of metolazone and other diuretics on potassium excretion. Clin. Pharmacol. Ther. 15:397-405, 1974.
8. Eggena, P., Barrett, J.D., Sambhi, M.P. et al: Validity of comparing the measurements of angiotensin I generated in human plasma by radioimmunoassay and bioassay. J. Clin. Endocrinol. 39:865-870, 1974.
9. Barrett, J.D., Eggena, P. and Sambhi, M.P.: Measurement of the blood levels of circulating angiotensin I and II. In press.
10. Sambhi, M.P., Eggena, P., Barrett, J.D. et al: A circulating renin activator in essential hypertension. Circ. Res. 36 and 37 (suppl. 1):28-37, 1975.
11. Tarazi, R.C., Dustan, H.P. and Frohlich, E.: Long-term thiazide therapy in essential hypertension. Circulation 41:709-717, 1970.
12. Laragh, J.H.: Vasoconstriction. Volume analysis for understanding and treating hypertension: The use of renin aldosterone profiles. Amer. J. Med. 55:261-274, 1973.
13. Bravo, E.L., Tarazi, R.C. and Dustan, H.P.: β-adrenergic blockade in diuretic-treated patients with essential hypertension. N. Engl. J. Med. 292:66-70, 1975.
14. Sambhi, M.P., Eggena, P., Barrett, J.D. et al: Propranolol interaction with metolazone induced alterations in renin system and blood pressure in essential hypertension (to be published).
15. Catt, K.J., Cain, M.D., Coghlan, J.P. et al: Metabolism and blood levels of angiotensin II in normal subjects, renal disease, and essential hypertension. Circ. Res. 26 (suppl. 2):177-193, 1970.

Discussion

Moderator: Dr. F. Gross

Dr. Kirkendall: I would like to ask Dr. Sambhi if he was able to identify any of their nonresponders to thiazide therapy on the basis of other hemodynamic characteristics, particularly pulse rate? Some patients who have a very rapid pulse rate do not respond well to thiazide diuretics. I wonder if, in more carefully controlled studies, such association was seen.

Dr. Sambhi: This question was asked of me yesterday by Dr. Lund-Johansen. My response was that people who are busy studying that many parameters of renin angiotensin system usually neglect to look at simple things like heart rate. We have not looked at this parameter, but I intend to try to retrieve that from our clinical records.

Dr. Kincaid-Smith: I have just a brief question for Dr. Sambhi. What was the dose of hydrochlorothiazide?

Dr. Sambhi: Fifty milligrams twice a day.

Question: I would like you to explain the rather curious elevation of the renin substrate in your study in one of the groups. Have you noticed any difference between the two groups in terms of changing hematocrit or protein? Assuming that there was one group that was more hemoconcentrated than the other one, could you explain some of this rise of renin substrate, or what is your explanation for the change in renin substrate?

Dr. Sambhi: We did not look at hematocrit. However, I would feel fairly confident that the magnitude of change in renin substrate that we saw and that achieved statistical significance in our patients could not be explained by a slight change in hematocrit.

Dr. Freis: You did not show us any data on this, but I think you said that the body weight was reduced more and that the sodium excretion was greater with hydrochlorothiazide. Is that correct?

Dr. Sambhi: Yes, reduction in body weight was significant in patients on hydrochlorothiazide only. The sodium excretion resulting from the chronic use of the two diuretics, however, statistically did not differ from each other.

Dr. Freis: If so, this would demand an explanation for the greater antihypertensive effect of metolazone which would be different from its diuretic effect and I wondered whether you had any thoughts on that.

Dr. Sambhi: Yes, the body weight was on a slide which I did not show because of time limitation. The reduction in body weight achieved significance only in case of patients who were on thiazides at the third month. The patients on metolazone had almost returned to their control weight by the third month. The changes in sodium, 24 hours sodium excretion, I hesitate to place equal reliance on that, although we did measure sodium and creatinine ratios and we only accepted those 24 hour urines that had respectable sodium:creatinine ratios. Likewise, by the third month, the sodium excretion tended to return to control levels in patients on metolazone. Now, you are quite right: If I were to speculate, I would have to say that there is a different mechanism of antihypertensive action of metolazone. We suggest that it has something to do with changes in renin reactivity index that we demonstrated in this study and that indicate a reduction in the overall activity of the renin angiotensin system and perhaps not in the circulation itself because it is difficult to explain it on the basis of changes in angiotensin II blood levels, at least from the data which we have shown. But it might be important in critical tissues, perhaps in the vascular wall or in the intrarenal tissues, that such change may be mediating the antihypertensive effect of this compound. But that is purely a speculation.

Dr. Gross: What is the half-life of metolazone as compared to hydrochlorothiazide and its duration of action? Has it a long prolonged duration of action, like, for example, chlorothalidone?

Dr. Sambhi: Yes, it is used only once a day and it certainly has a longer effect. But perhaps the information on half-life could come from some more knowledgeable people in the audience. Is there someone here in the audience today who could answer the question on half-life of metolazone?

Dr. Giering: The half-life has been found to be about eight hours for metolazone. The duration of diuretic action is approximately 12-24 hours in a single dose of 5 mg which is approximately comparable to 50 mg of hydrochlorothiazide.

Dr. Johnston: Dr. Sambhi, can you tell us whether the patients were on a fixed sodium intake, because I noticed that the nonresponders to the hydrochlorothiazide, in fact, did not increase their hematocrit; whereas, those who responded, did increase their hematocrit. Do you think that those who failed to respond to the chlorothiazide diuretic did not have a negative sodium balance and a reduction in their plasma and extracellular volume?

Dr. Sambhi: I did not show any data on alterations in hematocrit. No, the sodium intake was not fixed. These patients were outpatient subjects who were studied as outpatients with no control at all on their diet. So our only recourse was to measure the 24-hour urine sodium output, which did not differ in nonresponders versus responders.

Dr. Streeten: I wondered whether Dr. Sambhi has an explanation for the surprising finding that the patients treated with metolazone showed an increase in plasma renin activity, an increase in plasma renin substrate, and yet no change in A II. I wonder whether this failure of metolazone to raise A II might be due to the effect he has described on the renin reactivity index, or perhaps to a change in the metabolism of A II or conceivably to an effect on the converting enzyme?

Dr. Sambhi: Obviously, our conclusions were that if you reduce the reactivity index, or in other words reduce the renin and substrate reactivity, then that is what you will do. You will diminish the end product (A I) generation. So we would tend to explain this on the basis that, despite the significant elevation of renin itself, and in one group of patients, an increase in renin substrate, the reactivity declines so much that the end product generation would significantly decrease. So that is how we have explained this effect. However, the possibility of changes in A II metabolism or converting enzyme, that you raise, cannot be ruled out. As I said, these changes in renin angiotensin system may or may not be related to the antihypertensive effect. If the antihypertensive effect is dependent upon these changes of renin angiotensin system, it may conceivably be dependent upon changes in the circulating system, then it has to be some sort of rate phenomenon. In other words, the rate at which the receptors perceive the repetitive vasoconstrictor stimulus of angiotensin, they could be more susceptible to rate than concentration. Or, alternately, the effect might be exerted locally at the tissue level.

I would like to add one other comment. In our studies, the design included the addition of potassium routinely. We gave potassium routinely to all of our patients on both diuretics.

Longitudinal Study of Plasma Renin Activity in Hypertensive Patients Under Antihypertensive Treatment Including Diuretics

A. Zanchetti, M.D., G. Leonetti, M.D., A. Morganti, M.D., L. Terzoli, M.D., E. Schwarz, M.D., M. Manfrin, M.D. and M. Bernasconi, M.D.

A revival of interest for the various effects of antihypertensive drugs on plasma renin activity (PRA) and, whenever possible, on renin release stems from recent evidence that elevated plasma concentrations of angiotensin can play a pressor role, as witnessed by the hypotensive role of agents which block the action of the renin-angiotensin system in several cases of human [1-3] and experimental hypertension [4]. The suggestion has also been made [5, 6] that lowering of PRA may be one mechanism of the hypotensive action of agents like alpha-methyldopa or clonidine, or at least interpreted as an advantageous side effect. On the other hand, it has been considered that the renin stimulating properties of drugs like diuretics and direct vasodilators may lead to a kind of self-limitation of the hypotensive action of these drugs. Indeed, evidence that this may be true for vasodilators has been brought out by Pettinger and Mitchell [7], who showed that the high renin levels caused by minoxidil do play a vasoconstrictor role, because infusion of the angiotensin antagonist, saralasin, signifi-

A. Zanchetti, M.D., G. Leonetti, M.D., A. Morganti, M.D., L. Terzoli, M.D., E. Schwarz, M.D., M. Manfrin, M.D. and M. Bernasconi, M.D., Istituto di Ricerche Cardiovascolari and Istituto di Patologia Medica I, Universitá di Milano, and Centro per le Ricerche Cardiovascolari del C.N.R. Milan, Italy.

cantly lowered blood pressure in minoxidil-treated hypertensive patients, but had little further hypotensive effect after addition of propranolol had reduced the plasma renin levels.

Until recently, however, and with few exceptions, most of the available information on the interactions between PRA and antihypertensive drugs was derived from acute or short-term administration; and even more scanty and confused was the evidence about possible interactions when various antihypertensive agents are administered, an issue of some interest because treatment of hypertension is still carried out in most centers by multidrug regimens.

The renin-stimulating action of diuretic agents is worth some detailed comment, as they are such an important part of most antihypertensive regimens. There is no doubt that diuretics are strong and prompt stimulators of renin release. Current work by our group has shown that in two groups of outpatients receiving 50 and 100 mg chlorthalidone daily, respectively, and followed up at weekly or biweekly intervals, PRA had considerably risen at the end of the first week and then leveled off at these increased values for at least 13 weeks, which was the length of this study. Figure 1 summarizes the response of one patient: the PRA increase parallels a reduction in body weight, and there is also an increase in urinary aldosterone.

The two main problems, however, are (1) how long the stimulation of renin by diuretic treatment may last and (2) whether it is influenced by simultaneous administration of other antihypertensive drugs having opposite action on renin release. The two problems have either been little studied or been given contrasting responses. In particular the length of the renin-stimulating effect of diuretics has been reported differently by different groups of authors. For instance, Bourgoignie et al [8] have reported that PRA was increased after acute exposure to a thiazide diuretic for less than three weeks, but returned to normal when treatment was prolonged for more than two months. This does not agree with our experience, as the study we just mentioned above clearly indicates that in our patients the stimulating action continued unabated for at least three months. Johnston et al [9] found variable responses in patients receiving a thiazide in combination with other drugs for three to six months: half of the subjects had an increase while the other half showed small decreases. On the whole, compari-

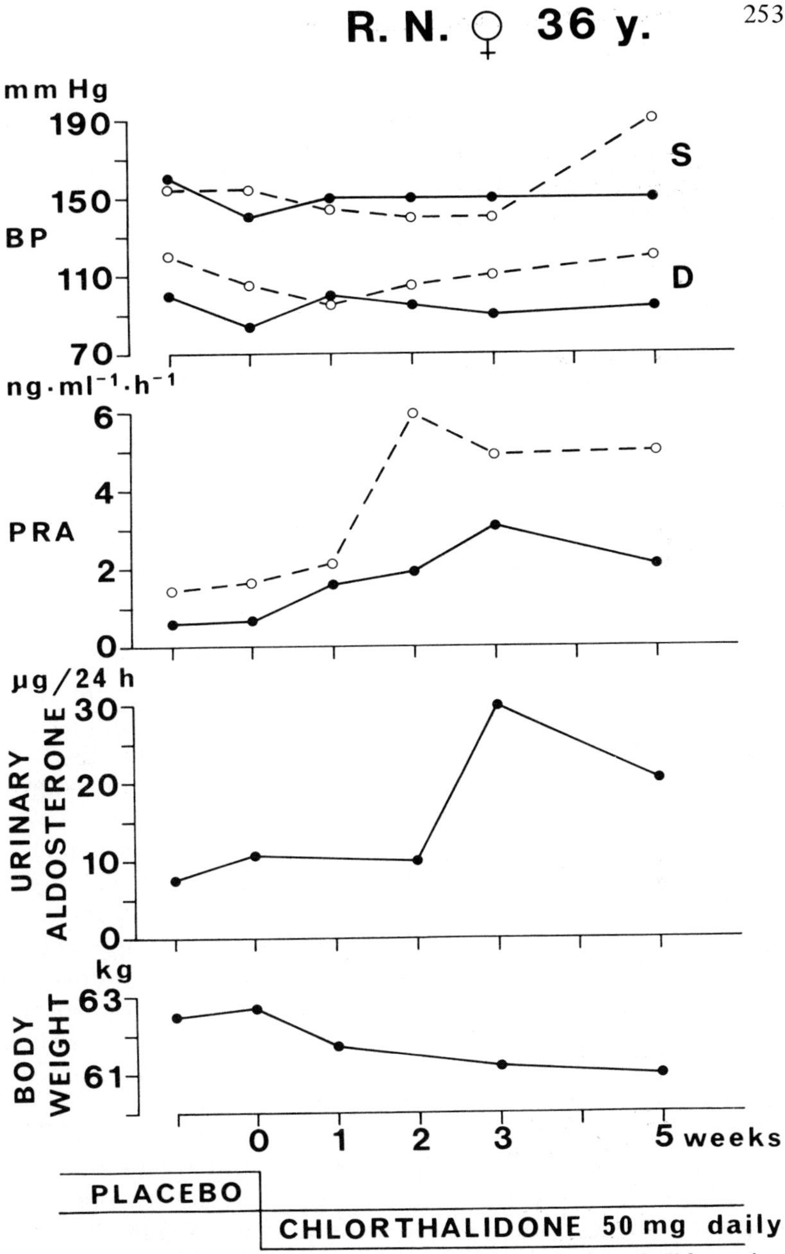

FIG. 1. Responses to chronic administration of chlorthalidone in a hypertensive patient. From above downwards: BP, systolic (S) and diastolic (D) blood pressure, supine (filled circles) and standing (hollow circles); PRA, plasma renin activity, supine (filled circles) and standing (hollow circles); urinary aldosterone (daily excretion); and body weight.

son of plasma renin in a group of untreated hypertensives and in a group of chronically treated ones gave no difference whatsoever. On the other hand, Vaughan et al [10] maintain that the renin-stimulating action of diuretic agents still continues unabated after several months of treatment, and the Cleveland group finds raised levels after three to six months of continuous diuretic treatment [11] and a decrease in plasma renin when the diuretic is stopped [12].

To clarify the problem, we have started a follow-up study of a group of 79 essential hypertensive patients receiving a combined drug regimen variable from subject to subject, but always including chlorthalidone. All the subjects were studied during the second to fourth week from the beginning of treatment, and a part of them could be seen again at a later time, varying from 3 to 12 months. PRA was measured (1) after the patient had been lying supine for two hours, (2) after active standing upright for two hours, and (3) after intravenous injection of 40 mg furosemide.

Figure 2 summarizes data from 79 patients during the acute part of the study. Standing mean arterial pressure decreased from 140 to 110 mm Hg; PRA was found significantly increased both in the supine posture and during upright standing. The increment on standing also became greatly exaggerated during acute antihypertensive therapy.

Figure 3 summarizes the findings in the 29 patients that could be followed both acutely and chronically. It will be seen that the increase in renin in the supine posture, after furosemide and particularly in the standing position, was not entirely maintained during the late portion of the study. Interestingly enough, blood pressure was on the average not so well controlled during chronic treatment as during acute treatment in these outpatients. The group of subjects was therefore split into two subgroups: the first one including patients (n = 18) whose mean arterial pressure was reduced to the same degree in both phases of the study, the second one including those patients (n = 11) whose blood pressure had returned practically to pretreatment values. It can be seen from Figure 4 that in both groups standing PRA was lower in the chronic as compared to the acute phase. However, in the group in which the hypotensive effect has late disappeared, there was evidence

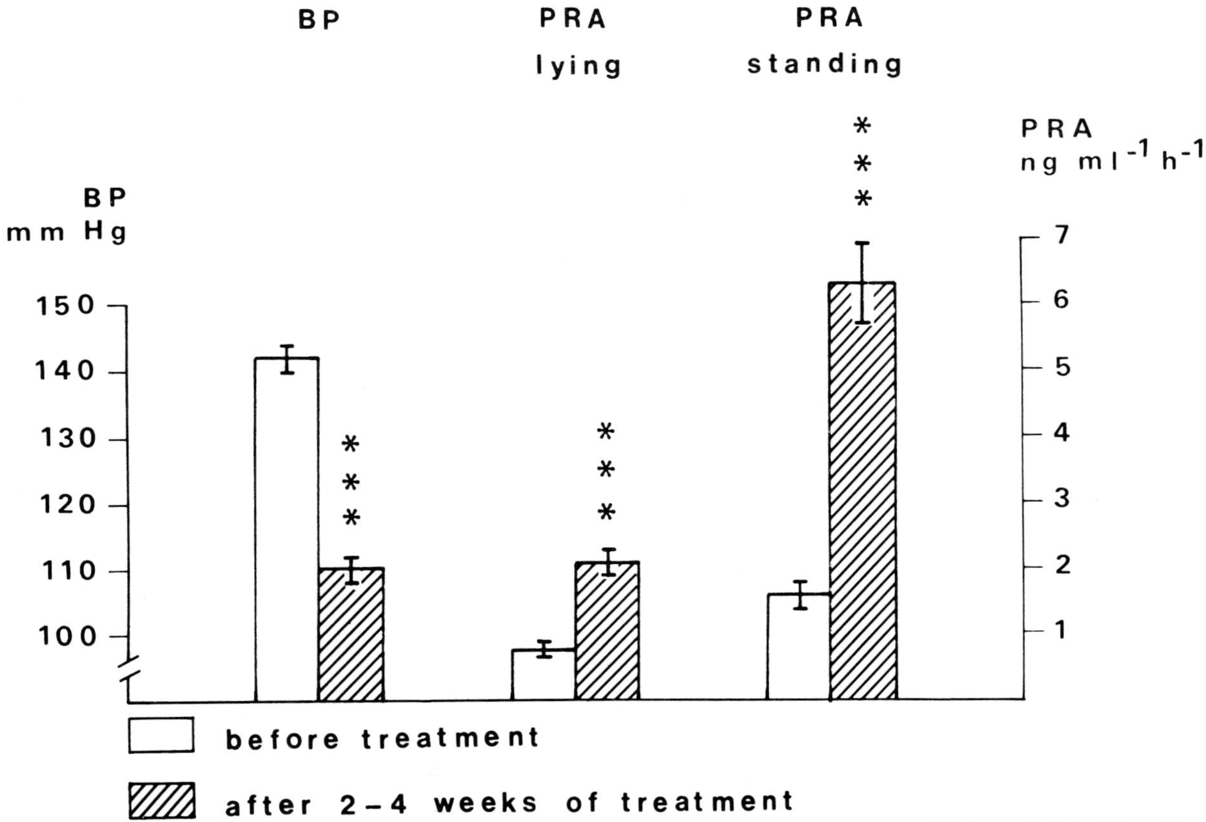

FIG. 2. Changes in mean arterial pressure (PB, *left*) and in plasma renin activity (PRA, *right*) in 79 patients treated for two to four weeks with a combined antihypertensive treatment including chlorthalidone. Open areas before treatment, shaded areas after treatment. The histograms and the bars represent means and standard errors of the mean. The three asterisks indicate that the differences between pre- and posttreatment means are statistically significant at the $p < 0.001$ level.

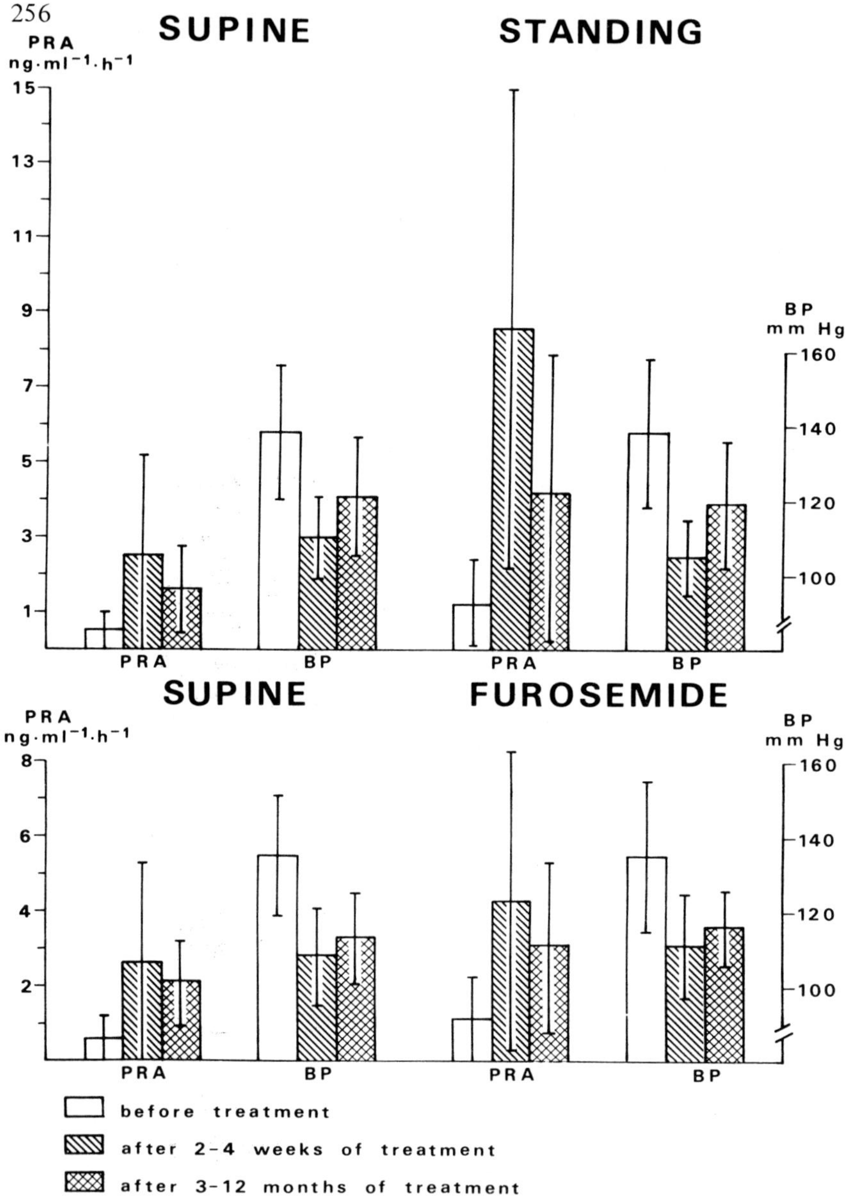

FIG. 3. Changes in plasma renin activity (PRA, *scale on left*) and in mean arterial pressure (BP, *scale on right*) in 29 hypertensive patients studied before treatment (open histograms) after two to four weeks of antihypertensive treatment (shaded histograms) and after 3-12 months of treatment (cross hatched histograms). Means and standard deviations.

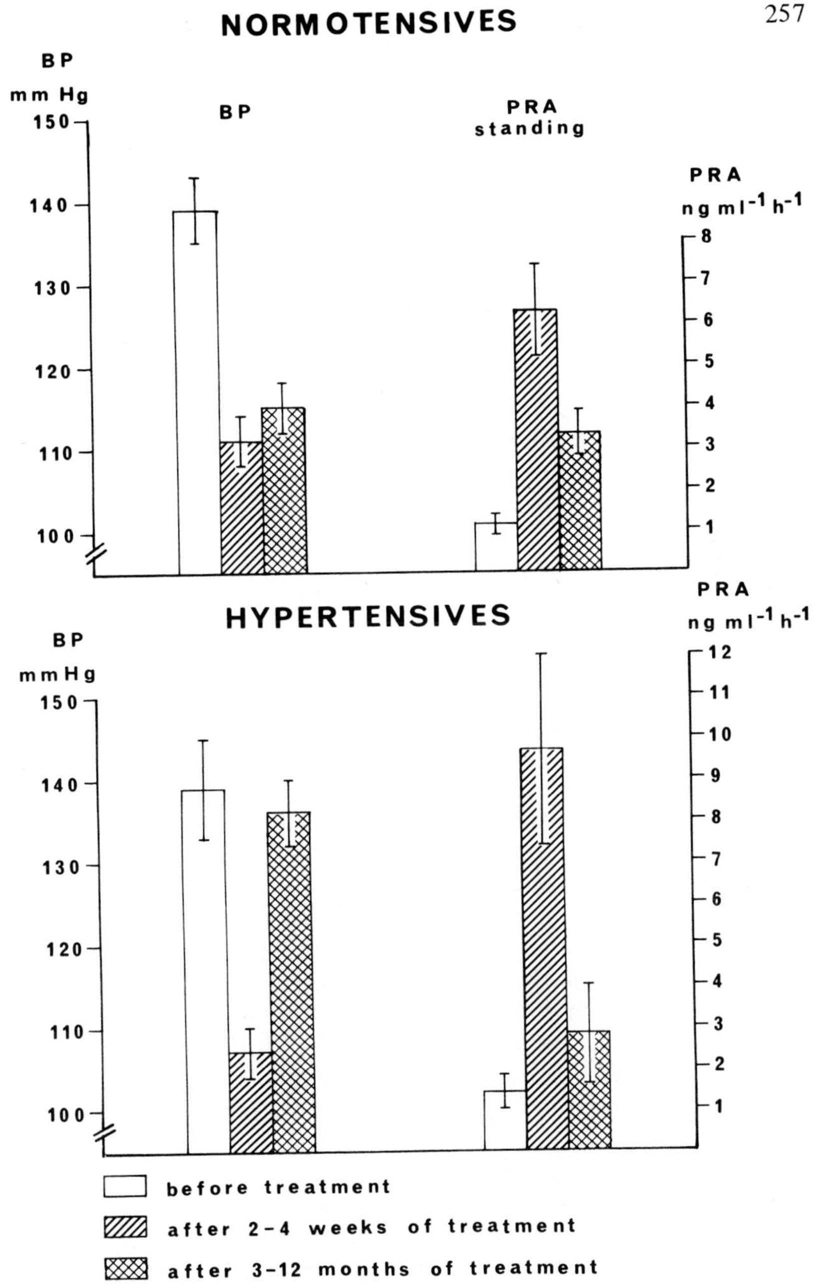

FIG. 4. Changes in mean arterial pressure (BP, *left*) and standing plasma renin activity (PRA) in 18 treated hypertensive patients who maintained good blood pressure control both during the acute (shaded histograms) and the chronic period of therapy (crossed hatched histograms) (upper half of the figure: Normotensives) and in 11 treated hypertensive patients, whose blood pressure control was good acutely but lost chronically (lower part of the figure: Hypertensives).

of a more complete normalization of the renin response: lowering of standing PRA was more marked and values statistically undistinguishable from pretreatment were also found in the supine posture and after furosemide. On the other hand, in the patients with a maintained hypotensive response, renin stimulation was damped but not exhausted. Indeed, standing PRA was still somewhat raised above pretreatment values, though not so markedly as during the very first weeks, and supine and furosemide values were still equally elevated in the chronic as in the acute phase of treatment in these patients. Supine values represent unstimulated renin release, furosemide values represent a response to a mild stimulus, while standing values are the response to a rather strong stimulus. Apparently the decreased renin-stimulating action of chronic antihypertensive therapy shows itself, at the beginning, only when the juxtaglomerular cells are tested with a strong renin-releasing stimulus. The more marked and earlier exhaustion of renin stimulation in patients in which the hypotensive response to treatment wanes may be the consequence of the renin-inhibitory action of raised arterial pressure, but is more probably due to worse compliance of these subjects to the recommended therapy.

It seems therefore that the renin-stimulating action of diuretics is gradually tuned down during chronic administration, but that in patients responsive to treatment the exhaustion of the renin-stimulating action is not very quick.

Our data, being collected in patients under combined therapy, give also some hints on which may be the effect of renin-suppressive drugs like α-methyldopa and clonidine when combined with chlorthalidone. The upper part of Figure 5 shows that pretreatment PRA, in the supine and standing postures, and after furosemide, was equal in the three groups of patients receiving (1) chlorthalidone with reserpine, (2) chlorthalidone plus reserpine and alpha-methyldopa, and (3) chlorthalidone plus reserpine, alpha-methyldopa and clonidine. After two to four week treatment, the group having higher renin levels was the one receiving chlorthalidone associated with reserpine only: the other two groups had slightly but consistently smaller PRA elevations. This suggests that alpha-methyldopa and clonidine have a renin-suppressing action, but that in front

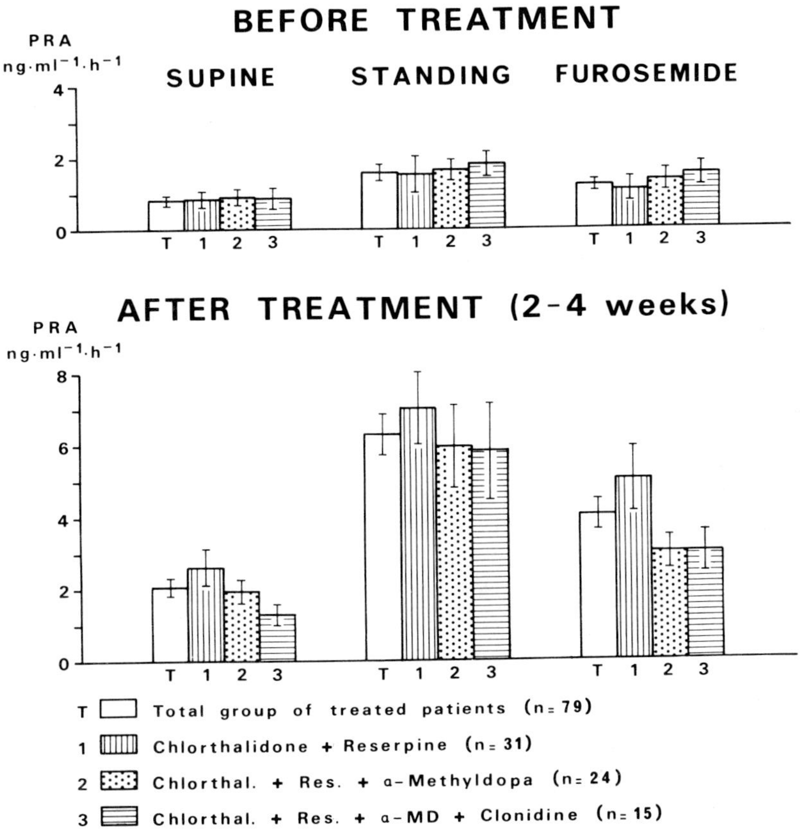

FIG. 5. Plasma renin activity (PRA) before treatment (*above*) and after two to four weeks of treatment (*below*) with various combinations of drugs, as indicated in the figure.

of the strong stimulation by the diuretic this inhibiting action can only play a minor role.

This observation opens the problem as to whether βadrenoreceptor blocking agents can exert their renin-suppressive influence when renin release has been stimulated by diuretic agents. Bravo et al [11] have reported that little or no decrease in PRA can be obtained when a 160 mg daily dose of propranolol is added to chronic diuretic therapy. This has been taken to demonstrate that renin release under chronic salt depletion is not neurally mediated. The problem of the mechanisms mediating renin release in response to salt depletion is controversial. Stella and Zanchetti [13] have shown in cats that acute salt depletion caused by a moderate dose of furosemide (0.75 mg/kg) releases renin only from an innervated kidney, but that much greater doses (6.0 mg/kg) also act on denervated kidneys. We have also shown that when hypertensive subjects receive 40 mg furosemide intravenously, a dose comparable weight to weight to 0.75 mg/kg dose in cats, renin release is entirely and easily blocked by even low plasma concentrations of propranolol [14], thus suggesting that the mechanism is neural. The mechanisms of renin release during chronic salt depletion, however, may be different from those responsible for acute depletion: the evidence available from animal experiments is controversial, a number of authors claiming that the mechanism is exclusively [15, 16] or predominantly [17] nonneural, other authors claiming that it is basically neural [18]. We are investigating this problem now and have only preliminary results available. It appears, however, that propranolol can antagonize PRA stimulation by chronic diuretic therapy, though this inhibition is not so complete and often occurs at higher propranolol plasma concentrations than those inhibiting the response to acute furosemide administration. An example is shown in Figure 6. Likewise, administration of a diuretic for a few consecutive days in propranolol-treated patients can break through the renin-suppressing action of the β-blocker and raise renin (Fig. 7), though probably not to the higher values that would have occurred without pre-existing propranolol.

The final problem is whether plasma renin levels caused by chronic diuretic treatment are sufficiently elevated to play a pressor role. No clear answer has been provided to this question, since to our knowledge the effect of blocking peptides, such as saralasin, has never been tested in hypertensive patients before and after prolonged administration of diuretics. Certainly, data from most of the available studies suggest that plasma renin is not as high during chronic diuretic therapy as in the cases under minoxidil reported by Pettinger and Mitchell. Until this information becomes available, it cannot be ruled out that diuretics may be potentially harmful agents in hypertensive patients with very high renin. In some patients with malignant

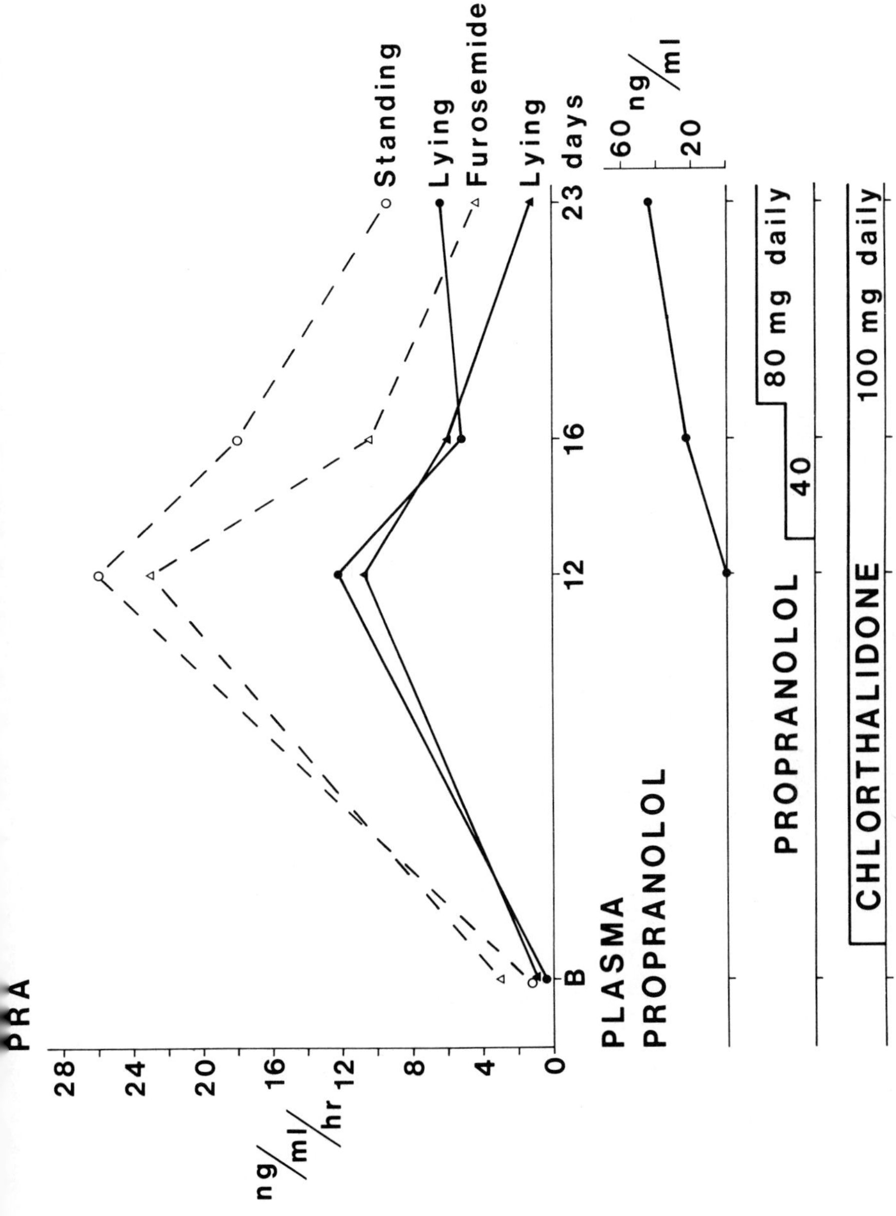

FIG. 6. Plasma renin activity in the lying and standing positions, and after an intravenous injection of 40 mg furosemide in a hypertensive patient receiving chlorthalidone first and then chlorthalidone plus propranolol.

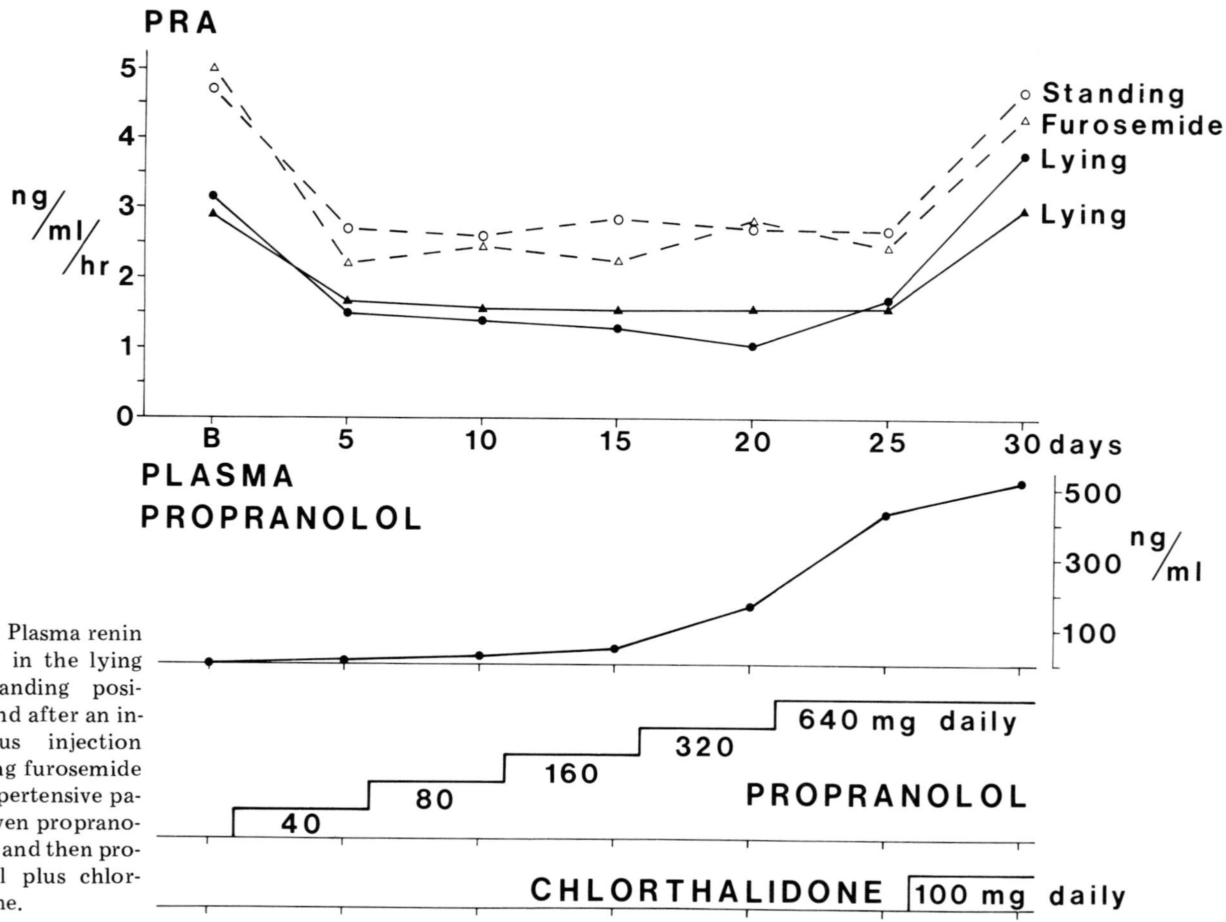

FIG. 7. Plasma renin activity in the lying and standing positions and after an intravenous injection of 40 mg furosemide in a hypertensive patient given propranolol first and then propranolol plus chlorthalidone.

hypertension high renin might indicate sodium depletion, and a further depletion is likely to aggravate the initial disturbance. Except in obviously depleted subjects, however, before renouncing the potentialities of diuretic therapy in a high renin patient with severe hypertension, we should remember the miserable perspective of the severely hypertensive patients before thiazide administration was introduced to potentiate the action of hypotensive drugs.

References

1. Brunner, H.R., Gavras, H., Laragh, J.H. et al: Angiotensin II blockade in man by Sar^{1}- ala^{8}-angiotensin II for understanding and treatment of high blood pressure. Lancet 2:1045, 1973.
2. Gavras, H., Brunner, H.R., Laragh, J.H. et al: The use of angiotensin-converting enzyme inhibitor in the diagnosis and treatment of hypertension. Clin. Sci. Molec. Med. 48 (suppl. 2):57, 1975.
3. Johnson, J.G., Black, W.D., Vukovich, R.A. et al: Treatment of patients with severe hypertension by inhibition of angiotensin converting enzyme. Clin. Sci. Molec. Med. 48 (suppl. 2):53, 1975.
4. Davis, J.O.: The use of blocking agents to define the functions of the renin-angiotensin system. Clin. Sci. Molec. Med. 48 (suppl. 2):3, 1975.
5. Laragh, J.H.: Vasoconstriction-volume analysis for understanding and treating hypertension: The use of renin and aldosterone profiles. Am. J. Med. 55:261, 1973.
6. Weidmann, P., Hirsch, D., Maxwell, M.H. et al: Plasma renin and blood pressure during treatment with methyldopa. Am. J. Cardiol. 34:671, 1974.
7. Pettinger, W.A. and Mitchell, H.C.: Renin release, saralasin and the vasodilator-beta-blocker drug interaction in man. N. Engl. J. Med. 292:1214, 1975.
8. Bourgoignie, J.J., Catanzaro, F.J. and Perry H.M., Jr.: Renin-angiotensin-aldosterone system during chronic thiazide therapy of benign hypertension. Circulation 37:27, 1968.
9. Johnston, C.I., Anavekar, N., Chua, K.G. et al: Plasma renin and angiotensin levels in human hypertension following treatment. Clin. Sci. Molec. Med. 45:287, 1973.
10. Vaughan, E.D., Laragh, J.H., Gavras, I. et al: Volume factor in low and normal renin essential hypertension: Treatment with either spironolactone or chlorthalidone. Am. J. Cardiol. 32:522, 1973.
11. Bravo, E.L., Tarazi, R.C. and Dustan, H.P.: βadrenergic blockade in diuretic-treated patients with essential hypertension. N. Engl. J. Med. 292:66, 1975.
12. Tarazi, R.C., Dustan, H.P., Frohlich, E.D. et al: Plasma volume and chronic hypertension. Arch. Intern. Med. 125:835, 1970.

13. Zanchetti, A. and Stella, A.: Neural control of renin release. Clin. Sci. Molec. Med. 48 (suppl. 2):215, 1975.
14. Leonetti, G., Mayer, G., Morganti, A. et al: Hypotensive and renin suppressing activities of propranolol in hypertensive patients. Clin. Sci. Molec. Med. 48:491, 1975.
15. Gotshall, R.W., Davis, J.O., Shade, R.E. et al: Effects of renal denervation on renin release in sodium depleted dogs. Am. J. Physiol. 225:344, 1973.
16. Brennan, L.A., Mulcahy, J.J., Carretero, O.A. et al: Effect of chronic sodium depletion in dogs with denervated kidneys and hearts. Am. J. Physiol. 227:1289, 1974.
17. Brubacher, E.S. and Vander, A.J.: Sodium deprivation and renin secretion in unanesthetized dogs. Am. J. Physiol. 214:15, 1968.
18. Mogil, R.A., Itskovitz, H.D., Russel, J.H. et al: Renal innervation and renin activity in salt metabolism and hypertension. Am. J. Physiol. 216:693, 1969.

Double-Blind Crossover Study of Propranolol and Spironolactone in Hypertension and Plasma Renin Measurements in Relation to Therapeutic Effects

Gordon S. Stokes, M.D., F.R.A.C.P.,
Michael A. Weber, M.B.B.S., James V. Smith, B.Sc.
and Judith M. Gain, S.R.N.

The vasoconstriction-volume analysis of hypertension [1] is an attractive hypothesis which offers a theoretical basis for predicting therapeutic responsiveness of hypertensive patients to antihypertensive drugs by reference to plasma renin levels. Some support for this hypothesis has been provided by several studies which have shown correlations between the pretreatment levels of plasma renin activity and responses to spironolactone [2-4] or propranolol [5]. However, these results have been obtained using protocols in which elements of either patient selection, observer bias, or both, could not be excluded.

While it is evident that at extreme ends of the spectrum of hypertension low-renin volume-dependent conditions such as primary aldosteronism respond specifically to diuretics and high-renin vasoconstrictor states such as renovascular hypertension respond to propranolol, it has not been established that the plasma renin level can serve in other cases as a valid marker

---

This work was supported by grants from the National Heart Foundation of Australia, the Australian National Health & Medical Research Council, G. D. Searle (Australia) Pty. Ltd. and I.C.I. Australia Ltd.

Gordon S. Stokes, M.D., F.R.A.C.P., Michael A. Weber, M.B.B.S., James V. Smith, B.Sc. and Judith M. Gain, S.R.N., Cardio-Renal Unit, Medical Research Department, Sydney Hospital, Sydney, Australia.

of the contributions of volume and vasoconstrictor factors. Hence, there is a need to further explore the relevance of renin measurements to the routine investigation of unselected hypertensive patients presenting for evaluation prior to treatment.

The present study was designed to determine the usefulness of several different standardized renin tests in predicting patients' responses to treatment with propranolol or spironolactone. Most patients had received no previous antihypertensive therapy and were selected only with respect to their blood pressure readings, which fell within a defined range of mild to moderate hypertension, and by their willingness to participate on a voluntary basis.

Patients and Methods

Thirty patients of Caucasian descent, with diastolic blood pressure between 101 mm Hg and 120 mm Hg, were referred from a community hypertension survey and gave their informed consent to participate in a double-blind trial lasting six months. In most subjects, there had been no previous exposure to antihypertensive drugs, for the hypertension had been newly discovered. Those previously treated had had no medications for at least a month before entering the trial. Two patients were withdrawn from the trial because of excessive placebo responses and one patient defaulted; thus, 27 patients, 10 females and 17 males, completed the trial. Their ages were between 24 and 60 years and weights between 52 and 100 kg (mean 74 kg). In all patients a detailed clinical assessment was made, including a full history, physical examination, chest x-ray, intravenous pyelogram, electrocardiogram, micro-urine and measurements of serum electrolytes, urinary catecholamines and creatinine clearance. In 24 patients the diagnosis of uncomplicated essential hypertension was made. In the other three there was pyelographic evidence of mild chronic pyelonephritis. Serum creatinine was 1.3 mg/dl or less in all cases.

Normal Volunteers

A group of 74 normal volunteers (mean age 36 years; 39 males and 35 females) with casual blood pressure readings less than 140/90, who were not taking oral contraceptives or other medications, contributed blood and urine samples to establish normal ranges for plasma renin activity.

Initial Measurements of Plasma Renin Activity (PRA) and Urinary Aldosterone Excretion

Blood samples for measurement of PRA were collected at 0930 hours in the erect posture using four different protocols in every patient: (a) without dietary restrictions and on the same day as the collection of a 24-hour specimen of urine for determination of sodium excretion, (b) following the intake of two 40 mg tablets of furosemide, one at 2100 hours the previous evening and the other at 0600 hours on the morning of the test, (c) after six days on a low sodium diet at home (nominally, 10 mEq/day), (d) after six days on the same diet, together with measured supplements of sodium chloride to bring the sodium intake up to 100 mEq/day. Urinary aldosterone excretion was also measured with the latter regimen. The degree of adherence to the low sodium diet was deemed acceptable in 21 patients, whose urinary sodium excretion on the day of renin measurement averaged 26 ± 4 (SE) mEq/d.

Plan of the Trial

The trial comprised a 2-week "run-in" placebo period followed by three 6-week treatment segments with 2-week "washout" placebo periods intervening, that is, 24 weeks in all. The active treatments were spironolactone (Aldactone, Searle, 100 mg tablets) in an initial dosage of three tablets (300 mg) per day (designated A) and propranolol (Inderal, Imperial Chemical Industries, 80 mg tablets) in an initial dosage of three tablets (240 mg) per day (designated I). A placebo tablet resembling Inderal was given with each active tablet of Aldactone and vice versa. In the remaining six-week treatment segment, two placebo tablets, counterfeits of Aldactone and Inderal, respectively, were administered. This segment is referred to as the placebo control period (designated C).

Patients were distributed by random allocation to three treatment sequences: ACI, IAC and CIA, such that there was an equal distribution of patients with low, intermediate and high PRA in each sequence.

The patient visited the trial clinic at two-week intervals. Blood pressure readings, lying and standing, were taken by two independent observers, then averaged by a third, who also recorded weight and resting pulse rate and collected blood samples for the determination of renin and electrolyte levels. Side effects and blood pressure control were then evaluated by a physician, who chose either to continue treatment with six tablets per day (three placebo plus three active or placebo) or to change to four or eight tablets per day if side effects were troublesome or blood pressure control inadequate. Side effects forced the complete withdrawal of an active medication after four weeks in four patients and after two weeks in one patient; placebos were given during the remainder of the treatment segments so affected. Care was taken that those involved with the management of the patients did not know the treatment sequence pertaining to each patient, which was determined by the pharmacist who dispensed the medications. At each visit, the patient was furnished with a fresh, coded supply of tablets (in excess of requirements) and returned those remaining from his previous supply, which were counted as a check on adherence to instructions.

Measurement of Blood Pressure

All blood pressure readings were made using London School of Hygiene and Tropical Medicine machines* which minimize observer bias by allowing covered mercury columns to be arrested and read after auscultation. Mean blood pressure was derived by adding one third of the pulse pressure to the diastolic pressure. The effects of treatment were assessed by comparing readings obtained during administration of active medication with those obtained during the placebo control period.

Laboratory Methods

Plasma renin activity was measured by radioimmunoassay after incubation of plasma for three hours at 37°C using the method of Haber et al [6] with modifications. These consisted of (a) buffering of plasma to pH 7.4 using 0.2 M tris

*Cinetronics Ltd., Mildenhall, Suffolk, U.K.

(hydroxymethyl) aminomethane acetate* and (b) following the 37° C incubation step by precipitation of plasma proteins with 67% ethanol.

Radio-iodinated angiotensin I was prepared and purified as described by Wilkinson et al [7]. The mean variation between duplicate assay results in 22 plasma samples (within-batch variability) was 9.2 ± 8.8 (SD)% and variation from the mean result for a quality control plasma included in each assay batch (between-batch variability) was 11.9 ± 9.7 (SD)%. The angiotensin standard used was Asp^1 Ile^5 Angiotensin I.† Urinary aldosterone excretion was determined by a double isotope technique [8]. Plasma concentrations of aldadiene (a metabolite of spironolactone) [9] and propranolol [10] were determined by fluorimetric methods.

Results

Effects of Treatment in the Double-blind Trial

The mean effects of treatment with spironolactone and propranolol are shown in Figure 1. Spironolactone, in a dose averaging 280 mg/day, decreased body weight by 2.3 ± 0.4 (SE) kg ($p < 0.001$) and mean blood pressure (standing) from 120 ± 2 mm Hg to 108 ± 2 mm Hg ($p < 0.001$). Pulse rate was increased by 2.5 ± 2 beats/min ($p < 0.1$) and plasma potassium by 0.47 ± 0.07 mEq/1 ($p < 0.001$). PRA rose from 1.2 to 7.6 ng/ml/hr ($p < 0.001$).

Propranolol, 220 mg/day, reduced mean blood pressure to a level of 104 ± 2 mm Hg ($p < 0.001$) without significant changes in body weight or plasma potassium level. Pulse rate fell to an average of 64 beats/min ($p < 0.001$) and PRA to a mean level of 0.7 ng/ml/hr ($p < 0.005$).

There was an insignificant degree of correlation between the decrease in PRA and the antihypertensive response to propranolol ($r = 0.26$; $p > 0.1$). Also, there was no significant relationship between the change in pulse rate with propranolol and the antihypertensive response ($r = 0.21$).

The mean decrease in recumbent blood pressure during treatment with propranolol was 14 ± 2 mm Hg. There was no

*Sigma Chemical Co., St. Louis, Mo.
†Schwarz-Mann Lot No. Y2375.

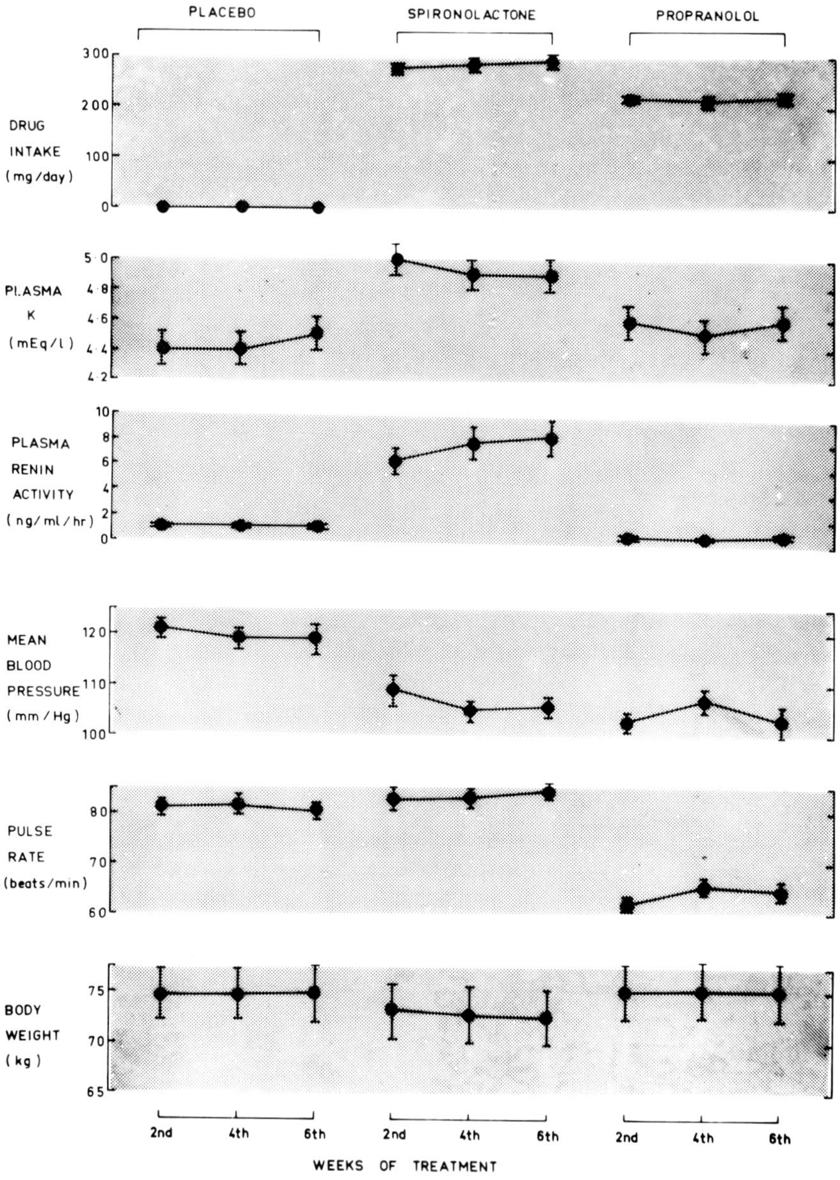

FIG. 1. Mean effects (±S.E.) of treatment with placebo, spironolactone and propranolol, given in a randomized double-blind crossover design in 27 hypertensive patients. There was a two-week placebo washout phase between each six-week treatment period.

orthostatic effect with this drug. The antihypertensive response to propranolol was maximal within the first two weeks of treatment. At the end of two weeks of treatment with spironolactone, the blood pressure reduction assessed from erect readings (10.4 mm Hg) was greater than that found in the recumbent posture (4.4 mm Hg). The orthostatic effect then diminished. For the last four weeks of treatment, mean blood pressure averaged 109 mm Hg during recumbency and 107 mm Hg in the erect posture.

The plasma concentration of the spironolactone derivative, aldadiene, which was measured after two weeks of therapy in 25 patients, averaged 16.0 ± 1.5 (SE) μg/100 ml and showed a low but significant degree of correlation ($r = 0.41$, $p < 0.05$) with the intake of spironolactone (per kilogram) as assessed by tablet returns. The plasma concentration of propranolol after the first two weeks of treatment with that drug averaged 137 ± 16 (SE) ng/ml (in 27 patients). No significant relationship was found between the intake and plasma concentration of propranolol.

Pretreatment Renin and Aldosterone Values

These are shown in Table 1. With a diet containing 100 mEq sodium per day, the mean value for PRA in the 27 patients was not significantly different from that in a group of 18 normal subjects (1.6 ± 0.2 (SE) ng/ml/hr and 2.0 ± 0.3 ng/ml/hr, respectively). Likewise, mean PRA after sodium depletion was not significantly different from that in normal subjects.

The results of stimulation of plasma renin levels by furosemide were variable. In nine patients challenged on two occasions, the percentage variation between the two results was 52 ± 18(SE)%, which was significantly greater than the assay variability. Comparison within patients showed that furosemide caused a significant increase in PRA above the levels obtained with 100 mEq sodium intake ($p < 0.005$), but was a less effective stimulus than sodium depletion ($p < 0.005$). The mean value after furosemide in patients was significantly lower than that in a group of 18 normal controls (2.7 and 4.5 ng/ml/hr, respectively; $p < 0.02$).

A nomogram showing the relationship between PRA and urinary sodium excretion in 69 normal subjects is shown in Figure 2. All coordinates for 21 patients (two or three values each) plotted on the nomogram fell within the normal range. However, in each of five patients, two values fell outside or on the limits of this range (Fig. 3), thus identifying four patients as "low-renin" cases (no. 11, 14, 16, 18 in Table 1) and one (no. 24) as a "high-renin" case. Results for furosemide-stimulated plasma renin activity in these cases (Table 1) were compatible with their position on the nomogram. A further patient (no. 15), whose solitary nomogram point lay just below the normal limit, had high PRA after furosemide and thus was not classified as "low-renin."

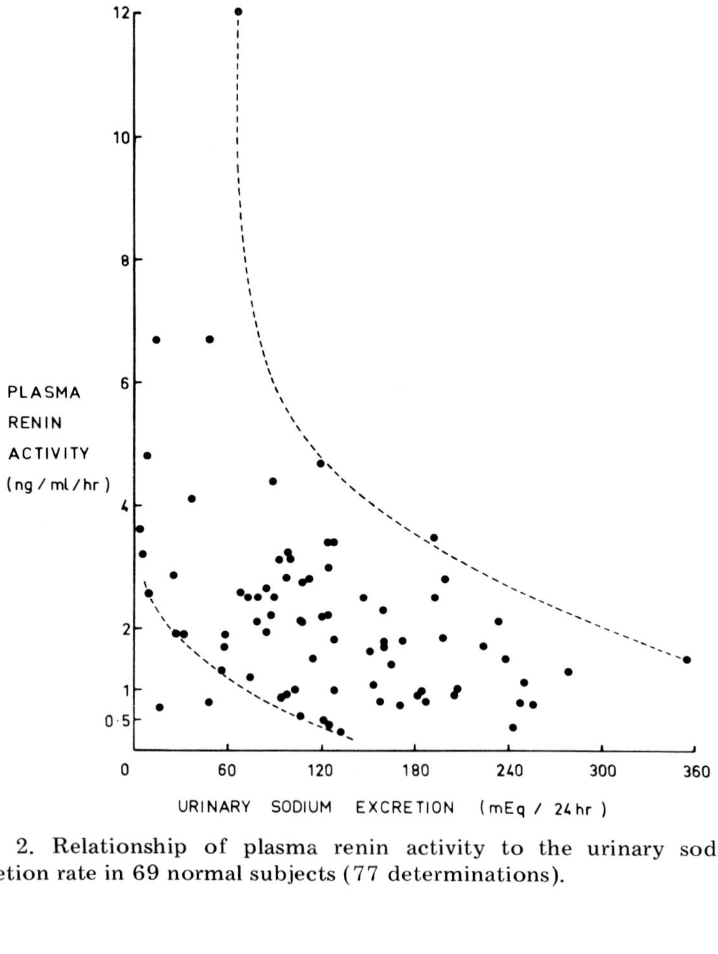

FIG. 2. Relationship of plasma renin activity to the urinary sodium excretion rate in 69 normal subjects (77 determinations).

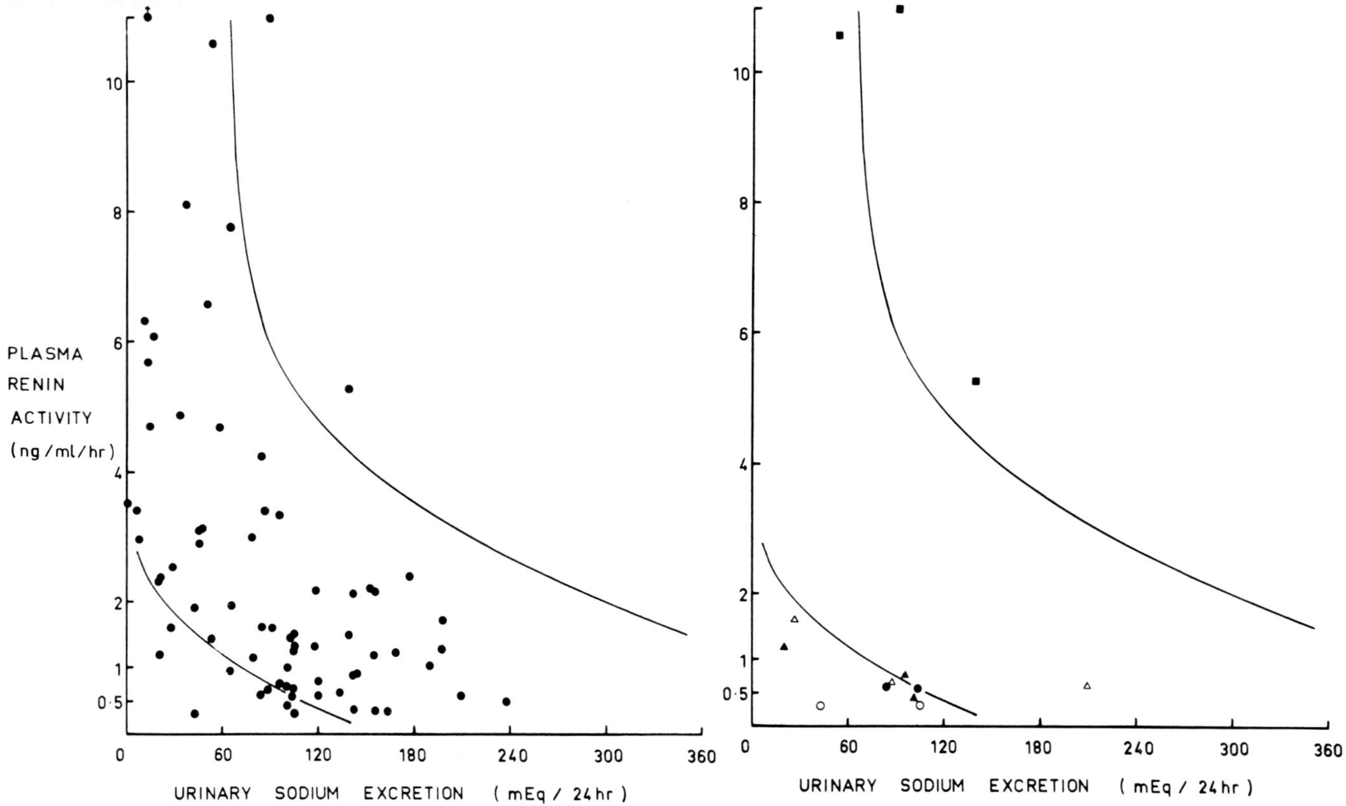

FIG. 3. *Left panel*, Relationship of plasma renin activity to the urinary sodium excretion rate in 27 hypertensive patients (71 determinations). The curves define the limits of the normal control population as shown in Figure 2. *Right panel*, Five patients categorized as "low-renin" or "high-renin" cases are shown separately, each represented by a different symbol.

Table 1. Pretreatment Data and Changes in Weight and Blood Pressure With Treatment in 27 Patients

No.	Sex	Age	Plasma Renin Activity (ng/ml/hr): 100 mEq Na Intake	Plasma Renin Activity (ng/ml/hr): 10 mEq Na Intake	Plasma Renin Activity (ng/ml/hr): Furosemide	Urinary* Aldosterone (μg/d)	Spironolactone: Change† in Mean Blood Pressure (mm Hg)	Spironolactone: Change in Weight (kg)	Propranolol: Change† in Mean Blood Pressure (mm Hg)
1	M	47	1.9	8.2	2.4	n.a.	− 15	− 1.4	− 9
2	F	37	0.6	4.7	1.0	3.7	− 28	− 6.5	− 22
3	F	40	1.5	3.1	3.1	8.5	+ 1	− 1.1	− 16
4	M	52	1.9	7.8	3.2	12.1	+ 2	− 2.7	− 20
5	M	60	3.1	6.3	1.9	7.0	− 4	− 4.4	− 10
6	F	57	1.6	2.3	0.8	4.9	− 32	− 6.2	− 24
7	F	36	1.3	2.5	3.0	7.4	+ 6	− 4.3	+ 7
8	F	50	0.4	3.4	2.3	6.1	− 27	− 1.7	− 12
9	M	59	1.2	n.a.	2.5	10.1	− 18	− 1.2	− 31
10	M	46	0.9	4.9	4.2	5.5	− 16	− 1.3	− 7
11	M	41	0.8	1.2	0.6	10.8	− 8	− 1.3	− 4
12	M	25	1.6	3.5	4.9	n.a.	− 12	− 3.0	− 14
13	M	49	0.4	2.4	5.5	8.5	− 7	− 3.0	− 11
14	M	56	0.3	n.a.	0.4	7.7	− 7	− 3.8	+ 4
15	M	41	1.4	n.a.	6.5	3.8	0	− 1.1	− 3
16	F	41	0.6	n.a.	1.0	8.0	− 18	+ 0.7	− 14
17	F	46	0.7	2.3	1.2	10.0	− 15	− 1.2	− 24
18	M	36	0.6	1.6	1.5	3.9	− 8	− 1.0	− 25
19	M	53	3.4	16.2	3.1	9.6	− 12	− 4.6	− 10
20	F	57	0.8	6.6	3.3	1.7	n.a.	n.a.	− 12
21	M	41	1.4	5.7	2.7	9.3	− 7	− 3.8	− 22
22	M	49	4.2	n.a.	1.8	4.5	+ 5	+ 0.9	− 7
23	M	29	0.9	6.1	1.9	7.6	+ 7	− 0.2	− 13
24	M	58	5.3	10.6	6.9	8.3	− 27	− 3.2	− 44
25	F	36	1.5	2.9	1.0	4.7	− 24	− 1.5	− 31
26	F	40	3.3	n.a.	1.8	18.5	− 2	− 2.0	+ 4
27	M	24	1.3	8.1	3.4	n.a.	− 11	− 0.6	− 24
Mean		45	1.6	5.3	2.7	7.6	− 10.7	− 2.3	− 14.6
S.E.		2	0.2	0.8	0.3	0.7	2.2	0.4	2.2

* Measured in relation to sodium intake of 100 mEq/d.

Urinary aldosterone excretion was within the normal range (3-20μg/d) in the 24 patients tested, including those with low renin values.

Relationships Between Initial Data and Effects of Treatment

Regression analyses of the relationships between initial values for PRA (Table 1) and averaged responses to treatment with spironolactone or propranolol did not reveal any significant correlations, nor were these responses significantly related to the initial rate of urinary aldosterone excretion ($r = -0.17$ to $+0.14$). However, there was a degree of correlation between pretreatment PRA and propranolol-induced changes in blood pressure at the end of two weeks of treatment. This reached a level of statistical significance only in the case of renin levels determined on a free diet (Table 2). No correlations were found between PRA and blood pressure decrements at four or six weeks.

Attempts were made to divide the patients into low- and normal-renin groups on the basis of furosemide-stimulated PRA. Only two patients had values less than the lowest value in the normal control group, which was 0.7 ng/ml/hr. Both these patients (no. 11 and 14) showed little response to spironolactone. If the lowest of the 18 values comprising the control range was excluded, the lower limit became 1.7 ng/ml/hr. Eight patients had values lower than 1.7 ng/ml/hr. The mean decrease in blood pressure with spironolactone in this subgroup was 18 mm Hg, which was significantly greater ($p < 0.025$) than that in the remainder of the hypertensive group (8 mm Hg). The decrease in blood pressure with propranolol, however, also

Table 2. Correlations Between Pretreatment PRA (x) and Propranolol-Induced Blood Pressure Responses (y)

x (PRA)	*y*	*Correlation Coefficient (r) of Relationship Between x and y*		
		at 2 Weeks	*at 4 Weeks*	*at 6 Weeks*
1. With free diet	Effect	– 0.60**	– 0.28	– 0.22
2. With 100 mEq Na intake	Effect	– 0.31	– 0.01	+ 0.04
3. With 10 mEq Na intake	Effect	– 0.42*	+ 0.12	– 0.04

** $p < 0.001$ * $0.05 < p < 0.1$

averaged 18 mm Hg in the low-renin subgroup, an effect which was slightly, but not significantly, greater than in the remainder.

Patients characterized as "low-renin" by the nomogram (Fig. 3) showed decreases in mean blood pressure averaging 10 mm Hg with both propranolol and spironolactone. These values did not differ significantly from responses in patients within the normal limits on the nomogram. The sole "high-renin" patient had a greater response to propranolol than any other patient, but also responded strongly to spironolactone.

Patients were ranked according to pretreatment PRA, and comparisons were made between the blood pressure responses to treatment at either end of the ranked series. Using the Wilcoxon rank-sum test, no significant differences were found between the low-renin and the high-renin ends of the series, although the antihypertensive effect of spironolactone appeared somewhat greater ($p > 0.05$, n.s.) in the seven patients with the lowest renin values than in the seven with the highest renin values (Fig. 4).

There was a significant correlation ($r = 0.57$; $p < 0.01$) between antihypertensive responses to spironolactone and propranolol (Fig. 5). The relative responsiveness of each patient to one or the other medication, irrespective of the initial severity of hypertension, was estimated by the distance of the relevant point in Figure 5 from the regression line. No significant relationship was found between these distances (taken with respect to sign) and initial PRA ($r = 0.23$; $p > 0.1$).

Side Effects of Therapy

At the end of each treatment segment the patients were questioned specifically regarding the symptoms numbered 1-11 in Table 3. Symptoms noted during a phase of active medication were discounted if they were also reported during the placebo phase. The last three symptoms in Table 3 were volunteered. Minor side effects, well known to be associated with spironolactone or propranolol, occurred in all patients. Those side effects severe enough to require reduction or suspension of active medication were, in the case of spironolactone, nausea (two patients), palpitations (one), dizziness (one) or muscle cramps (one); and in the case of propranolol, insomnia (two) or nausea (one). Soreness of the breasts was

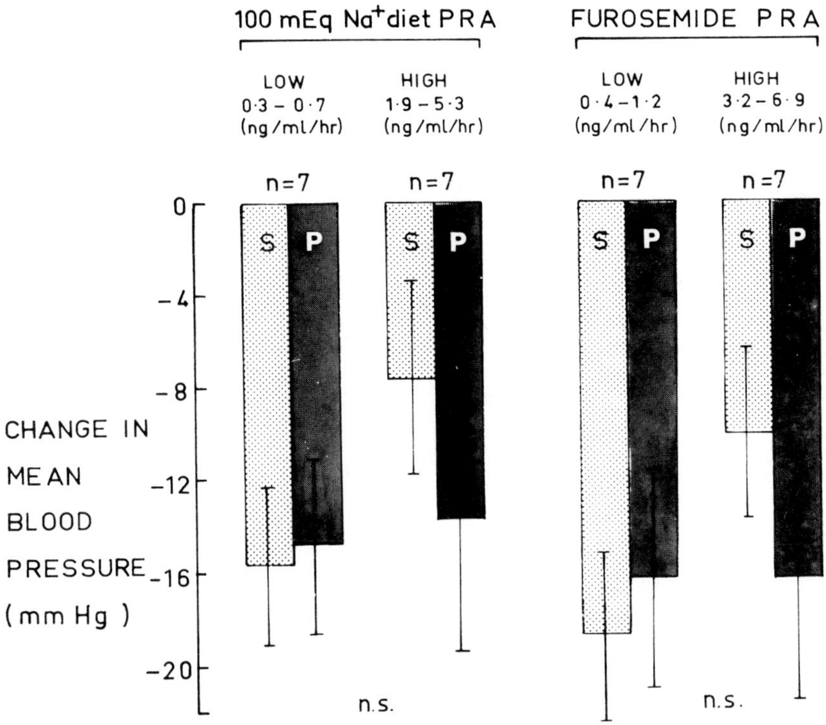

FIG. 4. Changes in mean blood pressure in relation to treatment with spironolactone (S) or propranolol (P) in subgroups defined by ranking patients according to pretreatment plasma renin activity. There were no significant differences in therapeutic responses between "low-renin" and "high-renin" subgroups (each of seven patients) at the extremities of the ranked series.

reported by three patients, but only one of these was a male. In his case, the symptom was first noted during propranolol treatment 12 weeks after finishing the spironolactone phase. Analysis of his plasma at that time showed no detectable level of aldadiene.

Discussion

In this double-blind crossover trial in patients with mild to moderate essential hypertension, no significant continuous relationship was found between the pretreatment levels of PRA

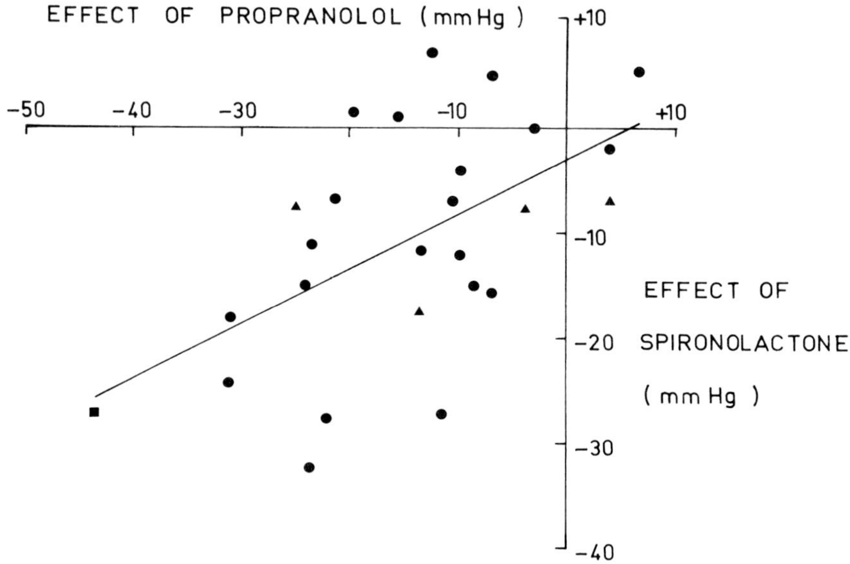

FIG. 5. Regression of antihypertensive effect of spironolactone on antihypertensive effect of propranolol in 27 hypertensive patients, classified by nomogram analysis (Fig. 3) as "low-renin" (▲), "high-renin" (■) or "normal-renin" (●). $Y = 0.52x + 3.0$; $r = 0.57$ ($p < 0.01$).

Table 3. Side Effects of Therapy

	Number of Patients	
	*Aldactone**	*Inderal†*
1. Dizziness or faintness	2	1
2. Nausea or indigestion	8	2
3. Diarrhea	0	2
4. Drowsiness or lassitude	6	6
5. Insomnia or disturbance of sleep rhythm	1	6
6. Nightmares	2	5
7. Depression	4	1
8. Soreness of breasts	1	2
9. Palpitations	4	1
10. Impotence	0	0
11. Wheezing or dyspnea	1	2
12. Paraesthesia	0	5
13. Cramps	4	0
14. Constipation	2	0

* spironolactone, 200-400 mg/day
† propranolol, 160-320 mg/day

and the chronic therapeutic effects of spironolactone or propranolol, whether the clinical protocol used for obtaining samples for determining PRA entailed administration of furosemide, a low-sodium diet, a sodium intake of 100 mEq/day or a free diet. This observation is in agreement with those of Hunyor et al [11] regarding spironolactone and Birkenhager et al [12], Hansson [13], Bravo et al [14], Dorhout Mees et al [15] and Leonetti et al [16] in regard to propranolol. It also agrees with our previous findings in an open study with propranolol [17]. A significant correlation was found between regular diet PRA and propanolol-induced decrements in blood pressure after two weeks, but not after four or six weeks of treatment; a similar trend, of lesser statistical significance, existed with regard to PRA on 100 mEq or low-sodium diets. These observations suggest that the early, but not the chronic antihypertensive response to propranolol could bear some relationship to pretreatment PRA.* However, no significant correlation could be found between the changes in PRA and changes in mean blood pressure with propranolol, reinforcing the impression gained from other studies [14, 18] that suppression of PRA is not the main mechanism by which beta-adrenergic blocking drugs reduce blood pressure.

There are certain factors which could disguise the presence of significant relationships between possible response-predictive parameters, such as PRA, and drug-induced changes in blood pressure.

Vagaries in the taking of medicine and variations in the absorption and metabolism of drugs are obvious difficulties. The plasma concentration of propranolol and the spironolactone derivative observed in patients in this study (mean levels 137 ng/ml and 16μg/100 ml, respectively) were for the most part within the ranges appropriate to the doses given which are about 100 ng/ml [19] and about 5-20μg/100 ml [9]. An attempt was made to monitor the patients' compliance in taking their medications and to increase their motivation in this regard by dispensing more than the requisite number of tablets and counting the remainder at the next visit. For the spironolactone phase of treatment, a low, but significant degree of correlation

*See observations of Corvol et al elsewhere in this volume.

was found between the net supply of medication and the plasma level of spironolactone derivative. Predictably, there was no significant relationship between plasma levels and drug intake during the propranolol phase [19].

Another factor which may interfere with the proper assessment of individual responses is a time-related change in the baseline from which specific therapeutic effects are measured. Common examples of this are the orientating reflex [20], the placebo response and diet-induced change in body weight. However, the design of the present trial, which included a placebo run-in phase, a placebo control period and randomization of treatment sequences, should have mitigated such problems.

A more subtle difficulty is the possibility that receptor sensitivity to endogenous angiotensin may vary from patient to patient [21], tending to obscure any relationship existing between initial PRA values and the blood pressure responses resulting from reduced renin-angiotensin activity. A similar problem arises when trying to predict therapeutic responses in terms of the vasoconstriction-volume hypothesis in low-renin states. An attempt to overcome this problem was made by quantitating the polarization of therapeutic responsiveness (toward either spironolactone or propranolol — see Figure 5) and determining its relationship to initial PRA levels. However, no significant association emerged from the use of this discriminant.

Previous workers have concentrated their attention on comparisons between low-renin and high-renin subgroups of patients, segregated by various strategies from hypertensive populations.

Thus, Carey et al [4], employing furosemide to stimulate PRA, identified patients with PRA below the normal range and compared their responses to spironolactone with those of patients having normal or high PRA. In a pilot study, we found the doses of furosemide which they used (totalling 120 mg at home, overnight) were too great for routine use in outpatients, for several subjects of the test arrived faint and exhausted from protracted nocturia. However, two doses of 40 mg given nine hours apart were found to produce a brisk effect in a group of normal subjects and this protocol was used in the present study.

Within-patient responses were found to be disappointingly variable. Nevertheless, the stimulatory effect of furosemide on PRA was shown to be significantly less in the patient group than in the normal controls. Disregarding one exceptionally low control value, eight of 27 patients were found to have furosemide-stimulated levels of PRA lower than the control range. The responses to spironolactone in these patients were significantly greater than in the remainder; however, they responded well to propranolol, too. In the former respect, but not the latter, our results are in partial agreement with those of Karlberg et al [22], who also carried out a crossover trial with spironolactone and propranolol. Using a method of analysis similar to theirs, we found that if the seven patients with the lowest initial renin values were compared with the seven having the highest values, the low-renin group response was the greater. However, this difference failed to reach the 5% level of significance by nonparametric testing, as did the smaller mean differences existing between larger subgroups at opposite ends of the renin scale. No differences at all were found in responsiveness to propranolol between low- and high-renin subgroups.

Use of a nomogram, as described by Bühler et al [5], separated off five patients with PRA distinctly higher or lower than the normal range. It is not surprising that only one patient was characterized as a high-renin case, since patients with very high PRA, who usually have severe or renovascular hypertension, were most uncommon in the Australian population from which the patients in the present study were sampled [23]. The relatively small number of low-renin patients, 15% (4 out of 27) compared to 28% in the series of Bühler et al [5], may be due to the presence in their study population of an appreciable proportion of black subjects, who have a much higher incidence of low-renin hypertension than white [24, 25]. The number of patients who were defined as potential propranolol responders or nonresponders by the criteria of Bühler et al [5] was too small for meaningful statistical analysis. However, it is noteworthy that although the solitary "high-renin" patient and two of the "low-renin" patients were classified correctly as a responder and nonresponders, respectively, the other two "low-renin" patients showed useful therapeutic responses to propranolol (Fig. 5).

Ultimately, the crucial question to be answered is whether PRA, determined by any simple protocol, should be used routinely in the clinic to predict patients' responses to therapy. Our findings suggest that in a Caucasian population, the proportion of patients in whom specific responses can be predicted by PRA is too small to justify the effort and expense involved. The subgroup of eight "low-renin" patients who were correctly classified by furosemide-stimulated PRA as spironolactone responders, also responded to propranolol, while only three of the five patients who could be clearly characterized by nomogram analysis were classified correctly. Thus, PRA appears to be a poor marker in predicting therapeutic responses by a vasoconstriction-volume analysis.

Summary

Twenty-seven patients in whom hypertension had been newly discovered by survey were treated with spironolactone, 200-400 mg/day for six weeks, and propranolol, 160-320 mg/day for six weeks, in a double-blind crossover trial. The antihypertensive effects of treatment, given in randomized sequences, were assessed by comparison with observations during a placebo period. Pretreatment levels of erect PRA were determined by four different protocols: in relation to the 24-hour urinary sodium excretion without dietary restriction; with furosemide stimulation; and at 100 mEq and 10 mEq levels of dietary sodium intake. No significant continuous relationships were found between pretreatment levels or treatment-induced changes in PRA and the chronic therapeutic effects of spironolactone or propranolol. A "low-renin" subgroup of eight patients, identified by the use of furosemide, was found to have increased responsiveness to spironolactone, but this drug also had useful antihypertensive effects in as many patients with normal or high PRA. No consistent differences were found in responses to propranolol between "low-renin" and "high-renin" subgroups. The results indicate that irrespective of the clinical protocol used for determining PRA, the proportion of Caucasian patients in whom specific antihypertensive effects could be predicted by PRA was too small to justify the routine measurement of initial plasma renin levels.

Acknowledgments

Our thanks are due to Mrs. L. Stoker, Mrs. E. Love, Mr. I. Thornell, Mrs. M. Marinkovic and Miss D. Lissner for technical assistance, to Searle (Australia) for aldadiene measurements and to the Biochemistry Department, Sydney Hospital (Dr. Frank Neale), for electrolyte measurements. We also thank Mrs. J. Gentle for arranging the diets and Dr. Helen Oates, Dr. R. Graham and Dr. R. Lewis for reviewing the manuscript.

This paper was prepared with the assistance of the physicians of the Cardiovascular Clinic, Sydney Hospital: Dr. G. E. Bauer, Dr. D. Jeremy, Dr. R. G. Lewis, Dr. I. McLachlan, Dr. S. Mitchell, Dr. G. Nyberg, Dr. J. Raftos and Dr. A. A. Young.

References

1. Laragh, J.H.: Vasoconstriction-volume analysis for understanding and treating hypertension. The use of renin and aldosterone profiles. Am. J. Med. 55:261, 1973.
2. Crane, M.G. and Harris, J.J.: Effect of spironolactone in hypertensive patients. Am. J. Med. Sci. 260:311, 1970.
3. Spark, R.F. and Melby, J.C.: Hypertension and low plasma renin activity: Presumptive evidence for mineralocorticoid excess. Ann. Intern. Med. 75:831, 1971.
4. Carey, R.M., Douglas, J.G., Schweikert, J.R. et al: The syndrome of essential hypertension and suppressed plasma renin activity. Arch. Intern. Med. 130:849, 1972.
5. Bühler, F.R., Laragh, J.H., Baer, L. et al: Propranolol inhibition of renin secretion: A specific approach to diagnosis and treatment of renin-dependent hypertensive diseases. N. Engl. J. Med. 287:1209, 1972.
6. Haber, E., Koerner, T., Page, L.B. et al: Application of a radioimmunoassay for angiotensin I to the physiologic measurements of plasma renin activity in normal human subjects. J. Clin. Endocrinol. Metab. 29:1349, 1969.
7. Wilkinson, R., Luetscher, J.A. and Nokes, G.W.: Iodination of angiotensin I for use in radioimmunoassay. J. Clin. Endocrinol. Metab. 33:545, 1971.
8. Coghlan, J.P. and Scoggins, B.A.: Measurement of aldosterone in peripheral blood of man and sheep. J. Clin. Endocrinol. Metab. 27:1470, 1967.
9. Gochman, N. and Gantt, C.L.: A fluorometric method for the determination of a major spironolactone (Aldactone) metabolite in human plasma. J. Pharmacol. Exp. Ther. 135:312, 1962.
10. Shand, D.G., Nuckolls, E.M. and Oates, J.A.: Plasma propranolol

levels in adults with observations in four children. Clin. Pharmacol. Ther. 11:112, 1970.

11. Hunyor, S.N., Zweifler, A.J., Hansson, L. et al: Effect of high dose spironolactone and chlorthalidone in essential hypertension: Relation to plasma renin activity and plasma volume. Aust. New Zeal. J. Med. 5:17, 1975.
12. Birkenhäger, W.H., Krauss, X.H., Schalekamp, M.A.D.H. et al: Antihypertensive effects of propranolol. Folia Med. Neerl. 14:67, 1971.
13. Hansson, L.: Beta-adrenergic blockade in essential hypertension. Effects of propranolol on hemodynamic parameters and plasma renin activity. Acta Med. Scand. Supplementum 550, pp. 1-40, 1973.
14. Bravo, E.L., Tarazi, R.C., Dustan, H.P. et al: Dissociation between renin and arterial pressure responses in beta-adrenergic blockade in human essential hypertension. Circ. Res. 36 and 37 (suppl. 1): 241, 1975.
15. Dorhout Mees, E.J., Geyskes, G.G., Vos, J. et al: Observations of the role of body fluid volumes and plasma renin activity in the management of hypertension. Arch. Int. Pharmacodyn. 214:335, 1975.
16. Leonetti, G., Mayer, G., Morganti, A. et al: Hypotensive and renin-suppressing activities of propranolol in hypertensive patients. Clin. Sci. Molec. Med. 48:491, 1975.
17. Stokes, G.S., Weber, M.A., Thornell, I.R. et al: Effects of acute and chronic administration of propranolol on blood pressure and plasma renin activity in hypertensive patients. *In* Edwards, K.D.G. (ed.): Drugs and the Kidney, Progress in Biochemistry and Pharmacology, 9, Basel: Karger, 1974, pp. 29-44.
18. Stokes, G.S., Weber, M.A. and Thornell, I.R.: β-blockers and plasma renin activity in hypertension. Br. Med. J. 1:60, 1974.
19. Shand, D.G.: Individualization of propranolol therapy. Med. Clin. N. Am. 58:1063, 1974.
20. Pickering, G.: High Blood Pressure, ed. 2. London: J. and A. Churchill Ltd., 1968, pp. 36-37, 395.
21. Pinto, B., Guasch, J. and Caralps, A.: Increased activity of a factor ("transferangiotensin") favoring the binding of angiotensin II to arterial wall in hypertension. Kidney International, 6:109, 1974.
22. Karlberg, B.E., Tegler, L. and Tolagen, K.: Essential hypertension: Therapeutic response to propranolol-spironolactone-placebo with reference to initial plasma renin levels. From Hypertension Symposium, Saltsjöbaden, Sept. 1974. Am. J. Med. (In press.)
23. Weber, M.A., Stokes, G.S., Moses, M. et al: Hypertension survey in a central city free chest X-ray clinic: The Sydney Hospital hypertension project. Med. J. Aust. 2:529, 1973.
24. Brunner, H.R., Laragh, J.H., Baer, L. et al: Essential hypertension: Renin and aldosterone, heart attack and stroke. N. Engl. J. Med. 286:441, 1972.
25. Kilcoyne, M.M., Thomson, G.E., Branche, G. et al: Characteristics of hypertension in the black population. Circulation 50:1006, 1974.

Discussion

Moderator: Dr. J. Genest

Dr. Johnston: Perhaps I should make a few comments, because the paper that I presented in Milan in 1972 has been twice misquoted. I like to think that this is so probably because it was edited in Italian. The first thing is that we did not demonstrate in that study that the fall in blood pressure correlated with the renin. What we did demonstrate was that patients treated with beta blockers had their blood pressure controlled and their plasma renin fell. I do not think that we would disagree with what Dr. Zanchetti has presented today, but there are important differences between your very well controlled study and our fairly random study of levels of plasma renin and angiotensin. For example, our patients were not on diuretics alone: Of the 176 patients, the vast majority received many other antihypertensive drugs.

Second, they had all been treated for at least three months, some for as long as up to two years, on a variety of drug regimes.

My third point is that they were mostly receiving chlorothiazide or cyclopentothiazide, because in our hands chlorthalidone at the dosage of 100 mg/day is fairly poisonous and we had to abandon one study because of extreme hypokalemia in the patients despite potassium supplements. Do you think that some of your high renin responses to the diuretic were achieved by stimulation by low plasma potassium?

Dr. Zanchetti: Of course, all of our patients also had their serum potassium measured. I do not have the statistical data with me today. There was some decrease in serum potassium but not to too low values. If I remember correctly they were on the average 3.8 or 3.9 mEq/L. All of our patients also received other drugs beyond chlorthalidone. The chlorthalidone dose varied among patients but seldom exceeded 50 mg/day. Certainly chlorthalidone is a stronger diuretic agent than are thiazides and this might explain why our renin stimulating effect was longer lasting than your study showed.

May I add that the paper you presented in Milan was not edited in Italy but in England. An Italian wouldn't have dared to change an Australian's English, but an Englishman was certainly pleased to.

Effects of Antihypertensive Agents on Blood Pressure and Renin in Severe Experimental Renal Hypertension

Michael Fernandes, M.D., Gaddo Onesti, M.D., Roman Dykyj, Anne B. Gould, Ph.D., Roberto Fiorentini, M.D.,* Kwan E. Kim, M.D. and Charles Swartz, M.D.

Mechanisms responsible for the induction and maintenance of hypertension involve the interaction of several systems [1]. In experimental renal hypertension, multiple mechanisms have been proposed: activation of the renin-angiotensin system [2-6]; autoregulation [1, 4, 7, 8]; alterations in body fluid distribution [9, 10]; activation of the adrenergic nervous system [11]; secretion of a renal vasopressor factor other than renin [12-14]; and failure of the kidney to exert a vasopressor function [15, 16].

The therapeutic approach to hypertension has included (1) diuretics, (2) peripheral vasodilators and (3) inhibition of adrenergic transmission at different sites.

The precise effect of different antihypertensive agents on different pathophysiologic mechanisms remains uncertain in the majority of instances.

Supported by the National Institutes of Health Grant #1-RO-1-HL-14588 and The Southeastern Pennsylvania Chapter of the American Heart Association.

Michael Fernandes, M.D. Gaddo Onesti, M.D., Roman Dykyj, Anne B. Gould, Ph.D., Roberto Fiorentini, M.D., Kwan E. Kim, M.D. and Charles Swartz, M.D., The Division of Nephrology and Hypertension, Department of Medicine, Hahnemann Medical College and Hospital, Philadelphia, Pa.

*Present address: Istituto di Patologia Medica, Universita Cattolica, Rome, Italy.

Of all factors possibly responsible for renal hypertension, the renin-angiotensin system has been the one most widely studied. The effects of antihypertensive agents on renin release have also received considerable attention [17].

It is the purpose of the present study to investigate the effect of three different pharmacologic agents on the blood pressure and plasma renin concentration in a rat model of severe experimental renal hypertension.

For this purpose, the experimental model of total ligation of the aorta between the renal arteries was used. This model was selected because of the precise reproducibility of blood pressure elevation and renin patterns at its different phases [18]. This allows the comparison of the effect of each drug on renin and blood pressure during the onset, as well as early and chronic phases.

The pharmacologic agents studied were furosemide, hydralazine and propranolol.

Materials and Methods

Male Sprague-Dawley rats weighing 300-350 gm were used. They were maintained on standard Purina chow and tap water ad libitum.

Hypertension was produced by complete constriction of the aorta between the renal arteries just below the origin of the superior mesenteric artery. Arterial pressure (systolic, diastolic and mean) and heart rate were measured through an indwelling teflon-tygon catheter inserted in the left common carotid artery and exteriorized at the neck [18]. A miniature pressure transducer* and direct writing recorder† were used.

Blood pressure and heart rate were measured in the conscious unrestrained animal moving freely in the cage.

At the time of blood pressure recording, 1 ml of blood for renin determination was withdrawn from the arterial catheter into chilled heparinized tubes. Plasma renin concentration was determined by the method of Gould [19].

Following aortic constriction, animals were allocated to designated periods (days 3, 5, 12, 20, 30 and 40). Carotid

---

*RP-1500, Narco Biosystems, Houston, Tex.

†DMP 4A Physiograph Narco Biosystems, Houston, Tex.

cannulation was performed 24 hours before blood pressure and renin determinations were made.

Drug therapy was initiated 15 days prior to aortic constriction and continued thereafter until termination of the experiment.

Furosemide was administered in the drinking water in a concentration of 300 mg/liter. This dose was calculated to be 36 mg/kg/day.

Hydralazine was administered in the drinking water in a concentration of 250 mg/liter. The dose was calculated to be 30 mg/kg/day.

Propranolol was administered in two doses. The low dose (3 mg/kg/day) was administered in two intraperitoneal injections of 0.5 mg given 12 hours apart. Propranolol was also administered to another group in the drinking water (500 mg/liter). This dose was calculated to be 60 mg/kg/day.

Following blood pressure recording and withdrawal of blood for renin determination, the rats were weighed, sacrificed and examined for possible renal infarctions. Rats with evidence of renal infarction were not considered.

The heart was removed, the atria excised and the ventricles flushed with saline and then blotted dry. Wet weight of the ventricles was determined in a Mettler precision balance. Ventricular weight was expressed as milligrams per gram body weight.

Five groups of animals were studied: (1) a control group with no antihypertensive drugs; (2) a hydralazine group; (3) a furosemide group; (4) a group treated with low doses of propranolol; and (5) a group treated with high doses of propranolol.

Results

Treatment With Furosemide

Ligation of the aorta resulted in sustained increase in blood pressure. The increase in blood pressure recorded in the furosemide-treated group was significantly less than in the control animals at all phases (Table 1, Fig. 1A).

Heart rate in the two groups is reported in Table 1. At the baseline evaluation, heart rate was lower in the furosemide-treated group. It was similar in the two groups at days 3 and 5.

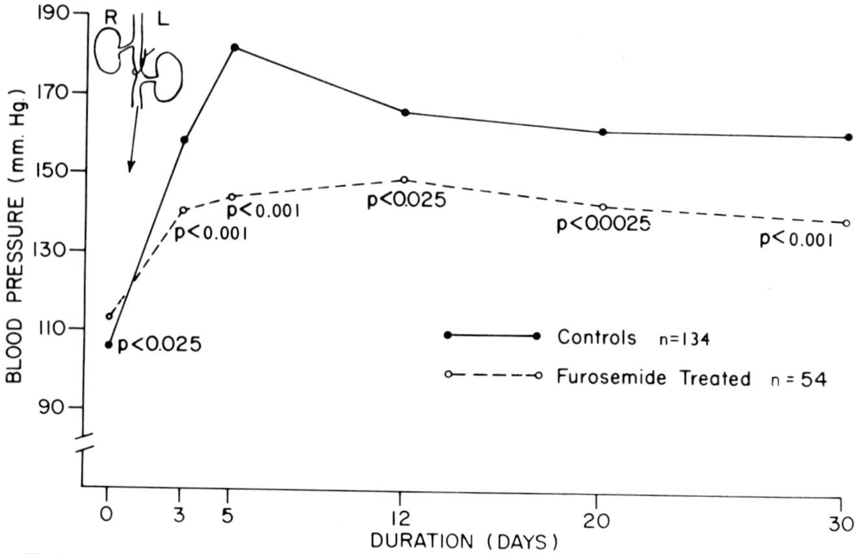

FIG. 1A. Effect of furosemide (36 mg/kg/day) on average mean arterial pressure in conscious renal hypertensive rats.

At days 12, 20 and 30, it was found again significantly lower in the treated group (Table 1).

Baseline peripheral plasma renin concentrations were similar in the two groups. In the untreated control, plasma renin concentration was significantly increased 3, 5 and 12 days after aortic ligation with maximum increase at day 5. Three, 5, 12 and 20 days after aortic ligation, plasma renin concentration was significantly lower in the furosemide-treated group. Thirty days after aortic ligation, plasma renin concentrations had returned to baseline; in addition, no differences between the two groups were detected (Table 1, Fig. 1B).

Treatment With Hydralazine

Baseline mean arterial pressures were similar in the hydralazine-treated and the control group. In the hydralazine-treated group, the increase in blood pressure which followed ligation of the aorta was significantly less than in the untreated control on days 3, 5, 12, 20 and 30 (Table 2, Fig. 2A). Moreover, on day 30 the mean arterial pressure in the

Table 1. Effects of Furosemide (36 mg/Kg/day) on Blood Pressure, Heart Rate and Plasma Renin Concentration in Conscious Renal Hypertensive Rats (C = Control, F = Furosemide-Treated)

Days After Aortic Ligation	*0*	*3*	*5*	*12*	*20*	*30*
Number	C = 20 F = 10	C = 21 F = 11	C = 25 F = 9	C = 24 F = 24	C = 24 F = 7	C = 20 F = 9
Mean arterial pressure (mm Hg)	C 106 ± 6.8	C 157 ± 18.69	C 182 ± 14.4	C 166 ± 20.15	C 161 ± 10.85	C 161 ± 10.62
	F 113 ± 11.9	F 140 ± 12.64	F 144 ± 12.82	F 149 ± 11.9	F 143 ± 16.36	F 134 ± 12.92
	$p < 0.025$	$p < 0.001$	$p < 0.001$	$p < 0.025$	$p < 0.0025$	$p < 0.001$
Heart rate (Beats/min)	C 408 ± 52	C 388 ± 13.6	C 424 ± 54.6	C 407 ± 51	C 391 ± 35	C 385 ± 42
	F 352 ± 67	F 375 ± 48	F 423 ± 34	F 355 ± 42	F 334 ± 34	F 353 ± 30
	$p < 0.125$	n.s.	n.s.	$p < 0.005$	$p < 0.001$	$p < 0.05$
Plasma renin concentration ($\times 10^{-4}$ G.U.)	C 0.92 ±0.37	C 3.68 ±0.75	C 8.68 ±6.1	C 3.02 ±2.0	C 1.68 ±0.82	C 0.95 ±0.4
	F 0.93 ±0.5	F 2.24 ±1.4	F 1.85 ±0.8	F 1.71 ±1.6	F 0.87 ±0.5	F 0.91 ±0.3
	n.s.	$p < 0.001$	$p < 0.001$	$p < 0.0125$	$p < 0.0125$	n.s.

Values are Means ± S.D.

hydralazine-treated group was not different from the baseline. Thus, hydralazine resulted in a return of blood pressure to normal at this phase.

Heart rate did not show any consistent differences in the two groups (Table 2).

In the hydralazine-treated group, ligation of the aorta resulted in a significant increase in peripheral plasma renin concentration at days 3 and 5. Such an increase, however, was much less pronounced than in the untreated controls (Fig. 2B). In contrast, at days 20 and 30, peripheral plasma renin concentration was higher in the hydralazine-treated group.

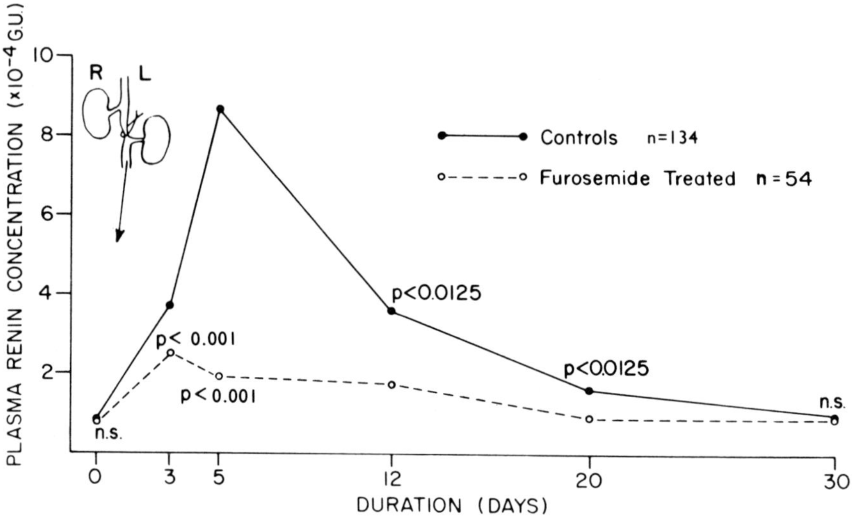

FIG. 1B. Effect of furosemide (36 mg/kg/day) on average plasma renin concentration in conscious renal hypertensive rats.

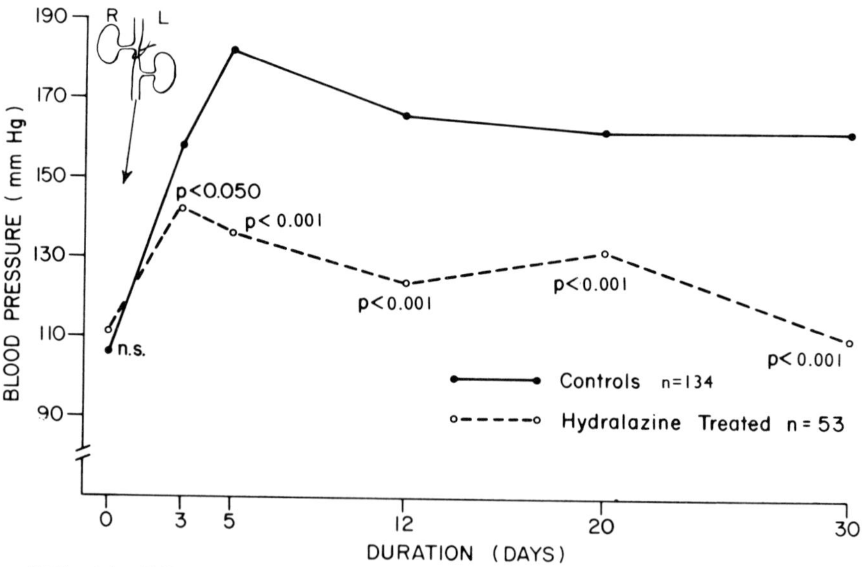

FIG. 2A. Effect of hydralazine (30 mg/kg/day) on average mean arterial pressure in conscious renal hypertensive rats.

Table 2. Effects of Hydralazine (30 mg/Kg/day) on Blood Pressure, Heart Rate and Plasma Renin Concentration in Conscious Renal Hypertensive Rats (C = Control, H = Hydralazine-Treated)

Days After Aortic Ligation	*0*	*3*	*5*	*12*	*20*	*30*
Number	C = 20 H = 11	C = 21 H = 7	C = 25 H = 6	C = 24 H = 13	C = 24 H = 12	C = 20 H = 5
Mean arterial pressure (mm Hg)	C 106 ± 6.8	C 157 ± 18.7	C 182 ± 14.4	C 166 ± 20.2	C 161 ± 10.8	C 161 ± 10.6
	H 111 ± 13.4	H 142 ± 13.13	H 137 ± 13.17	H 124 ± 17.3	H 132 ± 17.5	H 110 ± 10.8
	n.s.	$p < 0.05$	$p < 0.001$	$p < 0.001$	$p < 0.001$	$p < 0.001$
Heart rate (Beats/min)	C 408 ± 52	C 388 ± 13.6	C 424 ± 54.6	C 407 ± 51	C 391 ± 35	C 385 ± 42
	H 346 ± 38	H 374 ± 64	H 411 ± 39	H 448 ± 39	H 398 ± 56	H 404 ± 47
	$p < 0.0025$	n.s.	n.s.	$p < 0.0125$	n.s.	n.s.
Plasma renin concentration (× 10^{-4} G.U.)	C 0.92 ±0.4	C 3.68 ±0.8	C 8.68 ±6.1	C 3.02 ±2.0	C 1.68 ±0.8	C 0.95 ±0.4
	H 0.31 ±0.3	H 2.3 ±2.4	H 2.67 ±1.4	H 2.8 ±1.9	H 2.74 ±1.8	H 3.4 ±1.5
	$p < 0.001$	$p < 0.05$	$p < 0.025$	n.s.	$p < 0.025$	$p < 0.001$

Values are Means ± S.D.

Treatment With Propranolol (Low Dose)

Baseline mean arterial pressure was significantly higher in the propranolol-treated group as compared with the untreated animals (Table 3, Fig. 3A). Three, 5, 12 and 20 days after aortic constriction, mean arterial pressure was equally severe in the two groups. At day 30, mean arterial pressure was slightly but significantly higher in the treated group (Fig. 3A).

Heart rate did not show any consistent difference in the two groups.

Baseline peripheral plasma renin concentration was lower in the propranolol-treated group ($p < 0.005$) (Table 3, Fig. 3B).

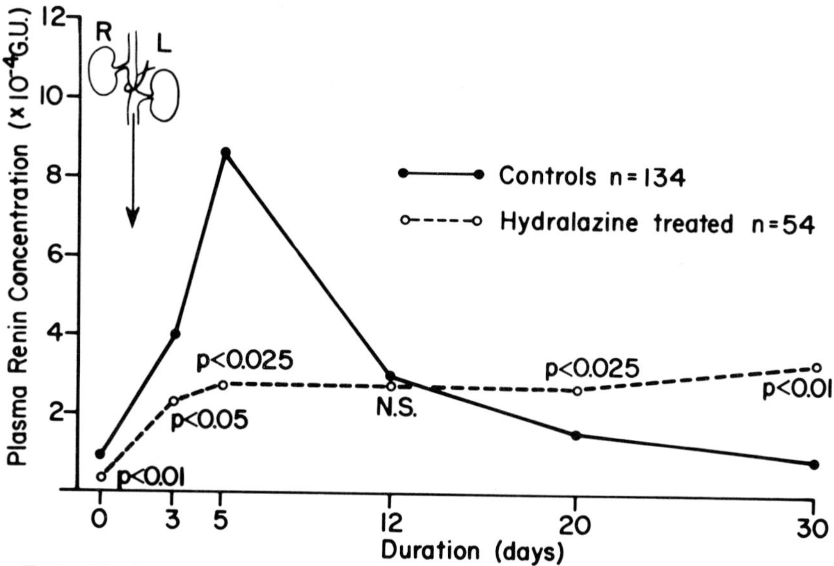

FIG. 2B. Effect of hydralazine (30 mg/kg/day) on average plasma renin concentration in conscious renal hypertensive rats.

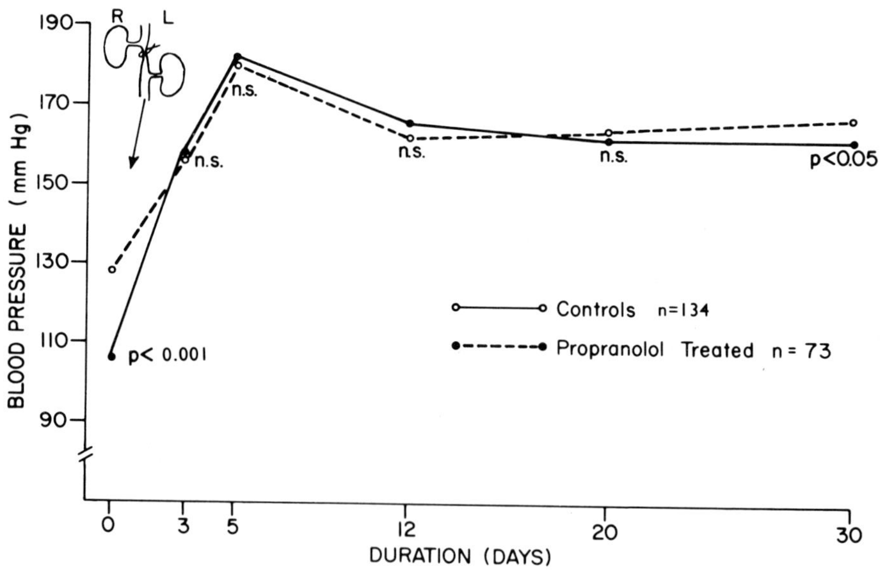

FIG. 3A. Effect of propranolol (3 mg/kg/day) on average mean arterial pressure in conscious renal hypertensive rats.

Table 3. Effects of Propranolol (3 mg/Kg/day) on Blood Pressure, Heart Rate and Plasma Renin Concentration in Conscious Renal Hypertensive Rats (C = Control, P = Propranolol-Treated)

Days After Aortic Ligation	*0*	*3*	*5*	*12*	*20*	*30*
Number	C = 20 P = 11	C = 21 P = 12	C = 25 P = 12	C = 24 P = 20	C = 24 P = 10	C = 20 P = 7
Mean arterial pressure (mm Hg)	C 106 ± 6.8	C 157 ± 18.69	C 182 ± 14.4	C 166 ± 20.15	C 161 ± 10.85	C 161 ± 10.62
	P 129 ± 7.9	P 157 ± 10.4	P 178 ± 14.4	P 162 ± 12.45	P 159 ± 22.5	P 170 ± 16.9
	$p < 0.001$	n.s.	n.s.	n.s.	n.s.	$p < 0.05$
Heart rate (Beats/min)	C 408 ± 52	C 388 ± 13.6	C 424 ± 54.6	C 407 ± 51	C 391 ± 35	C 385 ± 42
	P 395 ± 40	P 333 ± 75	P 385 ± 51	P 400 ± 41	P 354 ± 47	P 355 ± 64
	n.s.	$p < 0.0025$	$p < 0.025$	n.s.	$p < 0.015$	n.s.
Plasma renin concentration ($\times 10^{-4}$ G.U.)	C 0.92 ±0.4	C 3.68 ±0.8	C 8.68 ±6.1	C 3.02 ±2.0	C 1.68 ±0.8	C 0.95 ±0.4
	P 0.55 ±0.3	P 2.68 ±2.3	P 4.55 ±2.2	P 2.86 ±2.0	P 2.11 ±1.6	P 1.30 ±0.7
	$p < 0.005$	$p < 0.05$	$p < 0.025$	n.s.	n.s.	n.s.

Values are Means ± S.D.

Aortic ligation resulted in an increase in peripheral plasma renin concentration in both groups at days 3, 5, 12 and 20. The magnitude of renin increase was much less in the propranolol-treated group as compared to the untreated controls during the early phase at days 3 and 5. At day 30, peripheral plasma renin concentrations had returned to baseline values in both groups. In addition, no differences between the two groups were recognized at this phase.

Treatment with Propranolol (High Dose)

Baseline mean arterial pressure was significantly higher in the propranolol-treated group (Table 4, Fig. 4A). The increase

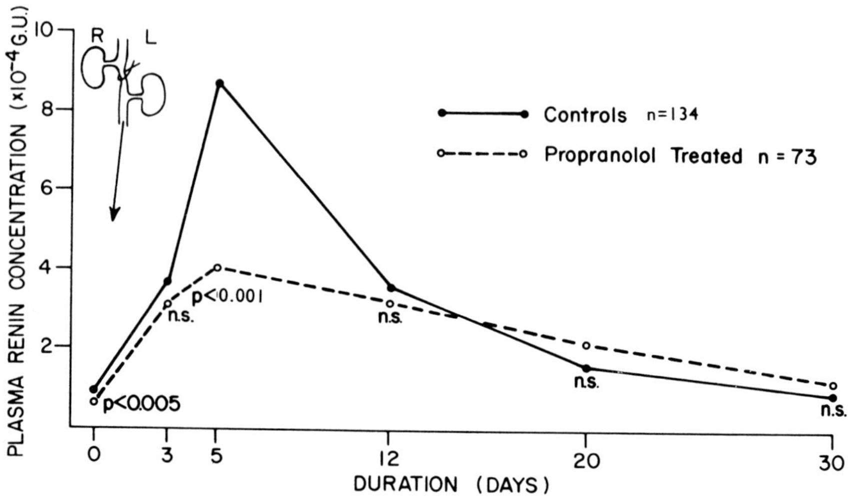

FIG. 3B. Effect of propranolol (3 mg/kg/day) on average plasma renin concentration in conscious renal hypertensive rats.

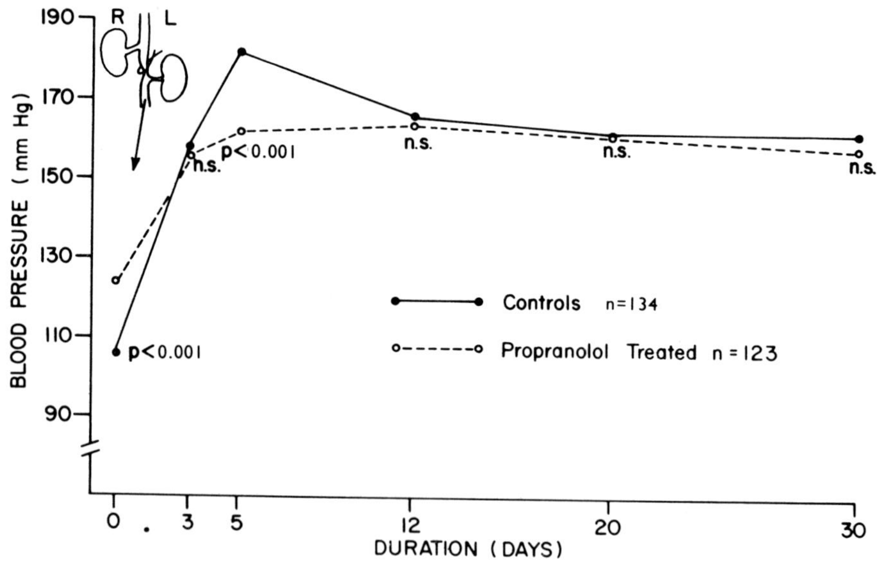

FIG. 4A. Effect of propranolol (60 mg/kg/day) on average mean arterial pressure in conscious renal hypertensive rats.

Table 4. Effects of Propranolol (60 mg/Kg/day) on Blood Pressure, Heart Rate and Plasma Renin Concentration in Conscious Renal Hypertensive Rats (C = Control, P = Propranolol-Treated)

Days After Aortic Ligation	*0*	*3*	*5*	*12*	*20*	*30*
Number	C = 20 P = 18	C = 21 P = 12	C = 25 P = 32	C = 24 P = 23	C = 24 P = 31	C = 20 P = 7
Mean arterial pressure (mm Hg)	C 106 ± 6.8	C 156 ± 18.7	C 182 ± 14.4	C 166 ± 20.2	C 161 ± 10.9	C 161 ± 10.6
	P 124 ± 10.7	P 158 ± 12	P 162 ± 16.4	P 165 ± 16.1	P 161 ± 15.6	P 152 ± 19.7
	$p < 0.001$	n.s.	$p < 0.001$	n.s.	n.s.	n.s.
Heart rate (Beats/min)	C 408 ± 52	C 388 ± 13.6	C 424 ± 54.6	C 407 ± 51	C 391 ± 35	C 385 ± 42
	P 362 ± 55	P 333 ± 20.6	P 365 ± 58.6	P 398 ± 43	P 373 ± 54	P 330 ± 31
	$p < 0.01$	$p < 0.01$	$p < 0.001$	n.s.	n.s.	$p < 0.0025$
Plasma renin concentration ($\times 10^{-4}$ G.U.)	C 0.92 ±0.4	C 3.68 ±0.8	C 8.68 ±6.1	C 3.02 ±2.0	C 1.68 ±0.8	C 0.95 ±0.4
	P 0.54 ±0.3	P 3.51 ±0.8	P 4.49 ±3.8	P 3.25 ±1.9	P 2.21 ±1.4	P 1.38 ±0.6
	$p < 0.005$	n.s.	$p < 0.001$	n.s.	n.s.	n.s.

Values are Means ± S.D.

in blood pressure which followed aortic ligation was equally severe in the propranolol-treated group at all phases with the exception of day 5. At this phase mean arterial pressure had increased to 182 ± 14.4 mm Hg in the untreated group, but to only 162 ± 16.4 mm Hg in the propranolol-treated group ($p < 0.001$) (Table 4, Fig. 4A).

Heart rate was lower in the propranolol-treated group at all phases (Table 4).

Baseline peripheral plasma renin concentration was lower in the propranolol-treated group ($p < 0.005$) (Table 4, Fig. 4B). Aortic ligation resulted in an increase in peripheral plasma renin concentration in both groups at days 3, 5, 12 and 20. The

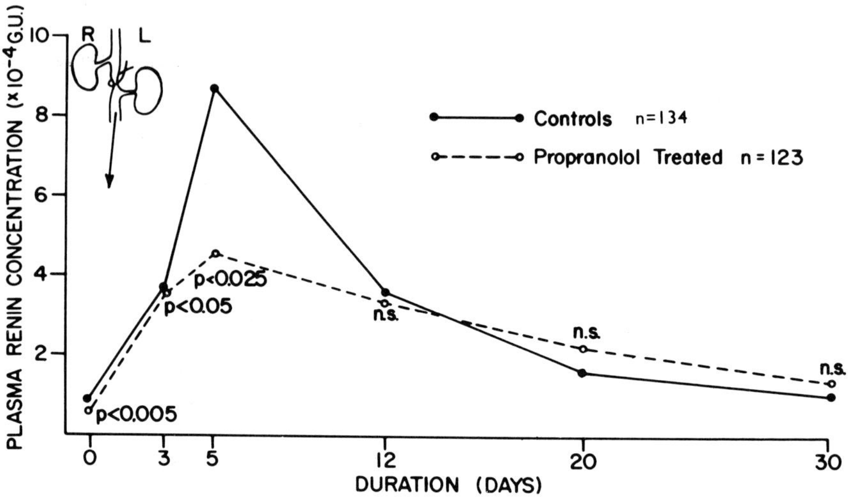

FIG. 4B. Effect of propranolol (60 mg/kg/day) on average plasma renin concentration in conscious renal hypertensive rats.

magnitude of renin increase was much less in the propranolol-treated group as compared to the untreated controls during the early phase at days 3 and 5.

Effect of Propranolol on Cardiac Hypertrophy

Propranolol was administered at the dose of 60 mg/kg/day for 15 days before aortic ligation and continued thereafter for the duration of the study. Mean arterial pressure and ventricular weight/body weight ratio before aortic ligation and 20 and 40 days thereafter are reported in Figure 5.

Baseline mean arterial pressure was slightly higher in the propranolol-treated group. Baseline ventricular weight/body weight ratio was similar in the two groups.

Twenty days after aortic ligation, mean arterial pressure was increased in both groups to the same degree. Ventricular weight/body weight ratio was slightly higher in the untreated group.

Forty days after aortic ligation, mean arterial pressure remained equally severe in both groups; ventricular weight/body weight ratio was significantly higher in the untreated group; 4.45 mg/gm versus 3.43 mg/gm ($p < 0.001$).

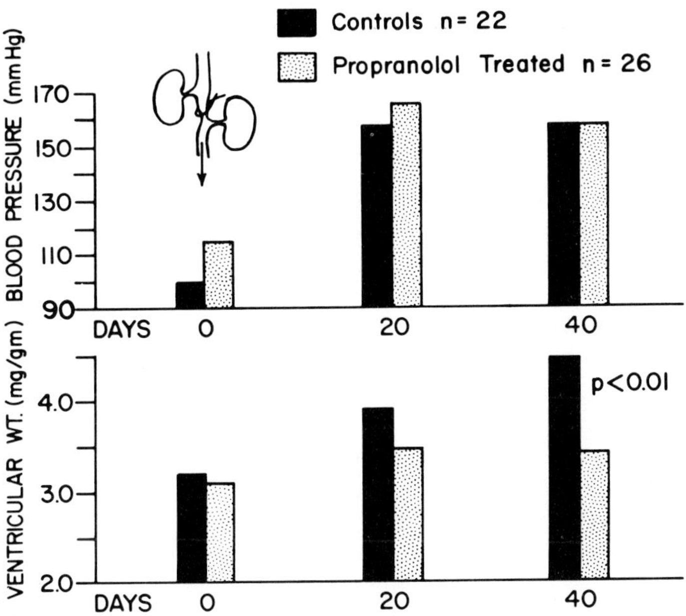

FIG. 5. Effect of propranolol (60 mg/kg/day) on ventricular weight (mg/gm body weight) in severe renal hypertensive rats.

Discussion

The experimental model of severe renal hypertension employed in this investigation is characterized by a precise reproducibility of blood pressure and renin at different phases. Therefore, it offers the opportunity of assessing the effects of different pharmacologic agents on blood pressure and renin at each phase [18]. Thus, not only can drug effects be established, but pathophysiologic conclusions may also be derived from the drug effects.

Administration of furosemide (36 mg/kg/day) effectively reduces the blood pressure at all phases. During the early phase of this type of experimental renal hypertension, the increase in renin which follows aortic ligation is significantly blunted by furosemide treatment. The most dramatic difference in renin between furosemide and control group is seen five days after aortic constriction. This phase is characterized by highest plasma renin levels in the untreated model. Administration of thiazide diuretics in man and in the experimental animal is known to stimulate renin release [20-23]. Also, administration of furosemide is a strong stimulus to renin release [24-27]. In our experiment, a seemingly paradoxical blunting of the renin response to aortic ligation was seen in rats treated with furosemide (36 mg/kg/day) for two weeks prior to the initiation of the observation and throughout the duration of the study.

In the present study, long-term pretreatment and treatment with furosemide were carried out. Although it is well accepted that acute or short-term administration of furosemide results in decrease in blood volume and renin stimulation, the long-term effects of this diuretic on blood volume, systemic hemodynamics and renin are not established. Furthermore, the mechanisms of antihypertensive action of furosemide remain to be determined [28, 29].

Concomitantly with the relative suppression of renin, a significant and persistent decrease in hypertension was produced in the present model. The reasons for this effect of furosemide on renin cannot be explained at this time.

Hydralazine effectively reduced mean arterial pressure in this experimental model. The increase in plasma renin concentration, which follows aortic ligation, was minimized but not abolished by hydralazine administration. At days 3 and 5, renin was much lower in the hydralazine-treated group than in the untreated controls. This finding is in contrast with the well-known renin stimulatory effect of acute administration of hydralazine [17, 30]. It would appear that chronic hydralazine administration reduces both blood pressure and renin in the early phase of this model of experimental hypertension.

Thus, both furosemide and hydralazine, when administered chronically, decrease blood pressure and renin in the early phase, despite their known renin-stimulating ability when administered acutely. In a clinical setting also characterized by high blood pressure and higher renin, administration of combination of drugs (some of which are renin stimulators) resulted in a concomitant decrease of renin and blood pressure [31]. Thus, it is postulated that in this experimental model elevation of renin and blood pressure are concomitant phenomena, not necessarily associated by a cause-effect relationship.

In the chronic phase of this model, hydralazine administration resulted in sustained blood pressure reduction to normotensive levels associated with a peripheral plasma renin concentration significantly higher than the untreated controls (days 20 and 30). Thus, the effects of prolonged administration of hydralazine on renin vary significantly with the different pathophysiologic mechanisms operating at different phases.

Low doses of propranolol (3 mg/kg/day), administered for two weeks before the initiation of the observations and continued throughout the duration of the study, minimized but did not abolish the increase in renin which occurs three and five days after aortic ligation. Despite this significant suppression of renin by propranolol, the blood pressure was equally severe in treated and untreated animals at days 3, 5, 12 and 20. At day 30, the blood pressure was actually higher in the propranolol-treated animals. It should also be noted that baseline blood pressure (before aortic ligation) was higher in the group pretreated with propranolol. With this low dose, heart rate was lower during the early (days 3 and 5) and late (day 30) phases.

High doses of propranolol (60 mg/kg/day), administered for two weeks before the initiation of the observations and continued throughout the duration of the study, exerted on renin the same effect as the low dose (3 mg/kg/day). Thus, the increase in propranolol dose did not result in any additional suppression of renin. Also, the effects of "low" and "high" doses of propranolol on heart rate were similar. "High" doses of propranolol did not affect the blood pressure on days 3, 12, 20 and 30. On day 5, however, the blood pressure was 10% lower than in the untreated controls.

In the present model of severe renal hypertension, propranolol at the doses used was unable to prevent the onset and to affect the progression of blood pressure elevation with the only exception of a mild blood pressure reduction at day 5 with the high dose. These data demonstrate a marked dissociation between the effect of propranolol on renin and heart rate and on blood pressure. Such a dissociation has been seen in hypertensive patients [32].

Failure of beta-adrenergic blockers to prevent the onset of spontaneous hypertension in the rat has been used to demonstrate that the initial increase in cardiac output is not essential for the development of hypertension [33]. It is possible that this consideration may apply to the present experimental model. This interpretation must remain speculative until the sequence of hemodynamic events in this model is elucidated.

It is interesting to note that propranolol significantly protected against cardiac hypertrophy without reducing blood pressure. This finding supports the concept that blood pressure elevation might not be the sole factor contributing to cardiac hypertrophy [34, 35].

As the severity of the initial renin level is minimized by propranolol (without effect on blood pressure), it is postulated that the renin-angiotensin system might play a biochemical role in enhancing myocardial hypertrophy [35].

The protective effect of propranolol against myocardial hypertrophy requires further investigation and suggests important potential usefulness in hypertensive heart disease.

Acknowledgments

The authors acknowledge with thanks the invaluable technical assistance of Messrs. Luis and Jose Maldonado. Ms. Janice Levy performed the renin determinations. The studies were conducted during the tenure of Dr. Michael Fernandes as Pfizer Research Fellow.

They also appreciate the efficient assistance of Mrs. Reene Ruiz in the preparation of this manuscript.

References

1. Guyton, A.C., Coleman, T.G. and Granger, H.J.: Circulation, overall regulation. Ann. Rev. Physiol. 34:13, 1972.
2. Scornik, O.A. and Paladini, A.C.: Angiotensin in blood levels in dogs with experimental renal hypertension. Am. J. Physiol. 201:526, 1961.
3. Koletsky, S., Rivera-Velez, J.M., Marsh, D.G. et al: Relation of renal arterial pressure to activity of renin-angiotensin system in renal hypertension. Proc. Soc. Exp. Biol. Med. 125:96, 1967.
4. Bianchi, G., Tilde Tenconi, L. and Lucca, R.: Effect in the conscious dog of constriction of the renal artery to a sole remaining kidney on hemodynamics, sodium balance, body fluid volumes, plasma renin concentrations and pressor responses to angiotensin. Clin. Sci. 38:741, 1970.
5. Pals, D.T., Masucci, F.D., Denning, G.S., Jr. et al: Role of the pressor action of angiotensin II in experimental hypertension. Circ. Res. 29:673, 1971.

6. Carretero, O.A. and Bujak, B.: Role of angiotensin in benign and malignant experimental hypertension. Life Sci. 9:1097, 1972.
7. Ledingham, J.M. and Cohen, R.D.: Changes in extracellular fluid volume and cardiac output during the development of experimental renal hypertension. Canad. Med. Ass. J. 90:292, 1964.
8. Ledingham, J.M. and Pelling, D.: Cardiac output and peripheral resistance in experimental renal hypertension. Circ. Res. 20 and 21/2, 187, 1967.
9. Lucas, J. and Floyer, M.A.: Renal control of changes in the compliance of the interstitial space: A factor in the etiology of renoprival hypertension. Clin. Sci. 44:397, 1973.
10. Lucas, J. and Floyer, M.A.: Changes in body fluid distribution and interstitial tissue compliance during the development and reversal of experimental renal hypertension in the rat. Clin. Sci. Molec. Med. 47:1, 1974.
11. de Champlain, J.: The influence of sodium in relation to experimental hypertension. *In* Onesti, G., Kim, K.E. and Moyer, J.H. (eds.): Hypertension: Mechanisms and Management. New York and London: Grune and Stratton, 1973, p. 147.
12. Eide, I. and Aars, H.: Renal hypertension in rabbits immunized with angiotensin II. Scand. J. Clin. Lab. Invest. 25:119, 1970.
13. MacDonald, G.J., Louis, W.J., Renzini, V. et al: Renal-clip hypertension in rabbits immunized against angiotensin II. Circ. Res. 27:197, 1970.
14. Grollman, A. and Krishnamurty, V.S.R.: A new pressor agent of renal origin: Its differentiation from renin and angiotensin. Am. J. Physiol. 221:1499, 1971.
15. Fasciolo, J.C.: Accion del rinon sano sobre la hipertension arterial por isquemia renal. Rev. Soc. Argent. Biol. 14:15, 1938.
16. Muirhead, E.E., Leach, B.E., Byers, L.W. et al: Antihypertensive function of the renal medulla. *In* Onesti, G., Kim, K.E., and Moyer, J.H. (eds.): Hypertension: Mechanisms and Management. New York and London:Grune and Stratton, 1973, p. 731.
17. Kuchel, O. and Genest, J.: Effect of antihypertensive drugs on renin release. *In* Onesti, G., Kim, K.E. and Moyer, J.H. (eds.): Hypertension: Mechanisms and Management. New York and London: Grune and Stratton, 1973, p. 411.
18. Fernandes, M., Onesti, G., Weder, A. et al: Experimental model of severe renal hypertension. J. Lab. Clin. Med. (In press.)
19. Gould, A.B., Skeggs, L.T. and Ka, J.R.: Measurement of renin and substrate concentration in human serum. Lab. Invest. 15:1802, 1966.
20. Mogil, R.A., Itskovitz, H.D., Russell, J.H. et al: Renal innervation and renin activity in salt metabolism and hypertension. Amer. J. Physiol. 216:693, 1969.
21. Vander, A.J.: Direct effect of potassium on renin secretion and renal function. Am. J. Physiol. 219:455, 1970.
22. Tarazi, R.C., Dustan, H.P. and Frohlich, E.D.: Long-term thiazide threapy in essential hypertension. Circulation 41:709, 1970.

23. Acchiardo, S., Dustan, H.P. and Tarazi, R.C.: Similar effects of hydrochlorothiazide and spironolactone on plasma renin activity in essential hypertension. Circ. Res. 24:103, 1972.
24. Fraser, R., James, V.H.T., Brown, J.J. et al: Effect of angiotensin and of furosemide on plasma aldosterone, corticosterone, cortisol, and renin in man. Lancet 2:989, 1965.
25. Brown, T.C., Davis, J.O. and Johnston, C.I.: Acute responses in plasma renin and aldosterone secretion to diuretics. Am. J. Physiol. 211:437, 1966.
26. Rosenthal, J., Boucher, R., Nowaczynski, W. et al: Acute changes in plasma volume, renin activity, and free aldosterone levels in healthy subjects following furosemide administration. Canad. J. Physiol. Pharmacol. 46:85, 1968.
27. Meyer, P., Menard, J. Papanicolau, N. et al: Mechanism of renin release following furosemide diuresis in rabbit. Am. J. Physiol. 215:908, 1968.
28. Tarazi, R.C.: Diuretic drugs: Mechanisms of antihypertensive action. *In* Onesti, G., Kim, K.E. and Moyer, J.H. (eds.): Hypertension: Mechanisms and Management. New York and London: Grune and Stratton, 1973, p. 251.
29. Cannon, P.J.: Clinical use of diuretics in hypertension. *In* Onesti, G., Kim, K.E. and Moyer, J.H. (eds.): Hypertension: Mechanisms and Management. New York and London: Grune and Stratton, 1973, p. 261.
30. Bozovic, L. and Castenfors, J.: Effect of hydralazine and pentolinium on renin release. Acta Med. Scand. Suppl. 472, 224, 1967.
31. McAllister, R.G., Van Way, C.W. III, Dayani, K. et al: Malignant hypertension: Effect of therapy on renin and aldosterone. Circ. Res. 28-29 (suppl 2):160, 1971.
32. Zanchetti, A., Leonetti, G., Morganti, A. et al: Correlation between renin-suppressive and hemodynamic effects of beta-adrenoreceptor blocking agents. *In* Onesti, G., Fernandes, M. and Kim, K.E. (eds.): Control of Blood Pressure by Central Nervous System. New York and London: Grune and Stratton. (In press.)
33. Pfeffer, M.A., Frohlich, E.D., Pfeffer, J.M. et al: Pathophysiological implications of the increased cardiac output of young spontaneously hypertensive rats. Circ. Res. 34 and 35/1, 235, 1974.
34. Masson, G.M.C., McCormack, L.J., Dustan, H.P. et al: Hypertensive vascular disease as a consequence of increased arterial pressure. Am. J. Pathol. 34:817, 1958.
35. Sen, S., Tarazi, R.C., Khairallah, P.A. et al: Cardiac hypertrophy in spontaneously hypertensive rats. Circ. Res. 35:775, 1974.

Effect of Propranolol on Plasma Renin Activity, Renal Renin, and Brain and Adrenal Isorenins in the Rat

G. P. Guthrie, Jr., M.D., A. Dornier, M.D., R. Boucher, Ph.D., O. Kuchel, M.D., J. M. Rojo-Ortega, M.D., W. Nowaczynski, D.Sc. and J. Genest, C.C., M.D.

The beta-adrenergic blocking agents, most notably propranolol, have been established in the past 12 years as effective antihypertensive drugs [1, 2]. Yet the mechanism of this therapeutic effect remains controversial, especially relative to the renal renin-angiotensin system. Although chronic propranolol therapy may lower the plasma renin activity of hypertensive patients [3, 4], much evidence, to be briefly reviewed later, suggests that the suppression of renin secretion is not responsible for this antihypertensive action. To further explore the relationship between chronic propranolol administration and renin, the renal content and plasma activity of this enzyme were

---

The work reported from our laboratories was generously supported through a group grant given by the Medical Research Council of Canada to the multidisciplinary research group on hypertension at the Clinical Research Institute of Montreal.

G. P. Guthrie, Jr., M.D., Research Fellow;* A. Dornier, M.D., Research Fellow*; R. Boucher, Ph.D., Senior Researcher* and Professor of Medicine, University of Montreal; O. Kuchel, M.D., Senior Researcher* and Professor of Medicine, University of Montreal and McGill University; J. M. Rojo-Ortega, M.D., Senior Researcher*; W. Nowaczynski, D.Sc., Senior Researcher* and Professor of Medicine, University of Montreal and McGill University; J. Genest, C.C., M.D., Scientific Director* and Professor of Medicine, University of Montreal and McGill University, Canada.
*Clinical Research Institute of Montreal, Canada.

measured in groups of rats receiving two dose levels of the drug. Furthermore, since an antihypertensive effect mediated by a central nervous system action of the drug has been proposed [5], the effect of the drug on brain isorenin activity was measured as well as on adrenal isorenin content.

Materials and Methods

Three groups of Sprague-Dawley rats weighing 200-250 gm were studied: (a) a control group of 11 rats which received 0.2 ml of isotonic saline intraperitoneally 3 times daily for 15 days (group 1), (b) 12 rats which received dl-propranolol hydrochloride (Inderal®)* at 6 mg/kg of body weight per day in three divided doses in 0.2 ml of saline for 15 days (group 2); and (c) 12 rats which received propranolol at 30 mg/kg/day in three divided doses in 0.2 ml of saline for 15 days (group 3). The rats were maintained on Purina chow and received tap water ad libitum.

Systolic blood pressures were measured under light ether anesthesia by the tail cuff technique one hour after propranolol administration on the 7th and 15th day of the experiment. Heart rates were measured from pulse readings. On the 15th day, the rats were anesthetized with sodium pentobarbital (60 mg/kg intraperitoneally) and aortic blood was immediately centrifuged at 4°C and 10,000 rpm for ten minutes and the plasma was frozen at −20°C. Kidneys, adrenal glands and brains were also immediately frozen.

Plasma renin activity was measured by the rat bioassay of Boucher [6] with a 15-hour plasma incubation period. Kidneys were homogenized at 0°C, 1 gm of the homogenate was diluted in 200 ml bidistilled water and 0.1 ml was employed for the renal renin content by the method mentioned above. Isorenin from brain frontal cortex and whole adrenal glands were measured by a modification of the above method [7].

Results

No significant differences in weight or blood pressure were found between the three groups. The pulse was decreased in

---

*Supplied by Richard Davies, Ayerst Co., Montreal.

groups 2 and 3 receiving propranolol and more so in group 3 receiving the higher dose (Fig. 1). No significant differences were found in adrenal isorenin activity (Fig. 2), frontal cortex renin activity (Fig. 3) or renal renin content (Fig. 4). The mean plasma renin activity was slightly decreased in the rats receiving propranolol at 6 and 30 mg/kg/day and was significant ($p<0.05$) only for group 2 (Fig. 5).

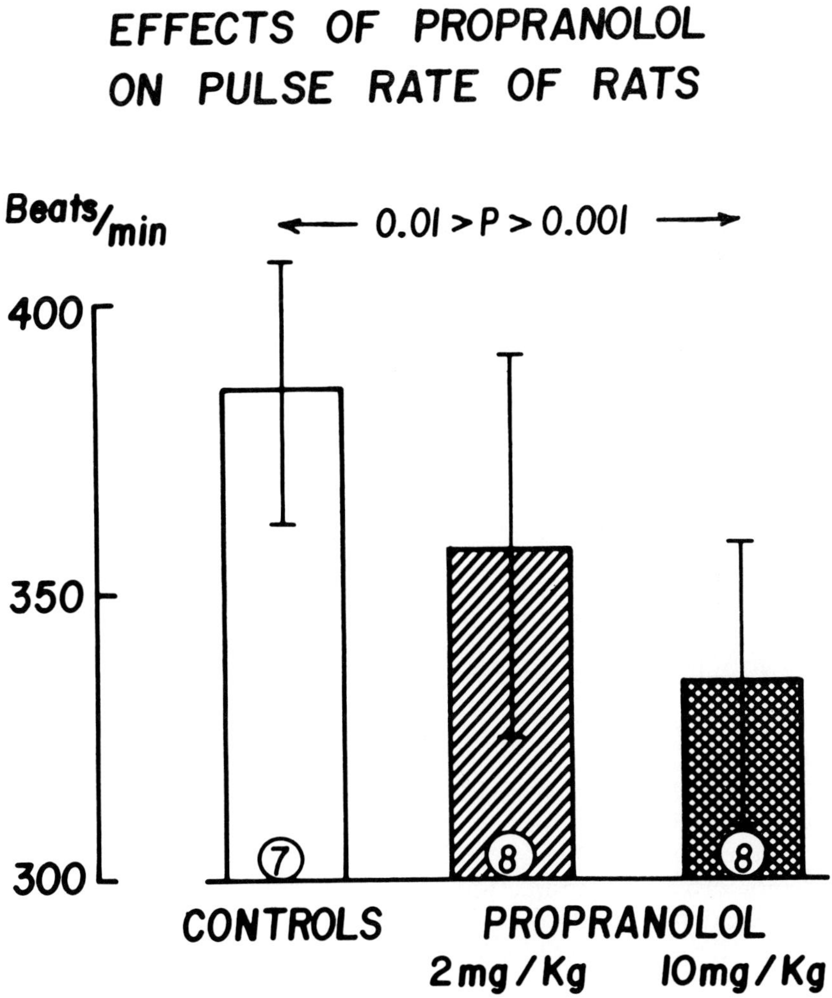

FIGURE 1.

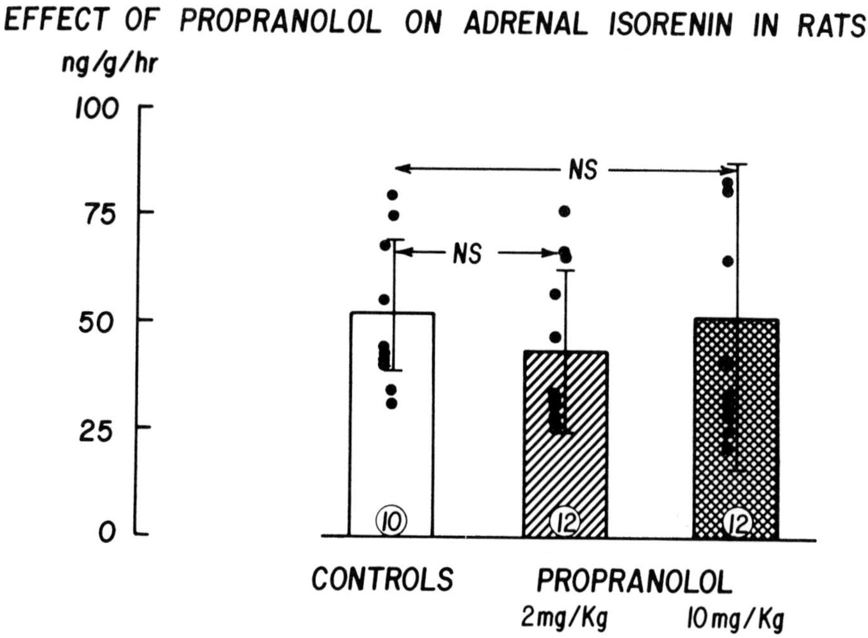

FIGURE 2.

Closer examination of groups 2 and 3 revealed that the plasma renin activity responded in two distinct fashions. Ten of the 24 rats had total suppression of the plasma renin activity, four of 12 at the lower dose and six of 12 at the higher dose. No significant difference in plasma renin activity was noted between controls and the 14 other rats in both groups that did not exhibit suppression to an undetectable level.

Discussion

Several lines of investigation have suggested that angiotensin may participate in cerebral mechanisms of blood pressure regulation [8]. Although this circulating peptide may exert a pressor effect by interaction with the area postrema or other area lacking a blood-brain barrier [9], the presence of angiotensin II in the cerebrospinal fluid [10], itself a pressor agent via interaction with suprapontine structures [11], appears to be generated by the intrinsic isorenin present in brain tissue [7,

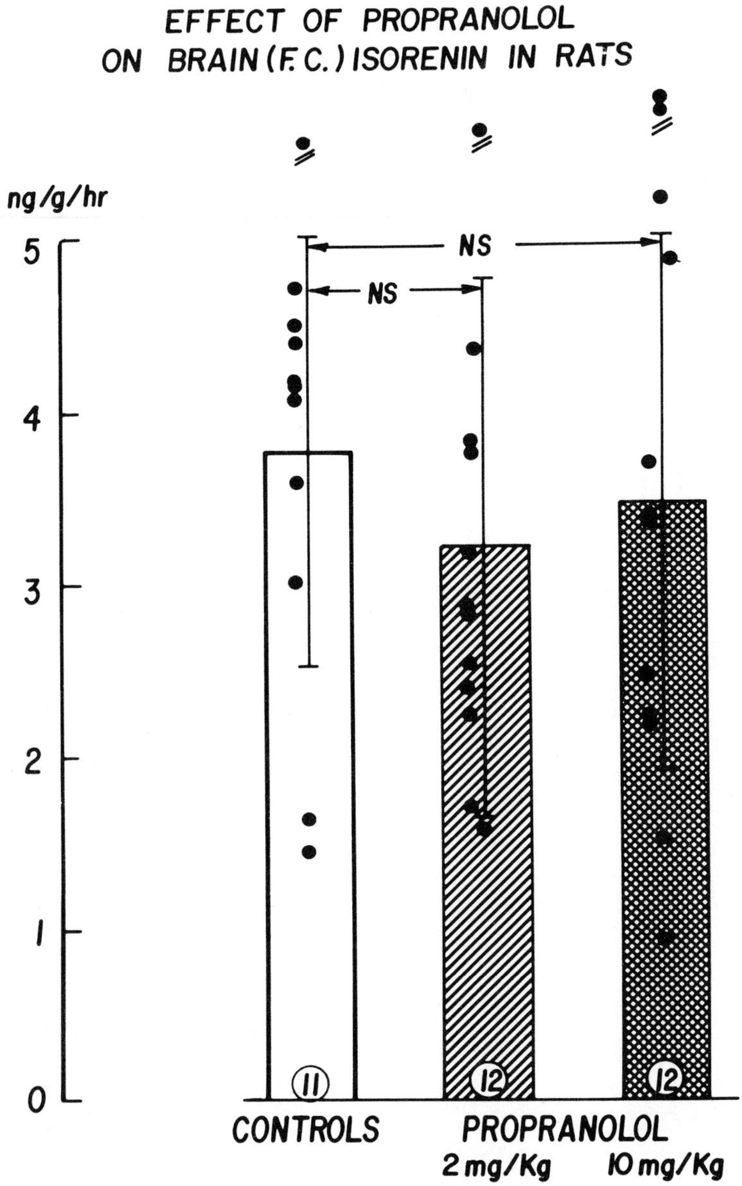
EFFECT OF PROPRANOLOL
ON BRAIN (F.C.) ISORENIN IN RATS
ng/g/hr
5
4
3
2
1
0
NS
NS
11
12
12
CONTROLS
PROPRANOLOL
2 mg/Kg
10 mg/Kg

FIGURE 3.

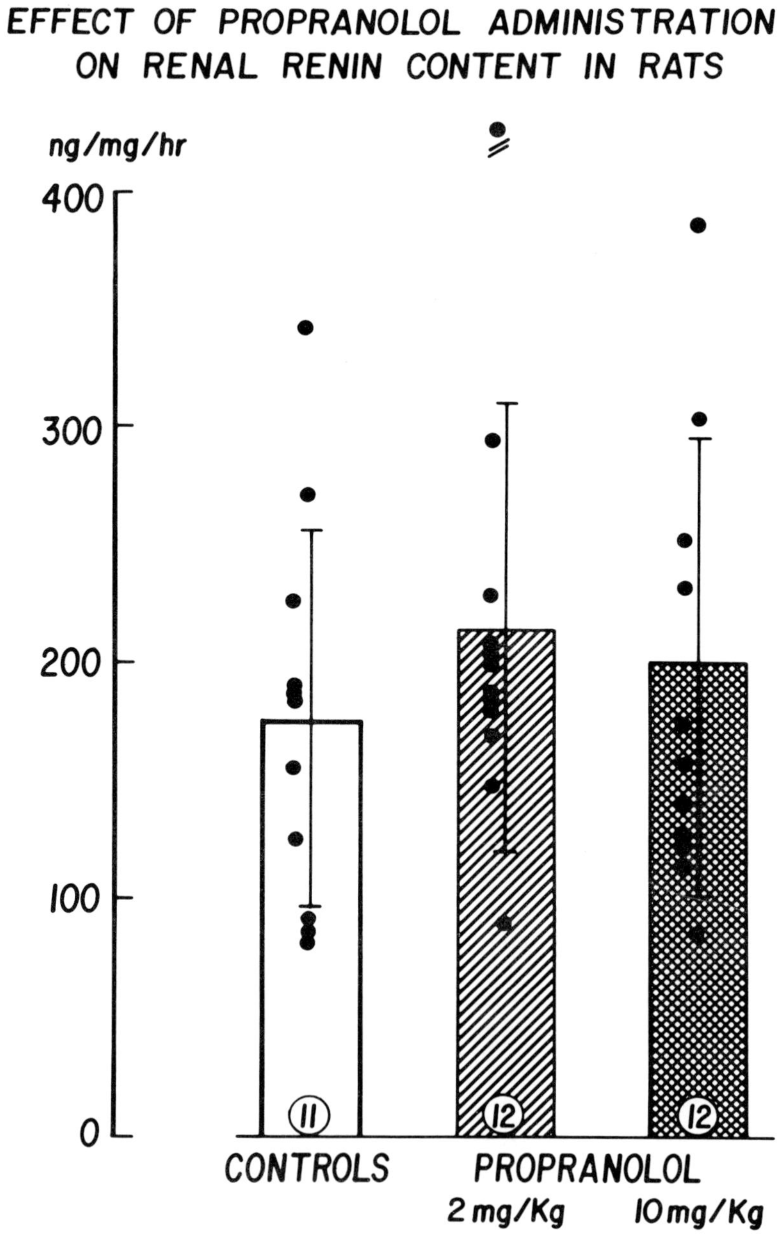
EFFECT OF PROPRANOLOL ADMINISTRATION
ON RENAL RENIN CONTENT IN RATS
ng/mg/hr
400
300
200
100
0
11
12
12
CONTROLS
PROPRANOLOL
2 mg/Kg
10 mg/Kg

FIGURE 4.

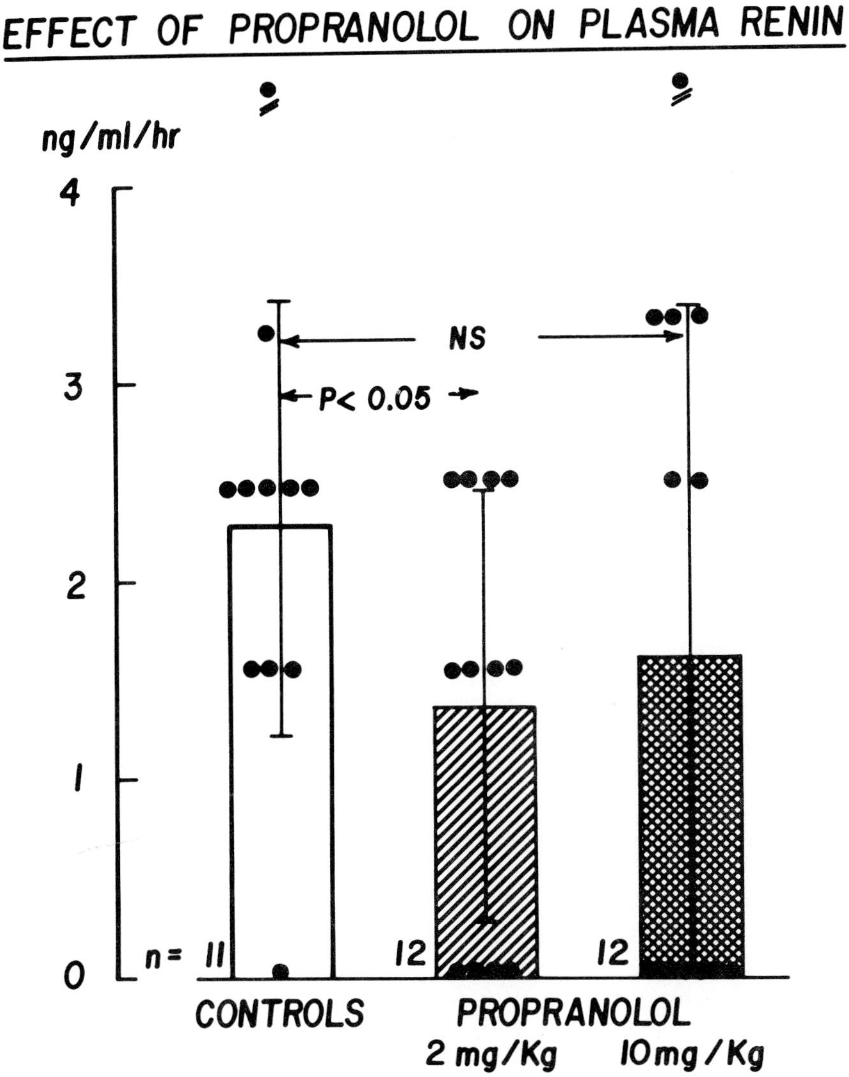
EFFECT OF PROPRANOLOL ON PLASMA RENIN
ng/ml/hr
4
3
2
1
0
NS
P< 0.05
n= 11
12
12
CONTROLS
PROPRANOLOL
2 mg/Kg
10mg/Kg

FIGURE 5.

10]. Whereas a central antihypertensive action of propranolol has been proposed [12], our findings make unlikely an effect on brain isorenin activity as an involved mechanism. However, distal interaction of propranolol on angiotensin stimulation of central vasomotor centers is not excluded by these findings.

Adrenal isorenin, capable of in situ generation of angiotensin II, has been postulated as having a role in physiologic and pathologic mechanisms of aldosterone production in animals and man [13]. As the activity of this enzyme is also unaffected by chronic propranolol administration in the rat, observations of smaller declines in plasma aldosterone levels than in plasma renin activity in essential hypertensive patients receiving chronic propranolol therapy [14, 15] may be related to unsuppressed adrenal isorenin, although such an explanation is speculative.

Although plasma propranolol levels were not measured in this study, the significant depression of heart rate indicates that effective beta blockade was achieved, and Forman and Mulrow [16] have shown comparable doses of parenteral propranolol (2 mg/kg) yield plasma concentrations of greater than 200 ng/ml for over six hours in the spontaneously hypertensive rat.

The lack of a hypotensive effect of propranolol in normal rats has been previously reported [17], and its effect in various hypertensive rat models has been variable. Several investigators [17-19] have reported that oral propranolol prevents the onset of hypertension in young spontaneously hypertensive rats, but is without effect on the established hypertensive state of the older animal [16, 19]. Similarly, the drug appears to blunt the development of rat DOCA-salt hypertension, but is ineffective after its onset. That DOCA-salt hypertension is associated with depressed plasma renin activity [20], yet is prevented by propranolol, illustrates a disparity between an antirenin and antihypertensive effect of the drug in the rat.

Although experimental manipulations causing acute variations in the plasma renin activity may not be reflected by changes of renin concentration in renal tissue, most chronic stimuli such as sustained volume expansion or contraction do show parallel changes in the renal content and plasma activity of renin [21]. Under such conditions, the amount of renin extractable from renal tissue directly reflects the requirements. Modulation of renin synthesis, storage and release in the chronic state appears to be primarily a function of the pressure-sensing mechanism at the juxtaglomerular apparatus, which can override influences on renin secretion by adrenergic mechanisms. The recent demonstration by Hanson et al [22] that propranolol does not significantly suppress the plasma renin activity in dogs with chronic thoracic inferior caval constriction and ascites and by Bravo et al [23] that the drug does not abolish the elevated renin values seen in humans on prolonged thiazide therapy supports this concept of the dominance of volume mediated control of renin secretion in the chronic state. Our finding that the plasma renin activity is inconsistently suppressed and that renin renal content is unchanged in normal rats implies that net renal renin synthesis and storage is unaffected by propranolol and that renin is available for release by other mechanisms.

With the risk of extending an interpretation of our findings in normotensive rats to hypertensive humans, we believe these results tend to support the concept that the antihypertensive effect of chronic propranolol administration does not depend upon or result from chronic suppression of the plasma renin activity. Buhler et al [14] have proposed that propranolol exerts its antihypertensive effect by its specific antirenin activity from evidence of correlation of these two effects. Other groups have also noted such a positive correlation with this and similar drugs (Fig. 6). However, a larger number of studies have

POSITIVE CORRELATION BETWEEN ANTIHYPERTENSIVE AND RENIN-SUPPRESSION EFFECTS OF β-BLOCKERS IN HUMAN HYPERTENSION

DRUG	REFERENCES
PROPRANOLOL	BUHLER ET AL. (1972a,b)
PROPRANOLOL, PRACTOLOL, OXPRENOLOL, TIMOLOL, PRINDOLOL, ICI 66082	BUHLER ET AL. (1975)
PRINDOLOL	JOHNSTON ET AL. (1973)
ICI 66082	ABERG (1974)
ALPRENOLOL	CASTENFORS ET AL. (1973)

FIGURE 6.

observed a dissociation between the antirenin and antihypertensive actions of the beta-blockers (Fig. 7).

First, Prichard and Gillam [3] have noted the delay of several days before an antihypertensive effect is seen, in contrast to the relatively prompt observation of renin suppression after propranolol therapy as noted by Michelakis and McAllister [4] and Tarazi and Dustan [24]. Such a time lag may result from the delay in attainment of sustained effective plasma propranolol levels since Chidsey et al [25] have shown that a longer plasma half-life of the drug is seen during chronic than acute administration. Second, suppression of the plasma renin activity occurs at lower doses of beta-blockers than those required for antihypertensive activity, shown most clearly by Leonetti et al [26] (Fig. 8). Third, several studies have not confirmed the correlation between suppression of the plasma renin activity and blood pressure response. Bravo et al [23] have shown that propranolol is ineffective in suppressing the chronic hyperreninemia in hypertensive patients from chlorothiazide administration despite its antihypertensive effect. And finally, Amery et al [27] and Esler [28], using the cardioselective beta-1 antagonists ICI 66082 and practolol, respectively,

DISSOCIATION BETWEEN ANTIHYPERTENSIVE AND RENIN-SUPPRESSING EFFECTS OF β-BLOCKERS IN HUMAN HYPERTENSION

NATURE OF DISSOCIATION	DRUG	REFERENCES
1 - TEMPORAL (↓PRA BEFORE ↓BP)	PROPRANOLOL	PRICHARD & GILLIAM (1969) MICHELAKIS & McALLISTER (1972) TARAZI & DUSTAN (1972)
2 - DOSE DEPENDENT (↓PRA LOWER DOSE THAN ↓BP)	PROPRANOLOL	MICHELAKIS & McALLISTER (1972) LEONETTI ET AL. (1975)
3 - CORRELATIVE (DEGREE OF ↓PRA ↮ DEGREE OF ↓BP)	PROPRANOLOL	TARAZI & DUSTAN (1972) HANSSON (1973) MAGGIORE ET AL. (1975)
	PROPRANOLOL, RO3-4787 PROPRANOLOL,PRINDOLOL	GEORGE ET AL. (1975) MORGAN ET AL. (1975)
	PROPRANOLOL(+THIAZIDE) PROPRANOLOL,PRINDOLOL	BRAVO ET AL. (1975) STOKES ET AL. (1974)
4 - BETA-RECEPTOR SELECTIVITY (? ↓BP BY β_1 BLOCKADE, ↓PRA BY β_2 BLOCKADE)	ICI 66082 PRACTOLOL	AMERY ET AL. (1974) ESLER (1974)

FIGURE 7.

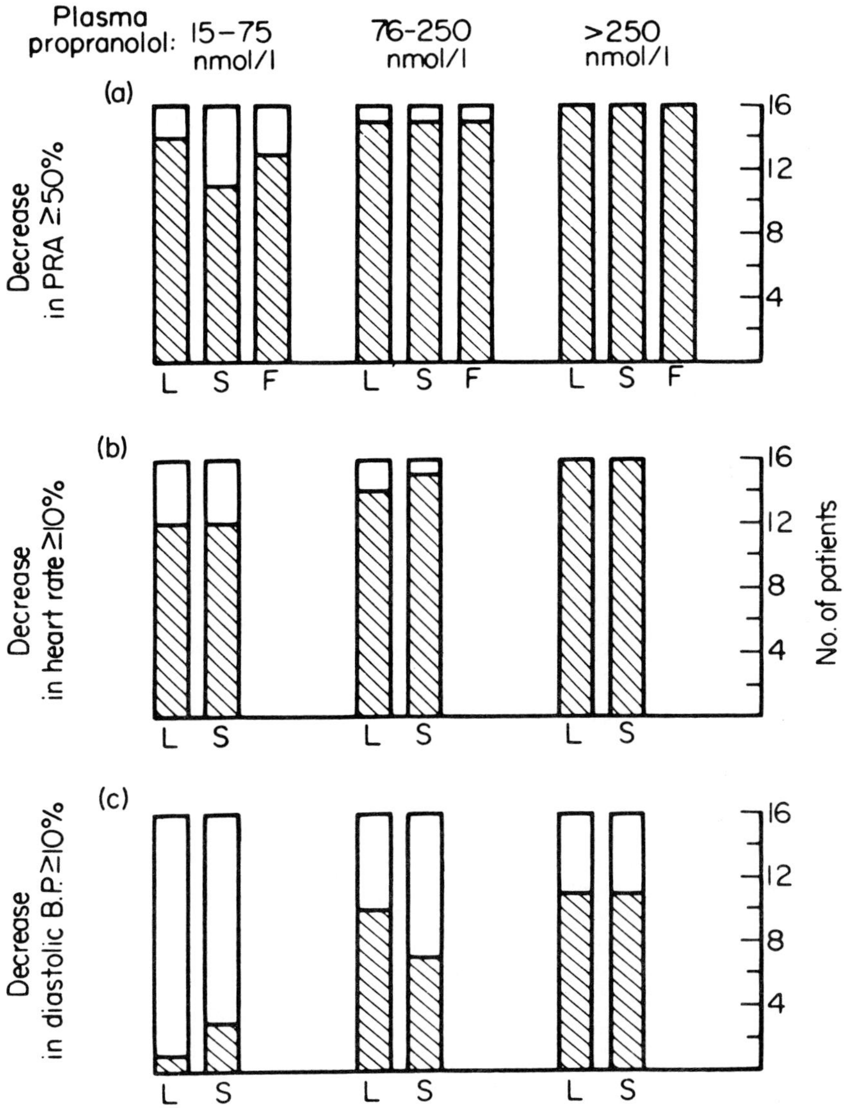

FIG. 8. Incidence of decrease in plasma renin activity, heart rate and diastolic blood pressure at low (15-75 nmol/1), intermediate (76-250) and high (>250) plasma propranolol concentrations in 16 essential hypertensive patients. (L=lying, S=standing, F=after IV furosemide; nmol/ 1÷3.8=ng/ml.) (Reprinted with permission from Leonetti et al [26].)

have shown effective antihypertensive responses without suppression of the plasma renin activity, although conflicting results have been reported by Aberg [29] and Buhler [30] using the same agents. Similarly, Weber et al [31] have concluded that renin release is mediated by a beta-2 receptor using various beta-adrenergic antagonists in the rabbit. Assaykeen [32] reached similar conclusions using specific agonists in the dog.

In conclusion, that long-term propranolol therapy causes inconsistent plasma renin suppression and unchanged renin renal content in the rat implies unchanged long-term renin synthesis and storage and supports the concept that chronic suppression of renin release is not the primary antihypertensive action of the beta-blockers.

References

1. Prichard, B.N.C. and Gillam, P.M.S.: Use of propranolol (Inderal) in treatment of hypertension. Br. Med. J. 2:725, 1964.
2. Zacharias, F.J., Cowen, K.J., Presst, J. et al: Propranolol in hypertension: A study of long-term therapy 1964-70. Am. Heart J. 83:755, 1972.
3. Prichard, B.N.C. and Gillam, P.M.S.: Treatment of hypertension with propranolol. Br. Med. J. 1:7, 1969.
4. Michelakis, A.M. and McAllister, R.G.: Effect of chronic adrenergic receptor blockade on plasma renin activity in man. J. Clin. Endocrinol. Metab. 34:386, 1972.
5. Lewis, P.J., Meyers, M.G., Reid, J.L. et al: Mechanism of beta-blockade hypertension. N. Engl. J. Med. 288:689, 1973.
6. Boucher, R., Veyrat, R., de Champlain, J. et al: New procedures for measurement of human plasma angiotensin and renin activity levels. Canad. Med. Ass. J. 90:194, 1964.
7. Ganten, D., Marquez-Julio, A., Granger, P. et al: Renin in dog brain. Am. J. Physiol. 221:1733, 1971.
8. Ferrario, C.M., Gildenberg, P.L. and McCubbin, J.W.: Cardiovascular effects of angiotensin mediated by the central nervous system. Circ. Res. 30:257, 1972.
9. Scroop, G.C. and Lowe, R.D.: Efferent pathways of the cardiovascular response to vertebral artery infusions of angiotensin in the dog. Clin. Sci. 37:605, 1969.
10. Ganten, D., Hutchinson, J.S. and Schelling, P.: The intrinsic brain iso-renin-angiotensin system in the rat; Its possible role in central mechanisms of blood pressure regulation. Clin. Sci. Molec. Med. 48:265s, 1975.

11. Severs, W.B., Daniels, A.E., Smookler, H.H. et al: Interrelationship between angiotensin II and the sympathetic nervous system. J. Pharmacol. Exp. Ther. 153:530, 1966.
12. Day, M.D. and Roach, A.G.: Central adrenoreceptors and the control of arterial blood pressure. Clin. Exp. Pharmacol. Physiol. 1:347, 1974.
13. Ganten, D., Ganten, U., Kubo, S. et al: Influence of sodium, potassium and pituitary hormones on iso-renin in rat adrenal glands. Am. J. Physiol. 227:224, 1974.
14. Buhler, F.R., Laragh, J.H., Baer, L. et al: Propranolol inhibition of renin secretion. A specific approach to the diagnosis and treatment of renin-dependent hypertensive diseases. N. Engl. J. Med. 287:1209, 1972.
15. Buhler, F.R., Laragh, J.H., Vaughan, E.D. et al: Antihypertensive action of propranolol. Am. J. Cardiol. 32: 511, 1972.
16. Forman, B.H. and Mulrow, P.J.: Effect of propranolol on blood pressure and plasma renin activity in the spontaneously hypertensive rat. Circ. Res. 35:215, 1975.
17. Vavra, I., Tom, H. and Greselin, E.: Chronic propranolol treatment in young spontaneously hypertensive and normotensive rats. Canad. J. Physiol. Pharmacol. 51:727, 1973.
18. Folkow, B., Lundgren, Y. and Weiss, L.: The effect of prolonged propranolol treatment on blood pressure and structural design of the resistance vessels in young spontaneously hypertensive rats. Acta Physiol. Scand. 14:8A, 1972.
19. Conway, J., Darwin, K., Hilditch, A. et al: Effect of propranolol on blood pressure in normal and hypertensive rats. Clin. Sci. Molec. Med. 48:101s, 1975.
20. Pettinger, W.A., Marchelle, M. and Augusto, L.: Renin suppression by DOC and NaCl in the rat. Am. J. Physiol. 221:1071, 1971.
21. Gross, F.: Renin stores in the kidney and plasma renin activity. *In* Fisher, J.W. (ed.): Kidney Hormones. New York:Academic Press, 1971, pp. 93-116.
22. Hanson, R.C., Davis, J.O. and Freeman, R.H.: Effects of propranolol on plasma renin activity in conscious dogs with thoracic inferior vena caval constriction or renal artery constriction. Fed. Proc. 34:834, 1975.
23. Bravo, E.L., Tarazi, R.C. and Dustan, H.P.: β-adrenergic blockade in diuretic-treated patients with essential hypertension. N. Engl. J. Med. 292:66, 1975.
24. Tarazi, R.C., Dustan, H.P., Frohlich, E.D. et al: Plasma renin and arterial pressure response to propranolol. Circulation, 46 (suppl. 2): 70, 1972.
25. Chidsey, C.A., Morselli, P., Bianchetti, G. et al: Studies on the absorption and disposition of propranolol in hypertensive patients during therapy. Circulation 52:313, 1975.
26. Leonetti, G., Mayer, G., Morganti, A. et al: Hypotensive and renin-suppressing activities of propranolol in hypertensive patients. Clin. Sci. Molec. Med. 48:491, 1975.

27. Amery, A., Billiet, L. and Fagard, R.: Beta-receptors and renin release. N. Engl. J. Med. 290:284, 1974.
28. Esler, M.D.: Effect of practolol on blood pressure and renin release in man. Clin. Pharmacol. Ther. 15:484, 1974.
29. Aberg, H.: Plasma renin activity after the use of a new beta-adrenergic blocking agent (ICI 66082). Int. J. Clin. Pharmacol. 9:98, 1974.
30. Buhler, F.R., Marbet, G., Patel, U. et al: Renin-suppressive potency of various beta-adrenergic blocking agents at supine rest and during upright exercise. Clin. Sci. Molec. Med. 48:61s, 1975.
31. Weber, M.A., Stokes, G.S. and Gain, J.M.: Comparison of the effects on renin release of beta adrenergic antagonists with differing properties. J. Clin. Invest. 54:1413, 1975.
32. Assaykeen, T.A.: Evidence for β_2-adrenergic receptor mediation of renin release in dogs. Endocrinology 92:A-192, 1973.

Bibliography

Castenfors, J., Johnssen, H. and Oro, L.: Effect of alprenolol on blood pressure and plasma renin activity in hypertensive patients. Acta Med. Scand. 193:189, 1973.

George, C.F., Lewis, P.J., Steiner, J.A. et al: A comparison of propranolol and compound RO3-4787 in the treatment of arterial hypertension in man. Clin Sci. Molec. Med. 48:65s, 1975.

Hansson, L.: Beta-adrenergic blockade in essential hypertension. Acta Med. Scand. suppl. 550, 1973.

Johnston, C.I., Anavekar, N., Chua, K.G. et al: Plasma renin and angiotensin levels in human hypertension following treatment. Clin. Sci. Molec. Med. 45:287s, 1973.

Maggiore, Q., Biagini, M., Zoccali, C. et al: Long-term propranolol treatment of resistant arterial hypertension in hemodialyzed patients. Clin. Sci. Molec. Med. 48:73s, 1975.

Morgan, T., Carney, S. and Roberts, R.: Changes in plasma renin activity and blood pressure after acute and chronic administration of β-adrenergic receptor blocking drugs. Clin. Sci. Molec. Med. 48:81s, 1975.

Stokes, G.S., Weber, M.A. and Thornell, I.R.: Beta-blockers and plasma renin in hypertension. Br. Med. J. 1:60, 1974.

Discussion

Moderator: Dr. F. Gross

Dr. Doyle: I would like to ask Dr. Onesti how he interprets his data? Does he agree with my interpretation that an elevated plasma renin represents simply a response to the raised blood pressure? In fact, what you have demonstrated is that you keep the blood pressure down by some rather unusual means, such as hydralazine or furosemide, and we will not go into how those work. The blood pressure stays down and the plasma renin does not go up. When you fail to reduce the blood pressure with a drug like propranolol, which is allegedly a specific preventive of renin release, you do not. Now, the other point which I believe is very significant — in that particular model it is very common, indeed, to get changes in malignant hypertension in the top kidney. Did you find any difference in the incidence of fibrin in blood vessels in the kidney in the various treatment groups?

Dr. Onesti: The interpretation that an elevated plasma renin represents simply a response to the blood pressure is one of the intellectual options that I had. It is our "easy way out," but I still favor it. The other consideration is that in the experiments which I described we have pretreated the animal for two weeks before we constricted the aorta. We have not yet established the effect of those pharmacologic agents on renin and blood pressure *after* the induction of the hypertension. This could be a completely different thing.

We are now referring to this model as severe renal hypertension. In a number of cases, we find the histologic changes of malignant hypertension in the kidney (the contralateral kidney) and in the mesenteric vessels.

I cannot speak yet on the morphologic changes in the arteries after treatment.

Dr. Gross: Dr. Onesti, when you say that these animals are pretreated for two weeks with furosemide, then you should start in this group with a higher renin.

Dr. Onesti: Yes, but this is not the case with the dose of furosemide employed (36 mg/kg/day). By using higher doses of furosemide we observe, however, a strong stimulation of renin. On higher doses of furosemide, presumably because of natriuresis, the renin is stimulated as expected.

Dr. Gross: So these animals get the negative sodium balance.

Dr. Onesti: Those on higher doses of furosemide definitely do.

Dr. Mulrow: Dr. Onesti, I would like to offer a possibility that might explain why propranolol failed to lower the blood pressure in your hypertensive rats and yet protected against development of left ventricular hypertrophy. It is this: The half-life of propranolol in the rat is short. It is about 100 minutes. The rat is a nocturnal animal. Rats are taking most of their propranolol at night. The propranolol blood levels are higher at night. As a result, they are having nocturnal control of the blood pressure, but by the time we experimenters get around to measuring the blood pressure during the day it is not as low as one might expect and it would be low at night.

Dr. Onesti: At the beginning of the study we also thought of that. We have done blood pressure measurements in the early morning hours and in the afternoon. There is no significant difference in blood pressure at different hours when propranolol is administered chronically.

Dr. Kincaid-Smith: First, I want to ask Dr. Onesti a question: What is the secret of his success in keeping his rats alive for so long? Using the same model, we have had a much higher mortality. Second, I wish to comment on our experiments and morphologic studies on the blood vessels in a rat with a transparent back chamber. A control area showing blood vessels in the transparent chamber before hypertension is induced is compared with the same area immediately after ligating the aorta. A dramatic alteration develops in the blood vessels.

Dr. Onesti: We also had an extremely high mortality with this model, until we talked to Dr. M. Rojo-Ortega in Montreal.* He taught us the following things: (1) Only Sprague-Dawley rats are to be used for this technique of aortic constriction because

---

*Rojo-Ortega, J.M. and Genest, J.: A method for production of experimental hypertension in rats. Canad. J. Physiol. Pharmacol. 46:83, 1968.

the Wister rat has a much weaker myocardium and dies from cardiac failure after the aortic ligation. (2) Manipulation of the aorta must be minimized in order to preserve lumbar vessels inervating the medulla. No periaortic dissection. (3) We must use animals of a weight of at least 250-300 gm.

Dr. Corvol: We have recently developed an experiment which is very similar to that described by Dr. Onesti. We used an acute constriction, not a complete ligature of the aorta between the two renal arteries. Blood pressure and plasma renin concentration were measured every ten minutes after aortic constriction. After 30 minutes, the aorta was unclipped and the same measurements performed again. Propranolol was absolutely unable to prevent this hypertension although propranolol quickly suppressed the rise in plasma renin concentration in this experiment. However, we thought that this represented really a renin-dependent hypertension because the administration of the converting enzyme inhibitor completely suppressed the rise in blood pressure. It is difficult to interpret these data, but I think that the plasma renin concentration we are measuring at the present time may not reflect very well the action of angiotensin II on the smooth vascular receptor.

Dr. Onesti: I would like to comment about the difference between complete occlusion of the aorta at this level versus simple narrowing. We tried both models. We are now using complete ligation because it gives us a greater reproducibility on a day-by-day basis of blood pressure, heart rate and renin.* There is a certain variability of the onset and severity of hypertension depending upon the degree of constriction.

Dr. Hollifield: This comment is to Dr. Guthrie. Drs. Campbell and Pattinger several years ago reported that any type of anesthesia can result in elevation of plasma renin activity. Our own studies have been done in dog, rat, rabbit — all indicate that propranolol can fairly quickly lower the plasma renin activity to a much greater degree than you have shown. I wonder if your results with the poor suppression of plasma renin activity might not be due to the fact that you have used light ether anesthesia as the method of preparing your animals before blood drawing. We routinely use a guillotine post-

*Fernandes, M., Onesti, G., Weder, A. et al: Experimental model of severe renal hypertension. J. Lab. Clin. Med. (In press.)

decapitation as the method of collecting blood for plasma renin activity or concentration.

Dr. Guthrie: You are quite right, Dr. Hollifield. In fact, we used two types of anesthesia: (1) light ether anesthesia for blood pressure measurement, and (2) sodium pentabarbital before they were sacrificed, and I realize that both are stimuli to renin release. But the point is that despite these stimuli, plasma renin was variably suppressed and renal renin content was unchanged. I think that is the main point of my talk, that renal renin content did not change at all.

Effects of Dietary Sodium, Diuretics and Hypertension on Renin and Kallikrein

C. I. Johnston, M.D., P. G. Matthews, M.D.
and E. Dax, M.D.

Introduction

Kallikreins are enzymes which act upon a plasma α_2 globulin, kininogen, to produce kinins. They are found both in the plasma and secretory glands including the kidney. Kinins including bradykinin, a nonapeptide, are the most powerful known vasodilators and also cause diuresis and natriuresis when infused into man.

Recently changes in urinary kallikrein excretion have been reported to occur during sodium balance and in hypertensive states. However, the reports are conflicting for whereas Adetuyibi and Mills [1] and Carretero and Oza [2] showed a decrease in urinary kallikrein excretion associated with a low salt diet and a positive correlation between urinary sodium excretion and kallikrein excretion, Geller et al [3] demonstrated a rise in urinary kallikrein excretion associated with a low salt diet in both rats and man [4, 5]. Margolius et al [6, 7] also found decreased urinary kallikrein excretion in rats with experimental hypertension and patients with essential hypertension. They also postulated that changes in urinary kallikrein excretion were positively related to the level of salt-retaining hormones.

Renin is also an enzyme found in the kidney which acts upon a plasma α_2 globulin to produce an active polypeptide,

---

C. I. Johnston, M.D., P. G. Matthews, M.D. and E. Dax, M.D., Department of Medicine, Monash University, Prince Henry's Hospital, Melbourne, Australia.

angiotensin. Angiotensin is the most potent vasoconstrictor known and may be antidiuretic. The renin-angiotensin system has also been shown to be involved in both sodium homeostasis and hypertensive states. Recently Wong et al [8] have demonstrated a very close correlation between bradykinin levels and renin activity and angiotensin during both acute sodium loading and the upright posture in man.

This report further examines and establishes the relationship between the renin-angiotensin system and urinary kallikrein excretion during high and low sodium intakes in rats and during the development of experimental renal hypertension in the rat.

Methods

Male Sprague Dawley rats weighing 120-150 gm were used. One group of eight rats was fed on a normal diet for 5 days, followed by a low sodium diet for 28 days. A second group of eight rats was fed a normal diet for 5 days followed by the same diet with 2% saline in place of distilled water for drinking for 28 days. A further group of five rats were alternatively fed for five-day periods with a normal diet, a high salt intake, a low salt intake, followed by a normal diet and a high salt diet.

For the first ten days and the 28th day, the first two groups were placed in individual metabolic cages and their food and water intake measured and their urine collected for measurement of volume, sodium, potassium and kallikrein content. The group of five rats with changing salt balance were maintained in metabolic cages throughout the experimental period.

To produce a natriuresis without sodium loading, four rats were placed in individual metabolic cages and their urine volume, sodium potassium and kallikrein excretion measured over four hours. Following this, they were injected with 2 mg frusemide (Hoechst) intraperitoneally and these parameters measured again over four hours. Five rats given 0.1 ml dextrose intraperitoneally served as controls and blood was drawn for plasma renin and angiotensin before and after the diuretic.

Ten rats kept on an ad libitum diet and water intake underwent a unilateral nephrectomy. Ten other rats had a renal clip (0.2 mm id) placed on their left renal artery (2K Goldblatt rats) and ten other rats had left renal artery stenosis (1K

Goldblatt rats) and contralateral nephrectomy performed. Twenty-eight days later five 2K and five 1K Goldblatt animals that had developed stable severe hypertension together with five unilateral nephrectomized rats were placed in individual metabolic cages. Their urinary volume, sodium, potassium and kallikrein excretion and plasma renin activity were measured. Blood pressure was measured in conscious, lightly restrained rats by the method of Friedman and Freed [9].

Plasma renin was measured by a competitive binding radioimmunoassay [10] and plasma angiotensin by radioimmunoassay [11].

Kallikrein Incubation and Bradykinin Radioimmunoassay

Urinary kallikrein was measured by an enzyme kinetic method employing radioimmunoassay of generated bradykinin. 50μl of urine diluted 1:50 was incubated with 100μl of acid heated dog plasma [12] as a source of kininogen and 100μl of Tris HCl buffer pH 8.2 containing 0.01 M 1,10 phenantholine, 0.01 M Na EDTA and 0.1% neomycin. The mixture was incubated at 37°C for 30 minutes and the reaction stopped by adding 2 vol of cold absolute ethanol. The bradykinin generated was measured in a 20μl aliquot by radioimmunoassay [13, 14].

Bradykinin-specific antibodies were raised in rabbits by repeated injections of bradykinin (Sandoz) coupled to human serum albumin by gluteraldehyde condensation. ^{125}I Tyrosine ^{8} bradykinin was produced by the method of Greenwood and Hunter [15] using tyrosine ^{8} bradykinin obtained from New England Nuclear. Bradykinin (BRS 640, Sandoz) was used as standards and separation of free from the antibody bound ^{125}I bradykinin performed by the double antibody method.

Results

Kallikrein Incubation and Bradykinin Radioimmunoassay

A typical standard curve for the bradykinin radioimmunoassay is shown in Figure 1. The assay had a sensitivity of 50 pg of bradykinin, crossreacted with kallidin (lysyl bradykinin) but did not crossreact to the peptides vasopressin, oxytocin or angiotensin. The intra-assay variability was 4.0% and the interassay variability was 10.2%.

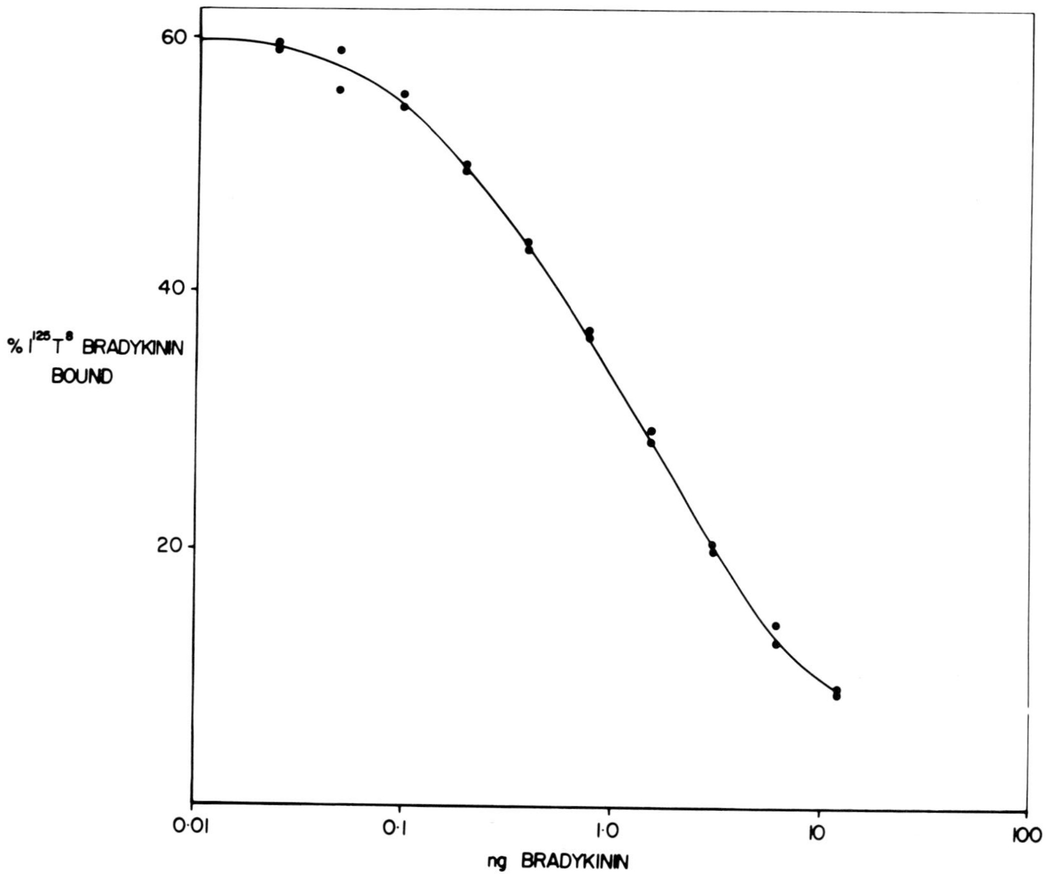

FIG. 1. Standard bradykinin radioimmunoassay curve showing displacement of antibody-bound $^{125}I\ T^8$ bradykinin by increasing quantities of unlabeled bradykinin.

When increasing volumes of rat urine were incubated with the semi purified dog kininogen there were proportional increases in the bradykinin produced. There was also a linear increase in bradykinin formation with time up to 60 minutes of incubation. Recovery of added bradykinin (50 ng) was 98.2 ± 2.8% (n = 10).

Changes in Sodium Balance

The changes in urinary sodium and kallikrein excretion, plasma renin activity and plasma angiotensin in normals, sodium-loaded and sodium-depleted rats on the fifth day is shown in Table 1. In sodium loading there was a significant and rapid fall in urinary kallikrein from control levels of 89.15 ± 8.96μg BK hr^{-1}/day to 14.09 ± 2.16μg BK hr^{-1}/day ($p < 0.001$) on the first day which was maintained until day 5. This was associated with rises in sodium excretion and falls in plasma renin and plasma angiotensin. In sodium depletion there was an initial rise in urinary kallikrein excretion on the second day to 98.37 ± 16.3μg BK hr $^{-1}$/day to levels of 52.4 ± 14.09μg BK hr $^{-1}$/day on the fifth day. These insignificant changes in urinary kallikrein were associated with significant rises in plasma renin and angiotensin (Table 1).

Table 1. Urinary Sodium and Kallikrein Excretion and Plasma Renin Activity and Plasma Angiotensin During the Control Period and After Five Days of Sodium Loading or Sodium Depletion

	Urinary Sodium Excretion mEq/day	*Urinary Kallikrein Excretion µgBK hr $^{-1}$/day*	*PRA ng ml $^{-1}$hr $^{-1}$*	*Plasma Angiotensin pg ml $^{-1}$*
Normals n = 16	0.48 ± 0.05	89.15 ± 8.96	22.9 ± 1.7	75.0 ± 18.0
Sodium loaded n = 8	27.4* ± 2.9	25.17* ± 6.76	2.6* ± 0.6	19.5* ± 2.1
Sodium depleted n = 8	0.07* ± 0.07	52.4 ±14.1	46.5* ± 3.7	171.2* ± 23.2

Values are means ± ISEM

*p < 0.001.

After 28 days of sodium loading the urinary kallikrein, plasma renin and angiotensin were still significantly depressed. However, in sodium-depleted rats there was now a significant rise in urinary kallikrein levels to 171.37 ± 25.79μg BK hr $^{-1}$/day ($p < 0.001$) associated with a maintained elevation in plasma renin and angiotensin (Table 2).

The changes in urinary sodium and kallikrein excretion in the five rats subjected to sequential loading and depletion is illustrated in Figure 2. This shows that urinary kallikrein is rapidly depressed during sodium loading and gradually increases on sodium depletion though not to elevated levels in five days. Urinary kallikrein could not be correlated with changes in urinary volume, sodium or potassium excretion, although high urinary sodium excretion was associated with low kallikrein excretion and conversely low sodium with high kallikrein. Urinary kallikrein excretion was however closely correlated to plasma renin activity (Fig. 3) and plasma angiotensin ($r = 0.73$, $p < 0.01$).

Acute Natriuresis With Frusemide

The changes in urinary sodium excretion, plasma renin activity and urinary kallikrein excretion are depicted in Figure 4. Frusemide was associated with a natriuresis and, in contrast to sodium loading, a rise in urinary kallikrein and plasma renin,

Table 2. Urinary Sodium and Kallikrein Excretion, Plasma Renin and Plasma Angiotensin After 28 Days of Sodium Loading or Sodium Depletion

	Urinary Sodium Excretion mEq/day	*Urinary Kallikrein Excretion μgBK hr⁻¹/day*	*PRA ng ml⁻¹ hr⁻¹*	*Plasma Angiotensin pg ml⁻¹*
Normals n = 16	0.48 ± 0.05	89.15 ± 8.96	22.9 ± 1.7	75.0 ±18.0
Sodium loaded n = 8	11.06 ± 1.02	54.7* ± 14.3	10.3 ± 2.1	39.6 ± 3.6
Sodium depleted n = 7	0.29 ± 0.06	171.37* ± 25.79	29.1 ± 5.2	81.8 ±11.5

Values are means ± ISEM.

*$p < 0.005$.

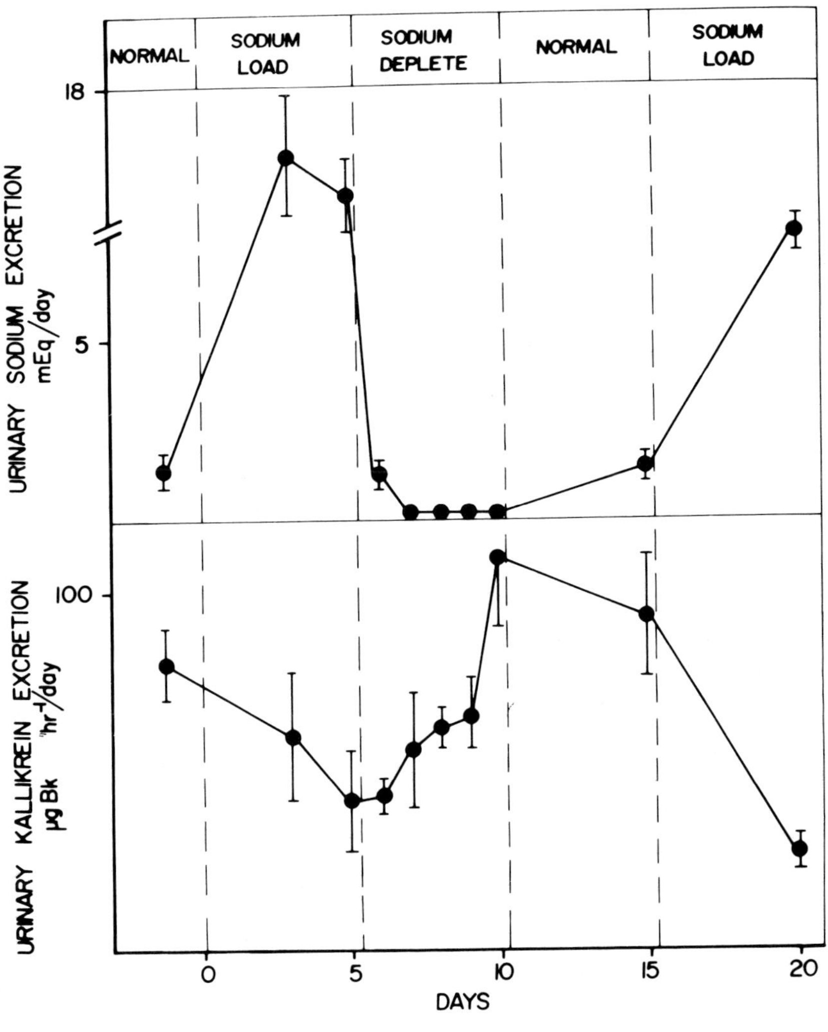

FIG. 2. Changes in urinary sodium excretion and urinary kallikrein excretion in five normal rats when placed on a normal, a high salt and a low salt intake.

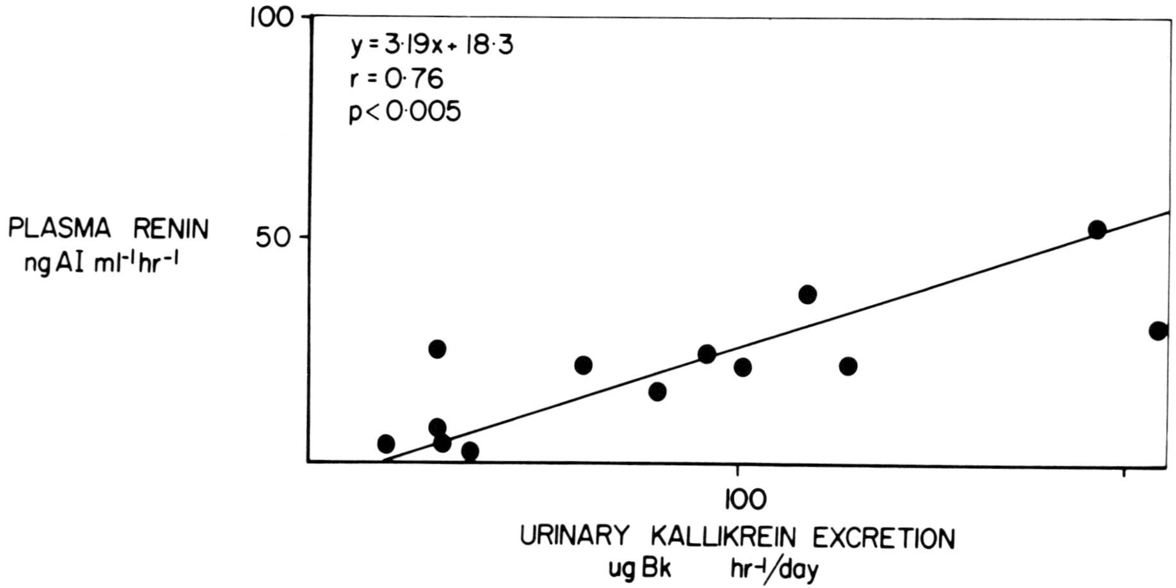

FIG. 3. Relationship between plasma renin and urinary kallikrein excretion in individual rats on normal, high and low sodium intake.

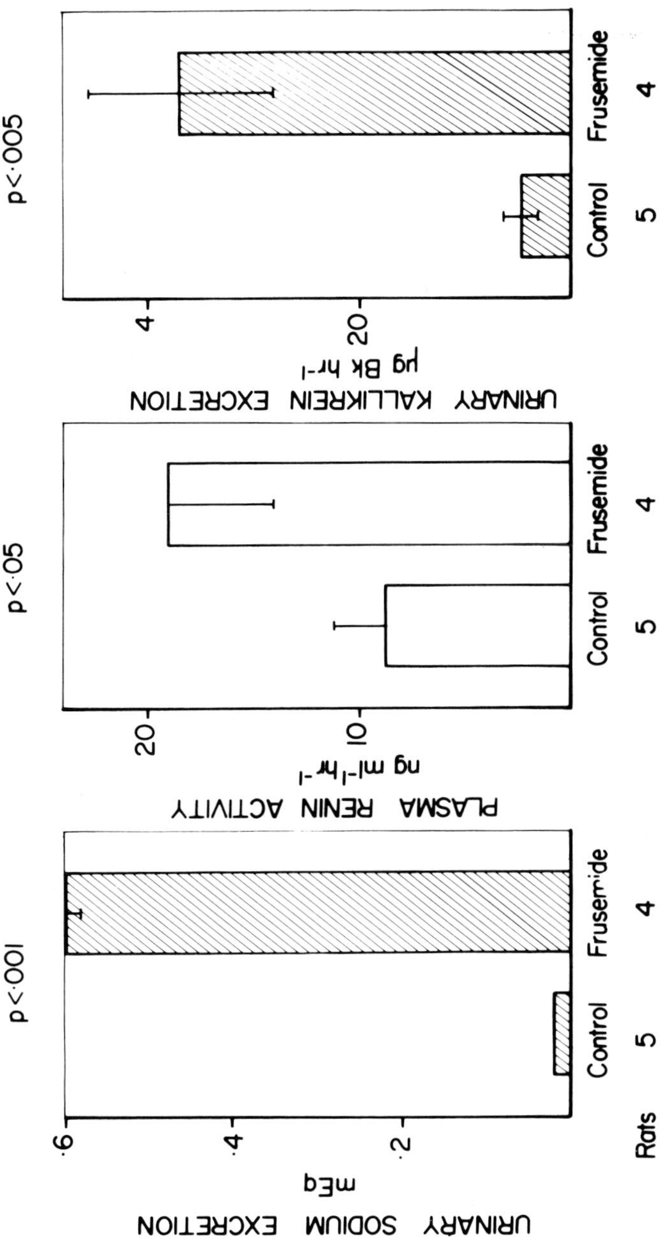

FIG. 4. Urinary sodium excretion, plasma renin activity and urinary kallikrein excretion in a four-hour period in four rats after 2 mg frusemide intraperitoneally, compared to control animals.

thus again maintaining the direct relationship between kallikrein excretion and plasma renin rather than sodium excretion.

Experimental Renal Hypertension

Rats with unilateral renal artery clipping (2K Goldblatt) developed hypertension associated with elevated plasma renin levels and a significant increase in urinary kallikrein excretion to 215.2 ± 24.2 ($p < 0.005$ v normals v unilateral nephrectomized animals). Animals with left renal artery stenosis and contralateral nephrectomy (1K Goldblatt), however, had normal levels of plasma renin and normal urinary kallikrein excretion rates (Fig. 5).

Discussion and Conclusions

The renin-angiotensin system and the kallikrein-kinin system both appear to be involved in sodium homeostasis. Our results do not support those of Adetuyibi and Mills [1] or Carretero and Oza [2] who suggested that urinary kallikrein excretion was related to renal sodium excretion. However, they do confirm those of Geller et al [3] and Margolius et al [4, 5] who showed that urinary kallikrein rose in rats and man when sodium depleted. The results reported here are also very similar to results published by Wong et al [8] in man. These workers showed that in saline loading plasma bradykinin fell in parallel with plasma renin and angiotensin and rose in conjunction with rises in plasma renin and angiotensin when sodium-loaded individuals assumed the upright posture.

The relationship of urinary sodium excretion and urinary kallikrein is very similar to the inverse relationship between plasma renin and sodium excretion. In general, low sodium excretion as in sodium depletion is associated with high renal kallikrein excretion whereas high sodium excretion is associated with low renal kallikrein excretion. The relationship between urinary kallikrein was a hyperbolic one similar to that seen between plasma renin and sodium excretion [16]. However, urinary sodium excretion can be dissociated from kallikrein excretion in acute situations. Thus, in acute sodium depletion urinary sodium falls rapidly, but urinary kallikrein does not rise until after several days [4, 5]. A more striking dissociation is

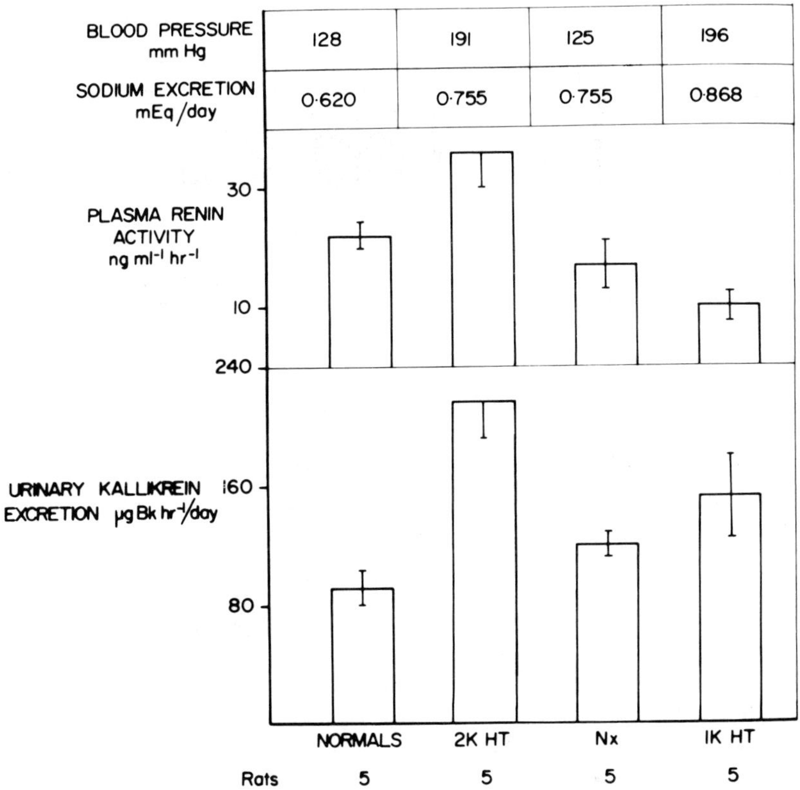

FIG. 5. Blood pressure, sodium excretion, plasma renin activity and urinary kallikrein excretion in normal rats, rats with left renal artery stenosis (2KHT), unilateral nephrectomized rats (Nx) and rats with left renal artery stenosis and unilateral nephrectomy (IKHT).

observed during acute natriuresis produced by frusemide. The natriuresis produced by this diuretic is associated with a very marked increase in kallikrein excretion, in marked contrast to the fall in kallikrein excretion seen in the natriuresis accompanying sodium loading. However, the natriuresis caused by frusemide is associated with a rise in plasma renin. In these studies we observed close and parallel changes in plasma renin and angiotensin and urinary kallikrein excretion.

The situation of urinary kallikrein excretion in hypertension appears more complex. Urinary kallikrein excretion has been shown to be reduced in man with essential hypertension [4, 5, 17] and in renal hypertensive rats [2, 6, 7, 18]. However, it has been reported to be high in spontaneously hypertensive and DOCA hypertensive rats [6, 7] and in patients with pheochromocytoma and primary aldosteronism [6, 7]. In this study 1K Goldblatt hypertensive rats had normal urinary excretion levels of kallikrein, whereas 2K Goldblatt hypertensive rats had elevated levels of urinary kallikrein. This is interesting as it has been shown that the plasma renin and angiotensin levels and probably also aldosterone levels differ in these two experimental models. One Kidney Goldblatt hypertensive rats have normal renin levels whereas 2K Goldblatt hypertensive animals have elevated levels of renin and angiotensin [19]. This observation was confirmed in this study and again illustrates the close relationship between plasma renin and urinary kallikrein.

It would appear therefore that in both sodium balance (Table 3) and hypertension, kallikrein excretion is directly related to plasma renin. However, as plasma renin and aldosterone are also closely related, it is possible that the changes in kallikrein excretion are related to changes in mineralocorticoid activity. This would be supported by the changes in DOCA salt hypertension, primary aldosteronism and escape from mineralocorticoids (Table 4).

Table 3. Relationships Between Urinary Kallikrein Excretion, Plasma Renin and Aldosterone to Sodium Balance and Excretion

	Sodium Balance		
	Sodium Depletion	*Sodium Load*	*Diuretics*
Sodium balance	↓	↑	↓
Renin	↑	↓	↑
Aldosterone	↑	↓	↑
Kallikrein	↑	↓	↑

Table 4. Relationship Between Plasma Renin and Aldosterone in Two Kidney Goldblatt Hypertension (2KHT), One Kidney Goldblatt Hypertension (1KHT), Essential Hypertension and Primary Aldosteronism

	Hypertensive States			
	2KHT	1KHT	EHT	PÅLDO
BP	↑	↑	↑	↑
Sodium balance	↓	↑	=	↑
Renin	↑	=	=↓	↓
Aldosterone	↑	=	=↑	↑
Kallikrein	↑	=↓	↓	↑

Acknowledgments

We would like to thank Mrs. J. Leversha for expert technical assistance. This study was supported by a grant in aid from the National Heart Foundation of Australia. Dr. G. Matthews is a National Health and Medical Research Postgraduate Medical Scholar.

References

1. Adetuyebi, A. and Mills, I.H.: Relation between urinary kallikrein and renal function, hypertension and excretion of sodium and water in man. Lancet 2:203-207, 1972.
2. Carretero, O.A. and Oza, N.B.: Urinary kallikrein, sodium metabolism and hypertension. *In* Sambhi, M.P. (ed.): Mechanisms of Hypertension. Amsterdam:Excerpta Medica, 1973.
3. Geller, R.G., Margolius, H.S., Pisano, J.J. et al: Effects of mineralocorticoids, altered sodium intake and adrenalectomy on urinary kallikrein in rats. Circ. Res. 31:857-861, 1972.
4. Margolius, H.S., Horwitz, D., Geller, R.G. et al: Urinary kallikrein excretion in normal man. Circ. Res. 35:812-819, 1974.
5. Margolius, H.S., Horwitz, D., Pisano, J.J. et al: Urinary kallikrein excretion in hypertensive man. Circ. Res. 35:820-825, 1974.
6. Margolius, H.S., Geller, R., De Jong, W. et al: Altered urinary kallikrein in rats with hypertension. Circ. Res. 30:358-362, 1972.
7. Margolius, H.S., Geller, R.G., De Jong, W. et al: Urinary kallikrein excretion in hypertension. Circ. Res. 30, II - 125 - II - 131, 1972.

8. Wong, P.Y., Talamo, R.C., Williams, G.H. et al: Response of the kallikrein-kinin and renin angiotensin systems to saline infusion and upright posture. J. Clin. Invest. 55:691-698, 1975.
9. Friedman, M. and Freed, S.C.: Microphonic manometer for indirect determination of systolic blood pressure in the rat. Proc. Soc. Exp. Biol. Med. 70:670-672, 1949.
10. Johnston, C.I., Mendelsohn, F. and Caseley, D.: Plasma renin determination employing a radioimmunoassay of angiotensin. Proc. Aust. Soc. Med. Res. 2:271-272, 1969.
11. Johnston, C.I., Mendelsohn, F.A.O. and Doyle, A.E.: Metabolism of angiotensin II in sodium depletion and hypertension in humans. Circ. Res. 30 (suppl. II):203-213, 1972.
12. Horton, E.W.: The estimation of urinary kallikrein. J. Physiol. 148:267-282, 1959.
13. Spragg, J., Austen, K.F. and Haber, E.: Production of antibody against bradykinin: Demonstration of specificity by complement fixation and radioimmunoassay. J. Immunology, 96:333-341, 1966.
14. Mashford, M.L. and Roberts, M.L.: Determination of human urinary kinin levels by radioimmunoassay using a tyrosine analogue of bradykinin. Biochem. Pharm. 20:969-973, 1971.
15. Greenwood, F.C. and Hunter, W.M.: The preparation of ^{131}I labelled human growth hormone of high specific radioactivity. Biochem. J. 89:114-123, 1963.
16. Laragh, J.H., Sealey, J. and Brunner, H.R.: The control of aldosterone secretion in normal and hypertensive man: Abnormal renin aldosterone patterns in low renin hypertension. Amer. J. Med. 53:649-663, 1972.
17. Margolius, H.S., Geller, R., Pisano, J.J. et al: Altered urinary kallikrein excretion in human hypertension. Lancet 2:1063-1065, 1971.
18. Croxatto, H.R. and San Martin, M.: Kallikrein-like activity in the urine of renal hypertensive rats. Experientia 26:1216-1217, 1970.
19. Hutchinson, J.S., Matthews, P.G., Dax, E. et al: Plasma renin and angiotensin levels in experimental hypertension in the rat. Clin Exp. Pharmacol. Physiol. suppl. 2, pp. 83-88, 1975.

Bibliography

Matthews, P.G. and Johnston, C.I.: Urinary kallikrein excretion and renal sodium handling. Proc. VIth International Congress of Nephrology, Abstract No. 127 (1975).

Discussion

Moderator: Dr. F. M. Bumpus

Dr. Williams: I have two questions to ask of Dr. Johnston: We had trouble with our data in explaining two questions that maybe you could help with. Since under all of the circumstances you described aldosterone was rising, Margolius has suggested that it is aldosterone and the K producing the changes in the urinary kallikrein and not sodium and the renin-angiotensin system. Do you have any data that could dissociate those two responses?

The second question is this: I would assume from your studies in the rat that you would suggest that people with essential hypertension have lower urinary kallikrein probably because they have lower levels of renin activity.

Dr. Johnston: As regards the first point, as to whether it is mineralocorticoids or not, I do not have any data and I purposely have not done the type of experiments that Margolius and Geller did. But it does not in our hands relate at all to the urinary potassium excretion or any change in potassium. I think it is very interesting that about three groups now have reported in essential hypertension urinary kallikrein is low. Obviously, it would be nice if those patients were the very patients who had low renins because it would be an easy way for screening hypertensives to take the 24-hour urinary specimen.

Dr. Vallotton: Dr. Johnston, there is another point common to the renin-angiotensin system and the kallikrein-bradykinin system: it is the converting enzyme and bradykinin potentiating factor. Do you have any data on the effect of the SQ20881 on kallikrein and renin when measured simultaneously?

Dr. Johnston: No, it has not been available in Australia.

Dr. Gross: Dr. Johnston, it is now more than 30 years ago that E. Schlittler, in the research laboratories of CIBA Limited, found that kallikrein excretion in the urine was reduced in patients with essential hypertension. It was E. Wollheim who first claimed that a substance — he called it depressan — was reduced in hypertension. The hypothesis that hypertension was a consequence of the reduction of a depressor agent was good, but the only fault with Wollheim's theory was that he did not believe that it was kallikrein whose excretion in the urine was diminished. This, however, as you have shown, and as others have shown as well, is true.

Dr. Johnston: Yes, of course, it would be nice if we could show that in hypertension kallikrein was less and this could be one of the reasons why their blood pressure was up.

Dr. Bumpus: Of course, the source of the urinary kallikrein is different from the plasma. So there are two separate things there, possibly.

Dr. Streeten: That is exactly what I was going to say. As far as I know, the two enzymes are quite distinct in pH optima. So it is a little difficult to extrapolate from the one to the other unless there is any known connection between the two systems, of which there appears to be no evidence at present.

Effect of Diuretics on the Function of the Juxtaglomerular Apparatus in the Normal Kidney and During Experimental Acute Renal Failure

Klaus Thurau, M.D.

The level of arterial blood pressure is a multifactorial event. Among other parameters, however, the extracellular volume of the body, in particular its sodium chloride content, is one of the major determinants for blood pressure.

The preservation of a given extracellular volume requires that the enormous volume, which is filtered at the glomerular site, be maintained for the organism through tubular reabsorption, a process which depends to a large extent upon active transport by the tubular cells and which, in effect, is a volume-conserving mechanism. Because of the dependence of tubular volume reabsorption upon cell metabolism, the tubular cells can conserve filtered fluid quantitatively only when filtration rate does not exceed the reabsorptive capacity of the nephron, but is in balance with it. The compatibility of these two processes, ie, filtration and active reabsorption, is described as tubuloglomerular balance. This property of the nephron, which is believed to be mediated via the renin-angiotensin system, has received much attention during the last few years.

Under antidiuretic conditions, there is almost perfect tubuloglomerular balance, which results in a minimal urinary volume loss, whereas some degree of imbalance is established under conditions of volume expansion and during the action of diuretics, resulting in an increased urinary loss of volume and

Klaus Thurau, M.D., Department of Physiology, University of Munich, Germany.

salt and consequently in a reduction of extracellular volume. However, both processes, glomerular filtration and tubular reabsorption, are energetically independent of each other, since the force driving the formation of filtrate is the blood pressure and the energy for reabsorption originates from the metabolism of the tubular cells. Therefore, it is of particular interest to consider which mechanisms exist to tie these two primarily independent processes together, so that balance results, and how diuretics and extracellular volume expansion interfere to the effect that imbalance and increased urinary volume loss occur.

Tubuloglomerular Feedback

More than ten years ago, first experimental data were obtained indicating that the glomerular filtration rate of a single nephron unit is affected by the NaCl content in the tubular fluid at the macula densa segment [1, 2]. This segment is located at the end of Henle's loop, where the nephron has anatomical contact with its own glomerulus forming the cellular complex of the juxtaglomerular apparatus. Since then, much evidence has accumulated showing that the juxtaglomerular apparatus is an important structural prerequisite for tubulo-glomerular balance, as recently reviewed by Thurau and Mason [3]. The immediate signal for the operation of the feedback is the NaCl concentration in the tubular fluid at the macula densa. According to recent data of Schnermann [4], the chloride ion might be responsible for initiating the reaction. The NaCl concentration at the macula densa, as assessed by early distal tubular fluid analysis, has been found to increase with increasing delivery of fluid out of the proximal convolution [5-7]. At the same time, glomerular filtration rate of the nephron under study falls [7, 8]. Hence, the functional characteristics of the loop of Henle are such that changes in tubular fluid flow rate are translated into changes in NaCl concentration at the end of the loop, thereby establishing a flow rate dependent signal at the juxtaglomerular apparatus. This signal triggers a mechanism in the juxtaglomerular apparatus, which adjusts the rate of glomerular filtrate to that level which approximates the reabsorptive capacity of the nephron up to the macula densa segment. Hence, one determinant of the rate of glomerular filtrate is the tubular reabsorptive capacity itself.

It is most likely that the changes in single nephron glomerular filtration rate, resulting from the macula densa signal, are caused by vascular reactions in the region of the glomerular arterioles. When glomerular capillary pressure is assessed using the stop flow pressure technique of Gertz, while increasing the perfusion rate through the loop of Henle, it can be demonstrated that glomerular capillary pressure decreases [8, 9]. Such changes in glomerular filtration dynamics do not occur when the loop of Henle is perfused with Na-free, isosmotic mannitol at rates higher than normal. This indicates that it is the change in NaCl rather than changes in perfusion pressure or perfusion rate which triggers the feedback mechanism.

The vascular reactions of the glomerular arterioles, which are governed by the tubuloglomerular feedback system, appear to be associated with varying degrees of renin activity in the vascular region of the juxtaglomerular apparatus. The localization of renin within the juxtaglomerular apparatus, which is part of a single nephron unit, permits the functional autonomy of a single nephron to establish tubuloglomerular balance. When the NaCl concentration in the tubular fluid at the macula densa of the single nephron is increased from its naturally low value of 20-40 to 140 mM, which is associated with a reduction in filtration rate, the attached juxtaglomerular apparatus shows a highly significant increase in renin activity from 14.1 ± 9.0 to 35.7 ± 18.8 ng/0.1 ml/h, as shown in Figure 1 [10]. This activation does not occur when mock distal fluid is used as perfusate. When the normally low NaCl concentration at the macula densa is reduced further to almost zero, using isosmotic mannitol, activation of renin does not occur and even a slight decrease is apparent.

The renin activity in single juxtaglomerular apparatuses is also increased when NaCl concentration in the tubular fluid at the macula densa is elevated in the course of experimental acute renal failure, induced by temporary renal ischemia or uranyl nitrate [11, 12]. Under those conditions NaCl concentration in the tubular fluid at the macula densa is increased as a result of reduced tubular reabsorptive capacity of NaCl. This increased

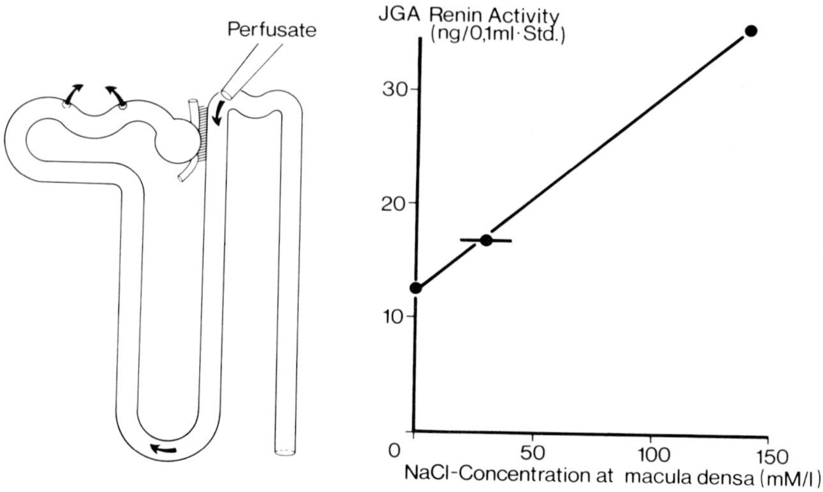

FIG. 1. *Left*, Schematic representation of the retrograde perfusion technique for changing intratubular fluid composition at the macula densa. *Right*, Correlation between NaCl concentration at the macula densa and renin activity in the microdissected JGA. The value indicated by ——●—— represents JGA renin measurements from nephrons without experimental perfusion of the macula densa, which were perfused naturally by glomerular-borne tubular fluid. (From Thurau et al [10].)

juxtaglomerular apparatus renin activity is again associated with a low glomerular filtration rate, such as normally found during experimental acute renal failure.

The data of Stowe and Schnermann [13] are consistent with the assumption that locally formed and acting angiotensin causes the changes in glomerular filtration dynamics. They found that the reduction in glomerular capillary pressure, as a result of stimulating the macula densa, is weakened when angiotensin II antagonists or converting enzyme inhibitors are given. Furthermore, the decrease in single nephron filtration rate resulting from a macula densa stimulus is almost completely abolished in volume expanded DOCA rats, in which the juxtaglomerular apparatus renin content is reduced [14].

Interference of Tubuloglomerular Feedback by Diuretics

Diuretics inhibit tubular reabsorption in various segments of the nephron. However, a reduction in tubular volume reabsorption alone is not sufficient to produce a diuresis, since the existence of a fully functioning tubuloglomerular feedback restricts glomerular filtration rate to prevent volume loss. Therefore, to act successfully, a diuretic, in addition to its inhibition of tubular NaCl reabsorption, must interfere with the tubuloglomerular feedback system. This in effect leads to tubuloglomerular imbalance allowing the kidney to maintain a high glomerular filtration rate at reduced tubular NaCl reabsorption and, hence, a brisk diuresis, as illustrated in Figure 2.

This action of diuretics has been investigated [15-18]. The NaCl concentration in the tubular fluid at the macula densa increases during the action of diuretics. However, the reduction in GFR, normally observed in a kidney not exposed to diuretics, is not apparent (Fig. 3). When early distal Na concentration is increased to 105 mEq by temporary renal ischemia or by furosemide and hydrochlorothiazide, a reduction in GFR is pronounced only in the postischemic model and not during the action of diuretics (Fig. 4). Hence, natriuretic agents are capable of breaking the feedback loop. This action of

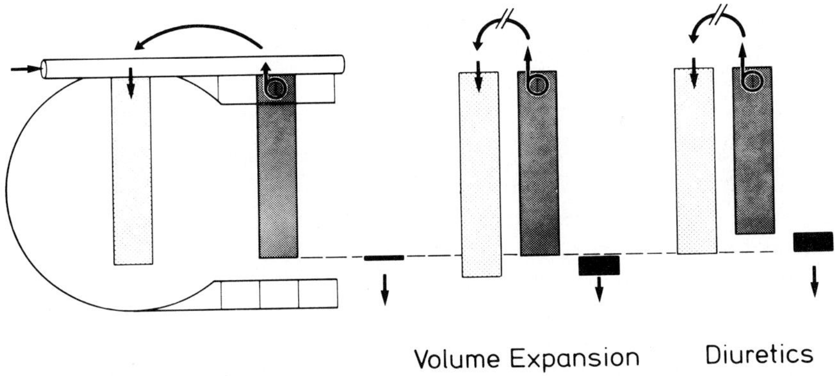

FIG. 2. Principles of interference with the gain of the tubuloglomerular feedback mechanism, allowing the kidney to maintain a diuresis. *Left*, The function of the feedback (↙⌒) couples GFR (↓, light column) to the tubular reabsorption (↑, dark column), leaving a minimal volume for excretion (↓, black column). *Middle*, During volume expansion, reabsorption is maintained, but because of reduction in JGA renin activity, rendering the feedback less sensitive to a given NaCl stimulus, GFR is increased and hence urine volume rises. *Right*, Diuretics reduce tubular reabsorption and interfere with the action of NaCl at the macula densa, allowing GFR to be maintained, thus permitting high urine output.

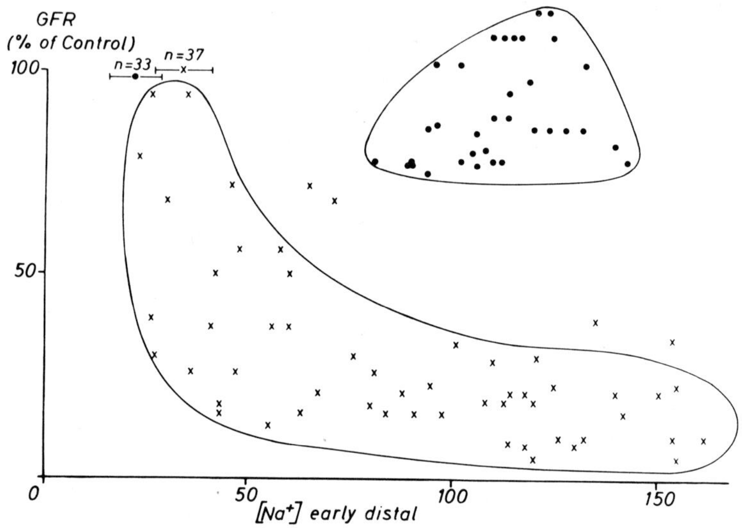

FIG. 3. Glomerular filtration rate, as % of control, as a function of early distal sodium concentration in the rat kidney after the administration of furosemide and after renal ischemia. The symbols with a number indicate control values for both groups with standard deviation and number of control measurements. Furosemide = (.), postischemic = (x). (From Horster, Nagel and Thurau, unpublished.)

diuretics has been studied recently in more detail by Wright and Schnermann [17]. When the macula densa is stimulated in a normal nephron, the single nephron filtration rate is reduced, as expected. However, when the stimulus is presented to the macula densa in the presence of diuretics in the tubular fluid, such as furosemide, triflocine or ethacrynic acid, the reduction in filtration rate no longer occurs (Fig. 5). This indicates that diuretics interfere with the ability of the NaCl receptors at the macula densa to perceive the signal.

The same inhibitory effect of furosemide upon the feedback mechanism, as found in the normal nephron, can also be demonstrated in nephrons with experimentally reduced reabsorptive capacity, showing the functional characteristics of acute renal failure [18]. When 140 mM NaCl is applied to the macula densa, single nephron GFR is low. However, when

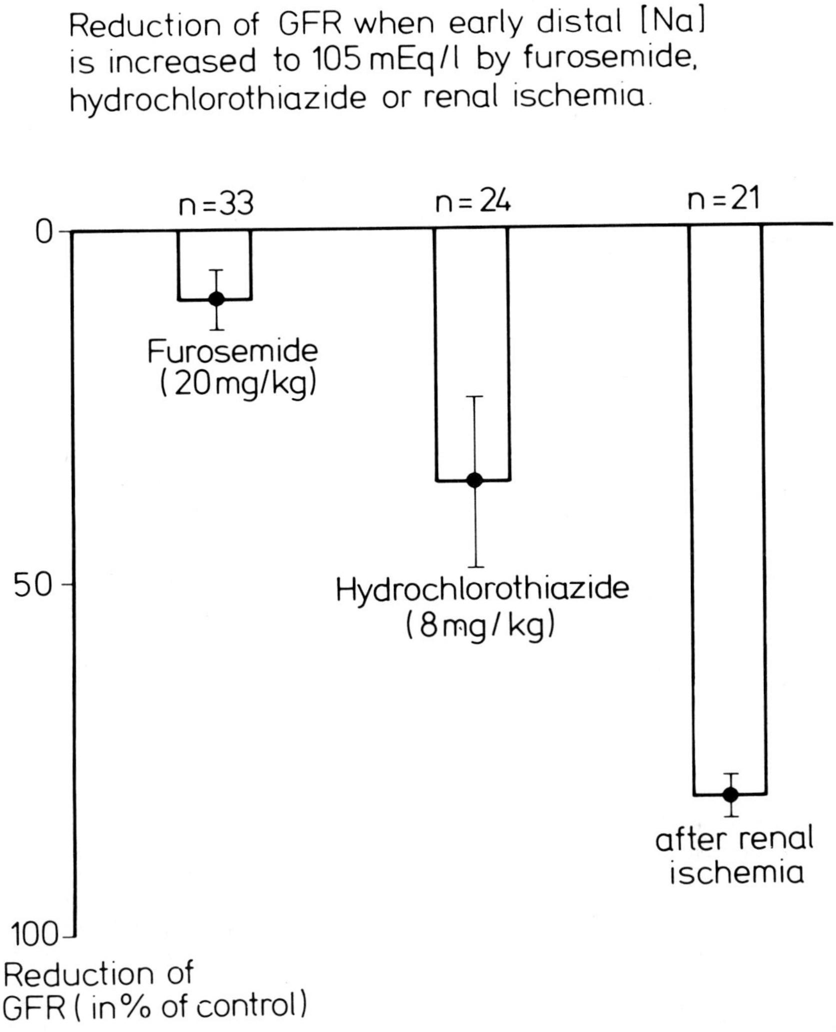

FIG. 4. The rate of reduction of whole kidney GFR when early distal sodium concentration is increased to 105 mEq/l by furosemide, hydrochlorothiazide or renal ischemia. (From Horster, Nagel and Thurau, unpublished.)

furosemide is included in the perfusate of the macula densa segment, GFR increases as if NaCl concentration at the macula densa were low (Fig. 6).

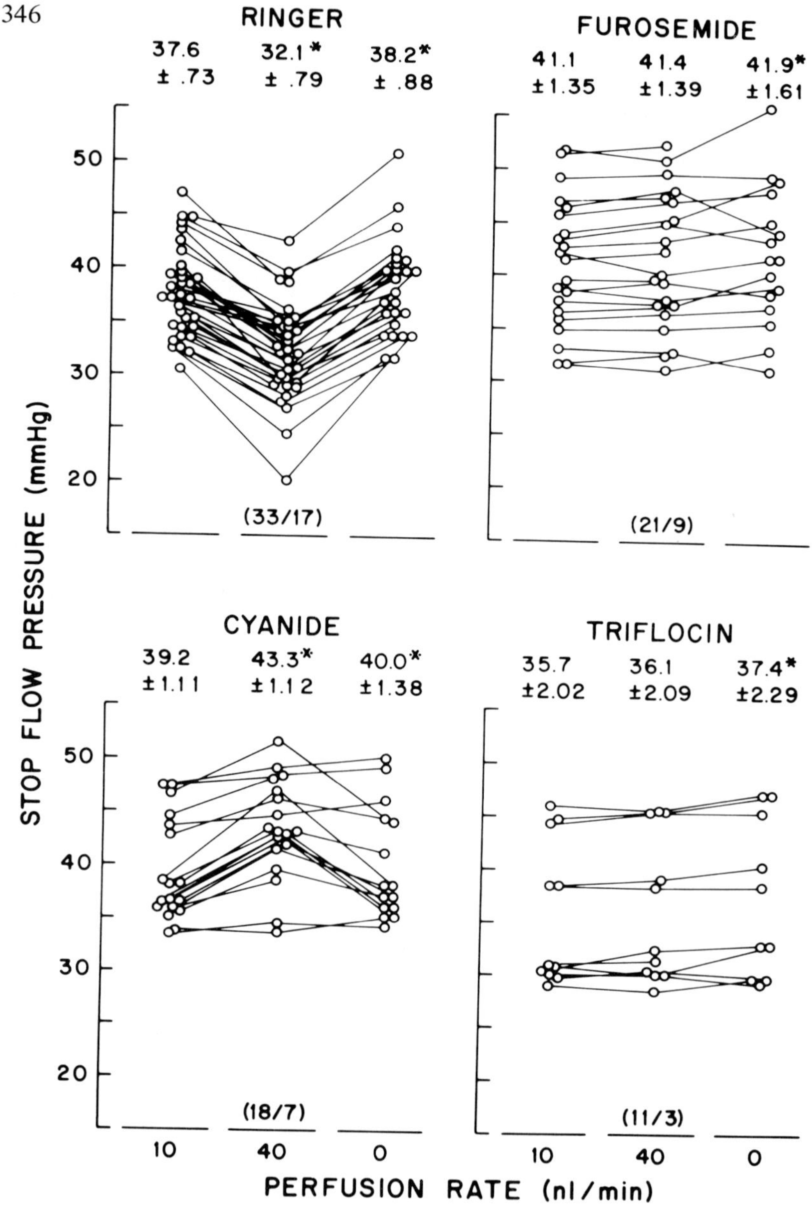

FIG. 5. Effect of loop perfusion rates and diuretics and cyanide on proximal stop flow pressure as a measure for glomerular capillary pressure. The reduction in stop flow pressure as a result of increased macula densa stimulation (40 nl/min) found in controls is abolished when transport inhibitors are included in the perfusate. Courtesy of Wright and Schnermann [17].

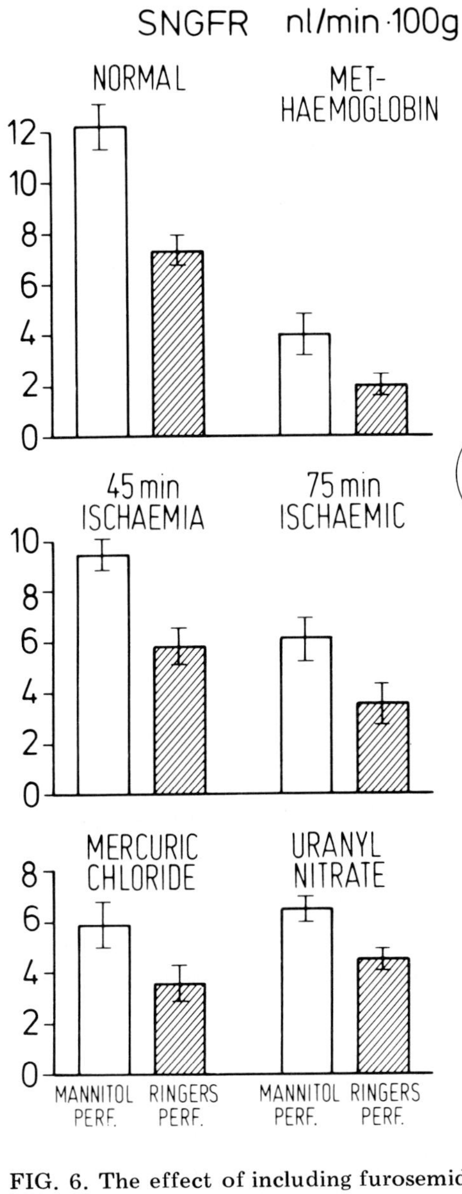

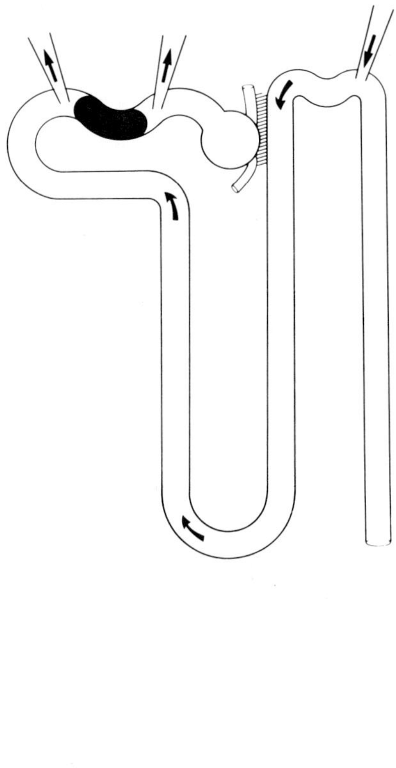

FIG. 6. The effect of including furosemide (10^{-4}) into the Ringer solution perfusing the loop of Henle of kidneys during experimental acute renal failure upon single nephron filtration rate. Hatched columns: Ringer perfusion. Open columns: Ringer and furosemide perfusion. Acute renal failure was produced by temporary renal ischemia, methaemoglobin, mercuric chloride and uranyl nitrate [18-20].

These data show that the natriuresis, induced pharmacologically by diuretics, results not only from inhibition of tubular NaCl reabsorption, but also from simultaneous interference with the feedback control of GFR, thereby establishing tubuloglomerular imbalance. This appears to be valid especially for those diuretics which exert their inhibiting effect upon tubular NaCl reabsorption primarily upon the proximal convolution and the loop of Henle up to the macula densa. Other diuretics, which primarily act upon NaCl and volume reabsorption beyond the macula densa, ie, in the distal convolution and collecting duct, may exert their diuretic effect even without interfering with the tubuloglomerular feedback mechanism.

This type of interference with the effectiveness of the tubuloglomerular feedback mechanism is pharmacologically induced. Another type of interference with the feedback is equally important and may be considered as a more physiological mechanism to establish tubuloglomerular imbalance: during extracellular volume expansion by saline infusion or high salt intake, juxtaglomerular apparatus renin activity is decreased. This change is not explained by a decrease in the NaCl signal at the macula densa, as it remains unchanged [3]. Rather, it must be assumed that this variation in juxtaglomerular apparatus renin activity results from a signal which is directly related to the state of extracellular volume expansion. Little is known about the pathway of this modifying stimulus and further work will be needed to show whether neuronal or humoral factors are responsible or whether the function of the renin-producing cells in the juxtaglomerular apparatus is influenced directly by the state of extracellular volume expansion, as recently discussed [16].

It is apparent that the dependency of the juxtaglomerular apparatus renin activity on the state of extracellular volume expansion offers a mechanism by which the gain of the feedback system can be reset: in the high volume state the gain of the feedback control of GFR by the NaCl concentration at the macula densa is reduced because of the lowered juxtaglomerular apparatus renin activity, allowing for a high GFR [14, 21] and hence large urinary output (Fig. 7).

A description of the effectiveness of the tubuloglomerular feedback system, therefore, must distinguish between these two different types of interference, as illustrated in Figure 7: (1) by

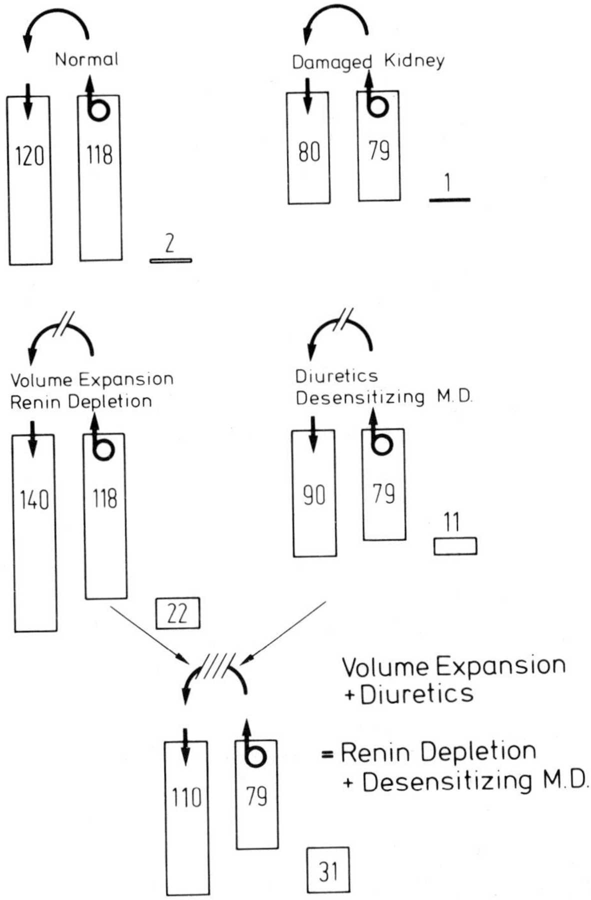

FIG. 7. Schematic illustration of the coupling between tubular reabsorption (↑) and GFR (↓) via the tubuloglomerular feedback mechanism (↙⌒↘). The numbers express volume movement in milliliters per minute. In the normal kidney with a reabsorptive rate of 118 ml/min, GFR is adjusted to 120 ml/min, leaving 2 ml/min as urine volume. In the damaged kidney with reduced reabsorption (79 ml/min), but intact feedback, GFR is reduced accordingly. The sensitivity of the feedback can be reduced (↙//↘) either by volume expansion, which lowers JGA renin activity and allows filtration rate to rise to supranormal values at a given reabsorption rate, or by some diuretics, which desensitize the macula densa to a given NaCl stimulus. In both cases tubuloglomerular imbalance occurs, resulting in a GFR, which is relatively too high for the existing tubular reabsorption. This imbalance leads to an increase in urinary volume. Both inhibitory effects upon the feedback may reinforce one another (↙///↘) during volume expansion (reduction in renin) and during simultaneous application of diuretics (desensitizing the macula densa). This combined action allows the kidney to excrete a larger fraction of filtered load.

changing the sensitivity of the macula densa to NaCl (diuretics) or (2) by changing juxtaglomerular apparatus renin activity independent of the NaCl at the macula densa (extracellular volume). The latter type of modulation of the feedback appears to be the means by which tubuloglomerular imbalance is achieved during the volume expanded state to allow the kidney to produce a NaCl diuresis.

References

1. Thurau, K. and Myle, M.: Mikropunktionsversuche zur Funktion des juxtaglomerulären Apparates in der Warmblüterniere. *In* Normale und pathologische Funktionen des Nierentubulus. Proc. 3 Symp. Ges. für Nephrol. Berlin 1964, Bern-Stuttgart:Hans Huber, 1965.
2. Thurau, K. and Schnermann, J.: Die Natriumkonzentration an den Macula densa-Zellen als regulierender Faktor für das Glomerulumfiltrat. Klin. Wschr. 43:410-413, 1965.
3. Thurau, K. and Mason, J.: The intrarenal function of the juxtaglomerular apparatus. *In* Guyton, A.C. and Thurau, K. (eds.): MTP International Review of Science, Kidney and Urinary Tract Physiology, Physiology Series 1 Vol. 6. Butterworths, London, and University Park Press, Baltimore, 1974, pp. 357-389.
4. Schnermann, J.: Regulation of single nephron filtration rate by feedback — facts and theories. Klin. Nephrol. 3:75, 1975.
5. Cortney, M.A., Nagel, W. and Thurau, K.: Micropuncture study of the relationship between flow rate through the loop of Henle and sodium concentration in the distal tubule. Pflüeger Arch. Ges. Physiol. 287:286-295, 1966.
6. Morgan, T. and Berliner, R.W.: A study by continuous microperfusion of water and electrolyte movements in the loop of Henle and distal tubule. Nephron 6:388-405, 1969.
7. Schnermann, J., Wright, F.S., Davis, J.M. et al: Regulation of superficial nephron filtration rate by tubulo-glomerular feedback. Pflüeger Arch. Ges. Physiol. 318:147-175, 1970.
8. Hierholzer, K., Müller-Suur, R., Gutsche, H.U. et al: Filtration in surface glomeruli as regulated by flow rate through the loop of Henle. Pflüeger Arch. Ges. Physiol. 352:315-337, 1974.
9. Schnermann, J., Persson, A.E.G. and Ågerup, B.: Tubuloglomerular feedback nonlinear relationship between glomerular hydrostatic pressure and loop of Henle perfusion rate. J. Clin. Invest. 52:862, 1973.
10. Thurau, K., Dahlheim, H., Grüner, A. et al: Activation of renin in the single juxtaglomerular apparatus by sodium chloride in the tubular fluid at the macula densa. Circ. Res. 30/31(II):182-II 186, 1972.
11. Vogt, Ch., Stowe, N., Dahlheim, H. et al: Mechanisms determining GFR after renal ischaemia. Pflüeger Arch. Ges. Physiol. 343, R 42, 1973.

12. Flamenbaum, W., Hamburger, R.J., Huddleston, M.L. et al: The initiation phase of experimental acute renal failure: An elevation of uranyl nitrate-induced acute renal failure in the rat. (To be published in Kidney Intern., Supplement on Acute Renal Failure, 1975.)
13. Stowe, N.T. and Schnermann, J.: Renin angiotensin mediation of tubuloglomerular feedback control of filtration rate. Fed. Proc. 33:347, 1974.
14. Schnermann, J., Hermle, M., Schmidmeier, E. et al: Impaired potency for feedback regulation of glomerular filtration rate in DOCA escaped rats. Pflüeger Arch. Ges. Physiol. 358:325-338, 1975.
15. Thurau, K.: Influence of sodium concentration at macula densa cells on tubular sodium load. Ann. N.Y. Acad. Sci. 139:388-399, 1966.
16. Thurau, K.: The juxtaglomerular apparatus: Its role in the function of the single nephron unit. *In* Modern Diuretic Therapy in the Treatment of Cardiovascular and Renal Disease. Amsterdam:Excerpta Medica, 1973.
17. Wright, F.S. and Schnermann, J.: Interference with feedback control of glomerular filtration rate by furosemide, triflocin, and cyanide. J. Clin. Invest. 53:1695-1708, 1974.
18. Mason, J. and Thurau, K.: The physiological mechanisms responsible for the adjustment of renal function during acute renal failure. Proc. VI Int. Congr. Nephrol., Florence, 1975.
19. Takabatake, T., Mason, J., Flamenbaum, W. et al: Micropuncture investigations in acute renal failure. *In* Nieren- und Hochdruckkrankheiten, Dustri-Verlag:Dr. K. Feistle, München, 1974.
20. Mason, J., Takabatake, T., Olbricht, Ch. et al: Tubuloglomerular feedback after renal ischaemia. Proc. XXVI Int. Congr. of Physiol. Sciences, New Delhi, 1974.
21. Dev, B., Drescher, C. and Schnermann, J.: Resetting of tubuloglomerular feedback sensitivity by dietary salt intake. Pflüeger Arch. Ges. Physiol. 346:263, 1974.

Discussion

Moderator: Dr. E. D. Freis

Dr. Doyle: Could you explain to me exactly how the GFR is reduced? In other words, what is the mechanism by which it is done. You say that there is 10 to 12 times the concentration of renin in the JG apparatus as in plasma, but the difficulty that I have is that if there is local production of angiotensin, if it is released anywhere, presumably it is released very close to the glomerulus, which is substantially free of smooth muscles, as far as I know. What data there are suggest that when renin is released from the kidney that you cannot detect any excessive renin in the efferent arteriole. Could you clarify that for me?

Dr. Thurau: The mechanism behind the formation of the glomerulus filtrate is presently under debate. Glomerular filtration rate may be altered by changing the effective filtration pressure or the glomerular plasma flow. Both models lead to the same net effect. I cannot answer which of these two models apply to the change in glomerular filtration rate induced by the feedback mechanism. All I would like to say is that the measurements of pressure in the proximal convolution indicate that glomerular capillary pressure is affected. As to the site of renin release, data from the Australian group indicate that renin is not released primarily into the blood at the site of the glomerular apparatus but rather enters the blood via the tissue or the lymphatics. That fits, I think, very well with the idea of a local action of these substances. From anatomical and histological studies it is well known that there are lymphatics in the area of the glomerular apparatus. Renin or angiotensin, which appears to be locally formed, apparently leaves the kidney via the lymphatics and the venous vessels but is not directly secreted into the blood which passes by JGA.

As I said, whether it is afferent vasoconstriction or a retraction of the glomerular capillaries, I do not know. But the fact is that the glomerular capillary pressure is reduced. There is, however, no evidence that this decrease in glomerular capillary pressure, which leads to the decrease in filtration rate, is due to a dilation of the efferent arteriole.

Dr. Kaplan: Dr. Thurau, is it possible, experimentally, to keep the early distal sodium concentration from increasing in the face of a diuretic agent to further show if the effect of the diuretic is a specific one?

Dr. Thurau: This is possible by retrograde perfusion from an early distal puncture site. The experimental approach is to increase first the sodium concentration and then to include the diuretics into the perfusate as I have shown it today. It appears to be more difficult to start off with the low sodium concentration which normally exists at that site because the stimulus to the macula densa is minimal and a further reduction of that stimulus by diuretics is difficult to detect in the response of the single GFR.

Dr. Sambhi: I have two questions for Dr. Thurau. Will you tell us your thoughts on how diuretics might disrupt this glomerulotubular balance, as you showed us in your data? If you consider one possibility as blocking the transport at the macula densa then should this effect be different with different diuretics? If you wish, will you comment in the light of your data, on the studies that we did that are well known to you, mainly that we gave diuretics and got a rise in renin. Then took off the diuretics and while the patients were getting repleted, we saw a further rise in renin, much higher than with diuretics. These experiments were somewhat similar to Dr. Denton's group in sheep, that while the sheep were repleting themselves, after sodium loss, their renin went up higher. At that period of repletion one can only surmise that the distal tubular sodium had to be very low because they were trying, very vigorously, to conserve sodium.

Dr. Thurau: Amiloride which primarily acts upon the distal tubule, beyond the macula, has little effect upon the feedback. Concerning the detailed mechanism of how diuretics disrupt the feedback, either it is a direct effect upon the luminal membrane permeability of the macula densa cells or upon the ion transport. This is still to be investigated. As to your findings about the increase in renin activity during the action of diuretics and the further increase during the repletion phase I am afraid I cannot answer your question. However, I should like to clarify one point: the peripheral renin you measure may be affected (1) by a macula densa mechanism and (2) a mechanism which is directly related to extracellular volume as I have discussed it last year in the Milan meeting. Hence, renin activity in the JGA is subject, at least, to two stimuli, one from the macula densa and one directly related to extracellular volume at a constant macula densa signal.

Dr. Catt: To return to the earlier point raised by Dr. Doyle about the way in which angiotensin II could operate locally to affect glomerular filtration, there have been two studies showing localization of angiotensin II in the renal glomerulus and mesangial cells. One of these reports employed tritiated angiotensin II* and the other used ^{125}I-angiotensin II.† The latter authors were able to correlate the extent of binding of angiotensin II to the isolated glomeruli with a change in the diameter of the glomeruli during exposure to angiotensin II in vitro. These results might offer some indication of the type of action which could be exerted locally by angiotensin II to alter glomerular filtration.

Dr. Thurau: I think we both agree that it is too early to take these measurements as to indicate that there is a local formation, but it is suggestive. I may mention another finding, which was obtained last year by Dr. Fred Mendelson when he was in our laboratory. He showed that the blood-free renal tissue contains angiotensin II. In other words, there is increasing evidence that the renal tissue is capable of forming intrarenally angiotensin II and our functional results would be consistent with such an intrarenal formation.

Dr. Denton: How do you conceive the feedback loop, whereby the contemporary level of angiotensin II in renal artery blood influences the rate of secretion of renin, actually works? The fact that we infuse angiotensin into the renal artery and inhibit the release of renin, which occurs during the early stages of sodium deficiency, and second, for example, it was shown earlier this morning that with P113 being infused into the sodium-deficient animal, you get a rise in renin because there is an opening of the loop of feedback of angiotensin on renin

---

*Osborne, M., Meyer, P., Droz, B. et al: C. R. Acad. Sci. (Paris) 276:2457-2460, 1960.

†Sraer, J.D., Sraer, J., Ardaillou, R. et al: Kidney Int. 6:241-246, 1974.

released by the kidney. I was just curious as to how you see this, structurally and functionally, working from your consideration of these various problems of the local level.

Dr. Thurau: We have not yet investigated the effect of infused angiotensin upon the feedback. But I have some reservation about the physiological meaning of such an experiment. If you infuse angiotensin II into the renal artery you get a very unphysiological distribution, even the medulla which probably never sees in its normal life angiotensin II receives this material. Second, all vascular segments are exposed to angiotensin II, the arterioles, the arteries, the veins, which normally, apparently, does not occur. That means that not only the vascular tree is affected but also the tubular function because tubular function results from the hemodynamics in the kidney. I think we have to leave that open.

Dr. Denton: I must admit I do not quite understand when you say unphysiological, insofar as there is a naturally contrived infusion of angiotensin going into the renal artery all the time, particularly in the sodium-deficient animal.

Dr. Thurau: Is this concentration the same as the concentration of inborn angiotensin II?

Dr. Denton: No. We endeavor to block the rise of renin which occurs in the early stages of sodium deficiency by infusing angiotensin II into the renal artery. You can calculate the appropriate levels. You can infuse at a rate which contrives a level of angiotensin II in renal arterial blood which is about the same as occurs in sodium deficiency. So you are working within the physiological range — not a pharmacological range.

Dr. Thurau: I have no answer. Is there any evidence that in the test tube angiotensin interferes with the renin activity?

Dr. Denton: I do not know the answer.*

---

*In vitro angiotensin I or II does not appear to cause product inhibition of the enzymatic activity of renin. — Editor

III

Effects on Renin-Angiotensin-Aldosterone Axis

Primary Aldosteronism: The Effects of Spironolactone Upon Adrenal Function and Morphology

J. W. Conn, M.D., D. L. Hinerman, M.D.
and E. L. Cohen, M.D.

It is generally agreed that spironolactone antagonizes the sodium retaining effects of aldosterone by competing with the hormone at its cellular receptor sites (kidney, sweat glands, lacrimal glands, salivary glands and intestine). From a physiological point of view, its major influence is via the kidney, where it inhibits aldosterone-mediated sodium reabsorption and aldosterone-mediated potassium secretion. The sodium diuresis thus induced results in contraction of extracellular fluid volume, stimulation of renin release and an increased production of aldosterone. Stimulation of the renin-angiotensin-aldosterone system is what one expects from any diuretic agent which results in a loss of sodium and water from the body. But we have observed an additional effect with spironolactone. We have found that this compound has a specific effect on the aldosterone-producing cells of the adrenal cortex, an effect which inhibits aldosterone production. We wish to discuss our

---

Supported in part by United States Public Health Service Grant No. HL-14520, National Heart and Lung Institute, National Institutes of Health; by Grant RR-42 from the General Clinical Research Centers Program of the Division of Research Resources, National Institutes of Health; and by research funds provided by the United States Veterans Administration to a VA Distinguished Physician.

J. W. Conn, M.D., Distinguished Physician, United States Veterans Administration, L. H. Newburgh University Professor of Internal Medicine (Emeritus), University of Michigan Medical School; D. L. Hinerman, M.D., Professor of Pathology; and E. L. Cohen, M.D., Professor of Internal Medicine, University of Michigan Medical School, Ann Arbor, Mich.

data dealing with this effect in patients with primary aldosteronism. We will observe not only the very striking morphological changes in the aldosterone-producing cells but also the accompanying alterations in serum and urinary aldosterone and in plasma renin activity (PRA).

Five years after the 17-spirolactone steroids and spironolactone came into clinical use, Janigan [1], studying autopsy material, described the occurrence of eosinophilic, laminated bodies within the cytoplasm of the cells of the adrenal glomerulosa zone in patients who, during life, had received these compounds for the management of various forms of edema. People with similar disorders, treated with other forms of diuretic therapy, failed to exhibit such bodies in their adrenal glands. Six years later these observations were confirmed and extended by Jenis and Hertzog [2] and Davis and Medline [3] with the aid of electron microscopy. These bodies consist of whorls of concentrically arranged endoplasmic reticulum containing a central core of lipid material. Within the cell they range from 2μ to 20μ in diameter and are found exclusively in the aldosterone-producing cells (glomerulosa cells) of the adrenal cortex. Careful search by Jenis and Hertzog [2] indicated that "spironolactone bodies" were not found in any other region of the adrenal gland or in any other organ of the body. All of the foregoing studies had been carried out on postmortem material. Fisher and Horvat [4] in prospective studies were able to produce similar bodies in the adrenal glomerulosa zone of rats to which spironolactone had been administered by gastric lavage for 3 and 12 weeks. They concluded that the spironolactone body probably represented a morphological expression of altered aldosterone production or secretion.

In a preliminary communication we [5]. reported the first studies concerning the formation of spironolactone bodies (SB) in living people. We had observed these bodies in adrenal tissue surgically removed from patients with primary aldosteronism who had received spironolactone preoperatively. Therefore, we proceeded with further studies in an attempt to relate the morphological changes to physiological changes in aldosterone production and in PRA. From such data we concluded, at that time, that spironolactone exerts a direct effect upon aldosterone-producing cells inhibiting the production and/or release of aldosterone and that the spironolactone body may reflect intense biosynthetic activity within the glomerulosa cell in response to the block in aldosterone biosynthesis induced by spironolactone. We also reported that in primary aldosteronism due to adenoma, the SB were confined to the tumor and absent in the glomerulosa zone of the adrenal cortex proper, with an occasional exception which we shall discuss. On the other hand, in cases with aldosteronism due to bilateral hyperplasia, the SB were found to be distributed equally in both adrenal glands throughout the glomerulosa, both in nodules and in the adrenal glomerulosa zone. Finally, it was found that the number of bodies formed under the influence of spironolactone was related to the duration of spironolactone administration rather than to the dose administered (150-400 mg/day).

The studies to be reported have been carried out on 23 cases of primary aldosteronism from whom adenomas have been removed and on 5 surgically treated cases with aldosteronism due to bilateral adrenal hyperplasia. All of the patients received spironolactone up to 12 hours before operation for various lengths of time and in daily dosages varying from 150 to 400 mg/day. Aldosterone and PRA were each measured by radioimmunoassay as described from this laboratory previously [6, 7]. The time of administration of spironolactone varied from 2 to 170 days preoperatively.

Morphological Studies

We shall describe the morphological appearance of SB, their location and the changes in their numbers in relation to duration of spironolactone administration. These bodies are easily seen and can be accurately counted under the ordinary light microscope. However, their appearance under the electron microscope, as reported by Jenis and Hertzog [2], is very striking. Figure 1, taken from their study, shows a typical spironolactone body within the cytoplasm of a glomerulosa cell. It is composed of whorls of concentric, tightly packed, agranular membranes with a lipid central core. These are whorls of smooth endoplasmic reticulum upon which it is known that enzymatic reactions occur in the biosynthesis of steroid

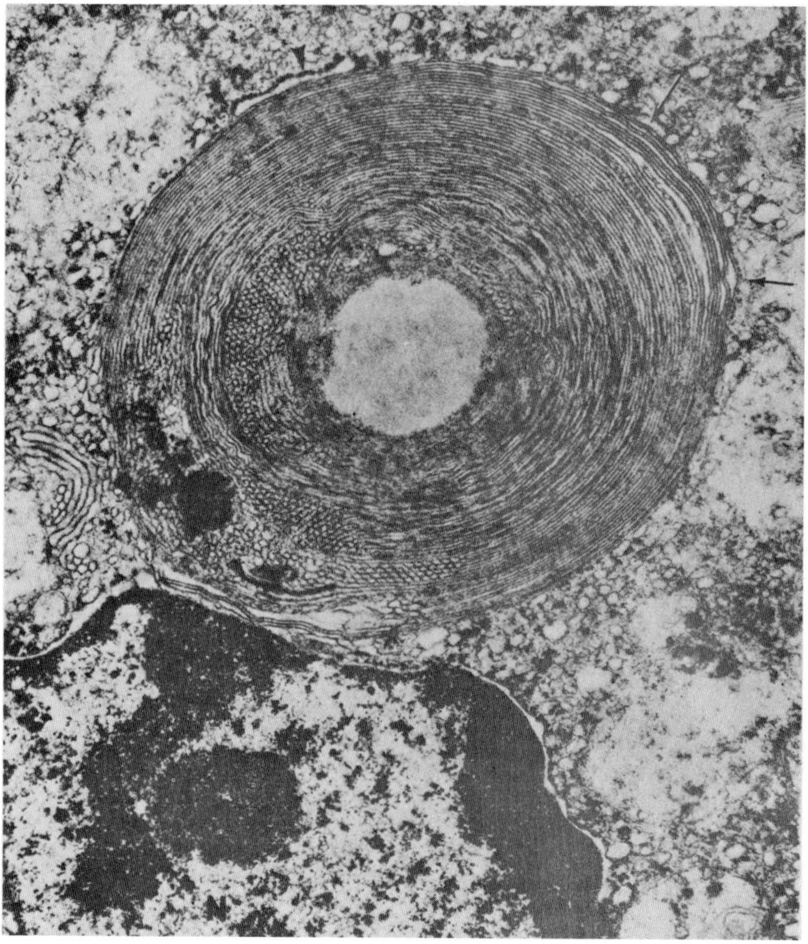

FIG. 1. Electron micrograph of a spironolactone body. (From Jenis and Hertzog [2]. Copyright 1969, American Medical Association.)

hormones [4, 8]. It has been shown by Giacomelli et al [8] that glomerulosa cells of rats, stimulated by low sodium intake, show increased amounts of smooth endoplasmic reticulum in the cytoplasm. But these accumulations do not resemble SB either in form or in extent. Those changes in the stimulated rat glomerulosa cells were, however, interpreted as evidence of increased intracellular enzymatic activities for the production of aldosterone.

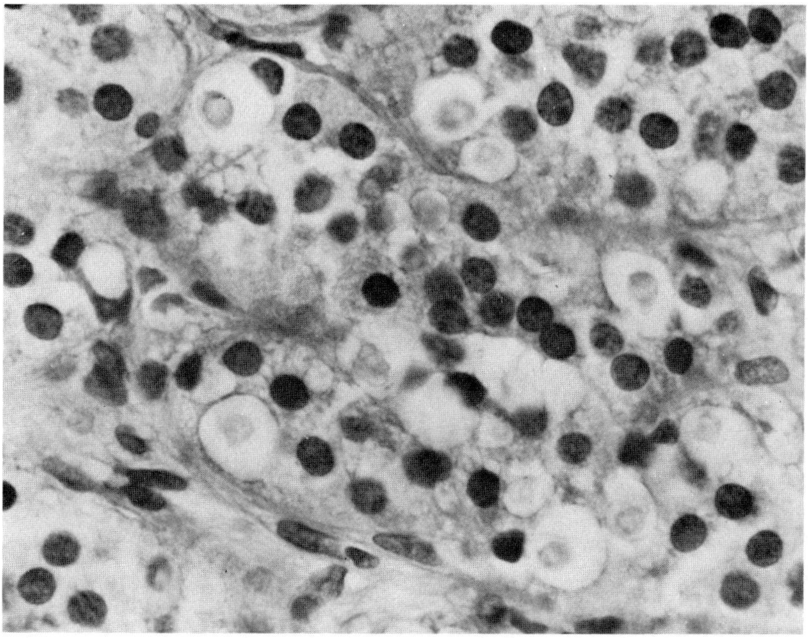

FIG. 2. Spironolactone bodies in a section from an aldosterone-producing tumor (bodies surrounded by a white halo) × 675.

Figure 2, from our own study, shows the appearance of SB by light microscopy. This is a section from an aldosterone-producing tumor. The bodies stain pink with eosin and are seen within a white halo. Figure 3 shows a section from the same tumor at lower power and indicates that SB are easily identified and counted. Figure 4 is a section from one of the adrenal glands of a patient with aldosteronism due to bilateral hyperplasia. In these patients the SB are distributed evenly throughout the glomerulosa cells of the hyperplastic glomerulosa and nodules, while in tumor cases these bodies are confined to the tumor and are unusual in the cells of the glomerulosa proper.

Figure 5 shows the life cycle of the spironolactone body as derived from counts of SB in the adenomas of 23 patients with proven primary aldosteronism. In each case spironolactone was administered until 12 hours before operation, but the *duration* of administration varied from 2 to 170 days. The average daily dose for each patient is recorded in parentheses. The ordinate indicates the spironolactone body count, the mean value

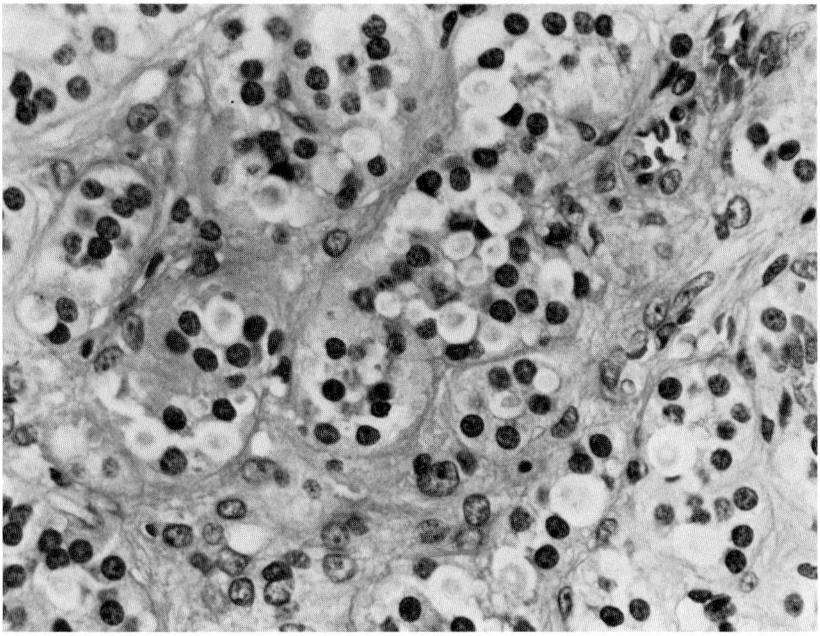

FIG. 3. Spironolactone bodies in a section from an aldosterone-producing tumor (× 350, the magnification for counting).

obtained from counting five random high power fields. The abscissa shows the duration of spironolactone administration before operation. As the points that you see were plotted, at first there appeared to be no relationship between duration of spironolactone treatment and the number of SB, since, for example, there was the same number at 10 days as at 90 days. But we soon realized that the peak counts were occurring between 40 and 60 days with a gradual and highly significant increase between 3 and 50 days. Following this a highly significant decrease from 50 days to 170 days occurred. Note that the counts follow the line in relation to time regardless of the dosage (150-400 mg/day) employed. Note, too, that SB do not occur until the patient has received the drug for at least three days. Observe, also, that at 100 and 110 days there are two *additional* cases that showed no SB. In these patients spironolactone had been discontinued 18 and 24 days prior to surgery. These two values were, of course, not computed in the

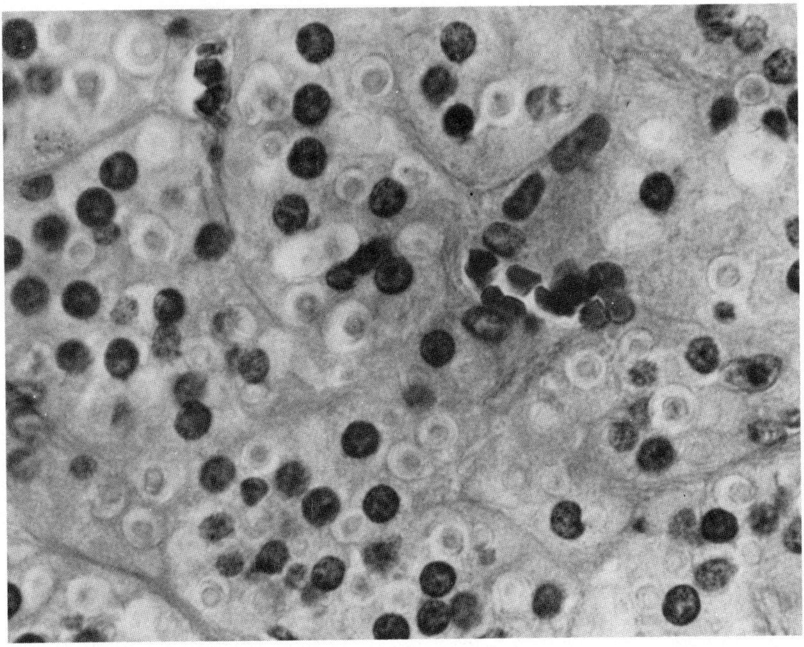

FIG. 4. Spironolactone bodies in a section of adrenal glomerulosa from a case of aldosteronism due to bilateral adrenal hyperplasia (× 675).

regression lines produced by the other 23. Thus, accelerating formation of SB occurred during the first 50 days and then they began to diminish in number with time. While still present at 170 days, there were only a few. In the five cases studied with bilateral hyperplasia, the life cycle of SB followed the same pattern, but there were too few patients to allow for separate statistical analysis. The regression lines are solely from the 23 patients with tumors who received spironolactone up to the time of operation.

Physiological Studies

It seemed important to determine, if possible, if there were any detectable functional changes in the renin-angiotensin-aldosterone system as SB were being formed rapidly. Therefore, we elected to study this system in detail during the first 20 days of spironolactone administration, with removal of the adenoma

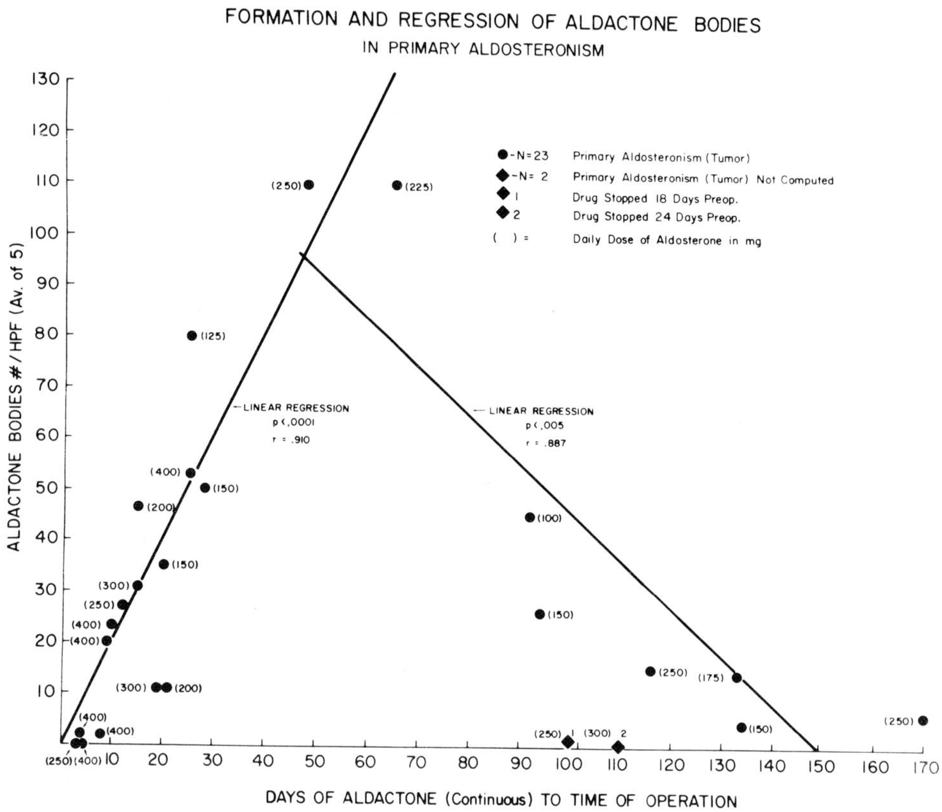

FIG. 5. The life cycle of spironolactone bodies based upon duration of spironolactone administration up to the time of operation and number of bodies found *in the tumor*.

immediately at the end of the short course of spironolactone. We had already observed in nine such patients a sharp *decrease* in aldosterone excretion for as long as 27 days after the beginning of spironolactone treatment. Those results will be shown subsequently. But we chose three patients for detailed study. They received spironolactone for 10, 11 and 20 days, respectively.

Figure 6 shows the results obtained on a patient who received 400 mg of spironolactone daily for the ten days preceding her operation. By the sixth day aldosterone excretion

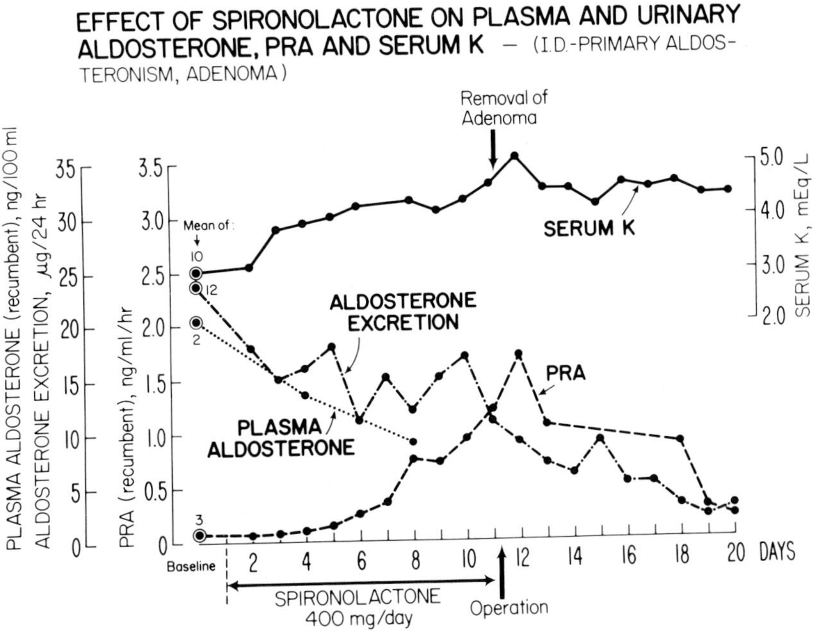

FIG. 6. The effect of spironolactone on plasma and urinary aldosterone, PRA and serum potassium in a case of aldosterone-producing adenoma.

had fallen to 50% of the mean baseline value. It then fluctuated at relatively low values for four days and, again, reached 50% of the average baseline level on the day before operation. By the eighth day of spironolactone, plasma aldosterone had fallen from 21.3 to 9.6 ng/100 ml. Plasma renin activity rose very slowly from very low levels to the lower part of the normal range by the day before operation. But, despite this very significant rise in PRA, aldosterone excretion was still 50% below baseline. Not only did aldosterone secretion fail to respond to a rise in PRA, but it also failed to respond to a rise of serum potassium from 3.0 to 4.6 mEq/L. After the adenoma had been removed, aldosterone excretion remained in the normal range for six days. In our experience this does not occur unless spironolactone is used preoperatively. Without the drug, aldosterone excretion drops precipitously to subnormal values (usually 1µg or less per day) within 24 to 48 hours, and it remains subnormal for several weeks and often for several months [9-12]. This is because the normal glomerulosa cells have not been receiving angiotensin II stimulation for years, ie, the time that primary aldosteronism has existed. Thus, as indicated by the aldosterone excretion rate in the first six postoperative days (Fig. 6), the normal glomerulosa zone has been awakened to activity by the increased PRA induced by the administered spironolactone. But this stimulus to aldosterone persisted for only a few days following cessation of the drug. By days 18, 19 and 20 aldosterone excretion is between 2μg and 3μg/day. PRA is also sluggish, falling quickly almost to preoperative levels. Removal of the tumor has unmasked the fact that the *normal* zona glomerulosa is producing some aldosterone in the immediate postoperative period (six days) but probably less than a similarly stimulated normal glomerulosa. If we assume that the normal glomerulosa had been partially activated by the day before operation, then tumor plus normal glomerulosa had resulted in total aldosterone excretion of 11μg (50% below baseline). This would mean that only 2μg came from the tumor on that day versus 24μg before spironolactone was given. It should be recalled that before the administration of spironolactone essentially all of the aldosterone produced was coming from the tumor [9-11]. Thus, when renin finally rose to levels which activated the normal glomerulosa cells, the tumor cells remained unresponsive to it. On the other hand, long-term spironolactone therapy in primary aldosteronism can, indeed, produce high values for both renin and aldosterone as will be shown shortly, but the aldosterone response is small in relation to the large rise in PRA. Table 1 presents additional data on electrolyte excretion and weight changes in the course of this patient's study.

Figure 7 shows, in another case, the same series of events (as described in the previous patient) during an 11-day period of spironolactone administration (400 mg/day). Urinary and plasma aldosterone fell, while PRA and serum potassium were rising. Again, aldosterone excretion fell to about 50% of the mean baseline value and plasma aldosterone fell from 53 to 27 ng/100 ml. But, in the postoperative period, in contrast to the previous case, this patient's normal glomerulosa cells were not even partially awakened by 11 days of preoperative treatment with spironolactone; very little, if any, aldosterone was contri-

Table 1. Primary Aldosteronism
Preoperative Treatment with Spironolactone (400 mg/Day) for 10 Days
Intake – Na – 120 mEq/24 h
K – 70 mEq/24 h

Date	Weight kg	Serum – mEq/L Na	K	Urine – mEq/24 h Na	K	PRA ng/ml/h Recumbent	Aldo. Excret. µg/24 h	Plasma Aldo. ng/100 ml
Nov.								
1	76.3	144	3.2	125	70	.14	23	18.9
2	75.5	142	3.0	159	74	.06	21	23.6
* 3	74.0	145	3.1	235	69	.06	18	
* 4	73.2	142	3.8	156	33	.07	15	
* 5	73.0	144	3.9	140	36	.10	16	13.5
* 6	72.9	145	4.0	121	42	.14	18	
* 7	72.5	144	4.2	138	48	.24	11	
* 8	71.7	–	–	144	61	.36	15	9.6
* 9	71.5	142	4.3	142	58	.75	12	
*10	71.2	143	4.1	132	61	.73	15	
*11	71.1	141	4.3	147	66	.92	17	
*12	71.0	138	4.6	96	47	1.20	11	
#13	72.3	142	5.1	126	68	1.70	9	
14	70.9	137	4.5	119	87	.96	7	
15	71.0	129	4.5	60	58	–	6	
16	70.3	138	4.2	52	54	–	9	
17	70.3	138	4.6	58	57	–	5	
18	70.1	143	4.5	63	52	–	5	
19	70.0	142	4.6	74	57	.87	3	
20	70.9	144	4.4	113	67	.27	2	
21	70.9	145	4.4	150	71	.20	3	

* – Spironolactone
# – Removal of adenoma

buted by the adrenals proper. Thus, in primary aldosteronism there is great variability in the depth of suppression of the renin-aldosterone system, and this contributes to the variability in time that it takes postoperatively to recover normal aldosterone secretion. This variability is illustrated for PRA in Table 2. In the ten adenoma patients shown, it is observed that in cases Nos. 1 and 6 severe suppression still exists after six weeks of administration of spironolactone. In addition, recovery of glomerulosa cell function lags considerably behind return of renin secretion [9-12].

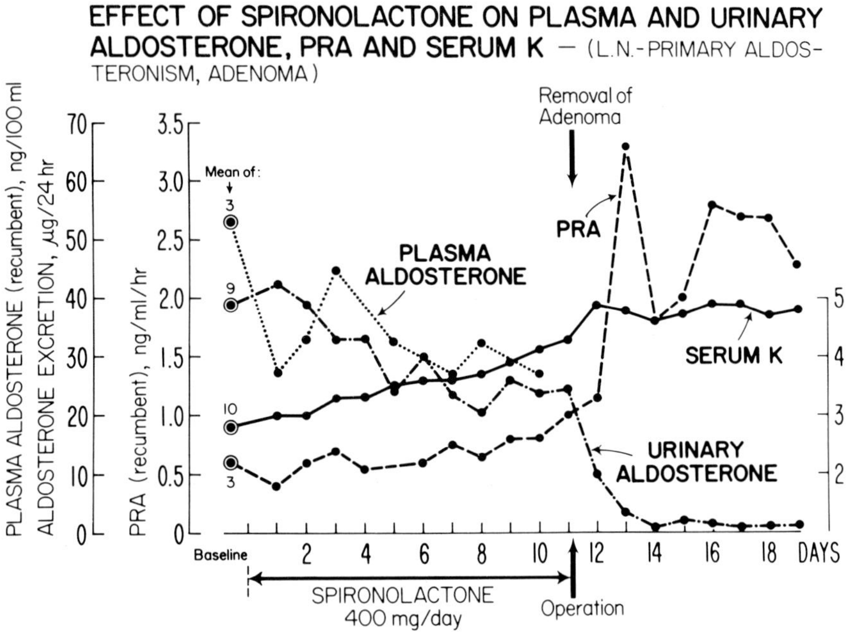

FIG. 7. The effect of spironolactone on plasma and urinary aldosterone, PRA and serum potassium in a case of aldosterone-producing adenoma.

Table 2. Primary Aldosteronism
Effect of Spironolactone on PRA
(2 hr upright, ng/ml/hr)

Case No.	*Diet – 120 mEq Na*	*120 mEq Na Aldactone 200 – 400 mg/Day* 10-14 Days	*6 Weeks*
1	.1	.4	.6
2	.1	1.9	
3	.1		9.6
4	.2	.6	9.9
5	.4		27.0
6	.5	.5	.7
7	.5	1.2	
8	.6	.1	
9	.8	6.8	
10	1.0	14.9	

Normal 7.7 ± 1.0 (SEM)

The next patient (Fig. 8) underwent a detailed study with spironolactone administration for 20 days before her operation. She received 400 mg of spironolactone daily for the first four days and 300 mg daily thereafter. It was our good fortune that we chose this patient for study because she telescoped in a short period of time various phenomena that usually require much more time to occur. Her aldosteronism was somewhat milder than that in the other two cases with serum potassium fluctuating between 3.6 and 4.0 mEq/L while on a diet containing 120 mEq/day of sodium. It is observed (Fig. 8) that upon administration of spironolactone, there was a short-lived, initial decrease in aldosterone excretion. With a tenfold increase of PRA (into the normal range) by day 12, aldosterone excretion came back only to baseline values. We interpret this to mean that the sharp increase in PRA has quickly awakened the mildly suppressed normal glomerulosa cells to secrete some aldosterone, covering up a continued partial block in aldosterone production by the tumor. There then ensued, on day 15 and beyond, a very large increase in PRA (142-fold above baseline) and aldosterone excretion went to twice its baseline values. This is what one often sees in tumor cases after six weeks of spironolactone therapy rather than 15 days. Note that in the postoperative period, aldosterone excretion was 16μg and 17μg/day on the second and third postoperative days and then gradually fell to 4.5μg/day on the tenth postoperative day. Thus, in the course of spironolactone administration, the normal glomerulosa cells were stimulated to produce a pretty good amount of aldosterone. This phenomenon appears to have been under way by the eighth day of spironolactone administration (day 12). This patient's response to spironolactone (probably because she was milder with a much less suppressed renin-aldosterone system) was to awaken her dormant normal glomerulosa cells much more rapidly than do most patients with primary aldosteronism.

Figure 9 summarizes the early changes (1 to 27 days) in aldosterone excretion induced by spironolactone in primary aldosteronism. The open circles represent the day of operation and the duration of time of spironolactone administration. It will be observed that in all 12 cases of primary aldosteronism there was a decrease in aldosterone excretion of from 25% to 83%. The longest period of reduced aldosterone production that

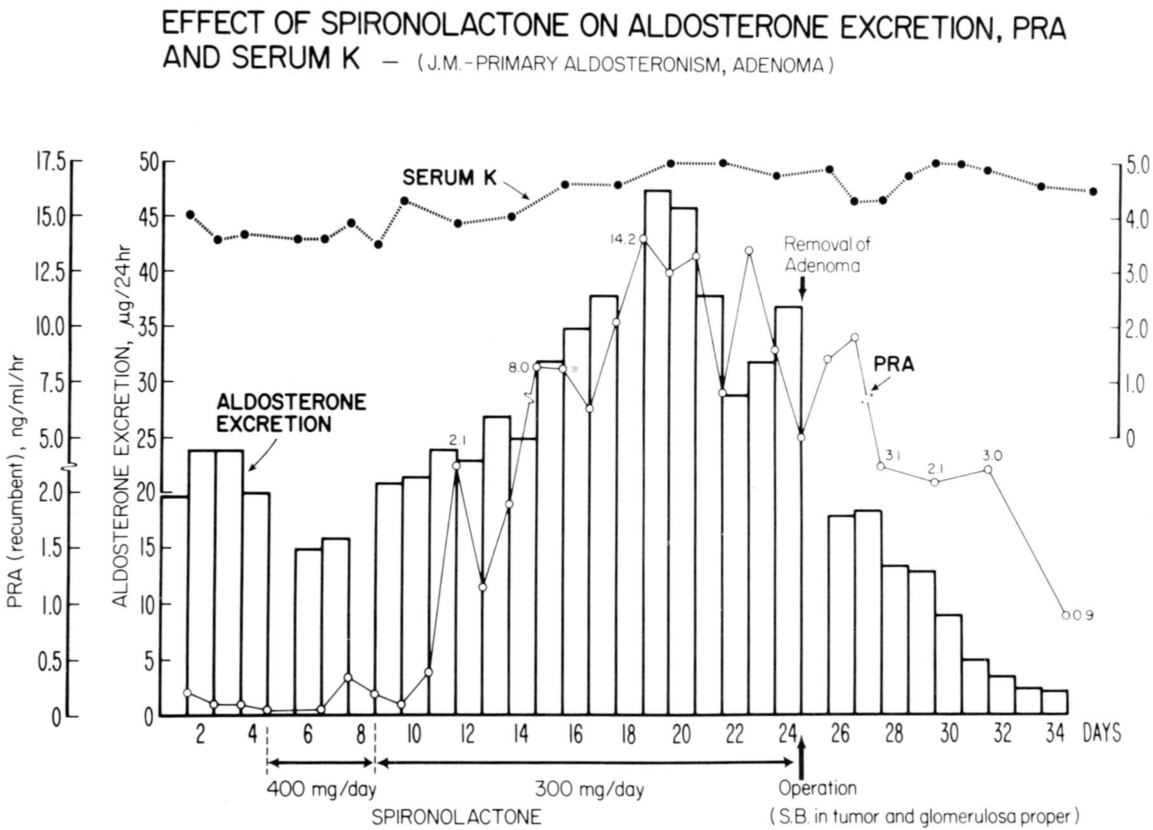

FIG. 8. Effect of spironolactone on aldosterone excretion, PRA and serum potassium in a case of aldosterone-producing adenoma.

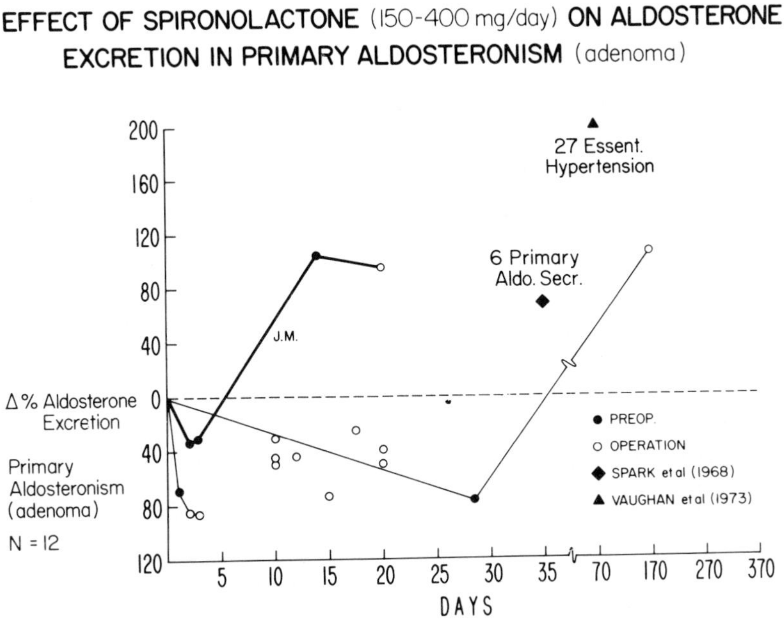

FIG. 9. Effect of spironolactone (given from 2 to 170 days up to the day of operation) upon aldosterone excretion in 12 patients with aldosterone-producing adenoma.

we observed was 27 days. Two patients operated upon at 20 days had aldosterone excretion rates 40% and 50%, respectively, below their baseline values. The patient represented by the heavy line is the one that we have just described in detail in Figure 8. At two and three days of spironolactone her aldosterone excretion was found to be 35% below baseline. By 14 days (day 18) the blocking effect of spironolactone was no longer evident and, at that time, aldosterone excretion was 100% above baseline while PRA had increased 142-fold. Thus, her aldosterone response at 14 days was similar to that of other patients with primary aldosteronism treated with spironolactone for six weeks [13] and somewhat lower than that of patients with essential hypertension treated with spironolactone for ten weeks [14]. It is clear then that in patients with primary aldosteronism, spironolactone results in an initial suppression of aldosterone production *by the tumor* as indicated by falling levels of both plasma and urinary aldosterone. Depending upon how long it takes to awaken the suppressed normal glomerulosa cells, this inhibition may be observed for as long as four months [15]. Usually, however, aldosterone excretion rises above baseline values by six weeks.

Comments

Correlation of Morphological and Functional Changes

There is no doubt that the whorls of endoplasmic reticulum observed in the aldosterone-producing cells are the direct result of administration of spironolactone. These whorls are not simply a reflection of greatly overfunctioning glomerulosa cells, because in the absence of spironolactone they do not occur. We have reviewed sections from 84 of our adenoma cases and 8 of our cases with bilateral hyperplasia that did not receive spironolactone, and in no instance was anything resembling a spironolactone body encountered. But when spironolactone is given in the presence of *actively secreting aldosterone-producing cells* SB are found; they are being formed very rapidly during the first 40 days of administration of spironolactone (Fig. 5), a period during which the fall in plasma and urine aldosterone is observed.

We have suggested [5] that spironolactone, in the doses usually employed clinically, induces a partial block in the biosynthetic pathway of aldosterone and that the spironolactone body is a morphological expression within the glomerulosa cell of an effort to overcome the block. That spironolactone can, indeed, inhibit steroidal biosynthesis of several corticosteroids in rat adrenal in vitro has recently been demonstrated by Erbler [16, 17].

Assuming that a partial block in aldosterone biosynthesis is responsible for the highly significant progressive increase in the number of SB during the first 40 days of continuous administration of this drug, it is important to recall that these counts apply to SB in the *adenomas* of these patients and that SB are only rarely observed in the glomerulosa cells of the adrenal proper in such patients. This important finding is helpful in interpreting the functional changes.

It has been well established by several investigators [9-12] that in primary aldosteronism due to adenoma, the glomerulosa cells of the adrenals themselves are producing little or no aldosterone and that they are in a severely suppressed functional state from which it is very difficult to arouse them for weeks or months after the adenoma has been removed, even when renin has returned to normal levels. If aldosterone biosynthesis is not occurring, these cells should show no effect of the introduction of a block into the biosynthetic pathway. On the other hand, the aldosterone-producing cells of the adenoma are very active and are functioning independently of the level of PRA and despite low levels of serum potassium. It is not surprising that upon administration of spironolactone, the block in aldosterone production should be seen quickly, both morphologically and functionally, in the adenomas of cases of primary aldosteronism. This syndrome, when due to adenoma, provides a unique opportunity to uncover the blocking action of spironolactone upon aldosterone-producing cells because the normal renin-angiotensin-aldosterone system is severely suppressed and is initially unresponsive to the sodium diuresis which the drug has induced (Table 2). Thus, the block in aldosterone production by the tumor remains uncovered until the renin-aldosterone system recovers sufficiently that it hides the block.* It seems significant (Fig. 8) that when aldosterone excretion was at its height (100% above baseline) PRA had risen to 142 times its baseline value, suggesting that the aldosterone-producing cells were responding suboptimally. A similar discrepancy, in similar patients given spironolactone for four weeks, has been noted by Kremer et al [19]. Mantero et al [20], studying a patient with an aldosterone-producing tumor, noted that four weeks of treatment with spironolactone (400 mg/day) resulted in a marked decrease in aldosterone excretion, ie, from 48μg to 58μg/day before treatment to

---

*It should be appreciated that except in a good radioimmunoassay system, spironolactone may interfere with aldosterone determinations, giving falsely elevated values. This may account for greatly elevated values [18] which have been reported in studies done before the advent of radioimmunoassays.

11μg/day to 20μg/day after treatment. A similar result has been reported recently by Sundsfjord et al [15]. In that case of primary aldosteronism, the previously markedly elevated aldosterone secretion rates and plasma aldosterone levels fell to normal values and remained there during four months of treatment with spironolactone. The tumor was then removed and complete cure was reported.

In normal people given spironolactone PRA rises rapidly and aldosterone secretion responds to that stimulus quickly (though, perhaps, suboptimally), thus covering up the partial underlying inhibition of aldosterone biosynthesis. Nevertheless, in this very situation SB do develop quickly. Such information is difficult to come by, since people with normal adrenals are not usually adrenalectomized after a week of spironolactone. However, a most cooperative patient scheduled to have a therapeutic adrenalectomy for metastatic cancer agreed to take spironolactone for one week before the operation. SB were present in the adrenals (Conn, 1975, unpublished data).

We have studied in detail only the first three weeks of spironolactone administration in primary aldosteronism in an effort to disclose the inhibition of aldosterone production. But there is an equally intriguing problem in the descending limb of the curve of SB. Patients who have had spironolactone for much longer periods of time have shown supernormal levels of both PRA and aldosterone and the number of SB in their adenomas has decreased gradually. We have not studied this area, namely, the compensatory mechanisms. Obviously, one of the compensatory mechanisms is represented by final awakening of the suppressed renin-aldosterone system which does occur on a more permanent basis with long-term preoperative spironolactone therapy. In the few such patients studied, occasional spironolactone bodies are observed in the glomerulosa cells of the normal part of the adrenal gland. But the virtual disappearance of SB from the adenoma itself as renin and aldosterone values rise above normal is an intriguing phenomenon. Perhaps SB formation stops because the cell has found a way to circumvent the block. Increased smooth endoplasmic reticulum would then recede. Only further investigations can answer such questions.

We have no data upon the accumulation of aldosterone precursors with which to suggest the site of a biosynthetic block. But if the SB is a manifestation of such a block, one may make an important inference (Fig. 10). These bodies are confined to aldosterone-producing cells and are not seen in normal fasciculata cells.* Since desoxycorticosterone and corticosterone biosynthesis proceeds in both zones, it seems likely that the block occurs beyond corticosterone, most likely in one or both of the final steps of aldosterone biosynthesis, ie, 18-hydroxylation of corticosterone and/or dehydrogenation of 18-hydroxycorticosterone to aldosterone. In this connection it seems significant that Vecsei et al [22] and Nicholls et al [23] have reported that aldosterone-producing adenomas have greatly elevated levels of 18-hydroxylase activity. This may be the site of inhibition by spironolactone.

In aldosteronism associated with bilateral hyperplasia, administration of spironolactone (five patients) for from 40 to 362 days resulted in a similar initial rise in SB followed after 50 days by a sharp reduction in their numbers. However, in this abnormality, the SB are evenly dispersed throughout the glomerulosa cells, both in the nodules and the adrenal proper. We have not studied the details of renin and aldosterone changes during early treatment with spironolactone in such patients. However, on the basis of the differences in the distribution of SB in this disorder, as compared with patients harboring an aldosterone-producing adenoma, we would conclude that the basic mechanisms of these two abnormalities are different. It is not surprising that an *adenoma* should be producing large amounts of aldosterone despite very low levels of renin and despite low levels of serum potassium. The virtual suspension of aldosterone production in the glomerulosa cells of the adrenal proper and the lack of SB formation there make for

*Some aldosterone-producing adenomas may be made up, in part, of cells which morphologically resemble fasciculata cells more than glomerulosa cells. Symington [21] has found that such cells contain some of the enzymatic machinery characteristic of both zones and terms them "hybrid cells." In such adenomas it is possible to observe spironolactone bodies in cells that look like fasciculata cells.

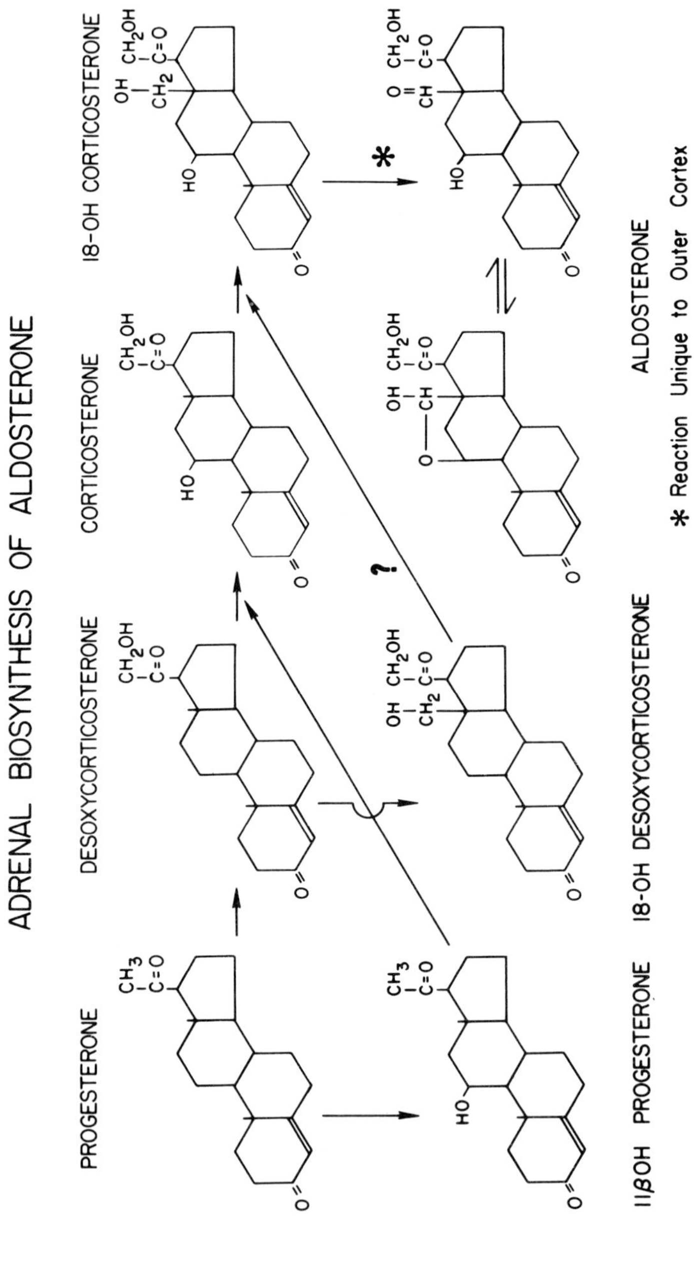

FIG. 10. Steps in the biosynthesis of aldosterone.

a very reasonable picture in the light of current knowledge. But in bilateral hyperplasia we also find what at first glance appears to be autonomous overproduction of aldosterone, since here, also, this is proceeding at low levels of PRA and serum potassium and normal levels of ACTH and serum sodium. But the analogy stops there because the glomerulosa cells of both of the hyperplastic adrenal glands are diffusely involved whether they are in nodules or in the hyperplastic adrenals proper. This diffuse distribution of SB suggests that the glomerulosa cells are very active and that they are receiving excessive stimulation from an, as yet, unidentified source. This may be the aldosterone-stimulating substance found in the blood of a patient with aldosteronism due to adrenal hyperplasia and *not found* in the blood of a patient with an aldosterone-producing adenoma [23]. It has previously been suggested that such a substance, other than ACTH, may be derived from the pituitary gland [24, 25].

Summary

Spironolactone bodies have been counted in adrenal tissue removed at surgery from 23 patients with primary aldosteronism (adenoma) and 5 patients with aldosteronism associated with bilateral adrenal hyperplasia. All had received spironolactone up until 12 hours preoperatively for various lengths of time. A high degree of correlation exists between the number of SB and the duration of spironolactone administration, the counts peaking at 50 days and diminishing thereafter almost to zero at 150 days. With daily amounts of spironolactone ranging from 170 to 400 mg, there is no correlation between numbers of SB and dose. The spironolactone body can be regarded as a specific marker of aldosterone-producing cells.

The rapid and progressive appearance of SB during the first three weeks of spironolactone administration coincides, in primary aldosteronism (tumor), with a sharp fall in urinary and plasma aldosterone. This suggests that spironolactone interferes with the biosynthesis of aldosterone in the adenoma and that the spironolactone body may be a manifestation of intense steroidal biosynthetic activity within the aldosterone-producing cells in response to this partial blockade. It is suggested that the block occurs in the final steps of aldosterone biosynthesis.

Spironolactone bodies are seen only occasionally in the suppressed glomerulosa cells of the adrenal proper in primary aldosteronism, even when they are very numerous in the adenoma. Since little or no aldosterone is being produced by these suppressed cells, one sees no evidence of a block in the biosynthetic pathway. Aldosteronism due to adenoma is unique in its ability to disclose the block in aldosterone biosynthesis induced by spironolactone. This is because for from several days to several months aldosterone cannot be produced in significant amounts by the glomerulosa cells of the adrenal proper which, otherwise, would tend to cover up the block. In people with normal adrenals a sharp rise in angiotensin II levels produces a prompt increase in aldosterone production which quickly hides any underlying partial block in aldosterone production. SB, nevertheless, are formed in such normal glomerulosa cells.

The distribution of SB in primary aldosteronism (adenoma) versus aldosteronism associated with bilateral hyperplasia suggests that these two disorders have different modi operandi, and that in the latter condition a factor other than the four known stimulators of aldosterone is operative.

References

1. Janigan, D.T.: Cytoplasmic bodies in the adrenal cortex of patients treated with spironolactone. Lancet 1:850, 1963.
2. Jenis, E.H. and Hertzog, R.W.: Effect of spironolactone on the zona glomerulosa of the adrenal gland: Light and electron microscopy. Arch. Pathol. 88:530, 1969.
3. Davis, D.A. and Medline, N.M.: Spironolactone (aldactone) bodies: Concentric lamellar formations in the adrenal cortices of patients treated with spironolactone. Am. J. Clin. Pathol. 54:22, 1970.
4. Fisher, E.R. and Horvat, B.: Ultrastructural features of aldosterone production. Arch. Pathol. 92:172, 1971.
5. Conn, J.W., Hinerman, D.L., Cohen, E.L. et al: Spironolactone (S) bodies (B) in primary aldosteronism (PA) and idiopathic aldosteronism (IA). Morphologic and functional relationships, abstracted. Clin. Res. 21:720, 1973.
6. Cohen, E.L., Grim, C.E., Conn, J.W. et al: Accurate and rapid measurement of plasma renin activity by radioimmunoassay. Results in normal and hypertensive people. J. Lab. Clin. Med. 77:1025, 1971.
7. Conn, J.W., Cohen, E.L., Lucas, C.P., et al: Primary reninism. Hypertension, hyperreninemia, and secondary aldosteronism due to renin-producing juxtaglomerular cell tumors. Arch. Intern. Med. 130:682, 1972.

8. Giacomelli, F., Wiener, J. and Spiro, D.: Cytological alterations related to stimulation of the zona glomerulosa of the adrenal gland. J. Cell Biol. 26:499, 1965.
9. Conn, J.W., Cohen, E.L. and Rovner, D.R.: Suppression of plasma renin activity in primary aldosteronism. Distinguishing primary from secondary aldosteronism in hypertensive disease. JAMA 190:213, 1964.
10. Conn, J.W., Rovner, D.R. and Cohen, E.L.: Natural history of recovery of the renin-angiotensin-aldosterone system following long-term suppression by aldosterone-secreting tumors. Program of the 47th meeting of The Endocrine Society, New York City (abstract), 1965, p. 60.
11. Biglieri, E.G., Slaton, P.E. and Silens, W.: Postoperative studies of adrenal function in primary aldosteronism. J. Clin. Endocrinol. 26:553, 1966.
12. Morimoto, S., Takeda, R. and Murakami, M.: Does prolonged pretreatment with large doses of spironolactone hasten a recovery from juxtaglomerular-adrenal suppression in primary aldosteronism? J. Clin. Endocrinol. 31:659, 1970.
13. Spark, R.F. and Melby, J.C.: Aldosteronism in hypertension: The spironolactone response test. Ann. Intern. Med. 69:685, 1968.
14. Vaughan, E.D., Jr., Laragh, J.H., Gavras, I. et al: Volume factor in low and normal renin essential hypertension: Treatment with either spironolactone or chlorthalidone. Am. J. Cardiol. 32:523, 1973.
15. Sundsfjord, J.A., Marton, P., Jorgensen, H. et al: Reduced aldosterone secretion during spironolactone treatment in primary aldosteronism: Report of a case. J. Clin. Endocrinol. 39:734, 1974.
16. Erbler, H.C.: Stimulation of aldosterone production in vitro and its inhibition by spironolactone. Naunyn Schmiedeberg Arch. Pharmacol. 273:366, 1972.
17. Erbler, H.C.: On the mechanism of the inhibitory action of the spironolactone SC 9376 (aldadiene) on the production of corticosteroids in rat adrenals in vitro. Naunyn Schmiedeberg Arch. Pharmacol. 277:139, 1973.
18. Salassa, R.M., Mattox, V.R. and Power, M.H.: Effect of an aldosterone antagonist on sodium and potassium excretion in primary hyperaldosteronism. J. Clin. Endocrinol. 18:787, 1958.
19. Kremer, D., Beevers, D.G., Brown, J.J. et al: Spironolactone and amiloride in the treatment of low renin hyperaldosteronism and related syndromes. Clin. Sci. Molec. Med. 45:213s, 1973.
20. Mantero, F., Armanini, D. and Urbani, S.: Antihypertensive effect of spironolactone in essential, renal and mineralocorticoid hypertension. Clin. Sci. Molec. Med. 45:219s, 1973.
21. Symington, T.: *In* Functional Pathology of the Human Adrenal Gland. Edinburgh and London: E. & S. Livingstone Ltd., 1969, p. 138.
22. Vecsei, P., Purjesz, I. and Wolff, H.P.: Studies on the biosynthesis of aldosterone in solitary adenoma and in nodular hyperplasia of the

adrenal cortex in patients exhibiting Conn's syndrome. Acta Endocrinol. (Kobenhavn) 62:391, 1969.
23. Nicholls, M.G., Espiner, E.A., Hughes, H. et al: Primary aldosteronism: A study in contrasts. JAMA 59:334, 1975.
24. Palmore, W.P. and Mulrow, P.J.: Control of aldosterone secretion by the pituitary gland. Science 158:1482, 1967.

Spironolactone Therapy in Primary Aldosteronism: Diagnostic and Therapeutic Implications

Arunabha Ganguly, M.D. and John A. Luetscher, M.D.

The entity of primary aldosteronism is generally defined as the triad of hypertension, hyperaldosteronism and suppressed plasma renin activity [1]. A vexing problem has been the distinction between patients with aldosterone-producing adenoma (APA) and those with similar clinical and laboratory findings, whose adrenal glands show either no morphological change or micronodular hyperplasia at surgery [2, 3]. These cases of idiopathic adrenal hyperplasia (IAH) were originally thought to be uncommon, but in most series today they approach 40%-50% of all patients with primary aldosteronism. The differential diagnosis between APA and IAH is important since adrenal surgery cures a majority of patients with APA [1]. Unilateral adrenalectomy or subtotal adrenalectomy in IAH seldom normalizes blood pressure, although it cures the potassium wasting [2-4]. Subtotal or total adrenalectomy may result in a worthwhile reduction in blood pressure in patients with IAH, but it entails serious problems in concurrent management of hypertension and adrenal insufficiency. Pathological diagnosis may be inconclusive when both adenoma and

---

This research was supported by grants from the National Institutes of Health HL-13917 and HL-17364. Dr. Ganguly held a fellowship under NIH Training Grant AM05021. Dr. Luetscher is the recipient of a Research Career Award (K6 AM 14176). Necessary facilities were provided by the General Clinical Research Center, Grant RR-70.

Arunabha Ganguly, M.D. and John A. Luetscher, M.D., Endocrine Division, Department of Medicine, Stanford University School of Medicine, Stanford, Calif.

7. Ganguly, A., Dowdy, A.J., Luetscher, J.A. et al: Anomalous postural response of plasma aldosterone concentration in patients with aldosterone-producing adrenal adenoma. J. Clin. Endocrinol. 36:401, 1973.
8. Ganguly, A., Melada, G.A., Luetscher, J.A. et al: Control of plasma aldosterone in primary aldosteronism: Distinction between adenoma and hyperplasia. J. Clin. Endocrinol. 37:765, 1973.
9. Melby, J.C.: Identifying the adrenal lesion in primary aldosteronism. Ann. Intern. Med. 76:1039, 1972.
10. Sundsfjord, J.A., Marton, P., Jorgensen, H. et al: Reduced aldosterone secretion during spironolactone treatment in primary aldosteronism: Report of a case. J. Clin. Endocrinol. 39:734, 1974.
11. Brown, J.J., Davies, D.L., Ferriss, J.B. et al: Comparison of surgery and prolonged spironolactone therapy in patients with hypertension, aldosterone excess, and low plasma renin. Br. Med. J. 2:729, 1972.
12. Spark, R.F. and Melby, J.C.: Aldosteronism in hypertension. The spironolactone response test. Ann. Intern. Med. 69:685, 1968.
13. Schambelan, M., Brust, N., Chang, B. et al: Aldosterone production in low renin hypertensive states: Response to spironolactone therapy. *In* Sambhi, M.P. (ed.): Mechanisms of Hypertension. Proceedings of an International Workshop Conference. International Congress Series no. 302. Excerpta Medica, 1973.

Discussion

Moderator: Dr. I. H. Page

Dr. Stokes: I would like to report a curiosity that we have observed in our patients with primary aldosteronism of which there were 12 in whom we have not seen bilateral nodular hyperplasia but only adenomas. We have used routinely for some years the test described initially by Lauler's group in which sodium loading is telescoped by giving a 2 liter sodium chloride load on two consecutive days. On each day 2 liters of 0.9 sodium chloride are given, and the effect on urinary aldosterone excretion is observed. In normal subjects or in patients with various forms of essential hypertension there is a suppression of the aldosterone level by this maneuver. Predictably, in half the patients with primary aldosteronism we have studied, there has been no such suppression. But the curiosity is that in the other half we have observed *a rise* in the urinary aldosterone level on the first day of sodium loading. I would be interested whether Dr. Luetscher or Dr. Conn has seen this and whether it might be of any use for differentiating the adenomatous disease from the hyperplasia.

Dr. Page: Thank you, Dr. Stokes. Any comments on that?

Dr. Luetscher: I have no experience with intravenous saline, but there have been a number of publications on this subject indicating that the intravenous saline loading test can be helpful in diagnosing primary aldosteronism. In analyzing data from patients with primary aldosteronism we were impressed by the variability of urinary aldosterone and more particularly of plasma aldosterone from hour to hour. We have not heard of increased aldosterone secretion following sodium loading, but there is considerable day-to-day variation in aldosterone excretion which makes measurements on particular days difficult to relate to experimental conditions. It is possible that saline suppression of aldosterone might not last throughout the 24-hour period. Hypertensive patients excrete the saline load very quickly. Plasma aldosterone might be very much depressed for a few hours after saline infusion, as Kem and others have described, yet the 24-hour measurement of aldosterone excretion could fail to reflect the brief suppression.

Dr. Mulrow: I have two comments for Dr. Conn. Regarding your comment that the return of aldosterone excretion to high levels in patients who were given aldactone prior to surgery may be related to the increase in plasma renin activity, the only suggestion I would make is that potassium may be just as important for renin since you know, certainly in animals, who are placed on low sodium diets and who have high renins and at the same time are potassium depleted, there is no increase in aldosterone, no increase in the glomerulosa width despite the fact that renin is elevated. But if you give potassium you can return that to normal.

Dr. Conn: I have no argument with that. I simply pointed out that despite the increase in renin and the increase in potassium there still was no early increase in aldosterone indicating the blocking action of aldactone.

Dr. Mulrow: My second comment is about the aldactone bodies and the implication where the biosynthetic block might be. At least from the histology, showing that aldactone affects the endoplasmic reticulum, there can be no implication of where the block may be since the last steps in biosynthesis occur in the mitochondria and the mitochondria show no histological abnormalities. Another possibility might be since certain drugs are metabolized by endoplasmic reticulum, particularly in the liver, that this is evidence that the zona glomerulosa is metabolizing the drug rather than any relationship between those bodies and the biosynthetic block.

Dr. Conn: I agree that we have no evidence to prove that the aldactone bodies represent a block in the biosynthesis of aldosterone. All that we say is that at the time the aldactone bodies are being formed aldosterone excretion and plasma aldosterone are falling, and there appears to be a direct relationship between those two phenomena.

Dr. Kaplan: Dr. Conn, you showed that the initial block of aldosterone biosynthesis could be overcome by a secondary rise in renin, turning on steroidogenesis in the rest of the adrenal, returning aldosterone levels back to or beyond the initial values.

Why doesn't spironolactone inhibit steroid synthesis in these cells as well?

Dr. Conn: I said earlier that I wanted you to remember the case in which we did find aldactone bodies in the normal glomerulosa. That was the patient that had a very great rise of 142 times baseline of renin and exhibited also excretions of 16 and 17 micrograms of aldosterone after the tumor was out. That patient did show aldactone bodies in the normal glomerulosa. Her glomerulosa was only mildly suppressed preoperatively. Incidentally, in the very early work with aldactone bodies it was pointed out that patients with edema treated with aldactone do get the aldactone bodies. The phenomenon is not confined to patients with aldosterone-producing tumors. I was very much interested in finding out how quickly a normal human adrenal would develop such bodies, but you cannot give aldactone to a person and then quickly take out his adrenals. But I had a very cooperative patient who was about to have an adrenalectomy for metastatic cancer and she agreed to take aldactone for one week before her operation. She had aldactone bodies in her adrenal gland at the end of that week. So that they do occur in normal adrenals. The prerequisite is that they must be actively aldosterone-producing cells.

Dr. Page: I thought you were going to say she volunteered.

Audience: It has ben reported, Dr. Conn, that aldactone does alter steroid biosynthesis. Is there any evidence for aldactone bodies in the testes of the animals, for example? The second question is: What would be the contribution of decreased aldosterone biosynthesis in lowering the blood pressure and restoring the normal sodium potassium levels in your patients?

Dr. Conn: I doubt that there are aldactone bodies in the testicles. Jenis and Herzog in 1969 found no sign of similar bodies in any other tissue in the body while there were many in the adrenal zona glomerulosa. Regarding the second question, if aldosterone biosynthesis is decreased, does that contribute to improvement in the patient, I doubt it since the peripheral effects of aldactone are probably already covering the aldosterone produced.

Dr. Dustan: I have a comment regarding an update of our own observations concerning the predictability of the cure of hypertension by surgery in patients with primary aldosteronism. We have continued to measure cardiac output in all patients preoperatively and continue to find that those with only slightly elevated peripheral resistance have relief of hypertension by surgical treatment. In contrast, the nonresponders have normal or reduced cardiac output and high peripheral resistance. Certainly we find it helpful to consider this type of hypertension as a hemodynamic abnormality (as all other hypertensions are) and assess it accordingly.

Dr. Vallotton: Dr. Conn mentioned the work of Erbler in Germany who, quite convincingly, showed that spironolactone inhibited biosynthesis of aldosterone in rats as well as in human beings without primary aldosteronism. Yet in a small series of subjects without primary aldosteronism, we have so far been unable to confirm the data. In each case an elevation of plasma as well as urinary excretion of aldosterone occurred under spironolactone. I wanted to ask if you had data on normal subjects and, second, if you think that because of the formation of these bodies in the adrenals spironolactone should not be given to patients with hypertension without primary aldosteronism.

Dr. Conn: That is a very good question. We have not studied normal people. If you give spironolactone to a normal person and you get a quick sharp rise of renin, and associated with it you get a rise in aldosterone, you do not know how high that patient's aldosterone would have been, without the aldactone, to a similar rise of renin. In other words, I think there is an underlying, partial block and that it is not possible to know what the normal response would have been to a similar rise in renin.

Dr. Gross: I should like to ask Dr. Conn if aldactone bodies are similar to those which have been observed after high doses of methylandrostinediol. These bodies stain very well with PAS. I wonder if aldactone bodies also stain with PAS?

Dr. Conn: I do not know that. The bodies are of lipoprotein makeup.

Dr. Gross: As far as I know they are in the zona glomerulosa and in the zona fasciculata.

The Role of Angiotensins in Aldosterone Release

F. M. Bumpus, Ph.D., M. C. Khosla, Ph.D. and E. L. Bravo, M.D.

Following the discovery in 1970 [1] that [8-Alanine]-angiotensin II had specific inhibitory properties toward angiotensin II, many other modifications of the eight position have been made to produce antagonists to the myotropic and pressor response to angiotensin II [2]. Our first approach was to make numerous modifications in position eight to obtain the best possible antagonist of angiotensin which did not possess agonist properties relating to catecholamine release, aldosterone release or myotropic activities. The next step was to produce analogs of angiotensin II which had good inhibitory properties, but which had increased in vivo half-lives. We knew that angiotensin was destroyed in plasma largely by aminopeptidases and it was our thought to modify the N-terminus to resist enzymatic degradation. While this latter effort was in progress Pals et al [3] synthesized and tested [Sar^1, Ala^8]-angiotensin II which has now come into great usage. Substitution of position one with sarcosine increased the potency of [Ala^8]-angiotensin II. We likewise have studied analogs with sarcosine in position one and have found that the introduction of sarcosine into the parent hormone itself gives to the molecule both a greater half-life and a greater binding to the receptor sites [4]. Introduction of other unnatural amino acids into this position has likewise given

This study supported in part by Grant HL 6835 from the National Heart and Lung Institute, National Institutes of Health, USPHS.

F. M. Bumpus, Ph.D., M. C. Khosla, Ph.D. and E. L. Bravo, M.D., Research Division, The Cleveland Clinic Foundation and The Cleveland Clinic Education Foundation, Ohio.

similar results. However, as yet in our laboratory the N-methylated series of amino acids have given the best results.

Introduction of various unnatural amino acids (eg, N-methyl amino acids) into other positions such as position four (tyrosine), which is subject to hydrolysis by chymotryptic-like enzymes, has not yet yielded agonists or antagonists with greater biological activities. The compounds that are discussed here are the three octapeptides now being used in several laboratories as well as a heptapeptide antagonist which seems to be rather specific for inhibiting aldosterone release from the adrenal cortex.

In Table 1 is presented a comparison of the antagonistic activities of [1-Sarcosine, 8-alanine]-, [1-Sarcosine, 8-isoleucine]- and [1-Sarcosine, 8-threonine] -angiotensin II on rat's blood pressure. The relative activities are expressed as dose ratios. [Sar^1, Thr^8]- and [Sar^1, Ile^8]-angiotensin II possess essentially similar activity, but both of these are considerably more potent than is the corresponding 8-alanine derivative. All three of these analogs possess slight pressor activity. Table 2 shows the pressor responses obtained in a rat at 3, 10 and 30 minutes. It is apparent that the 8-threonine derivative is considerably less of an agonist than are the other two. Table 3 shows the data obtained relating to experiments carried out by perfusion of the three analogs in a retrograde manner through the adrenal glands (M. Peach, unpublished results). It was observed that at rather low concentrations, [Sar^1, Ala^8]-angiotensin II invoked a rather high release of catecholamines. [Sar^1, Ile^8]-angiotensin II is much less potent as an agonist for the release of catecholamines, while the corresponding 8-threonine derivative did not release catecholamines even at 10^{-6} gm/ml

Table 1. Antagonistic Effect of Analogs of Angiotensin II Infusion in Rats (250 ng/kg/min) [12, 13]

Ang II Analog	*Ang II ED_{20} (ng) Before Infusion of the Analog*	*Ang II ED_{20} (ng) During Infusion of the Analog*	*Dose Ratio*
[Sar^1, Ala^8]- (P-113)	1.89 ± 0.19	14.16 ± 1.88	7.92 ± 1.21
[Sar^1, Ile^8]-	2.19 ± 0.15	52.37 ± 26.11	23.63 ± 6.87
[Sar^1, Thr^8]-	1.71 ± 0.26	44.55 ± 8.20	26.91 ± 3.30

Table 2. Comparative Initial Transient Pressor Activity Infusion in Rats (250 ng/kg/min) [12, 13]

Ang II Analog	*n*	*Rise in Blood Pressure mm Hg* 3 Min	10 Min	30 Min
[Sar^1, Ala^8]-(P-113)	9	15.11 ± 1.48	16.88 ± 1.87	17.44 ± 1.66
[Sar^1, Ile^8]-	11	17.81 ± 0.99	18.27 ± 1.72	14.81 ± 2.16
[Sar^1, Thr^8]-	15	9.46 ± 0.79	9.66 ± 2.00	9.20 ± 4.26

infused [5]. The latter two of these compounds acted as antagonists to the release of catecholamines when used at higher dose levels; in contrast, [Sar^1, Ala^8]-angiotensin II had no antagonistic properties at any of the levels used.

We have infused these three derivatives into salt-depleted dogs to determine both their abilities to inhibit aldosterone release and to determine whether or not they would possess agonist properties. Again, all three compounds are slight agonists; the 8-alanine derivative appears to have the highest agonist property, while the threonine compound had the lowest property. Blair-West et al [6] first observed that des-Asp^1-angiotensin II releases aldosterone from the adrenal gland on an equipotent basis to angiotensin II. It has been proposed that this may be the hormone that stimulates aldosterone synthesis and/or release. It may be formed from angiotensin II either by angiotensinase A in plasma or possibly by aminopeptidases in the adrenal gland itself. We felt that if this heptapeptide is a good agonist, then the introduction of isoleucine, alanine or

Table 3. Catecholamine Secretion From Perfused Cat Adrenals*

Agonist	*n*	*Dose Administered* 10^{-9}g	10^{-8}g	10^{-7}g	10^{-6}g	pA_2
Ang II	8	350 ± 90	850 ± 150	1650 ± 320	3350 ± 520	–
[Sar^1, Ala^8]-ang II	7	0	130 ± 15	375 ± 100	590 ± 75	No blockade up to 5×10^{-6} M
[Sar^1, Ile^8]-ang II	9	0	0	50 ± 10	175 ± 30	9.5
[Sar^1, Thr^8]-ang II	6	0	0	0	0	9.0

Data represent nanogram of epinephrine and norepinephrine released over basal secretion.
*M. Peach (unpublished results).

threonine in position seven or position eight of the octapeptides may possibly produce good antagonists for the release of aldosterone. This has proven to be correct.

Bravo et al [7] carried out the in vivo studies in male mongrel dogs weighing 20-25 kg. Following the operation to remove the right kidney and right adrenal gland under sterile conditions, the dogs were placed on a normal sodium and potassium diet and given daily intramuscular injections of dexamethasone (Decadron phosphate, 10 mg twice daily). After eight days, the dogs received 20 mg of dexamethasone intramuscularly one hour before surgery; anesthesia given was sodium pentobarbital (20 mg/kg). A femoral artery was catheterized and connected to a pressure transducer for continuous monitoring of arterial pressure. The remaining left kidney was removed and the left lumboadrenal vein was selectively cannulated by the method of Hume and Nelson. A loose ligature was then passed around the proximal end of the lumboadrenal vein as it drained into the inferior vena cava. During collection of adrenal venous blood, this ligature was tightened to facilitate venous drainage only through the catheter. For all experiments the studies were initiated 90-120 minutes following removal of the remaining kidney. Solutions for infusion were freshly prepared with normal saline and administered into peripheral veins through separate tubings at 1.0 ml/min with a constant infusion pump. Timed specimens of adrenal venous effluent (usually 10 ml) for steroid and electrolyte measurements were collected by drip and replaced each time with an equal amount of blood from a donor dog.

Both [Sar^1, Ile^8]-angiotensin II and [Sar^1, Ala^8]-angiotensin II have agonist properties as well as antagonist properties for aldosterone release and/or biosynthesis. The blockade of aldosterone with these two analogs appears to be at a higher dose level than observed with [Sar^1, Thr^8] derivative. Indeed, in experiments utilizing salt-depleted dogs of approximately five weeks duration, the octapeptides containing alanine or isoleucine in the eight position released aldosterone before they produced a blockade. Preliminary results indicate that [Sar^1 Thr^8] derivative had little or no agonist effect and had potent antagonistic activity on aldosterone formation in the dog. In comparing [Sar^1, Ile^8] analog against the des-Asp^1-angiotensin

II inhibitor, one notes a tremendous difference. Infusion of 200 ng/kg/min of the octapeptide inhibitor did not block the aldosterone release obtained by infusion of 20 ng/kg/min of angiotensin II. On the other hand, 200 ng/kg/min of des-Asp^1-[Ile^8]-angiotensin II almost completely blocked the release of aldosterone by this quantity of angiotensin II. Infusion of 20 ng/kg/min of angiotensin II gave approximately 20 mm Hg rise in blood pressure, which was not blocked by des-Asp^1-[Ile^8]-angiotensin II at a dose level of 200 ng/kg/min, but was completely blocked by [Sar^1, Ile^8]-angiotensin II at the same dose level.

Table 4 shows a comparison of the blockade of the octapeptide and heptapeptide by [Sar^1, Ile^8]-angiotensin II and the des-Asp^1-[Ile^8]-angiotensin II. The heptapeptide antagonist is 15-fold more potent than the octapeptide antagonist in the inhibition of aldosterone secretion whereas the octapeptide antagonist is far more potent as an inhibitor of myotropic activity. This strongly suggests the possibility that angiotensin III may be the hormone that releases aldosterone. To further test this hypothesis we infused poly-O-acetyl-seryl angiotensin II into a dog to determine both its effect upon blood pressure and aldosterone release. When infused at a level high enough to produce a 20 mm Hg rise in blood pressure the release of aldosterone was only about 10% of that noted from a similar vasopressor amount of angiotensin II itself. The specificity of this polymer for inducing a pressor response with very low aldosterone release suggests the possibility that angiotensin II

Table 4. Inhibition of Release of Aldosterone

	Agonist (Dogs)		*Antagonist (ng/kg/min)*	
	Pressor Response	*Aldosterone Secretion*	*To Inhibit Pressor Response**	*To Inhibit Aldosterone Secretion**
Angiotensin II	100	100		
[Des-Asp^1]-ang II	22	100		
[Sar^1, Ile^8]-ang II	1.2		40-80	3000
[Des-Asp^1, Ile^8]-ang II	0.4		800	200

*Ang II was infused at constant dose of 20 ng/kg/min in bilaterally nephrectomized ACTH-suppressed mongrel dogs.

must either be split before it can produce the response for aldosterone release or that this polymer, being considerably larger in molecular weight, cannot enter the cell as might angiotensin II in order to initiate the response. When comparing the activities of this polymer against angiotensin in a dog that has been prestimulated by angiotensin, there appeared to be no difference or very little difference in potencies of angiotensin II and poly-O-acetyl-seryl angiotensin II to release aldosterone. One interpretation of this result may be that angiotensin(s) may affect several points in the biosynthetic pathway of aldosterone and its release phenomenon. For example, in the prestimulated gland, the polymer being just as active as angiotensin may be effecting the release phenomenon or a small point in the biosynthetic pathway only; whereas in a nonstimulated adrenal gland either angiotensin II, the heptapeptide or the polymer may be required to enter the cell before stimulation can occur. These findings certainly suggest that angiotensin II receptors in adrenal cortex and vascular smooth muscle are functionally different.

These results show that (a) the octapeptide inhibitors have a high potency with respect to the blockade of the pressor or myotropic activity; (b) des-Asp^1 [Ile^8]-angiotensin II is a specific antagonist of the steroidogenic effect of angiotensin II and angiotensin III in the adrenal zona glomerulosa cells and (c) the heptapeptide des-Asp^1-angiotensin II may mediate part of the aldosterone-stimulating activity of angiotensin II. By utilizing compounds synthesized in our laboratories, Peach and Chiu [8] and Sarstedt [9] corroborated the above findings in the in vitro studies on isolated adrenal glomerulosa cells of the rats. In experiments comparing [Sar^1, Ile^8]-angiotensin II against the corresponding heptapeptide analog, des-Asp^1-[Ile^8]-angiotensin II, these authors observed that the heptapeptide derivative is at least ten times as potent in inhibiting angiotensin II-induced aldosterone as is the corresponding octapeptide inhibitor. Increasing the concentration tenfold of the two antagonists, the above investigators observed that the heptapeptide antagonist completely blocks angiotensin II-induced release of aldosterone while the octapeptide antagonist completely blocks the pressor response to angiotensin II. The reduction in aldosterone secretion from adrenal gland by these antagonists is mediated through blockade of angiotensins and does not effect the release stimulated by ACTH.

So far, a major emphasis has been to measure levels of renin and/or angiotensin I and II in the plasma, and only recently have people become interested in the measurements of angiotensin III. Goodfriend and Peach [10] have stated that angiotensin III has a shorter half-life than angiotensin II in plasma. This may also be true for the heptapeptide antagonist. As suggested by Blair-West et al [6], one must also consider the possibility of des-Asp^1-angiotensin I existing in plasma. The same plasma angiotensinase A that attacks angiotensin II will likewise remove aspartic acid from angiotensin I giving rise to a nonapeptide which has no pressor activity. This nonapeptide then should be acted upon by the converting enzyme in plasma or tissue to form angiotensin III. Upon this background we have synthesized the nonapeptide to determine whether or not it would cause a release of aldosterone. Tsai et al [11] have shown that this nonapeptide is a good substrate for the converting enzyme from porcine lung and plasma and, indeed, does give rise to angiotensin III as expected. In our laboratory preliminary experiments have shown that infusion of this nonapeptide into dogs stimulates aldosterone release with essentially no pressor response. This is extremely interesting because it suggests the possibility that the alternate pathway could be involved whereby the loss of aspartic acid from angiotensin I by plasma angiotensinase A or other aminopeptidases could lead to a direct effect upon sodium handling with essentially no vasopressor action. This aspect certainly needs further investigation.

References

1. Khairallah, P.A., Toth, A. and Bumpus, F.M.: Analogs of angiotensin II. II. Mechanism of receptor interactions. J. Med. Chem. 13:181, 1970.
2. Khosla, M.C., Smeby, R.R. and Bumpus, F.M.: Structure-activity relationship in angiotensin II analogs. *In* Page, I.H. and Bumpus, F.M. (eds.): Handbook of Experimental Pharmacology, vol. 37. Heidelberg:Springer-Verlag, 1974, p. 126.
3. Pals, D.T., Masucci, F.D., Denning, G.S., Jr. et al: Role of the pressor action of angiotensin II in experimental hypertension. Circ. Res. 29:673, 1971.

4. Hall, M.M., Khosla, M.C., Khairallah, P.A. et al: Angiotensin analogs: The influence of sarcosine substituted in position 1. J. Pharmacol. Exp. Ther. 188:222, 1974.
5. Khosla, M.C., Munoz-Ramirez, H., Hall, M.M. et al: Synthesis of angiotensin II antagonists containing N- and O-methylated-, and other amino acid residues. J. Med. Chem., 1976. (In press.)
6. Blair-West, J.P., Coghlan, D.A., Denton, J.W. et al: The effect of the heptapeptide (2-8) and hexapeptide (3-8) fragments of angiotensin II on aldosterone secretion. J. Clin. Endocrinol. 32:575, 1971.
7. Bravo, E.L., Khosla, M.C. and Bumpus, F.M.: Action of [1-Des(Aspartic acid), 8-isoleucine] angiotensin II upon the pressor and steroidogenic activity of angiotensin II. J. Clin. Endocrinol. 40:530, 1975.
8. Peach, M.J. and Chiu, A.T.: Stimulation and inhibition of aldosterone biosynthesis in vitro by angiotensin II and analogs. Circ. Res. 34 and 35 (suppl. 1):7, 1974.
9. Sarstedt, C.A., Vaughan, E.D., Jr. and Peach, M.J.: Selective inhibition by des-Asp^1-Ile^8-angiotensin II of the steroidogenic response to restricted sodium intake in the rat. Circ. Res. 37:350, 1974.
10. Goodfriend T.L. and Peach, M.J.: Angiotensin-three, [Des-Aspartic $acid^1$]-angiotensin II: Evidence and speculation for its role as an important agonist in the renin-angiotensin system. Circ. Res. 23 (suppl. 1):38, 1975.
11. Tsai, B.S., Peach, M.J., Khosla, M.C. et al: Synthesis and evaluation of [Des-Asp^1] angiotensin I as a precursor for [Des-Asp^1] angiotensin II ("Angiotensin III"). J. Med. Chem. 1975. (In press.)
12. Muñoz-Ramirez, H., Khosla, M.C., Bumpus, F.M. et al: Influence of the adrenal gland on the pressor effect and antagonistic potency of angiotensin II analogs. Eur. J. Pharmacol. 31:122, 1975.
13. Muñoz-Ramirez, H., Khosla, M.C. and Khairallah, P.A.: Evaluation of the antagonistic potency of [1-Sar, 8-Thr] angiotensin II in vivo. FASEB Proceedings Abst. No. 3113, 1975.

Effect of Angiotensin I, Angiotensin II and (Des-Asp^1)-Angiotensin II on Steroidogenesis in Isolated Fasciculata Cells From Bovine Adrenals

R. Hepp, M.D., A. Peytremann, M.D., A. M. Riondel, Ph.D. and M. B. Vallotton, M.D.

Peytremann et al [1] recently reported that angiotensin II (A II) is a potent stimulator of corticosteroid biosynthesis in isolated fasciculata cells from bovine adrenal glands. This effect of angiotensin II appears to be mediated through cyclic AMP. A stimulation of cortisol synthesis by angiotensin has been reported only in the beef [2, 3] and in the dog [4-6]. Since Blair-West et al [7] first demonstrated that the [2-8]-heptapeptide fragment of A II stimulated aldosterone secretion in ovine adrenals, other investigators have confirmed that [des-asp^1]-A II was a potent stimulus of aldosterone biosynthesis in vivo in the rat [8, 9] and in the dog [10] as well as in vitro with cat, dog or rabbit adrenal cells [11, 12]. These findings raised the question of a possible role of [des-asp^1]-A II as a physiological stimulus of steroid biosynthesis [13]. We therefore decided to study and compare the steroidogenic effect of A I, A II, [des-asp^1]-A II and [des-asp^1-arg^2]-A II on the fasciculata cells from bovine adrenals. These cells were chosen since they can be

---

Supported by grant No. 4485 and 3.2300.74 from the Swiss National Foundation for Scientific Research.

Presented in part at the Xth Acta endocrinologica Congress, Amsterdam, August 1975 (abstract No. 203).

R. Hepp, M.D., A. Peytremann, M.D., A. M. Riondel, Ph.D. and M. B. Vallotton, M.D., Division of Endocrinology, Department of Medicine, School of Medicine, University of Geneva, Hôpital Cantonal, Geneva, Switzerland.

obtained with 95% purity and represent a highly sensitive system [1]. Furthermore, we examined the effect of an inhibitor of the converting enzyme as well as of a structural analog antagonist of A II in order to answer the following questions: Does A II only stimulate steroidogenesis in this system or does its precursor A I, or its metabolites, [des-asp^1]-A II and [des-asp^1-arg^2]-A II, also influence steroid biosynthesis? Is A I converted to A II in fasciculata cells suspension and can a possible conversion from A I to A II be blocked by the converting enzyme inhibitor SQ 20′881? Does the structural analog [sar^1-ala^8]-A II inhibit the effects of A I, A II and [des-asp^1]-A II on steroid biosynthesis?

Materials and Methods

Isolated Fasciculata Cells

Fasciculata cell dispersions from bovine adrenal glands were prepared according to the method of Kloppenborg et al [14] as modified by Sayers et al [15]. In brief, bovine adrenal glands were obtained from a local slaughter-house and placed immediately on ice in KRBG*-buffer containing 500 mg albumin/100 ml. Slices of 0.5 mm were obtained with a Stadie-Riggs microtome. The second slices, representing mainly fasciculata, were used for the present experiments. The slices were mechanically dispersed by stirring with a siliconized glass rod in KRBG-buffer containing 250 mg/100 ml trypsin. Trypsin was then inactivated by adding lima bean trypsin inhibitor (100 mg/100 ml KRBG-buffer). The dispersed cells, after washing and centrifugation, were suspended in KRBG-buffer with 500 mg albumin/100 ml. Samples of 0.9 ml of this cell suspension were incubated in a shaking water bath at 37°C under an atmosphere of 95% O_2 and 5% CO_2. The appropriate additions of peptides (hormones, hormonal precursors or fragments and inhibitors) were made in 0.1 ml acid-albumin-saline. Each sample was incubated in triplicate. Unless otherwise stated, the incubation lasted 60 minutes. At the end of the incubation time, the samples were frozen until assayed.

---

*Krebs-Ringer Bicarbonate Glucose buffer.

Analytical Methods

Corticosteroids were determined by a protein-binding method [16]. By paper chromatography prior to assay it was found that cortisol represented approximately 60% and corticosterone 30% of the corticosteroids while aldosterone, measured by radioimmunoassay, accounted for only less than 1%. Immunoreactive angiotensin I and angiotensin II were determined by radioimmunoassays using antisera whose specificity has been thoroughly studied [17, 18]. Antibodies from antiserum raised against angiotensin I have less than 1% cross-reactivity with angiotensin II and practically none with smaller fragments. Antibodies from antiserum raised against angiotensin II, while not cross-reacting with angiotensin I, cross-react fully with both [des-asp^1]-A II and [des-asp^1-arg^2]-A II.

Materials

Asp^1-Ile^5-angiotensin I (A I) was obtained from Schwarz-Mann, Orangeburg, N.Y., and angiotensin II (A II) (Hypertensin®) from CIBA Pharmaceutical Products Inc., Basle. The [2-8]-heptapeptide or [des-asp^1]-A II and [3-8]-hexapeptide or [des-asp^1-arg^2]-A II were a gift of Dr. F.M. Bumpus, Cleveland, Ohio. The structural analog and antagonist of A II, [sar^1-ala^8]-A II was purchased from Eaton Laboratories, Norwich, N.Y. The nonapeptide (SQ 20′881), an inhibitor of the converting enzyme, was generously supplied by the Squibb Institute, Princeton, N.J. Synthetic [1-24]-ACTH (Synacthen®) was obtained from CIBA Pharmaceutical Products Inc., Basle. Trypsin and lima bean trypsin inhibitor were purchased from Worthington Biochemical Corp., Freehold, N.J.

Results

Steroid biosynthesis in isolated bovine fasciculata cells was stimulated by angiotensin II as well as by its precursor, A I, and its analog [des-asp^1]-A II (Fig. 1). The stimulation of steroid production was found to be dose-dependent for all three peptides. The dose-response curves for A II and [des-asp^1]-A II were superimposable, being characterized by a threshold between 10^{-9} and 10^{-8} M, a half maximal stimulation occurring at 5×10^{-8} M and a maximal 15- to 20-fold increase in steroid

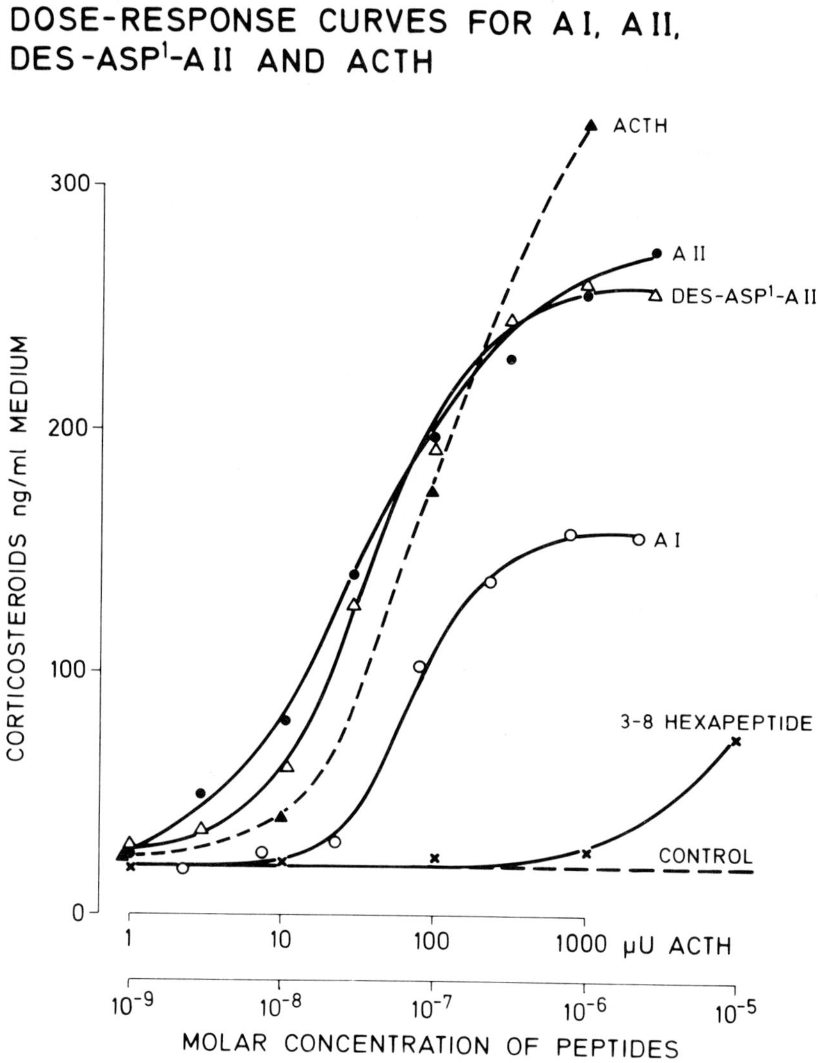

FIG. 1. Dose-response curves for A I, A II, [des-asp^1]-A II and ACTH on corticosteroid production by isolated bovine fasciculata cells.

production at 10^{-6} M. Although three to four times less potent than A II and [des-asp^1]-A II, A I displayed a definite effect with half maximal stimulation occurring at 5×10^{-8} M and a tenfold maximal increase of basal steroid production with 10^{-6} M. By contrast, [des-asp^1-arg^2]-A II stimulated steroid production only slightly at concentrations between 10^{-6} M and 10^{-5} M.

The time-course of corticosteroid production showed a significant increase already after ten minutes of exposure of the cells to A I, A II and [des-asp^1]-A II (Fig. 2). The steroid output increased steadily during the first 60 minutes, after which the increase became somewhat slower and finally tended to level off.

The recovery of immunoreactive A I from the medium at the end of the incubation period was almost identical whether it was incubated in the presence or in the absence of cells (Fig. 3). No generation of A II, heptapeptide or hexapeptide could be

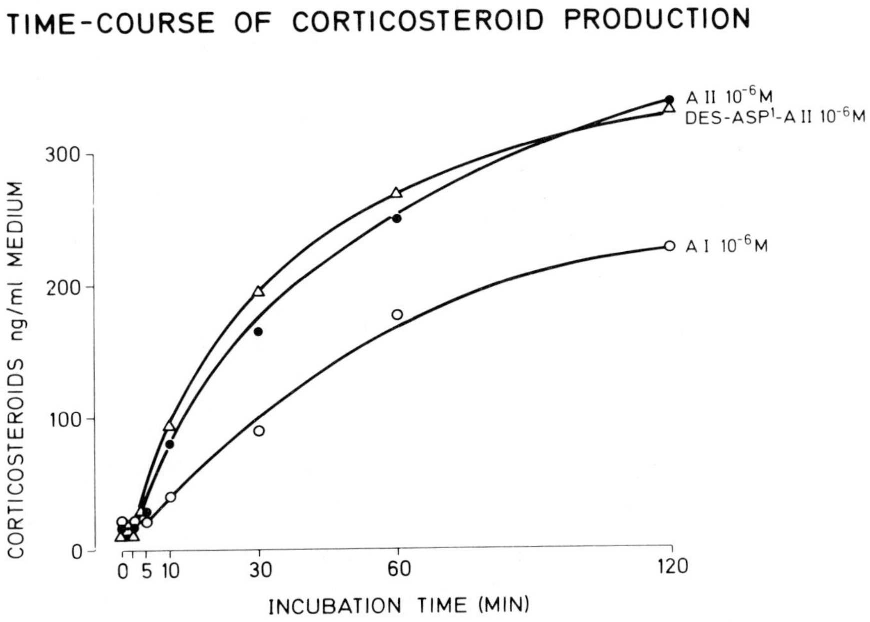

FIG. 2. Time-course of corticosteroid production by isolated bovine fasciculata cells in response to A I, A II and [des-asp^1]-A II.

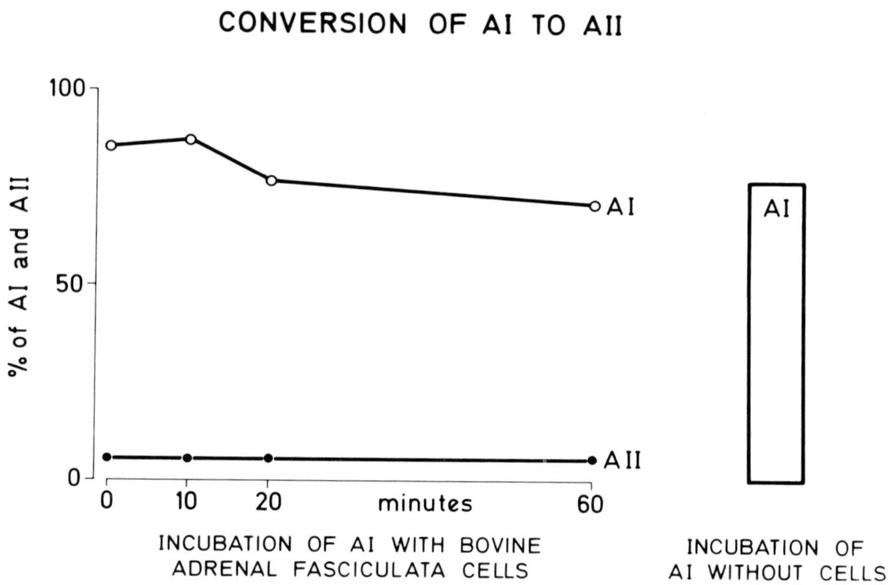

FIG. 3. Measurement of angiotensin I and II in the medium during incubation with adrenal fasciculata cells or after 60 minutes incubation without cells.

detected using an antiserum fully cross-reacting with these peptides in the radioimmunoassay for A II. Furthermore, when the converting enzyme inhibitor SQ 20′881 was added to the medium at concentrations ranging from 10^{-7} to 10^{-4} M, no significant alteration of steroid stimulation was observed with either A I, A II, [des-asp^{1}]-A II or ACTH (Fig. 4).

The structural analog of A II [sar^{1}-ala^{8}]-A II was found to inhibit the steroidogenic effect of A I, A II and the heptapeptide (Fig. 5). In the presence of [sar^{1}-ala^{8}]-A II at a concentration of 10^{-6} M, the dose-response curves for all three peptides were shifted to the right in a parallel manner. The maximal stimulations did not appear to be reduced significantly in the presence of the inhibitor. When the molar concentration of [sar^{1}-ala^{8}]-A II was modified between 10^{-9} to 10^{-5} M in the presence of each of the three peptides at a submaximal concentration (10^{-7} M), a dose-dependent inhibition of the steroidogenic effect was observed. The half-maximal inhibition

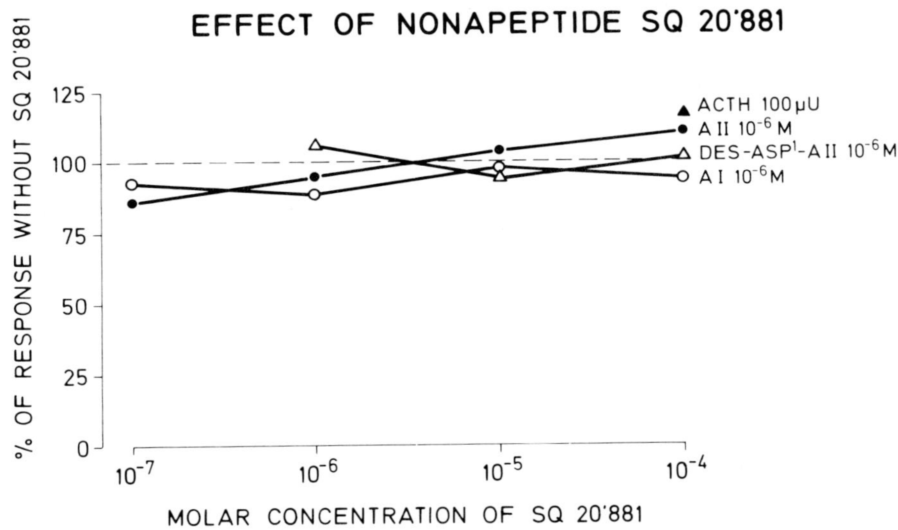

FIG. 4. Effect of increasing concentrations of SQ 20′881 on the steroidogenic action of A I, A II, [des-asp^1]-A II and ACTH on isolated bovine fasciculata cells.

(Fig. 6) of steroidogenesis was noted at a concentration of 4×10^{-7} M with A I and 1.2×10^{-6} with A II and 1.8×10^{-6} with [des-asp^1]-A II; [sar^1-ala^8]-A II did not affect the steroidogenesis induced by ACTH.

Discussion

The results of this study not only confirm the great sensitivity of isolated fasciculata cells from bovine adrenals to A II and ACTH [1], but also demonstrate an intrinsic steroidogenic activity for both the precursor of A II, A I, and its analog, [des-asp^1]-A II. Although A I is an active stimulator of steroid biosynthesis in this system, it possesses approximately half the intrinsic activity of A II and of the heptapeptide and behaves therefore as a partial agonist. It was important to assess if A I acted directly or only after its conversion to either A II or even to the heptapeptide. From the present results the following arguments support the concept that A I is an agonist in its own right. No significant conversion of A I to A II, heptapeptide or

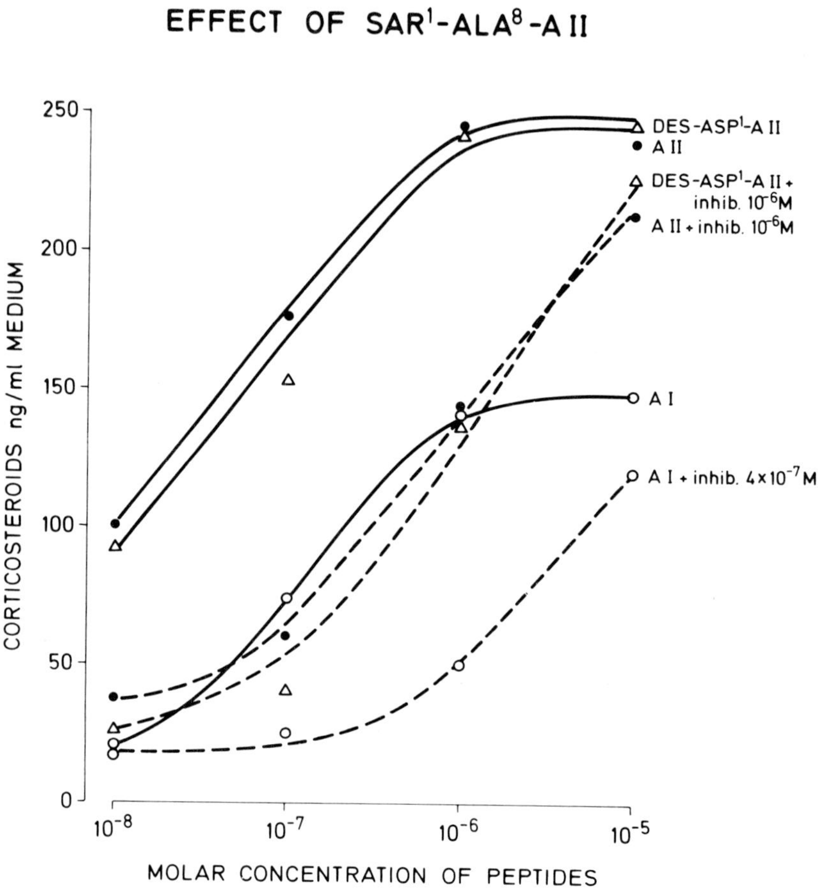

FIG. 5. Dose-response curves for A I, A II and [des-asp1]-A II on steroidogenesis given with (broken lines) and without (straight lines) [sar1-ala8]-A II. [sar1-ala8]-A II was added in concentrations known to inhibit 50% of the stimulatory effect of the angiotensins.

hexapeptide was found to take place during incubation; the recovery of A I is almost identical whether or not fasciculata cells were present in the medium and no generation of A II, heptapeptide or hexapeptide could be observed. In addition, the effect of A I on steroid biosynthesis was unaffected by the converting enzyme inhibitor SQ 20′881. This nonapeptide from *Bothrops jaracaca* is one of the most potent inhibitors of the converting enzyme and exhibits a prolonged effect in vivo. Therefore, it appears that A I has a direct intrinsic activity upon

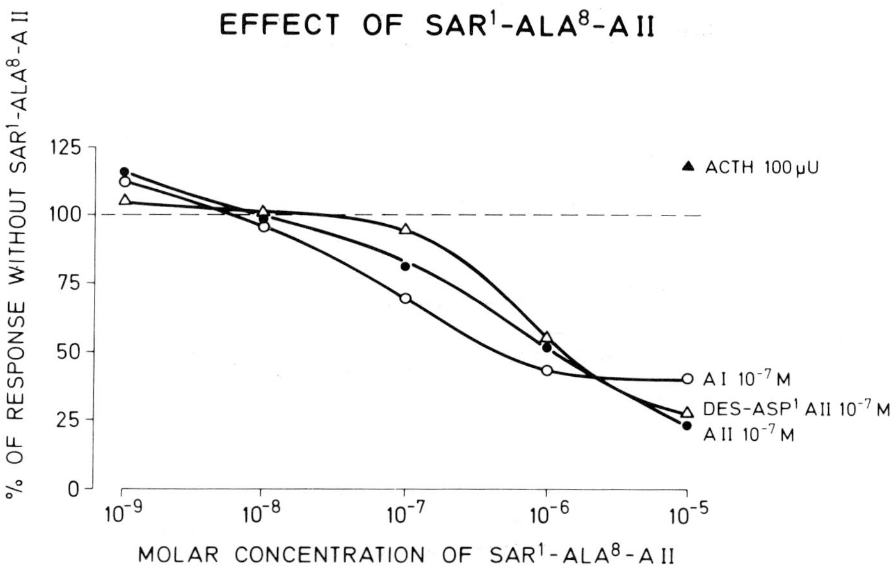

FIG. 6. Effect of increasing concentrations of [sar1-ala8]-A II on the steroidogenic action of A I, A II, [des-asp1]-A II and ACTH on isolated bovine fasciculata cells.

fasciculata cells from bovine adrenals. Thus, in addition to the adrenal medulla where it releases catecholamines [19] and the central nervous system [20-22] where it exerts a dipsogenic activity, the bovine adrenal cortex should be included among the target tissues able to respond to A I.

The heptapeptide [des-asp1]-A II is known to stimulate aldosterone synthesis [7-12] and to compete with A II for binding sites in glomerulosa cells [23, 24].

The effect of [des-asp1]-A II on steroidogenesis in isolated fasciculata cells is comparable to that of A II, the dose-response curves of both peptides being superimposable.

The inhibitor [sar1-ala8]-A II, one among many angiotensin analogs and antagonists substituted in position 1 and 8 [25, 26], when combined with A II and the heptapeptide, is able to displace the dose-response curves to the right in a parallel manner. The concentration of [sar1-ala8]-A II, required to produce a 50% inhibition of steroid production, is the same whether 10^{-7} M A II or 10^{-7} M heptapeptide is used as agonist; the ratio of the concentration of inhibitor over the concentration of agonist is 10:1. This inhibition appears to be of the competitive type and it is specific for angiotensin and its analog since ACTH-induced steroidogenesis remains unaffected. These data therefore suggest the presence of a common binding site for A II and the heptapeptide.

By contrast, the concentration of [sar^1-ala^8]-A II, required to block 50% of the steroid production induced with 10^{-7} M A I, is 2.5 times smaller (ratio of concentration of 4:1) than the concentration needed when the cells are stimulated with 10^{-7} M A II or heptapeptide.

It should be noted that in the adrenal medulla aliphatic 8-substituted analogs of A II, such as [ile^8]-A II (but not [ala^8]-A II), have been found to be effective inhibitors of A I- and A II-induced catecholamines release [27]. These data and other studies on smooth muscle receptor sites for the angiotensins suggest that on each of the target tissue angiotensin and some of its structural analogs are acting *via* the same binding site, but that these binding sites may differ from tissue to tissue [6, 10, 28-32]. Our own data and those of most of the investigators working with [sar^1-ala^8]-A II or other 8-substituted analogs of A II indicate that the inhibition observed is of the competitive type; [sar^1-leu^8]-A II may be an exception in not fulfilling the criteria for competitive inhibition [28].

In conclusion, the results of our experiments provide evidences that A I, A II and heptapeptide are all potent stimulators of steroid production in fasciculata cells from bovine adrenals, that A II and heptapeptide are equipotent in this system and that A I possesses an intrinsic activity in its own right without having to be converted to either A II or the heptapeptide. The possibility of conversion of A I to the nonapeptide [des-asp^1]-A I is not excluded and deserves further study.

Acknowledgments

The authors are indebted to Dr. F. M. Bumpus for a generous gift of the [des-asp^1]-angiotensin II and the [des-asp^1-arg^2]-angiotensin II and to the Squibb Institute for kindly supplying the nonapeptide SQ 20′881. They wish to thank Miss Christine Grillet and Mrs. Stéphane Fleury for their technical help, and Miss V. Nicolet for her secretarial assistance.

References

1. Peytremann, A., Nicholson, W.E., Brown, R.D. et al: Comparative effects of angiotensin and ACTH on cyclic AMP and steroidogenesis in isolated bovine adrenal cells. J. Clin. Invest. 52:835, 1973.
2. Kaplan, N.M. and Bartter, F.C.: The effect of ACTH, renin, angiotensin II, and various precursors on biosynthesis of aldosterone by adrenal slices. J. Clin. Invest. 41:715, 1962.
3. Kaplan, N.M.: The biosynthesis of adrenal steroids: Effects of angiotensin II, adrenocorticotropin, and potassium. J. Clin. Invest. 44:2029, 1965.
4. Carpenter, C.C.J., Davis, J.O. and Ayers, C.R.: Relation of renin, angiotensin II, and experimental renal hypertension to aldosterone secretion. J. Clin. Invest. 40:2026, 1961.
5. Slater, J.D.H., Barbour, B.H., Henderson, H.H. et al: Influence of the pituitary and the renin-angiotensin system on the secretion of aldosterone, cortisol, and corticosterone. J. Clin. Invest. 42:1504, 1963.
6. Bravo, E.L., Khosla, M.C. and Bumpus, F.M.: Vascular and adrenocortical responses to a specific antagonist of angiotensin II. Am. J. Physiol. 228:110, 1975.
7. Blair-West, J.R., Coghlan, J.P., Denton, D.A. et al: The effect of the heptapeptide (2-8) and hexapeptide (3-8) fragments of angiotensin II on aldosterone secretion. J. Clin. Endocrinol. 32:575, 1971.
8. Spielman, W.S., Davis, J.O., Freeman, R.H. et al: Stimulation of aldosterone by a heptapeptide fragment of angiotensin II in the rat, abstracted. Fed. Proc. 33:254, 1974.
9. Campbell, W.B., Brooks, S.N. and Pettinger, W.A.: Angiotensin II- and angiotensin III-induced aldosterone release in vivo in the rat. Science 184:994, 1974.
10. Lohmeier, T.E., Davis, J.O. and Freeman, R.H.: Des-Asp[1]-Angiotensin II: Possible role in mediating responses of the renin-angiotensin system (38840). Proc. Soc. Exp. Biol. Med. 149:515, 1975.
11. Peach, M.J. and Chiu, A.T.: Stimulation and inhibition of aldosterone biosynthesis in vitro by angiotensin II and analogs. *In* Hunt, J.C. (ed.): Hypertension XXII: Peptides, Lipids, Electrolytes, and Hypertension. Circ. Res. 34 and 35 (suppl. 1):1-7, 1974.
12. Chiu, A.T. and Peach, M.J.: Inhibition of induced aldosterone biosynthesis with a specific antagonist of angiotensin II. Proc. Nat. Acad. Sci. USA 71:341, 1974.
13. Goodfriend, T.L. and Peach, M.J.: Angiotensin III: (Des-Aspartic Acid[1])-angiotensin II. Evidence and speculation for its role as an important agonist in the renin-angiotensin system. Circ. Res. 36 and 37 (suppl. 1):1-38, 1975.
14. Kloppenborg, P.W.C., Island, D.P., Liddle, G.W. et al: A method of preparing adrenal cell suspensions and its applicability to the in vitro study of adrenal metabolism. Endocrinology 82:1053, 1968.
15. Sayers, G., Swallow, R.K. and Giordano, N.D.: An improved technique for the preparation of isolated rat adrenal cells: A sensitive,

accurate and specific method for the assay of ACTH. Endocrinology 88:1063, 1971.

16. LeClercq, R., Copinschi, G. and Franckson, J.R.M.: Le dosage par compétition du cortisol plasmatique. Modification de la méthode de Murphy. Rev. Franc. Etud. Clin. Biol. 14:815, 1969.
17. Vallotton, M.B.: Relationship between chemical structure and antigenicity of angiotensin analogues. Immunochemistry 7:529, 1970.
18. Vallotton, M.B.: Immunogenicity and antigenicity of angiotensin I and II. *In* Page, I. H. and Bumpus, F. M. (eds.): Angiotensin. Handbook of Experimental Pharmacology. New York:Springer-Verlag, 1974, vol. 37.
19. Peach, M.J.: Adrenal medullary stimulation induced by angiotensin I, angiotensin II, and analogues. Circ. Res. 28 and 29 (suppl. 2):11-107, 1971.
20. Soloman, T., Cavero, I. and Buckley, J.P.: Inhibition of the central pressor effects of angiotensin I and II. J. Pharm. Sci. 63:511, 1974.
21. Swanson, L.W., Marshall, G.R., Needleman, P. et al: Characterization of central angiotensin II receptors involved in the elicitation of drinking in the rat. Brain Res. 49:441, 1973.
22. Bryant, R.W. and Falk, J.L.: Angiotensin I as a dipsogen: Efficacy in brain independent of conversion to angiotensin II. Pharmacol. Biochem. Behav. 1:469, 1973.
23. Glossmann, H., Baukal, A.J. and Catt, K.J.: Properties of angiotensin II receptors in the bovine and rat adrenal cortex. J. Biol. Chem. 249:825, 1974.
24. Brecher, P.I., Pyun, H.Y. and Chobanian, A.V.: Studies on the angiotensin II receptor in the zona glomerulosa of the rat adrenal gland. Endocrinology 95:1026, 1974.
25. Regoli, D., Park, W.K. and Rioux, F.: Pharmacology of angiotensin. Pharmacol. Rev. 26:69, 1974.
26. Türker, R.K., Page, I.H. and Bumpus, F.M.: Antagonists of angiotensin II. *In* Page, I. H. and Bumpus, F. M. (eds.): Angiotensin. Handbook of Experimental Pharmacology. Berlin:Springer-Verlag, 1974, vol. 37.
27. Peach, M.J. and Ober, M.: Inhibition of angiotensin-induced adrenal catecholamine release by 8-substituted analogs of angiotensin II. J. Pharmacol. Exp. Ther. 190:49, 1974.
28. Rioux, F., Park, W.K. and Regoli, D.: I. Pharmacology of angiotensin antagonists. Canad. J. Physiol. Pharmacol. 51:108, 1973.
29. Regoli, D., Park, W.K. and Rioux, F.: II. Pharmacology of angiotensin antagonists. Canad. J. Physiol. Pharmacol. 51:114, 1973.
30. Steele, J.M. and Lowenstein, J.: Differential effects of an angiotensin II analogue on pressor and adrenal receptors in the rabbit. Circ. Res. 35:592, 1974.
31. Williams, G.H., McDonnell, L.M., Raux, M.C. et al: Evidence for different angiotensin II receptors in rat adrenal glomerulosa and rabbit vascular smooth muscle cells. Circ. Res. 34:384, 1974.
32. Mimran, A., Hinrichs, K.J. and Hollenberg, N.K.: Characterization of smooth muscle receptors for angiotensin: Studies with an antagonist. Am. J. Physiol. 226:185, 1974.

Discussion

Moderator: Dr. J. W. Conn

Dr. Catt: I would like to mention one or two results which are relevant to Dr. Bumpus' presentation. With regard to the effectiveness of the heptapeptide versus the octapeptide antagonists, our observations are quite different from those described by Dr. Bumpus and Dr. Bravo.

Figure 1 is a comparison of the inhibitory activities of these compounds, which were kindly given to us by Dr. Bumpus, upon angiotensin II-stimulated aldosterone production by isolated canine glomerulosa cells. The figure represents the 100% response to angiotensin II (10^{-9} M) and the inhibition (open circles) by increasing concentrations by [Sar^1, Ile^8] angiotensin II. The open squares illustrate the inhibitory effect of the [$Des\text{-}Asp^1$] antagonist on angiotensin II-induced aldosterone production. The bottom dashed line shows the intrinsic agonist activity of each of these two compounds. In this cell system, the [$Des\text{-}Asp^1$] antagonist is significantly less active as an inhibitor of angiotensin II than is the octapeptide antagonist. Furthermore, in regard to the view that conversion to the heptapeptide is an intermediate step in angiotensin II action, I agree that this is an attactive idea but, unfortunately, there is not one piece of direct evidence which has so far been produced to support this proposal.

Figure 2 shows two pieces of data which we find difficult to equate with the idea that the heptapeptide is an essential intermediate in the action of angiotensin II. The study illustrates the agonist effect of three peptides upon the dog adrenal cell production of aldosterone in vitro. The two superimposable curves on the left are the aldosterone responses to angiotensin II and [$Des\text{-}Asp^1$] angiotensin II, both peptides

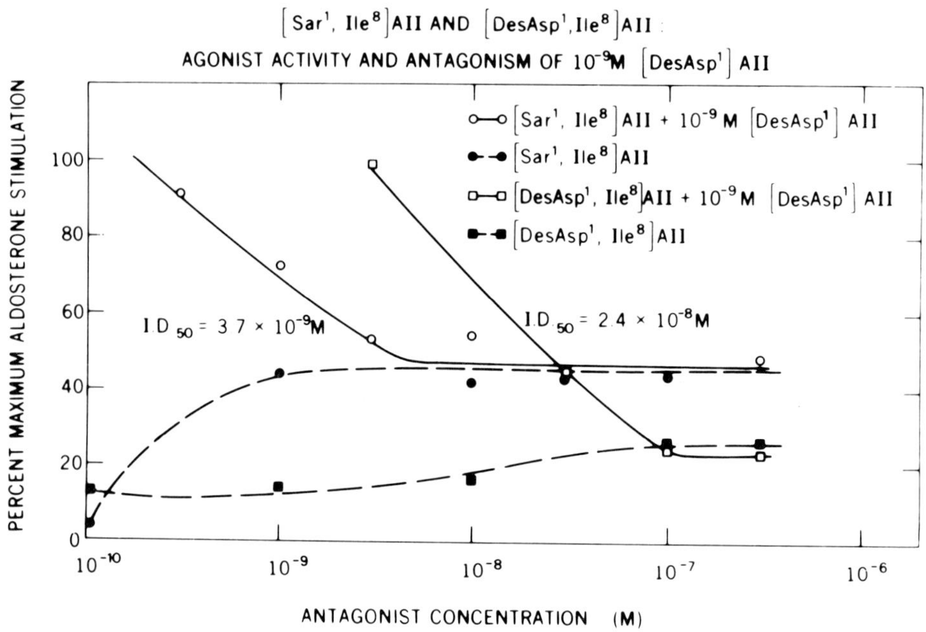

FIGURE 1.

showing identical potency as in receptor binding studies and in other reports of the aldosterone response to these agonists. This identical response means that angiotensin II would have to be *completely converted* to [Des-Asp1] angiotensin II in order to exert this effect, if formation of the heptapeptide is an essential intermediate step. Otherwise, if the [Des-Asp1] peptide is the obligatory intermediate, we should see less activity with angiotensin II than with the [Des-Asp1] compound. Second, [Sar1] angiotensin II, shown on the right hand side, is ten times more potent than angiotensin II upon aldosterone production. Yet, this compound has been proposed to be less susceptible to the N-terminal action of aminopeptidase, and should be less readily converted to the heptapeptide. Thus neither of these observations is in accordance with the notion that the heptapeptide is an important or essential intermediate in the action of angiotensin II on aldosterone production by the zona glomerulosa cell.

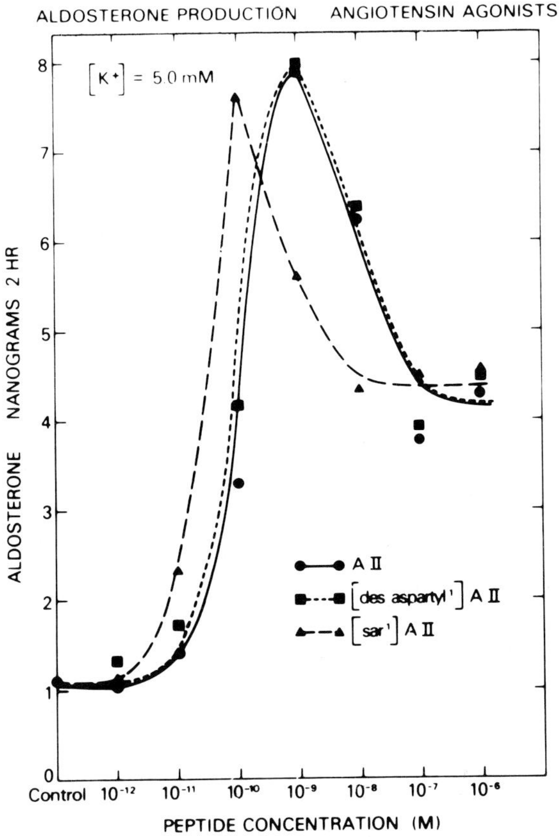

FIGURE 2.

Dr. Bumpus: I am really not trying to promote the idea that the heptapeptide is the true hormone for aldosterone release rather than angiotensin II. Whether or not it is called angiotensin III is immaterial. Our experiments have been designed to get information concerning the possible necessity for the lysis of aspartic acid for activity in the adrenal cortex. Plasma aminopeptidase A is specific for aspartic acid and glutamic acids and will not split sarcosine from [Sar^1] angiotension II or any of its derivatives. Pettinger has reported that aminopeptidase(s) occur in the adrenal gland but did not determine their specificities. It is entirely possible that more than one type of this enzyme occurs in the adrenal cortex. We are in the process of looking at the specificity of these.

Dr. Coghlan mentioned that one might consider sarcosine derivatives of angiotensin as analogues of the heptapeptide. An important determinant may be the side group of aspartic acid in position one. This hypothesis has not been tested. We have several derivatives, for example the N-methylisoasparagine compound to determine the importance of the side group in position one, in a derivative that would not be hydrolyzed by angiotensinase A.

Dr. Vallotton: There is complete agreement between Dr. Catt's data and our own: angiotensin II and the heptapeptide are equipotent in his as in our system.

Dr. Denton: I would be interested in your use of the term "release" rather than "secretion" in light of the fact, for example, that with the sodium-deficient sheep one can infuse radiolabeled corticosterone into the adrenal arterial supply and within a matter of 1.5 to 2.0 minutes we have radiolabeled aldosterone appearing in the adrenal venous effluent in the conscious animal. The amount of aldosterone you can extract from the adrenal in the Na-deficient animal would supply a minute or two secretion only. If you infuse aldosterone into the adrenal arterial supply you do not inhibit the adrenal secretion of the aldosterone. I was wondering against that background whether you care to elaborate further on the term "release" and the concept you have in mind. In relation to the remark perhaps this is an opportunity for us to thank Dr. Sambhi who made the heptapeptide available to us. I think it was 1968 and we sat on the data for two or three years before we published it. As you know we publish everything alphabetically, but in this instance I would like to remark that it was John Coghlan who put forward the hypothesis of conversion of nonapeptide to heptapeptide direct and the heptapeptide role as angiotensin III.

Dr. Bumpus: I really cannot comment much further on that subject. I assume that aldosterone moves across the plasma membrane by passive transport. In that case, your experiments strongly suggest that angiotensin does not affect release directly.

Unidentified: Dr. Bumpus, maybe I can give a little more direct countersupport for the notion, that is when you incubate the isolated glomerulosa cells with added aldosterone in the medium it does not seem to alter, at least, the rate of synthesis of conversion of triated B to triated aldosterone. Whether it alters the maximum production under those circumstances is obviously impossible to tell but it would appear to be, at least, somewhat unlikely that it alters the late step of aldosterone biosynthesis as opposed to what corticosterone does. Our experience is very similar to Dr. Catt's as far as the relative relationship of the heptapeptide analogue antagonists and the octapeptide antagonists. That is, if anything, the Ile analogue of the heptapeptide we find is less potent inhibitor of aldosterone in our isolated glomerulosa cell preparation and this, in part, is reflected in the fact that our response to P113 is considerably greater than yours being almost within the factor of 4 of molar potent as far as antagonist of angiotensin II as an agonist in our system. I am sure part of the differences are the relative sensitivity of the systems since our cell preparations, in a sense, lead to 250 picograms of angiotensin II per ml which is in the order of 10 to the minus 10 molar. And the P113 blocks the factor of 4 greater than that, that is 4 times 10 to the minus 9. So perhaps some of the differences are really where the sensitivities of the various systems are. But I would tend to agree with you that when we study any of the inhibitors in vivo we see a lot more intrinsic activity and a change in the relative agonist antagonistic properties of the compounds than we do when we study them in vitro, at least in the isolated glomerulosa or the isolated smooth muscle prep, whether it is stomach, uterus or vascular tissue. In conjunction with that I wonder if some of the differences that Dr. Vallotton showed in relationship to his beef adrenal study are, again, related to doses because the dose that you use producing blockade, for example, with P113, is 4 to 5 orders of magnitude different, I guess, than what we observed with the glomerulosa cell preparation. I wonder if you have any data looking at the same sort of phenomenon in the glomerulosa cell side of your preparation. I realize that it is probably heavily contaminated with the fasciculata cells and you may not be able to answer the question. But I wonder if some of the difference in response, or some of the responses you see, are really because you are using superpharmacologic doses of the compounds rather than closer to physiologic since all of us tend to use semipharmacologic doses when we study in vitro systems?

Dr. Bumpus: Results of Peach and co-workers are somewhat different from those of yours and Catt's. We have repeated Catt's findings showing an increased potency of [Sar^1] angiotensin II over the parent hormone in the isolated cell preparation. However, the in vivo results of Bravo show increased potency of the heptapeptide inhibitors. One may speculate that this may be explained by increased half-life of the heptapeptide. However, from the point of view of degradation of angiotensin II-(2-8)-heptapeptide itself, Peach reported that it was metabolized much more readily in the plasma than was angiotensin II.

Dr. Williams: Do you think that the fact that the animals were all anesthetized in some way influenced your results? Several reports have suggested anesthesia may have significant effects on the angiotensin system. In conjunction with the last study we have an A II antibody that is much better against A III than A II by a factor of about 30. Under those circumstances we would anticipate that if there was any significant increase in A III concentration, our A II values would be considerably higher than anyone else's. This is not the case.

Dr. Bumpus: I am aware of results from Glasgow that show the occurrence of angiotensin III. I believe they report about 80% as much angiotensin III as angiotensin II rat plasma. In rabbits and humans they report much less.

Dr. Thurau: Dr. Bumpus, you have indicated that nonapeptide makes better substrate for the converting enzymes than octapeptides. Now the question is, what type of converting enzyme did you use? The reason I am asking is that recent results from Dalheim showed that converting enzymes in the various organs are very different from each other with very different kinetics and characteristics. For example, the converting enzyme you can get from the kidney has a completely different pH optimum as compared to the converting enzyme of the plasma. It is not chloride dependent in reaction as is the converting enzyme in the plasma and the effect of EDTA is completely different. So it looks like we are dealing with a very different converting enzyme in various organs. The question is, what type of converting enzyme did you use?

Dr. Bumpus: Yes, converting enzymes from porcine lung and plasma were both tested. Peach has shown that the converting enzyme is more active toward the nonapeptide than the decapeptide.

Dr. Coghlan: I just want to make a few comments. First to Dr. Vallotton: You know we reported some time ago that we get very little stimulus when we infuse angiotensin I in vivo directly into the adrenal artery supply. There is another problem in that if we use in vitro preparations of sheep adrenal we do seem to get an effect of angiotensin II on cortisol secretion which is not seen in vivo, which I cannot explain. I would also like to come back to the question that Dr. Catt raised as to the role of the heptapeptide angiotensin III and comment on what Dr. Williams said in this regard. If the blood clearance rates of the angiotensin fragments are measured it is found that these are of the same order as angiotensin itself. This means that there are real concentrations of angiotensin III in arterial blood roughly equal in fact to those in venous. In some recent experiments that we have done the indications are that concentrations of angiotensin III are about 20%-30% of the angiotensin II concentration. So whether or not it is more active or whether or not it is an obligatory intermediate, it may still have an important role as an equipotent stimulus as Dr. Catt has shown. Certainly in the original publication we could not show that it was significantly more potent. I do not understand Dr. Williams' results, his use of his "unique" antibody. In fact, an antibody to fragments seems to me highly questionable as I think there is no doubt that 2-8 hepta, 3-8 hexpeptide do occur in venous blood.

Dr. Vallotton: I have no experience with angiotensin I infusion in vivo, but we have shown that angiotensin I does circulate in the blood. If angiotensin I has an effect on the zona glomerulosa as it has on the zona fasciculata, as we have demonstrated in bovine adrenals, then certainly the angiotensin I present in the blood could get access to the adrenal gland and exert its effect.

Competitive Antagonists of Angiotensin II: Inhibition of Receptor Binding and Aldosterone Production in Dispersed Adrenal Cells

K. J. Catt, M.D., Ph.D., S. Saltman, M.D., J. Douglas, M.D. and T. Kondo, M.D.

The development of angiotensin II analogues, which act as specific competitive antagonists of the actions of the parent peptide, has provided a valuable series of compounds for experimental studies and clinical research [1-5]. The availability of such antagonists has greatly improved the precision with which angiotensin-dependent processes can be identified during analysis of the physiological and biochemical characteristics of the renin-angiotensin system [6]. In addition, these compounds have been used to identify angiotensin-dependent hypertension in experimental animal models [7-9] and in certain patients with renal and essential hypertension [10, 11].

The most effective angiotensin II antagonists have been prepared by substitution of the C-terminal phenylalanine residue by aliphatic amino acids such as isoleucine, alanine and glycine [12]. Such 8-aliphatic analogues retain binding affinity for angiotensin II receptors in adrenal and smooth muscle cells, but evoke only a small target cell response, and can thus be employed to block the specific receptor sites in smooth muscle and adrenal cortex [13-15]. Substitutions at the N-terminus, particularly with sarcosine, have also been shown to enhance the antagonist potency of analogues modified in the 8 position.

K. J. Catt, M.D., Ph.D., S. Saltman, M.D., J. Douglas, M.D. and T. Kondo, M.D., Section on Hormonal Regulation, Reproduction Research Branch, National Institute of Child Health and Human Development, National Institutes of Health, Bethesda, Md.

The agonist activity of inhibitory angiotensin analogues is also determined by the nature of the C-terminal and N-terminal substituents. However, the extent to which such agonist properties are manifested may differ according to the experimental preparation and conditions which are employed to study specific responses to angiotensin II. For these reasons, it is important to establish the intrinsic biological properties of the antagonist peptides upon both receptor binding and target cell responses for angiotensin II. This objective has been approached in the adrenal gland by combined studies on the binding activity and steroidogenic effects of angiotensin II analogues in adrenal homogenates and dispersed cells from the zona glomerulosa.

Angiotensin II Receptors of the Adrenal Cortex

In previous studies on the interaction of ^{3}H- and ^{125}I-angiotensin II with particulate fractions of rat and bovine adrenal cortex, we have described the characteristics of receptors with high affinity, limited capacity and high specificity for angiotensin II and related peptides [16, 17]. The adrenal binding sites exhibited rapid kinetics of association and dissociation, and the binding process was found to be modified by sodium concentration [18] and by guanyl nucleotides [19]. The angiotensin II receptors have been shown to be situated in the plasma membrane of the adrenal cell, in common with the cellular location of receptors for other peptide hormones in their respective target tissues [20]. The highly selective uptake of angiotensin II and active derivatives by the particulate adrenal receptor preparation has indicated the potential value of this system for studies on the binding properties of angiotensin II derivatives [21, 22].

Competitive Binding Activity of Angiotensin II Analogues

The radioligand-receptor binding assay for angiotensin II, employing ^{125}I-labeled angiotensin II and homogenates of bovine adrenal cortex, has provided a useful method for direct evaluation of the binding properties of angiotensin analogues [21]. By this procedure, the relative binding activities of both agonist and antagonist derivatives can be determined from their potencies as competitive inhibitors of receptor binding of ^{125}I-angiotensin II. The radioligand-receptor assay procedure is relatively simple to perform, yet provides precise and biologically relevant estimates of the binding-inhibition potencies of angiotensin II derivatives. In general, agonist analogues of angiotensin II have shown competitive binding activities which are exactly proportional to their known relative biological activities upon aldosterone production by the zona glomerulosa. The native octapeptide, either [Asp^1] or [Asn^1] angiotensin II, and the [Des-Asp^1] heptapeptide were equipotent, while the [Des-Asp^1, Des-Arg^2] hexapeptide and the [Des-Phe^8] heptapeptide possessed less than 1% of the binding-inhibition activity of angiotensin II. In addition, the [Sar^1] derivative of angiotensin II, which is known to show about ten times the contractile activity of angiotensin II on the isolated rabbit aorta [23], was considerably more potent than the native octapeptide in the receptor binding assay. Angiotensin I exhibits about 5% of the binding activity of angiotensin II, in keeping with its low biological activity upon the adrenal cortex. Other angiotensin II fragments and biologically inactive analogues such as the [Phe^3, Tyr^8] octapeptide were devoid of significant binding-inhibition activity. However, it was of interest to note that even the C-terminal heptapeptide and tetrapeptide fragments of angiotensin II displayed a low degree of binding-inhibition activity and completely inhibited the combination of ^{125}I-angiotensin II with adrenal receptors when present in sufficiently high concentration. Such binding-inhibition activity was never seen with equally high concentrations of peptides unrelated to angiotensin II and suggests that the conformation of angiotensin II necessary for receptor binding is present in relatively small fragments of the molecule. Addition of other aminoacid residues greatly enhance the affinity of binding at the receptor site, and the presence of an aromatic C-terminal residue confers the ability to activate the receptors and evoke a target cell response, in this case steroidogenesis and aldosterone production. Another feature of interest in the agonist binding studies was the exactly similar potencies of the octapeptide and the [Des-Asp^1] heptapeptide. These peptides have been shown in several studies to exert identical steroidogenic activities upon the adrenal, even though the [Des-Asp^1] compound is consistently less active than angiotensin II upon smooth muscle contraction and blood pressure responses. The close correlation between the biological activities and binding characteristics of the various angiotensin II agonists provides compelling, though not absolute, evidence that the binding sites demonstrated in adrenal homogenates are indeed the functional receptors for angiotensin II. More direct evidence to confirm this view is provided by the combined binding and activation studies described below.

When angiotensin II antagonists were evaluated in the adrenal cortex radioligand-receptor assay, the binding-inhibition potencies of several derivatives were found to be generally correlated with their pA_2 values as antagonists of angiotensin II in smooth muscle [21]. Peptide analogues formed by C-terminal substitution with aliphatic residues such as isoleucine, alanine and glycine showed relatively high binding activities, which were considerably influenced by the nature of the N-terminal residue of the antagonist analogue. Thus, more basic N-terminal substituents such as guanidoacetic acid and sarcosine caused marked increases in the binding-inhibition potency of the [Ile^8]-substituted antagonists. Conversely, binding activity was abolished by introduction of acidic N-terminal residues such as succinic acid and pyroglutamic acid. The influence of the basicity of the N-terminal residue was also apparent in the binding studies with [Sar^1]-angiotensin II, which displayed increased binding potency in parallel with its increased agonist activity in vitro.

Of the C-terminal modifications evaluated by radioligand-receptor assay, binding-inhibition potency was highest for [Ile^8] derivatives and significantly lower for the [Leu^8], [Ala^8] and [Gly^8] compounds. The [D-Ile^8] derivative was almost devoid of binding activity and also showed extremely low antagonist activity in aortic smooth muscle. The relatively high binding-inhibition activity of the [Ile^8] derivative is consistent with the high potency of the [Ile^8] compounds as antagonists of angiotensin II. In terms of binding-inhibition activity and the pA_2 values in aortic smooth muscle, the [Sar^1, Ile^8] and [GAc^1, Ile^8] peptides would appear to be the most potent antagonists. Such an interpretation is consistent with the known activities of these compounds in terms of the dose-ratios required to inhibit the actions of angiotensin I in smooth muscle and adrenal cells. However, it has become apparent that the high binding affinity and antagonist activity of the [Ile^8] derivatives are accompanied by a significant degree of agonist activity. For this reason, the peptide analogues prepared by substitution with shorter chain aliphatic residues at the C-terminus have proven to be more satisfactory as competitive antagonists of angiotensin II.

The immunoreactivity of angiotensin II analogues was also of interest to compare with their binding activity in the adrenal receptor system. Since the C-terminal phenylalanine residue is an essential component of the antigenic site and is recognized by virtually all antisera raised against angiotensin II, it was not surprising that the 8-aliphatic substituent peptides showed no detectable cross-reactivity in the radioimmunoassay. This finding indicates that the loss of conformation produced by replacement of the C-terminal aromatic group by an aliphatic residue has a much more marked effect upon the antigenic site than upon the receptor binding site. Retention of immunoreactivity was only observed in angiotensin II analogues with C-terminal substituents such as tyrosine, tryptophane and thienylalanine.

The high immunoreactivity of the [Thienylalanine^8] substituted peptide is attributable to the considerable structural similarity of this residue to phenylalanine. The [Tal^8] derivative also showed high binding-inhibition potency in the radioligand-receptor assay, and despite its apparently high pA_2 value in the aortic strip, has behaved as an agonist upon aldosterone production during incubation with the isolated adrenal cells. This unusual compound merits more detailed study in a variety of angiotensin II target tissues and, in particular, should be further evaluated in smooth muscle.

Actions of Angiotensin II Analogues on Isolated Adrenal Cells

A convenient and highly sensitive system for studies on aldosterone production in vitro has been developed by the use of collagenase-dispersed dog adrenal cells and direct assay of aldosterone in the incubation medium [24, 25]. Such enzyme-dispersed cells are highly sensitive to angiotensin II and are of considerable value for studies on the actions of angiotensin agonists and antagonists [26]. The steroidogenic response of canine zona glomerulosa cells is consistently observed at physiological concentrations of angiotensin II, ie, 2 to 5 $\times$

10^{-11} M. The maximum aldosterone response of three to eight times the basal level is obtained with 3×10^{-10} M angiotensin II, and a decrease in steroid production occurs at angiotensin concentrations above 10^{-9} M. The aldosterone responses to angiotensin II and the [Des-Asp^1]-heptapeptide are identical, whereas the [Des-Asp^1, Des-Arg^2]-hexapeptide and the [Des-Phe^8]-heptapeptide are almost completely inactive. By contrast, the more potent agonist [Sar^1]-angiotensin II was about ten times more active than angiotensin II in stimulating aldosterone production, in keeping with its increased activity upon vascular smooth muscle.

The biological activities of a number of angiotensin II antagonists upon aldosterone production were also evaluated in the isolated canine glomerulosa cell preparation [22, 27]. In these studies, [Sar^1, Ileu^8] A II was found to be the most potent competitive antagonist of angiotensin II-stimulated aldosterone production, but was also a partial agonist at concentrations required to inhibit the steroidogenic effect of angiotensin II on dog adrenal cells. By comparison, [Sar^1 Ala^8] A II was significantly less potent than [Sar^1 Ileu^8] A II as a competitive inhibitor of angiotensin II-stimulated aldosterone production. The antagonist concentrations necessary to cause 50% inhibition of the aldosterone production induced by 10^{-9} M A II were 4×10^{-9} M for [Sar^1, Ileu^8] A II and 5×10^{-8} M for [Sar^1, Ala^8] A II; ie, the [Sar^1, Ile^8] derivative was about 12 times more active than [Sar^1, Ala^8] A II on a molar basis. However, [Sar^1, Ala^8] A II and [Sar^1, Gly^8] A II were found to be devoid of significant agonist activity upon adrenal cells and were therefore more completely effective antagonists of A II-stimulated aldosterone production by comparison with the [Ile^8] derivative. Both [Sar^1, Ala^8] and [Sar^1, Gly^8] A II produced complete inhibition of angiotensin II-stimulated aldosterone production at concentrations of 10^{-7} M and above. By contrast, the [Sar^1, Ile^8] antagonist never reduced aldosterone production to basal values, due to the intrinsic agonist activity of the [Ile^8] derivative. The observations suggest that increased length of the aliphatic side chain at the C-terminus of angiotensin II antagonists was accompanied by enhanced affinity for the receptor site and also by increased agonist activity of the analogue. The agonist activities of the [Ile^8], [Ala^8] and [Gly^8] peptides are illustrated in Figure 1.

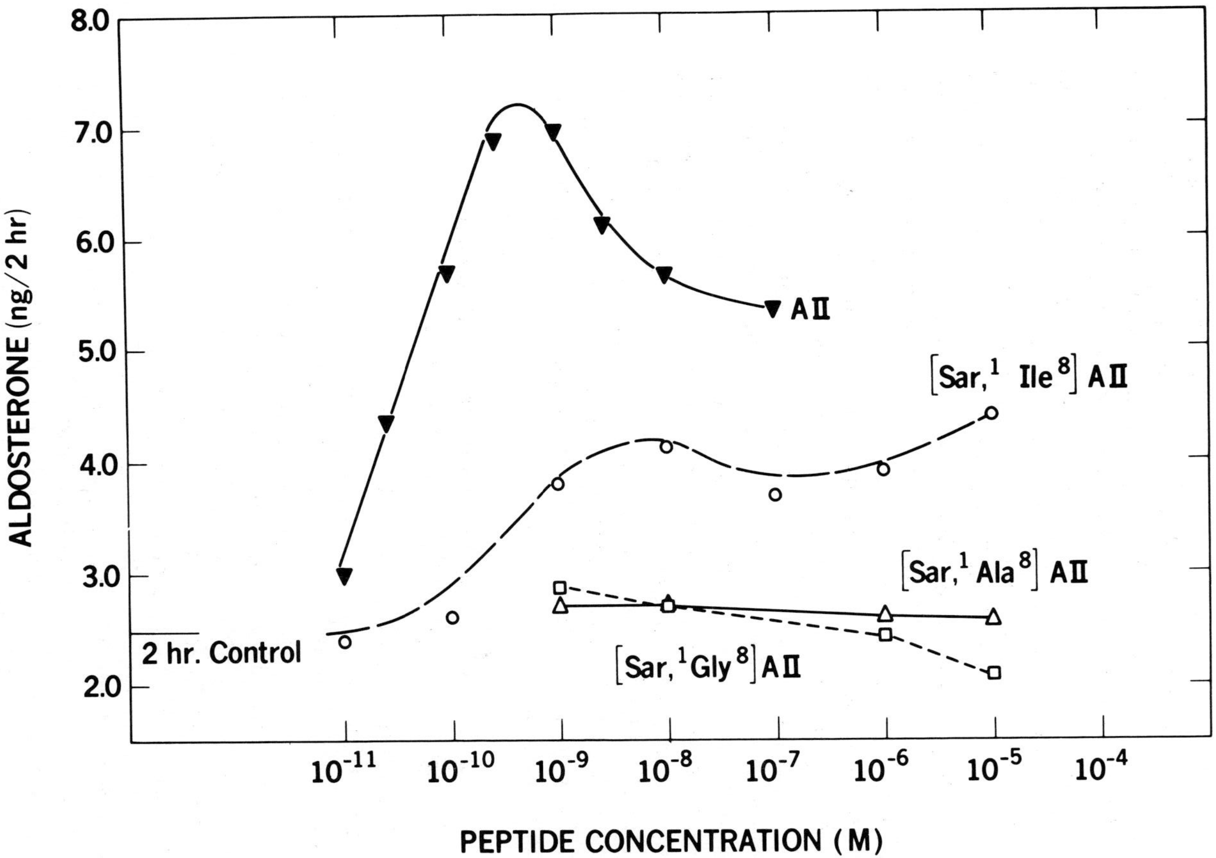

FIG. 1. Stimulation of aldosterone production in isolated adrenal cells by angiotensin II (A II) and the competitive antagonists [Sar^1, Ile^8], [Sar^1, Ala^8] and [Sar^1, Gly^8] angiotensin II.

The actions of angiotensin II and [Des-Asp[1]] A II upon aldosterone production were inhibited identically and completely by [Sar[1], Ala[8]] A II. [Sar[1] Ileu[8]] A II also inhibited aldosterone production by angiotensin II and [Des-Asp[1]] A II identically over the same concentration range. The heptapeptide antagonist [Des-Asp[1], Ileu[8]] A II was slightly more effective as an inhibitor of [Des-Asp[1]] A II than of the octapeptide (A II) agonist, but was a much less active antagonist than [Sar[1], Ileu[8]] A II as an inhibitor of the actions of both the heptapeptide and octapeptide agonists (Fig. 2). The antagonist activity of these analogues at the adrenal level, determined by the concentration required for 50% inhibition of maximum aldosterone secretion, correlated well with the pA_2 values measured upon isolated smooth muscle and also with the relative binding-inhibition potencies determined in a radioligand-receptor assay using bovine adrenal cortex homogenate. These observations have demonstrated that smooth muscle receptors and adrenal cortex receptors exhibit generally similar responses to angiotensin II antagonists and that the [Sar[1], Ala[8]] derivative of angiotensin II is a highly effective antagonist of the steroidogenic action of angiotensin II upon aldosterone production by the zona glomerulosa cells of the adrenal cortex.

Peptide Binding and Aldosterone Production by Isolated Adrenal Cells

The binding properties of angiotensin II receptors have also been examined in isolated cells prepared from the capsular layer of the canine adrenal gland [28]. In such cell preparations, the binding of angiotensin II and analogues could be directly compared with aldosterone production in vitro. The uptake of ^{125}I-angiotensin II by glomerulosa cells was specific, saturable and rapid, reaching a steady state of 45 min when cells were incubated at 37°C with physiological concentrations (10^{-11} M) of the labeled peptide. The intact cells were found to possess two orders of specific binding sites, a high-affinity group with Ka of $3.3 \times 10^9 M^{-1}$ which comprised 25%-33% of the total receptor population and a lower-affinity set with Ka of $2.5 \times 10^8 M^{-1}$. The binding and binding-inhibition activities of angiotensin II agonists and antagonists showed a high degree of

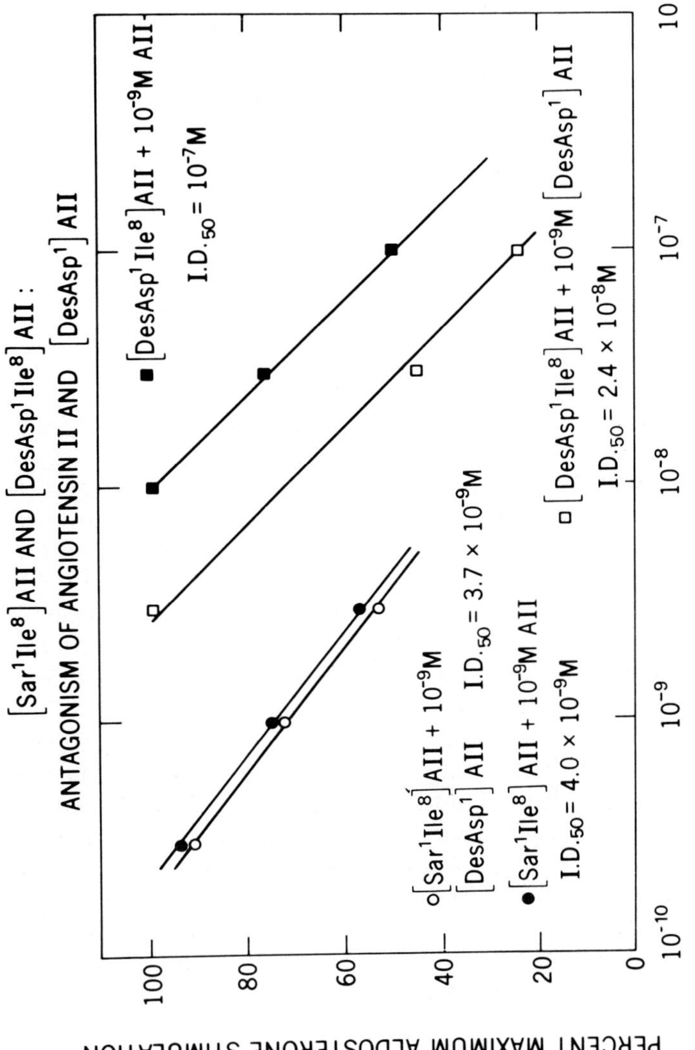

FIG. 2. Antagonist activities of [Sar[1], Ile[8]] and [Des-Asp[1], Ile[8]] angiotensin II upon aldosterone production by isolated adrenal cells incubated with angiotensin II and [Des-Asp[1]]-angiotensin II.

correlation with their biological activities upon the adrenal gland. Thus, angiotensin I displayed only 9% of the binding-inhibition potency of angiotensin II, and the [Des-Asp[1]] heptapeptide was equipotent with angiotensin II. The more highly active agonist, [Sar[1]] angiotensin II, was about seven times more potent than angiotensin II in binding-inhibition studies and was also found to exhibit an eightfold increase in affinity for the adrenal binding sites during kinetic and equilibrium binding studies ($Ka = 1.4 \times 10^{10} M^{-1}$). This increase in binding affinity was predominantly due to a marked increase in the association rate constant of the reaction between [Sar[1]] angiotensin II and the receptor sites. These characteristics of the [Sar[1]] derivative were reflected in the more rapid and higher binding of this agonist by cells incubated with equimolar concentrations of [Sar[1]] angiotensin II and angiotensin II.

The effects of the [Sar[1]] substitution upon binding affinity were also apparent during binding-inhibition studies with intact cells and angiotensin II antagonists (Fig. 3). Thus, the relative binding-inhibition potencies of typical antagonists in relation to angiotensin II as unity were [Sar[1] Ala[8]] angiotensin II — 0.5; [Des-Asp[1], Ile[8]] angiotensin II — 0.43; and [Sar[1], Ile[8]] angiotensin II — 3.1. Once again, the introduction of the [Sar[1]] residue caused a marked increase in the binding affinity of the peptide, in this case by about sixfold. These observations have provided direct evidence for the mechanism by which the [Sar[1]] substituted agonist and antagonist analogues exert higher biological activities than the corresponding peptides bearing [Asp[1]] as the N-terminal aminoacid residue. This action of sarcosine appears to be related to the charge of the N-terminal residue, since substitution of acidic residues has been shown to abolish binding to adrenal receptors, whereas the introduction of more basic groups, such as sarcosine and guanidoacetic acid, significantly increases the binding affinity and biological activity of the resulting derivatives.

Receptor Binding and Activation of Aldosterone Production

When simultaneous measurements of angiotensin II binding and aldosterone production were performed in isolated cells

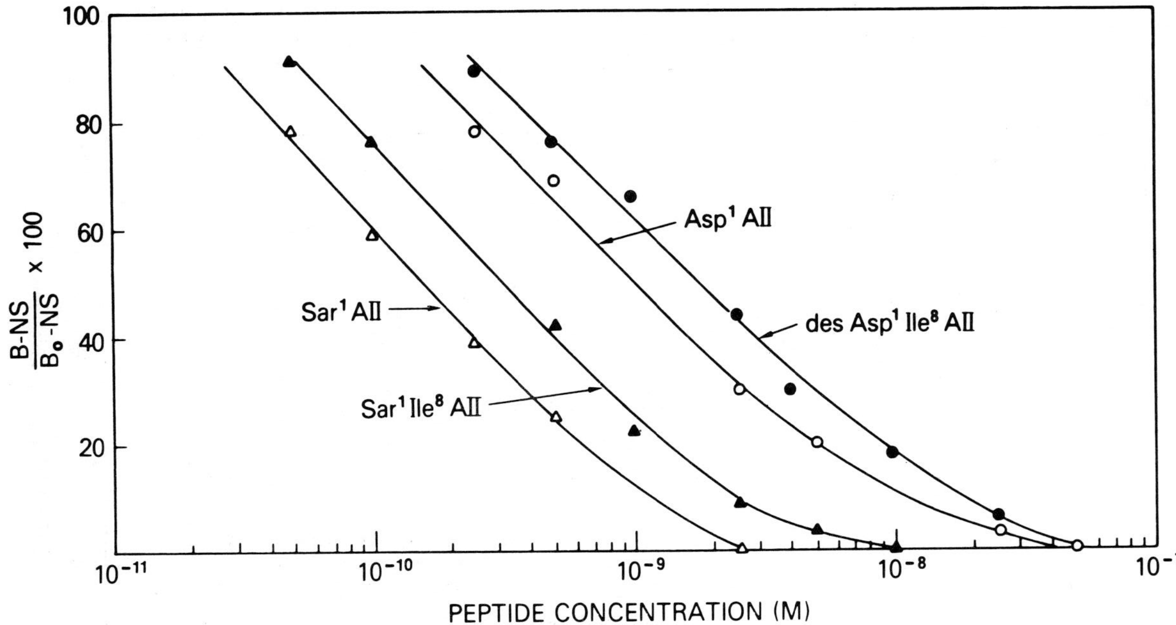

FIG. 3. Binding-inhibition curves obtained by incubation of dispersed adrenal glomerulosa cells with ^{125}I-angiotensin II and increasing concentrations of angiotensin II agonists and antagonists. The increased potency of the [Sar^1] derivatives is a consequence of increased binding affinity for the angiotensin II receptors.

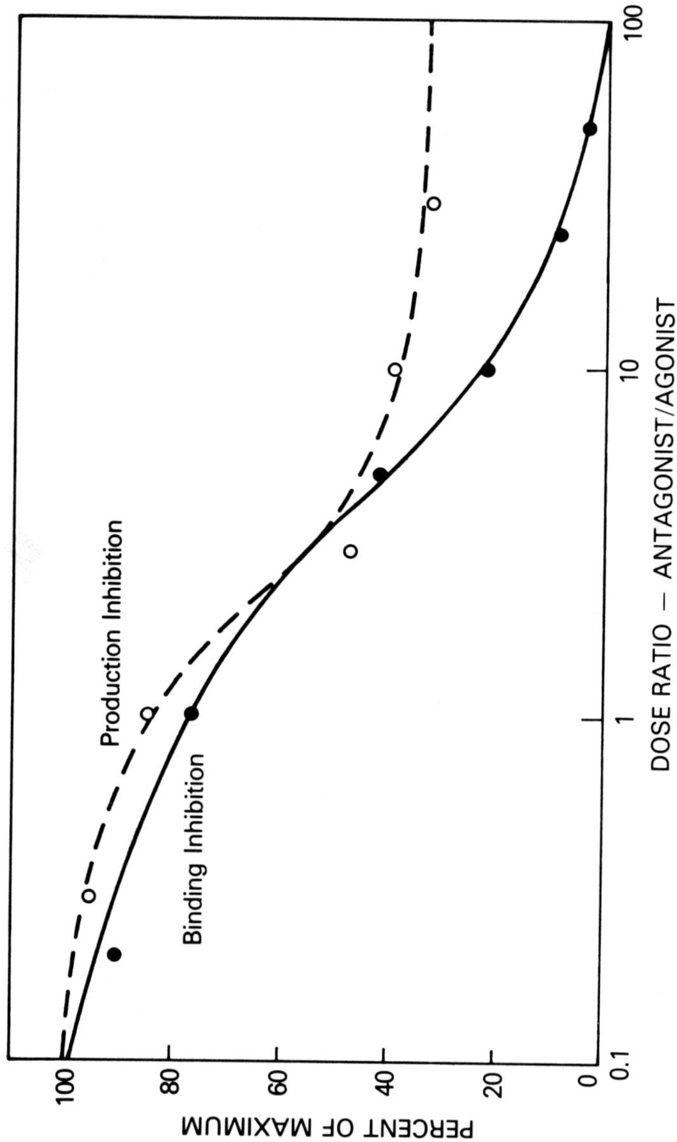

FIG. 4. Concomitant inhibition of angiotensin II binding and aldosterone production in isolated adrenal glomerulosa cells in the presence of increasing concentrations of [Sar[1], Ile[8]] angiotensin II.

prepared from the capsular layer of the canine adrenal gland, both binding and inhibition of binding of angiotensin II could be compared with aldosterone production [29]. Binding studies performed with intact adrenal cells have shown that the uptake of both agonists and antagonists of angiotensin was accompanied by commensurate changes in aldosterone production. Direct binding of angiotensin II by dispersed cells was correlated with increasing aldosterone production until about 25% of the receptor sites were occupied and then with the characteristic decrement in aldosterone production during further occupancy of receptors until saturation was reached.

Conversely, inhibition of angiotensin II binding to adrenal cells by antagonists could also be correlated with inhibition of the aldosterone response to angiotensin II. This effect is illustrated in Figure 4, which shows the concomitant reduction of both peptide binding and aldosterone production by increasing concentrations of the antagonist [Sar^1, Ile^8] angiotensin II. At higher concentrations of the antagonist, the agonist effect on aldosterone production becomes apparent, and the inhibitory effect on steroidogenesis does not exceed about 60% of the maximum response. The [Sar^1, Ala^8] antagonist is almost devoid of agonist activity and produces a more complete inhibition of both peptide binding and aldosterone synthesis. These correlations between angiotensin II binding and aldosterone production in isolated adrenal cells emphasize the biological significance of the angiotensin II binding sites and demonstrate their function as specific hormone receptors for angiotensin II and related peptides.

References

1. Marshall, G.R., Vine, W. and Needleman, P.: Specific competitive inhibitor of angiotensin II. Proc. Nat. Acad. Sci. USA 67:1624, 1970.
2. Turker, R.K., Yamamoto, M., Khairallah, P.A. et al: Competitive antagonism of 8-ala-angiotensin II to angiotensins I and II on isolated rabbit aorta and rat ascending colon. Eur. J. Pharmacol. 15:285, 1971.
3. Turker, R.K., Hall, M.M., Yamamoto, M. et al: A new long-acting competitive inhibitor of angiotensin. Science 29:1203, 1972.
4. Pals, D.T., Masucci, F.D., Sipos, F. et al: Specific competitive antagonist of the vascular action of angiotensin II. Circ. Res. 29:664, 1971.

5. Regoli, D., Park, W.K., Rioux, F. et al: Antagonists of angiotensin. Substitution of an aliphatic chain to phenyl ring in position 8. Rev. Canad. Biol. 30:319, 1971.
6. Davis, J.O.: Agents which block the action of the renin-angiotensin system. Circ. Res. 34:279, 1974.
7. Pals, D.T., Masucci, F.D., Denning, G.S.,Jr. et al: Role of the pressor action of angiotensin II in experimental hypertension. Circ. Res. 29:673, 1971.
8. Brunner, H.R., Kirshman, J.D., Sealey, J.E. et al: Hypertension of renal origin: Evidence for two different mechanisms. Science 174:1344, 1971.
9. Gavras, H., Brunner, H.R., Vaughan, E.D., Jr. et al: Angiotensin-sodium interaction in blood pressure maintenance of renal hypertensive and normotensive rats. Science 180:1369, 1973.
10. Brunner, H.R., Gavras, H. and Laragh, J.H.: Angiotensin II blockade in man by Sar^1-Ala^8-angiotensin II for understanding and treatment of high blood pressure. Lancet 2: 1045, 1973.
11. Streeten, D.H.P., Anderson, G.H., Freiberg, J.M. et al: Use of an angiotensin II antagonist (Saralasin) in the recognition of "angiotensinogenic hypertension." N. Engl. J. Med. 292:657, 1975.
12. Khosla, M.C., Smeby, R.R. and Bumpus, F.M.: Structure-activity relationship in angiotensin II analogs. *In* Page, I.H. and Bumpus, F.M. (eds.): Angiotensin. New York:Springer-Verlag, 1974, p. 126.
13. Johnson, J.A. and Davis, J.O.: Effects of a specific competitive antagonist of angiotensin II on arterial pressure and adrenal steroid secretion in dogs. Circ. Res. 32 (suppl. 1):1, 159, 1973.
14. Williams, G.H., McDonnel, L.M., Raux, M.C. et al: Evidence for different angiotensin receptors in rat adrenal glomerulosa and rabbit vascular smooth muscle cells. Circ. Res. 34:384, 1974.
15. Steele, J.M. and Lowenstein, J.: Differential effects of an angiotensin II analogue on pressor and adrenal receptors in the rabbit. Circ. Res. 35:529, 1974.
16. Catt, K.J., Glossmann, H. and Baukal, A.: *In* Sambhi, M.P. (ed.): Mechanisms of Hypertension, Amsterdam:Excerpta Medica, 1973, p. 200.
17. Glossmann, H., Baukal, A.J. and Catt, K.J.: Properties of angiotensin II receptors in the bovine and rat adrenal cortex. J. Biol. Chem. 249:825, 1974.
18. Glossmann, H., Baukal, A.J. and Catt, K.J.: Cation dependence of high-affinity angiotensin II binding to adrenal cortex receptors. Science 185:281, 1974.
19. Glossmann, H., Baukal, A.J. and Catt, K.J.: Angiotensin II receptors in bovine adrenal cortex. Modification of angiotensin II binding by guanyl nucleotides. J. Biol. Chem. 249:664, 1974.
20. Catt, K.J., Baukal, A., Ketelslegers, J.-M. et al: Angiotensin II receptors of the adrenal gland. Location and modulation by cations and guanyl nucleotides. Acta Physiol. Lat. Amer. 24:515, 1974.

21. Saltman, S., Baukal, A., Waters, S. et al: Competitive binding activity of angiotensin II analogues in an adrenal cortex radioligand-receptor assay. Endocrinology 97:275, 1975.
22. Catt, K.J., Saltman, S., Douglas, J. et al: Molecular pharmacology of angiotensin II receptors. *In* Walter, R. and Meienhofer, J. (eds.): Peptides: Chemistry, Structure and Biology (Proceedings of the Fourth American Peptide Symposium). Ann Arbor Science Publishers, 1975.
23. Hall, M.M., Khosla, M.D., Khairallah, P.A. et al: Angiotensin analogs: The influence of sarcosine substituted in position 1. J. Pharmacol. Exp. Ther. 188:222, 1974.
24. Fredlund, P., Saltman, S. and Catt, K.J.: Stimulation of aldosterone production by angiotensin II peptides in vitro: Enhanced activity of the (1-Sarcosine) analogue. J. Clin. Endocrinol. Metab. 40:746, 1975.
25. Fredlund, P., Saltman, S. and Catt, K.J.: Aldosterone production by isolated adrenal glomerulosa cells: Stimulation by physiological concentrations of angiotensin II. Endocrinology 97:1577, 1975.
26. Peach, M.J. and Chiu, A.T.: Stimulation and inhibition of aldosterone biosynthesis in vitro by angiotensin II and analogs. Circ. Res. 34-35 (suppl. 1): 7, 1974.
27. Saltman, S., Fredlund, P. and Catt, K.J.: Actions of angiotensin II antagonists upon aldosterone production by isolated adrenal glomerulosa cells. Endocrinology 98:884, 1976.
28. Douglas, J., Fredlund, P., Saltman, S. et al: Angiotensin II receptors of dog and rat adrenal cells: Relation of angiotensin binding to aldosterone synthesis. Endocrine Society 57th Annual Meeting, Abstract A 181, 1975.
29. Douglas, J., Saltman, S., Fredlund, P. et al: Receptor binding of angiotensin II and antagonists: Correlation with aldosterone production by isolated adrenal glomerulosa cells. Circ. Res. (In press.)

Effect of Angiotensin II Analogues on Aldosterone Secretion in Sodium-Deficient Sheep

J. R. Blair-West, M.Sc., Ph.D., J. P. Coghlan, Ph.D., D.Sc., D. A. Denton, M.B.B.S., H. D. Niall, M.D., B. A. Scoggins, M.Agr.Sc. (Cant.), Ph.D. and G. W. Tregear, B.Sc., Ph.D.

Introduction

The precise involvement of the renin-angiotensin system in the regulation of aldosterone secretion remains an enigma. This is with regard to both intrinsic basal secretion and increments produced by sodium restriction or sodium deficiency. The data challenging the acceptance of a simple cause and effect relationship between the contemporary level of angiotensin II in arterial blood and the rate of aldosterone secretion have been set out in recent reviews, as well as the data that have led to the wide acceptance of this commensurate causal relation as an established dogma [1, 2]. In addition to recent animal data, two recent clinical reports have described situations in which the two systems do not respond in concert. These are inappropriate ADH secretion [3] and starvation [4].

In 1971 our group demonstrated by adrenal arterial infusions in the conscious sheep that the 2-8 heptapeptide of

This work was supported by grants-in-aid from the National Health and Medical Research Council of Australia and the National Heart Foundation of Australia.

J. R. Blair-West, M.Sc., Ph.D., J. P. Coghlan, Ph.D., D.Sc., D. A. Denton, M.B.B.S., H. D. Niall, M.D., B. A. Scoggins, M.Agr.Sc. (Cant.), Ph.D. and G. W. Tregear, B.Sc., Ph.D., Howard Florey Institute of Experimental Physiology and Medicine, University of Melbourne, Parkville, Victoria, Australia.

angiotensin II — angiotensin III — was at least equivalent with angiotensin II in stimulating aldosterone secretion. Thus, additional issues were raised as to the formation of angiotensin III and its possible physiological role in control of aldosterone secretion [5].

Recently, several analogues of angiotensin II, said to be competitive inhibitors of angiotensin II, have been used experimentally, as well as a peptide which blocks the action of converting enzyme and thus prevents the formation of angiotensin II. The general usefulness of these analogues has been reviewed by Davis [6]. A considerable literature has already accumulated as these agents have been used to dissect the renin-angiotensin system. In regard to the adrenal zona glomerulosa it was initially difficult to see what major facts pharmacological blockage would reveal that had not already been disclosed by bilateral nephrectomy. On the other hand, the role of angiotensin II in normal blood pressure regulation and in hypertension was not well defined.

One important fact to emerge early was that the use of inhibiting analogues — 1 sar 8 ile, or 1 sar 8 ala — showed that the receptors for angiotensin II in vascular smooth muscle were not the same as in the adrenal [7-11].

The most controversial issue to date centers on the effect of high levels of 1 sar 8 ala, angiotensin II (P113) in animals following sodium restriction. Johnston and Davis [12] found very significant inhibition of aldosterone secretion could be achieved in the dog. In the anesthetized hypophysectomized sodium-restricted rat a significant fall could be produced but not to the basal levels [11, 13]. Steele and Lowenstein [7] were able at comparable doses of P113 to inhibit aldosterone secretion in the sodium-restricted rabbit but not to sodium-replete levels. These experiments in which peripheral blood aldosterone was measured may have been complicated by the impact of other cardiovascular effects on metabolic clearance rate, as well as the fact that P113 was a potent agonist even at low dosage.

There were evident advantages in using sheep with autotransplanted adrenal glands to examine further the effect of P113 on aldosterone secretion. The animals could be studied sodium replete and after controlled sodium depletion. The experiments could be done without the complication of anesthesia or surgery and the usual high ACTH secretion which follows. The inhibitor analogue could be administered locally into the adrenal arterial supply so that the sequelae of systemic infusion could be largely minimized. Finally, real sodium deficiency as distinct from simple reduction of dietetic intake could be easily contrived by parotid fistula so that the aldosterone secretion rate would be increased many times above basal. The data could then be set against the substantial knowledge already accrued on the regulation of aldosterone in the sheep, particularly with reference to the involvement of angiotensin II [1, 2]. Angiotensin II in circulating blood is essential for the normal increments in aldosterone secretion associated with sodium deficiency [14]. Angiotensin II does not biosynthetically mimic sodium deficiency in terms of incorporation of radiolabeled corticosterone into secreted aldosterone. Furthermore, in the Na-deficient animal following sodium replacement, aldosterone returns to replete levels faster than angiotensin II or even in the face of angiotensin II being sustained at high sodium replete levels by appropriate rate of infusion [1, 15]. In addition, aldosterone shows a highly significant increase in response to sodium deficiency when peripheral arterial blood angiotensin II is held in the normal sodium replete range by renal arterial infusion of angiotensin II. Also, in the Na-deplete animal nephrectomized 24 hours previously, aldosterone rises to the high Na-deficient range when angiotensin II is replaced by infusion which gives blood concentration in the Na-replete range only [15-19].

In the experiments which follow the protocols were broadly designed to provide the following data:

1. In the sodium-replete animal:
   a. the effect of the 1 sar 8 ala analogue alone
   b. the effect of the 1 sar 8 ala analogue on the incremental response in aldosterone secretion to either exogenous angiotensin II or angiotensin III — (2-8 heptapeptide).
2. In the sodium-deficient animal:
   a. the effect of the 1 sar 8 ala analogue on the increased aldosterone secretion.
   b. the effect of the 1 des 8 ile analogue on the increased aldosterone secretion.

Materials and Methods

Four sheep with single adrenal glands autotransplanted to a cervical carotid jugular skin loop were used exclusively for these studies [20-22]. Sodium depletion was produced when required by uncompensated loss of saliva for 48 to 72 hours from a permanent unilateral parotid fistula [23]. The techniques of local intra-adrenal arterial infusions and timed total adrenal venous collection using this preparation have been reported in detail previously [24]. The point to be emphasized is that materials can be introduced at physiological concentration locally into the arterial supply by continuous slow infusion, and that this preparation allows total collection of adrenal venous blood from an animal while conscious and undisturbed.

In the experiments reported here the putative inhibitory analogues saralasin acetate* (1 sar-8 ala angiotensin II or P113) or (1 des 8-ile angiotensin II) in normal saline were infused into the arterial supply of the adrenal at the rates indicated. Angiotensin II or 1-des angiotensin II in normal saline were infused into the jugular vein contralateral to the adrenal transplant at the rates shown for intravenous administration, otherwise into the carotid artery supplying the adrenal gland.

The total rates of secretion by the adrenal gland of cortisol corticosterone and aldosterone were calculated following analysis by double isotope dilution derivative assay [25]. Plasma $[Na^+]$ and $[K^+]$ were determined using a Technicon Autoanalyser. Renin was estimated by an enzyme kinetic procedure [26].

Results

The angiotensin II concentration in arterial blood of Na-replete sheep is 1.4 ± 1.1 ng/100 ml (n=41). With mild-severe Na deficiency it increased to 5-40 ng/100 ml. It may reach as high as 60-70 ng/100 ml [15, 17, 27]. Comprehensive clearance rate studies have shown that intravenous infusion of angiotensin II at 5-60μg/hr produced arterial blood angiotensin II concentration in the range 5-60 ng/100 ml — the Na-deficient

---

*Supplied by the Norwich Pharmacal Company, Norwich, N.Y.

range [28]. The blood flow of the autotransplanted adrenal in these experiments was between 500 and 1000 ml/hr, and the adrenal arterial concentrations of agonists and antagonists were contrived in the light of the measured physiological parameters instanced above.

Sodium-Replete Sheep

Close adrenal arterial infusions of P113 were made over a dose range of 1 → 300μg/hr. Figure 1 shows the results obtained when the infusion had continued for 15 to 30 minutes. At the highest dose a minor agonist effect is perhaps discernible. No

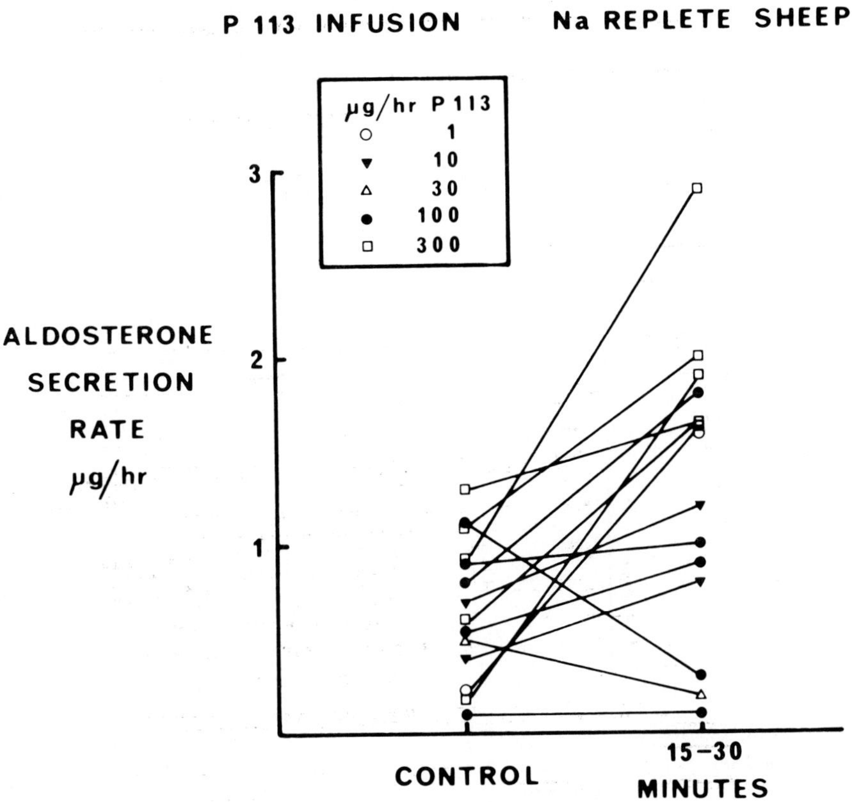

FIG. 1. The effect of 1 sar 8 ala angiotensin II infused into the adrenal artery of sodium-replete sheep.

meaningful or consistent changes were observed in cortisol secretion, plasma renin concentration or plasma $[Na^+]$ or $[K^+]$.

Figure 2 depicts experiments in which a series of intravenous infusions of angiotensin II were given at rates adequate to produce arterial blood levels of angiotensin II similar to those measured during Na deficiency. Samples were taken at approximately 15 minutes after start of the infusion. On another day under exactly comparable conditions a local arterial infusion of P113 at 10 or 100μg/hr was commenced 20 minutes prior to the systemic angiotensin II infusion. The P113 completely abolished the stimulating effect of the angiotensin II. The other relevant variables were not altered. The calculated ratio of P113 to angiotensin II in adrenal arterial blood was 100:1 or greater.

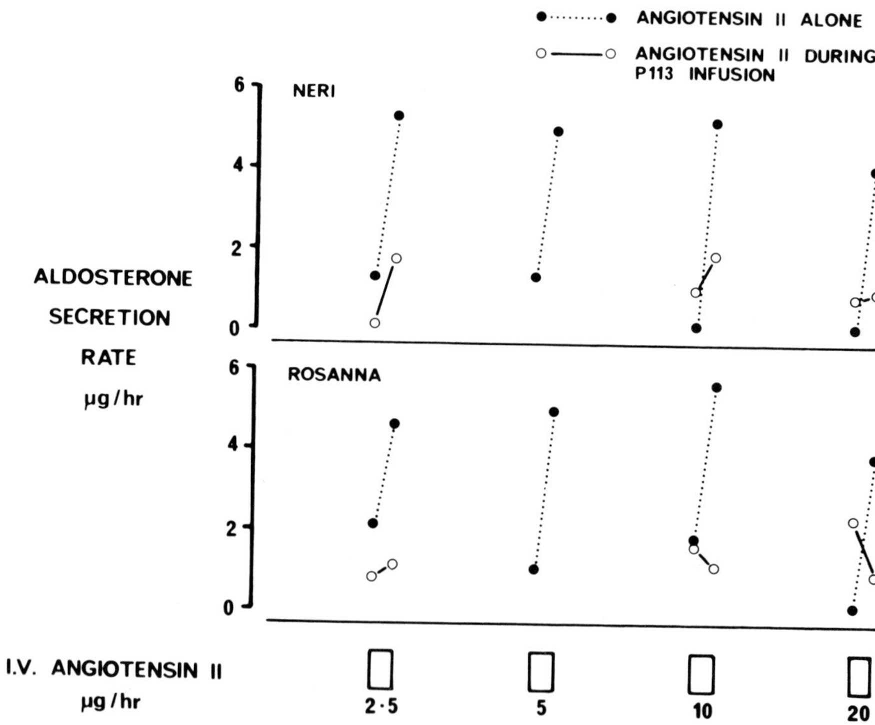

FIG. 2. The inhibition of systemic angiotensin II by 1 sar 8 ala angiotensin II infused into the adrenal. Neri (10μg/hr P113) Rosanna (100μg/hr P113)

Figure 3 shows similar experiments in which the stimulus used was the 2-8 heptapeptide, the effect of which was also abolished by P113 at 100μg/hr and 300μg/hr. In these experiments the heptapeptide was infused into the arterial supply at a rate to give 50-100 ng/100 ml, a level in the very highest range ever encountered for angiotensin II itself during sodium deficiency. The calculated ratio of P113 to angiotensin III in adrenal arterial blood was 200:1 or greater.

Sodium-Depleted Sheep

A series of stepwise local adrenal arterial infusions of P113 over a wide range of doses was made in moderately sodium-depleted sheep. Figure 4 shows an example in a single sheep,

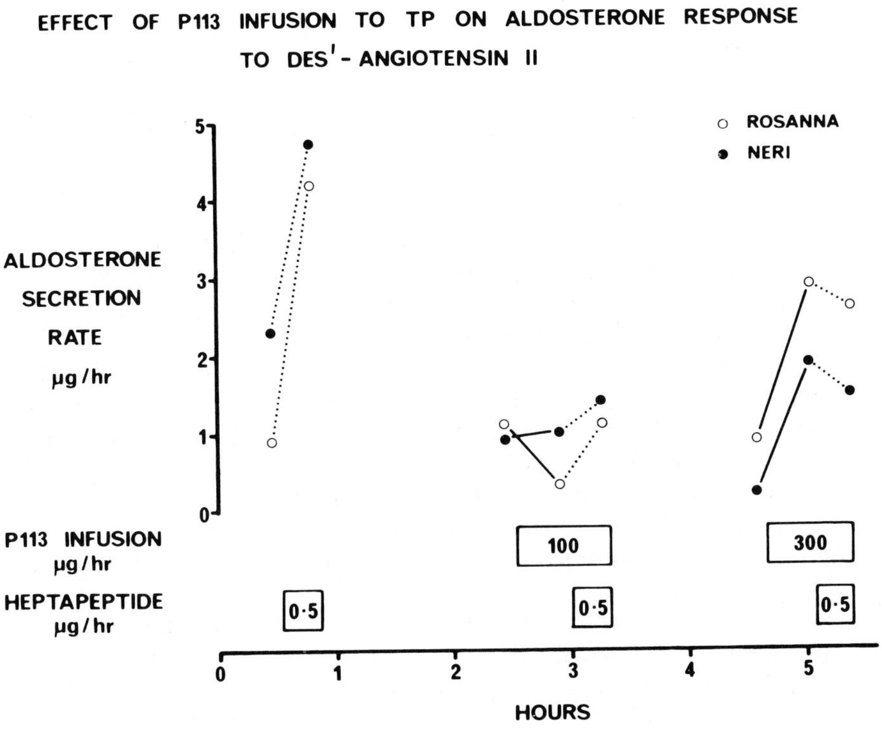

FIG. 3. The inhibition by 1 sar 8 ala angiotensin II into adrenal artery on arterial infusion of angiotensin III (2-8 heptapeptide).

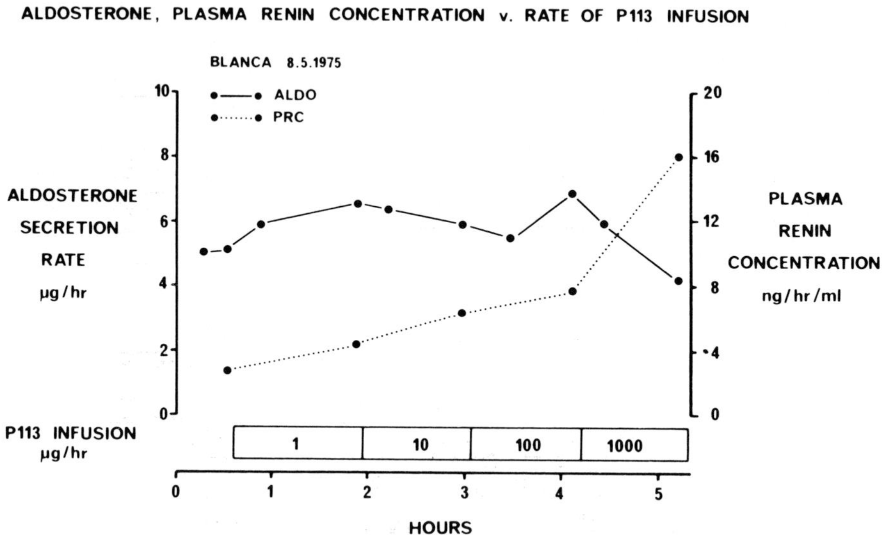

FIG. 4. Stepwise infusion of 1 sar 8 ala angiotensin II into the adrenal artery of moderately sodium-deficient sheep.

Blanca, where aldosterone secretion rate remained constant despite the very high infusion rates of P113, to the extent that eventually the recirculation of P113 had an effect on renal renin release. Figure 5 shows a similar experiment in Arnon. This type of response was fairly consistent at all times in this animal. When a P113 infusion was started, a fall in aldosterone secretion was seen at 15 minutes but then returned to normal over the next hour while the infusion continued, only to show a transient fall when the rate of P113 was further increased. The doses of P113 were calculated to be at least in the ratio to endogenous angiotensin of approximately 10, 100, 1000 and 10,000 to 1.

The change in aldosterone secretion rate produced after 15 minutes of P113 infusion for all dose levels used in the group of Na-deficient animals is shown in Figure 6. The mean values are joined by a solid line. Figure 7 shows the results at the one to two hour point of the infusion. Neither the values at 15 minutes or at two hours of these changes were statistically significantly different from the control values at any dose level when tested by paired t-test (Fig. 8).

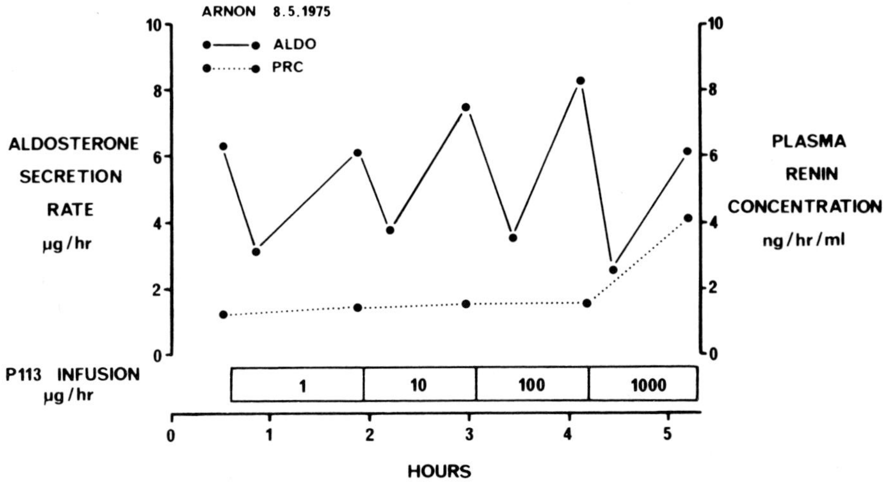

FIG. 5. Stepwise infusion of 1 sar 8 ala angiotensin II into the adrenal artery of moderately sodium-deficient sheep.

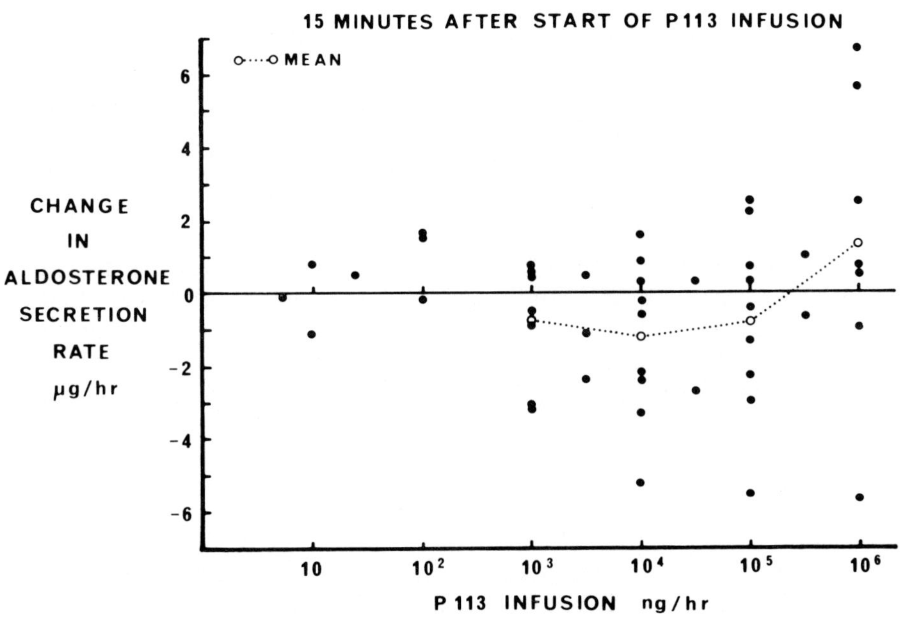

FIG. 6. Changes in aldosterone secretion in moderately sodium-deficient sheep at all dose levels after 15 minutes of infusion.

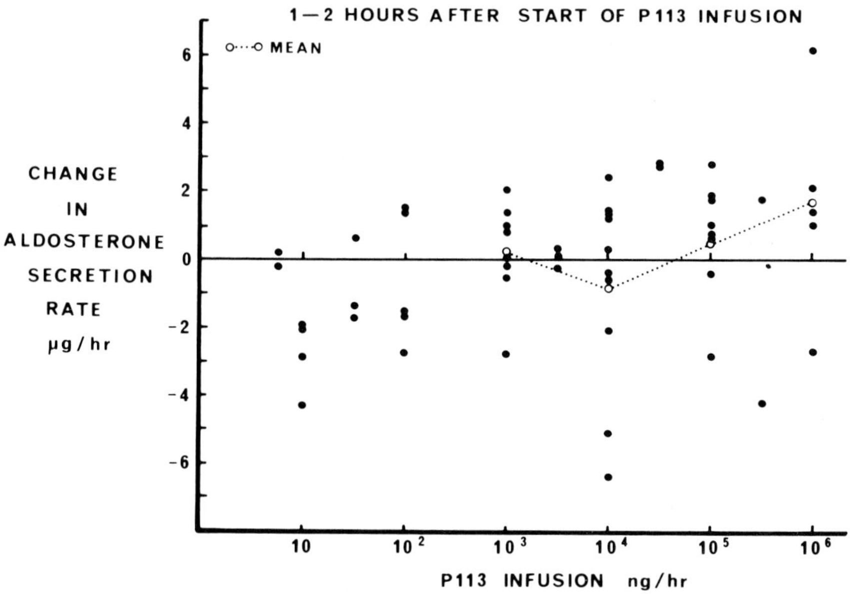

FIG. 7. Changes in aldosterone secretion in moderately sodium-deficient sheep at all dose levels after one to two hours of infusion.

Although renin levels increased at the highest doses illustrating that the recirculating analogue was affecting the angiotensin feedback on renin release, these changes were not large enough to have significantly altered the ratio of inhibition of arterial angiotensin II.

Figure 9 shows the effect of analogue 1 des 8 ile angiotensin II during sodium deficiency. This analogue did not reduce aldosterone secretion to near the replete range even at the highest infusion rates.

Consistently throughout all these experiments cortisol secretion and plasma [Na^+] and [K^+] were not significantly altered from control values.

Discussion

The results of these experiments are clear-cut. 1 sar 8 ala angiotensin II has a minor agonist effect on aldosterone secretion at high dosage. 1 sar 8 ala infusion will block the

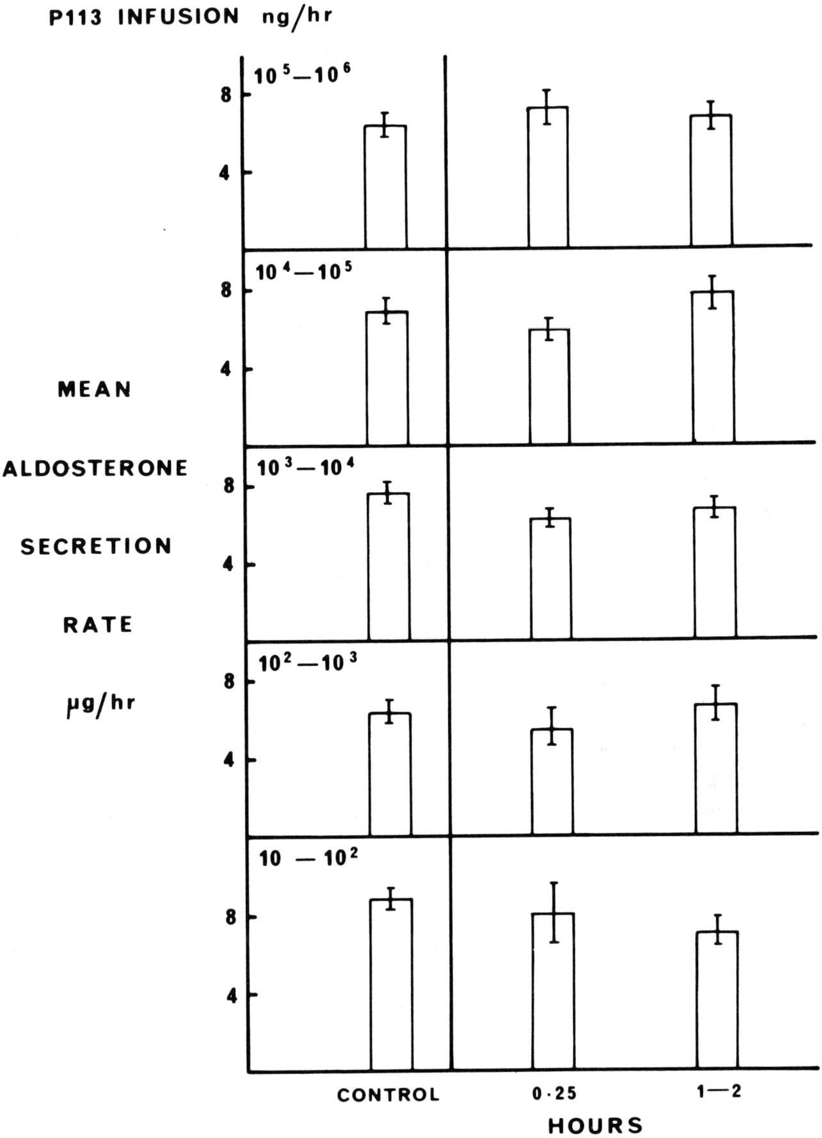

FIG. 8. Mean changes in aldosterone at different dose levels of 1 sar 8 ala angiotensin II at both 15 minutes and one to two hour point. None of these changes were significant.

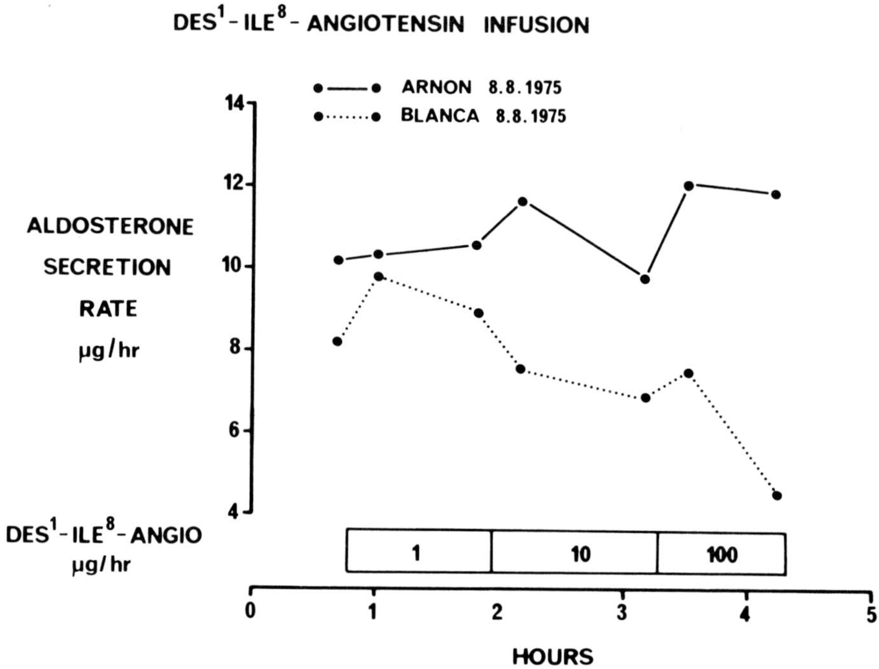

FIG. 9 A and B. The effect of 1 des-8 ile angiotensin II in the sodium-deficient sheep.

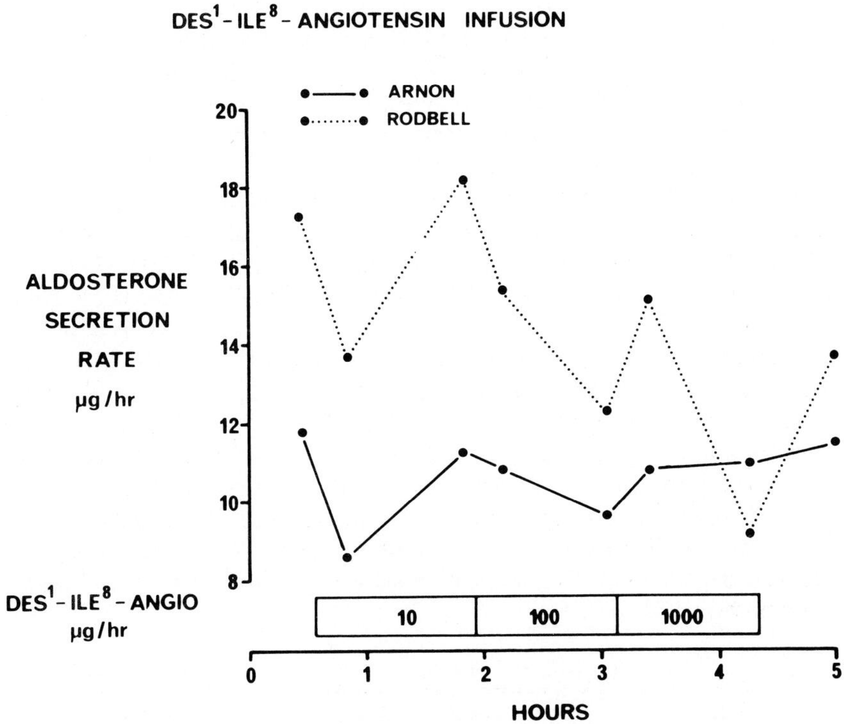
DES1-ILE8-ANGIOTENSIN INFUSION
ARNON
RODBELL
ALDOSTERONE
SECRETION
RATE
μg/hr
20
18
16
14
12
10
8
DES1-ILE8-ANGIO
μg/hr
10
100
1000
0
1
2
3
4
5
HOURS

FIGURE 9 B.

effect of either angiotensin II or angiotensin III when these are infused at rates which would lead to adrenal arterial blood levels in the upper part of the physiological range. The antagonist: agonist ratio used was greater than 100:1. During sodium deficiency, infusion rates of 1 sar 8 ala angiotensin at rates 10 to 100 times greater than these (ie, antagonist:agonist 5,000 to 10,000:1) did not consistently reduce the aldosterone secretion of the Na-deficient animal. To allow easy comparison between the experiments reported here, and others in the literature where systemic infusion has been used in vivo, or a specific molar concentration used with cell suspensions, a table of calculated local concentrations in the sheep has been included (Table 1). These calculations make no allowance for recirculation The blood clearance rate of 1 sar 8 ala angiotensin is known to be less than that of angiotensin II [29, 30]. If it is assumed that the blood clearance is only 20% of that for angiotensin II then once a steady state value is reached, recirculation would increase the concentrations estimated in Table 1 by 10%-20%. Making the same assumption in regard to blood clearance rate, a systemic infusion of 1 sar 8 ala angiotensin into the sheep at the rate — 6μg/kg/min reported by Johnston and Davis [12] as successful in the sodium-restricted dog — would give a systemic concentration of the analogue of the order of 700μg/l. Similar infusion rates on a body weight basis were used in the sodium-restricted rabbit by Steele and Lowenstein [7].

Table 1.

Infusion Rate P113 ng/hr	*Range Adrenal Blood Concentration**	*Molar Concentrations*
10	10-20 ng/l	$\cong 10^{-11} - 2 \times 10^{-11}$
3×10	30-60 ng/l	$\cong 3 \times 10^{-11} - 6 \times 10^{-11}$
10^2	100-200 ng/l	$\cong 10^{-10} - 2 \times 10^{-10}$
3×10^2	300-600 ng/l	$\cong 3 \times 10^{-10} - 6 \times 10^{-10}$
10^3	1.0-2.0μg/l	$\cong 10^{-9} - 2 \times 10^{-9}$
3×10^3	3.0-6.0μg/l	$\cong 3 \times 10^{-9} - 6 \times 10^{-9}$
10^4	10-20μg/l	$\cong 10^{-8} - 2 \times 10^{-8}$
3×10^4	30-60μg/l	$\cong 3 \times 10^{-8} - 6 \times 10^{-8}$
10^5	100-200μg/l	$\cong 10^{-7} - 2 \times 10^{-7}$
3×10^5	300-600μg/l	$\cong 3 \times 10^{-7} - 6 \times 10^{-7}$
10^6	1.0-2.0 mg/l	$\cong 10^{-6} - 2 \times 10^{-6}$

*Based on adrenal blood flow 0.5 l to 1.0 l per hour.

The two highest infusion rates used in the experiments described here in the sheep would straddle this range. In another study Chiu and Peach [31] showed that 1 sar 8 ile angiotensin II inhibited the effect of angiotensin II, or angiotensin III, on rabbit adrenal cell suspensions at 10^{-7} to 5×10^{-7}M. The effect inhibited involved molar concentration of angiotensin II greater than 10^{-8}M which is clearly supraphysiological. The physiological range of blood levels of angiotensin II in the sheep is 10^{-11} to 5×10^{-10}M. Furthermore, Chiu and Peach [31] showed that with angiotensin III, which appeared to have a higher affinity for adrenal cells, a ratio of antagonist:agonist greater than 50:1 was required for complete inhibition. For infused exogenous peptides in the sheep, the lowest ratio used was of the order of 100:1 which blocked the stimulation effect in the Na-replete animal of an infusion designed to produce the upper limit of the physiological range.

Allowing that a generous estimate of the angiotensin II level would be 200 ng/l in the sodium-deficient sheep [17], at the highest doses of 1 sar 8 ala angiotensin II the ratio of inhibitor to angiotensin II in adrenal arterial blood would have been 5,000 to 10,000:1. The same logic would apply to the experiments where the des asp 8 ileu angiotensin II was used without reducing aldosterone secretion to the sodium-replete range.

Blair-West et al [5] showed that in vivo angiotensin III was at least equivalent with angiotensin II in stimulating aldosterone secretion. This finding has been confirmed subsequently by others in the rat and dog, using in vivo preparations [11, 32, 33]. Experiments with adrenal cell suspension and using relative levels of blockade have suggested that the adrenal cell receptors have a higher affinity for angiotensin III than for angiotensin II [9, 10, 31, 32, 34-37]. Furthermore, there have been reports that the 1 des asp 8 ile analogue is a more potent inhibitor of aldosterone secretion [9, 10]. All this evidence supports the hypothesis raised initially by Blair-West et al [5] that the heptapeptide could have an important role in regulation of aldosterone secretion. Fredlund et al [38] have cautioned against a premature conclusion in regard to the role of angiotensin III.

No attempt has been made in the studies reported here to closely assess the effectiveness of P113 compared to des asp 8 ileu angiotensin II in terms of blockade of exogenous angiotensin II or angiotensin III. Both are effective inhibitors at infusion rates far below those which had no effect during sodium deficiency. These results must be set against the background that renal renin is known to be essential for continued aldosterone secretion during sodium deficiency in sheep [14]. Several explanations of the present findings are possible and these will have to be experimentally explored. (i) The action of angiotensin II on aldosterone secretion is reversed within one hour after cessation of an infusion [39, 40], so the time course of these experiments would appear to be adequate. (ii) It is possible that although blood-borne angiotensin II or angiotensin III was effectively blocked local production still occurred at a relatively inaccessible site. (iii) Because in the sheep aldosterone secretion increases with progressive Na deficiency, even though peripheral blood angiotensin II is held in the Na-replete range by renal arterial infusion of angiotensin II and it increases to Na-deficient levels in bilaterally nephrectomized animals infused with angiotensin II at rates to restore the blood level to the normal replete range [16, 19], the possibility must be entertained that the blockade with these analogues was not adequate to effectively reduce angiotensin II or III levels below the sodium-replete range. This seems unlikely. Alternatively, it is possible that because of the intrinsic agonist activity of the analogue, albeit low, that this was adequate to fulfill the permissive role angiotensin seems to play in relation to aldosterone secretion in the sodium-deficient sheep.

References

1. Coghlan, J.P., Blair-West, J.R., Denton, D.A. et al: Perspectives in aldosterone and renin control. Aust. New Zeal. J. Med. 2:178, 1971.
2. Blair-West, J.R., Coghlan, J.P., Denton, D.A. et al: Aldosterone regulation in sodium deficiency: Role of ionic factors and angiotensin II. *In* Page, I.H. and Bumpus, F.M. (eds.): Handbook of Experimental Pharmacology. Springer-Verlag, 1973, pp. 337-368.
3. Fichman, M.P., Michelakis, A.M. and Horton, R.: Regulation of aldosterone secretion in the syndrome of inappropriate antidiuretic hormone secretion. J. Clin. Endocrinol. Metab. 39:136, 1974.
4. Boulter, P.R., Spark, R.F. and Aiky, R.A.: Dissociation of the renin aldosterone system and refractoriness to the sodium retaining action

of mineralocorticoid during starvation in man. J. Clin. Endocrinol. Metab. 38:248, 1974.
5. Blair-West, J.R., Coghlan, J.P., Denton, D.A. et al: The effect of the heptapeptide (2-8) and hexapeptide (3-8) fragments of angiotensin II on aldosterone II on aldosterone secretion. J. Clin. Endocrinol. 32:575-578, 1971.
6. Davis, J.O.: Agents which block the action of the renin angiotensin system. Circ. Res. 34:279, 1974.
7. Steele, J.M. and Lowenstein, J.: Differential effects of an angiotensin II analogue on pressor and adrenal receptors in the rabbit. Circ. Res. 35:592, 1974.
8. Williams, G.H., McDonnell, L.M., Raux, M.C. et al: Evidence for different angiotensin II receptors in rat adrenal glomerulosa and rabbit vascular smooth muscle cell. Circ. Res. 34:384, 1974.
9. Bravo, E.L., Khosla, M.C. and Bumpus, F.M.: Action of [1 des(aspartic acid), 8 isoleucine] angiotensin II upon pressor and steroidogenic activity of angiotensin II. J. Clin. Endocrinol. Metab. 40:530, 1975.
10. Bravo, E.L., Khosla, M.C. and Bumpus, F.M.: Vascular and adrenocortical responses to a specific antagonist of angiotensin II. Am. J. Physiol. 228:110, 1975.
11. Davis, J.O.: The use of blocking agents to define the functions of the renin angiotensin system. Clin. Sci. Molec. Biol. 48:35, 1975.
12. Johnson, J.A. and Davis, J.O.: Effects of a specific competitive antagonist of angiotensin II on arterial pressure and adrenal steroid secretion in the dog. Circ. Res. 32 (Suppl. I):159, 1973.
13. Spielman, W.S. and Davis, J.O.: The renin angiotensin system and aldosterone secretion during sodium depletion in the rat. Circ. Res. 35:615, 1974.
14. Blair-West, J.R., Coghlan, J.P., Denton, D.A. et al: The effect of nephrectomy on aldosterone secretion in the conscious sodium-depleted hypophysectomised sheep. Aust. J. Exp. Biol. Med. Sci. 46:295-318, 1968.
15. Blair-West, J.R., Cain, M., Catt, K. et al: Aldosterone regulation and biosynthesis. International Congress Series 184. Proceedings 3rd International Congress Endocrinology 1968. Amsterdam: Excerpta Medica, 1969, pp. 276-285.
16. Blair-West, J.R., Coghlan, J.P., Cran, E.J. et al: Increased aldosterone secretion during sodium depletion with inhibition of renin release. Am. J. Physiol. 224:1409-1414, 1973.
17. Blair-West, J.R., Cain, M.D., Catt, K.J. et al: The dissociation of aldosterone secretion and systemic renin and angiotensin II levels during the correction of sodium deficiency. Acta Endocrinol. 66:229-247, 1971.
18. Blair-West, J.R., Cain, M.D., Catt, K.J. et al: Further facets of aldosterone regulation. *In* James, V.H.T. and Martini, L. (eds.): Hormonal Steroids. Amsterdam:Excerpta Medica, 1971, pp. 572-580.
19. Blair-West, J.R., Coghlan, J.P., Denton, D.A. et al: Current concepts in aldosterone control. *In* Scow, R.O. (ed.): International Congress

Series 273, Proceedings IVth International Congress Endocrinology. Amsterdam:Excerpta Medica, 1974, pp. 768-773.

20. McDonald, I.R., Goding, J.R. and Wright, R.D.: Transplantation of the adrenal gland of the sheep to provide access to its blood supply. Aust. J. Exp. Biol. Med. Sci. 36:83-96, 1958.
21. Denton, D.A., Goding, J.R. and Wright, R.D.: Control of adrenal secretion electrolyte-active steroids. Br. Med. J. II: 447-456 and 522-630, 1959.
22. Wright, R.D., Blair-West, J.R., Coghlan, J.P. et al: The structure and function of adrenal autotransplants. Aust. J. Exp. Biol. Med. Sci. 50:873-892, 1972.
23. Denton, D.A.: The study of sheep with permanent unilateral parotid fistulae. Quart. J. Exp. Physiol. 42:72-95, 1957.
24. Denton, D.A., Goding, J.R. and Wright, R.D.: The control of aldosterone secretion. Astwood, E.B. (ed.) Clin. Endocrinol. 1:373-391, 1960. New York: Grune & Stratton, Inc.
25. Coghlan, J.P., Wintour, M. and Scoggins, B.A.: The measurement of corticosteroids in adrenal vein blood of sheep. Aust. J. Exp. Biol. Med. Sci. 44:639-664, 1966.
26. Blair-West, J.R., Coghlan, J.P., Denton, D.A. et al: The renin/angiotensin-aldosterone system in sodium depletion. Med. J. Aust. 2:290-295, 1967.
27. Catt, K., Cain, M. and Coghlan, J.P.: Measurement of angiotensin II in blood. Lancet 2:1005-1007, 1968.
28. Cain, M.D., Catt, K.J., Coghlan, J.P. et al: Evaluation of angiotensin II metabolism in sheep by radioimmunoassay. Endocrinology 86:955, 1970.
29. Türker, R.K., Hall, M.M., Yamamoto, M.: New long lasting competitive inhibitor of angiotensin II. Science 177:1203, 1972.
30. Bumpus, F.M., Sen, S., Smeby, P.R. et al: Use of angiotensin II antagonists in experimental hypertension. Circ. Res. 32:150, 1973.
31. Chiu, A.T. and Peach, M.J.: Inhibition of induced aldosterone biosynthesis with a specific antagonist of angiotensin II. Proc. Nat. Acad. Sci. (U.S.A.) 71:341, 1974.
32. Campbell, W.B., Brooks, S.N. and Pettinger, W.A.: Angiotensin II and angiotensin III. Induced aldosterone release in vivo in the rat. Science 184:994, 1974.
33. Lohmeier, T.E., Davis, J.O. and Freeman, R.H.: Des-Asp^1-Angiotensin II: Possible role in mediating responses of the renin angiotensin system. Proc. Soc. Exp. Biol. Med. 149:515, 1975.
34. Peach, M.J. and Chiu, A.T.: Stimulation and inhibition of aldosterone biosynthesis in vitro by angiotensin II analogues. Circ. Res. 34 (suppl. 1):7, 1974.
35. Goodfriend, T.L. and Peach, M.J.: Angiotensin III: (Des Asp) Angiotensin II. Circ. Res. 36 (suppl. 1):38, 1975.
36. Bumpus, F.M. and Khosla, M.C.: Inhibition of the pressor and aldosterone releasing effects of angiotensin II. Clin. Sci. Molec. Med. 48:15, 1975.

37. Khosla, M.C., Smeby, P.R. and Bumpus, F.M.: On the selective antagonism of myotropic and steroidogenic activity of angiotensin II. *In* Walter, R. and Meunhofer, J. (eds.): Chemistry Biophysics or Biology of Peptides. Ann Arbor, Mich.:Ann Arbor Science Publishers, 1975.
38. Fredlund, P., Saltman, S. and Catt, K.J.: Stimulation of aldosterone production by angiotensin II peptides in vitro enhanced activity of the 1 Sar analogue. J. Clin. Endocrinol. Metab. 40:746, 1975.
39. Blair-West, J.R., Coghlan, J.P., Denton, D.A. et al: Humoral stimulation of adrenal cortical secretion. J. Clin. Invest. 41:1606-1627, 1962.
40. Blair-West, J.R., Coghlan, J.P., Denton, D.A. et al: Effect of variations of plasma sodium concentration on the adrenal response to angiotensin II. Circ. Res. 17:386-393, 1963.

Discussion

Moderator: Dr. J. W. Conn

Dr. Bumpus: We assume that our experiments on the dogs using the three derivatives are correct where we show a reduction of blood pressure with the threonine-8 derivative as compared with no drop in blood pressure immediately with the other two. Also, that the threonine derivative shows an immediate adrenal blockade in the salt-depleted dog, while the others do not. How does that affect your last hypothesis?

Dr. Coghlan: One of the things you mentioned with the threonine-8 analogue was that it had virtually no agonist activity. Is that true? This might really be the nub of the issue, in that as I said, the intrinsic agonist activity of the P113 is adequate to fill the permissive valve.

Dr. Vallotton: In Dr. Catt's presentation we saw that he was using very much the same range of concentration as we did. I have a question to ask Dr. Bumpus or Dr. Catt. Do you have any indication that angiotensinase A may be present in different concentrations in different tissues? If so it could explain, possibly, the differential effect one obtains with [Sar^1]-angiotensin II and [des-Asp^1]-angiotensin II on smooth muscle and on the adrenal cortex. Angiotensin II or its structural analogs may be degraded more quickly in one tissue than in another. Has anyone data on the distribution of angiotensin A?

Dr. Bumpus: Glenner and co-workers reported some years ago that aminopeptidase A occurs in the kidney. Whether or not that is the source of the plasma enzyme is not known. They appear to be identical. The specificity of the adrenal enzymes has not been determined.

Dr. Streeten: In human subjects we have found, as Dr. Coghlan so nicely showed for sheep, that saralasin has a mild agonistic effect on aldosterone production. We were able to bring this out first by infusing saralasin in the salt-loaded human subject. I am not sure what a salt-replete sheep is but I assume it just a sheep that is not salt overloaded but is eating its normal diet. I wonder whether Dr. Coghlan has tried salt loading his sheep. I would say too that in salt deficiency states in man or, at least, salt deprivation, which, as you pointed out, is slightly different, and also in situations where the renin-angiotensin system is spontaneously hyperactive such as in cirrhosis with ascites saralasin will reduce aldosterone blood levels. We have not excluded changes in clearances in these circumstances but they seem rather unlikely.

Dr. Coghlan: The sheep that I described as sodium replete had a sodium intake of 80 to 100 millimoles per day. I cannot really comment on your findings other than to say that in situations where the specific stimulus to aldosterone secretion is blood-borne angiotensin the experimental results would suggest that you can block the effect. What I am getting at is that aldosterone regulation is no doubt more complicated than was visualized at first. It is possible that aldosterone secretion can be stimulated by blood-borne angiotensin in some situations, but there are other mechanisms involved which we cannot block in sodium deficiency.

Dr. Corvol: Dr. Catt, did you make any binding studies with labeled angiotensin II inhibitors because one might expect some different binding kinetics with these inhibitors like saralasin.

Dr. Catt: We are currently labeling some antagonists to perform direct binding-inhibition studies, because in that way one can get a better idea of the true, intrinsic affinity in an homologous binding system. However, the normal use of these compounds is to antagonize angiotensin II at target cell receptors. Thus, their binding-inhibition activity in regard to competition with labeled angiotensin II is a more biologically relevant measure of relative binding activity, even though a more chemically correct binding affinity should be measured during competition studies with the antagonist itself.

Dr. Denton: As it is coming up in the discussion, I wonder if perhaps Dr. Bumpus might care to elaborate on the experimental conditions in these instances where the aldosterone secretion fell in the dog with angiotensin antagonist. Specifically, were these done under anesthesia? Was the renin measured before the induction of anesthesia and after the anesthesia to determine to what extent the inhibition that was being contrived was inhibition of the results of anesthesia and trauma or really due to the existing state of sodium deficiency? How was this produced, and how much sodium deficit was produced?

Dr. Bumpus: I cannot give all of the experimental details. Renin was measured and was considerably elevated. These are recent experiments and we don't have all the values. The first experiments were done under anesthesia, and this may well have an effect on renin release.

Dr. Williams: I wonder if the different responses of sodium deplete man and sodium deplete sheep are secondary to the differences in how depletion is produced rather than species differences.

Dr. Coghlan: Yes, to some extent I agree. I do not really see any great difference between the results in sheep and man. In man, it is simply that you have not been able to, or we have not been able to do the same extensive range of experiments and certainly not the same degree of sodium depletion. But I think because there is some confusion it is especially important to be specific about our definitions. That is why I choose to carefully spell out sodium deficiency in the sheep vis-á-vis sodium restriction in man because the restriction gives rise to much smaller sodium deficiency than we are using. I think if you want to examine the controls of aldosterone secretion then it is reasonable to but the response of the system with a graded stress — sodium deficiency of mild, moderate to severe, eg, 100-800 mmol negative. This is virtually never done in man. The experiments I reported today specifically examined the effect of the antagonists in moderate sodium deficiency. These experiments are not necessarily comparable with sodium-restricted man.

Effect of Antagonists of Angiotension II and Aldosterone Upon Plasma Levels of Adrenal Mineralocorticoids

P. J. Mulrow, M.D., R. Noth, M.D., S. Y. Tan, M.D., B. Forman, M.D. and A. Fernandez-Cruz, M.D.

Introduction

The purpose of this paper is to show the effects of two antihypertensive drugs on adrenal steroid production. The first part shows the effect of the angiotensin II antagonist P113, or saralasin, on aldosterone regulation in the dog and man, and the second part illustrates the effect of Aldactone (spironolactone) on plasma desoxycorticosterone levels.

Effect of P113 on Aldosterone Production

Dog studies. The experiments were designed to determine whether P113 is a specific antagonist for angiotensin II at the adrenal receptor site by investigating its effect upon aldosterone stimulation by angiotensin, ACTH or potassium infusions.

Male mongrel dogs were fasted overnight and received 4 mg of dexamethasone phosphate intramuscularly (IM) on the evening before and the morning of the experiment in order to inhibit ACTH release. After surgery to insert various cannula was completed, two separate infusions of saline with dexa-

---

Supported by USPH-H2-12758 and a grant-in-aid from Eaton Laboratories.

P. J. Mulrow, M.D., R. Noth, M.D., S. Y. Tan, M.D., B. Forman, M.D. and A. Fernandez-Cruz, M.D., Department of Medicine, Yale University School of Medicine, New Haven, Conn. Dr. Mulrow is currently Professor and Chairman, Department of Medicine, Medical College of Ohio, Toledo.

methasone phosphate 20μg/ml were started at a rate of 0.76 ml/min and continued for one hour. To these infusions the appropriate substances for the experimental studies were added. Two to three pairs of blood samples from the adrenal vein and femoral artery were collected at approximately ten-minute intervals during the control period before the experimental infusions. All shed blood was immediately replaced volume for volume with blood from a dexamethasone-treated dog whose volume was expanded with 1 liter of isotonic saline. Following control blood sampling, infusions with either P113, A II, ACTH or potassium were begun and continued for 30-60 minutes to obtain a steady state condition before two to three more samples of adrenal vein and femoral artery samples were obtained.

Results

In Figure 1 the data from four dogs are shown in which various doses of P113 were infused. There was no significant effect on aldosterone secretion at any of the doses. The blood pressure was slightly increased, but there was no dose-response relationship. Plasma potassium concentration was not significantly elevated, although there appeared to be a slight trend to higher concentrations with time. Total corticoids, not shown in this figure, did not change significantly and remained low; mean values were 0.49 control and 0.77, 0.55, 0.57, 0.43, 0.57μg/min at the five successive doses of P113.

Two control dogs with the saline-dexamethasone solution alone showed no consistent changes in aldosterone secretion rate or blood pressure with time.

In Figure 2 are summarized the changes in systolic blood pressure and aldosterone secretion from all P113 infusions as well as A II alone and A II plus P113 infusions. A II stimulated aldosterone secretion and elevated systolic blood pressure. When this same dose of A II was infused into dogs already receiving P113, both the increase in systolic blood pressure and aldosterone secretion could be prevented. The dose of P113 was occasionally altered to prevent any rise in blood pressure. Infusion of P113 alone had little consistent effect on aldosterone secretion, but did cause an increase in systolic blood

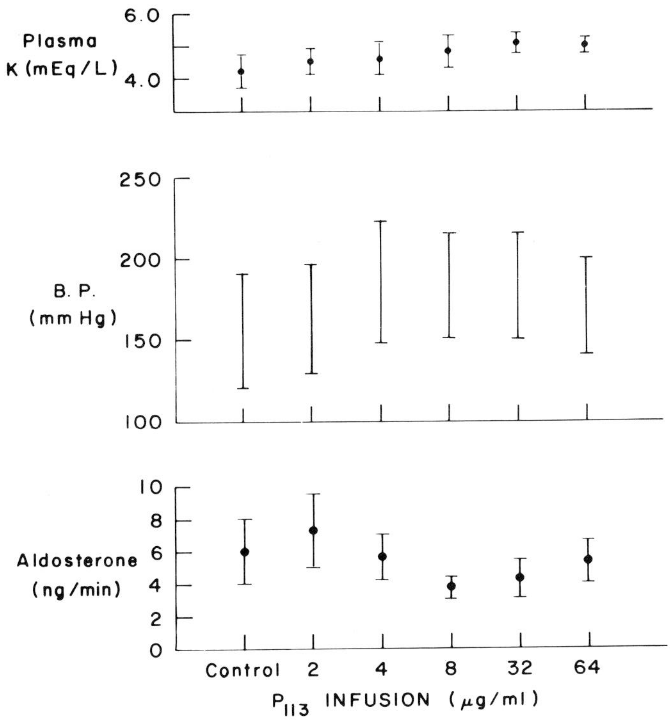

FIG. 1. The response of aldosterone secretion, blood pressure and plasma potassium to infusions of successively larger doses of P113 was studied in four nephrectomized, dexamethasone-suppressed dogs. The mean ±S. E. are shown for aldosterone and potassium, while the mean systolic and diastolic blood pressure is shown. The actual rate of P113 infusion is the concentration times the infusion rate of 0.76 ml/min. (Published in American Journal of Physiology. In press.)

pressure which is also demonstrated in Figure 1. Although P113 alone had no significant effect on aldosterone secretion when all the experiments were analyzed, four of the ten dogs did show a significant response to P113.

P113 and ACTH

In Table 1 it can be seen that P113 does not block the aldosterone stimulating effect of ACTH and, in some instances, appears to enhance its effect. There was also no consistent

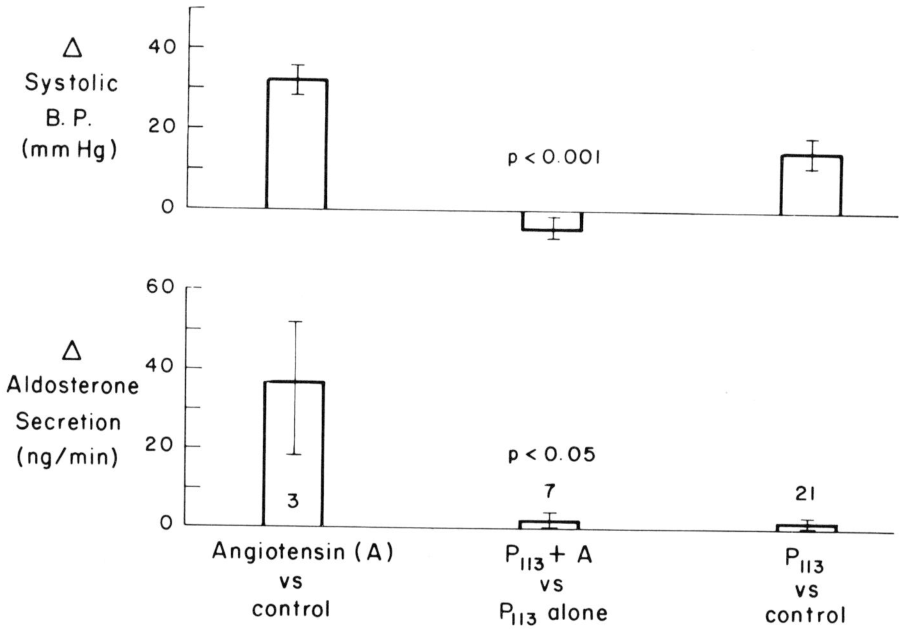

FIG. 2. The changes in systolic blood pressure and in aldosterone secretion following infusions of angiotensin II, P113, or angiotensin II plus P113 are shown. The angiotensin II dose was either 0.4μg or 0.8μg/min while the P113 dose was at least ten times this dose or adjusted higher to completely block the pressor response to angiotensin II. Angiotensin vs. control indicates the change in secretion or blood pressure when angiotensin was infused compared to the values during the control period in the same dog. P113 + A vs. P113 alone compares the responses when P113 was infused alone with the response when angiotensin (0.4μg or 0.8μg/min) was infused simultaneously. P113 vs. control compares the responses during the P113 and the control period in the same dogs. N indicates the number of dogs in each group, except for P113 vs. control when all infusions of P113 were averaged. Some dogs received more than one infusion of P113. Means ± S.E. are shown. The p values represent the values when the effects of P113 + angiotensin infusions are compared with the effect of angiotensin alone. (Published in American Journal of Physiology. In press.)

Table 1. Effect of P113 on Aldosterone Secretion Rate (ng/min) in Response to ACTH

Dose ACTH mu	*0*	*10*	*50*	*100*	*500*	*2000*
Dog #69						
Control	2.3					
ACTH			15.4		16.7	12.7
ACTH + P 113			14.9		17.9	16.1
Δ			− 0.5		+ 1.2	+ 3.4
Dog #71						
Control	4.0					
ACTH		4.1		22.9		43.1
ACTH + P 113		16.8		21.7		34.8
Δ		+12.7		− 1.2		− 8.3
Dog #72						
Control	1.1					
ACTH		1.7				84.4
ACTH + P 113		14.9				30.9
Δ		+13.2				−53.5

effect of P113 on the ACTH-induced rise in corticoid secretion. ACTH stimulated corticoid secretion and P113 did not prevent the rise.

P113 and Potassium

Figure 3 demonstrates a typical experiment. Infusion of P113 alone increased the secretion rate of aldosterone and the rate increased further when a KCl infusion was added. When the P113 was stopped, aldosterone secretion rose slightly, probably as a result of the rise in plasma K+ concentration. When a P113 infusion at twice the previous concentration was started, there was no significant decrease in aldosterone secretion. Corticoid secretion showed no consistent changes throughout this and other KCl and P113 experiments.

A summary of the results from four dogs is shown in Figure 4. P113 infusion did not inhibit the aldosterone stimulation by KCl infusions. The KCl increased plasma potassium which continued to rise throughout the experiments. When the P113

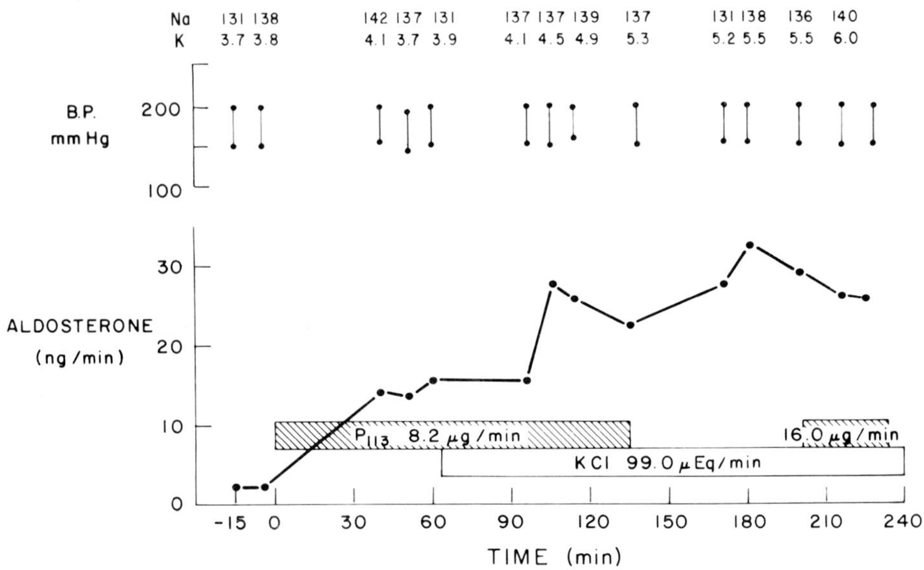

FIG. 3. Results from a representative 20 kg male dog. The time of P113 infusion is indicated by the longitudinal cross-hatched bars and the potassium chloride infusion by the open bar. The last P113 infusion began immediately after the third from last aldosterone secretion rate. Plasma (NA) and (K) are expressed in mEq/liter. The systolic and diastolic BP are shown. (Published in American Journal of Physiology. In press.)

was stopped, plasma K+ continued to rise and aldosterone rose as well. The reintroduction of the P113 infusion at twice the original concentration did not lower aldosterone secretion, but, in fact, the secretion rate continued to increase.

Discussion

Removal of the renin-angiotensin system by nephrectomy should make more tissue receptor sites available to circulatory angiotensin II and thus the animal more sensitive to infusions of angiotensin II, or to the agonistic effect of P113. In our study, P113 had a mild agonistic action on blood pressure, but no significant action on aldosterone secretion, although in an occasional dog, P113 did have a mild stimulating action. Other investigators have noted a mild agonistic action on blood pressure under certain circumstances [1, 2].

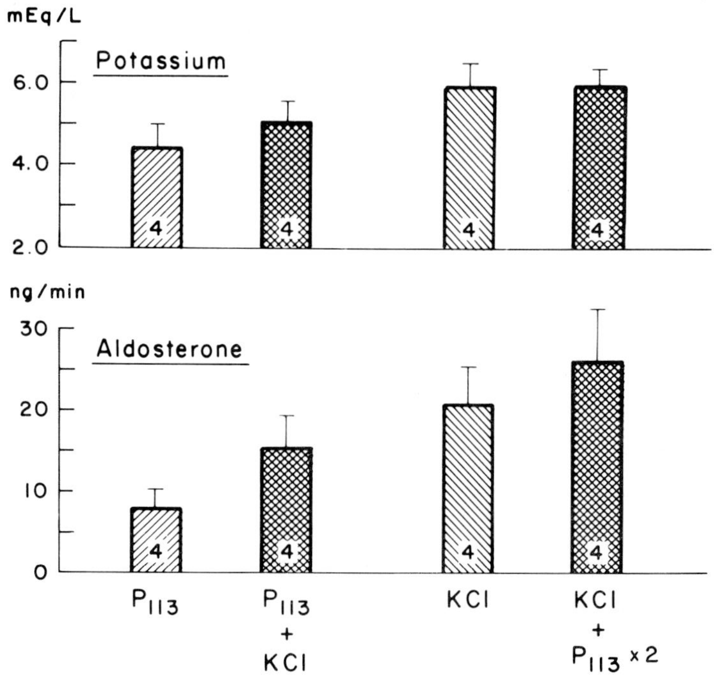

FIG. 4. Summary of results from four dogs. The separate bars indicate the aldosterone secretion rates and plasma potassium concentration during the P113 infusion alone, the initial P113 and KCl simultaneous infusions, when P113 was stopped and the KCl infusion continued and when P113 at twice the initial concentration was added to the KCl infusion (KCl and P113 × 2). The infusion rates of P113 and KCl are the same as illustrated in Figure 3. The mean ± SE are shown. These were calculated from the total number of samples (9 to 12) in each period. The numbers in the bars are the number of dogs. (Published in American Journal of Physiology. In press.)

The present in vivo experiments clearly establish that P113 is a specific adrenal inhibitor of angiotensin II and does not block the stimulation of aldosterone secretion by ACTH or potassium and confirms the results of Peach et al [3] from in vitro studies.

Human Studies

These studies were designed to investigate the effect of P113 upon aldosterone and blood pressure in normal man. Six human volunteers on either a normal sodium diet containing 170 mEq/day or a low sodium diet of 10 mEq/day were admitted to the Clinical Research Center on the morning of the experimental day. The subjects were supine for one to two hours before starting the P113 infusion. Blood pressure was recorded every two to five minutes during the control, P113 infusion and the postinfusion or recovery period. Blood for BUN, electrolytes, plasma renin activity and aldosterone measurement was withdrawn at the end of each period. After the postinfusion or recovery period, the subjects became ambulatory, and at the end of 30 minutes, the P113 infusion was restarted and continued for one hour, at which time the infusion was stopped and the postinfusion period continued for one hour.

Results

The effect of P113 on blood pressure and pulse rate while subjects were on a normal or low sodium diet is shown in Figure 5. The P113 infusion occurred during the fifth day of the 10 mEq sodium diet. In subjects on a normal sodium diet, P113 had no effect on blood pressure in either the supine or standing position. The pulse rate rose after the subjects became ambulatory and did not increase further during the P113 infusion.

In the subjects on the 10 mEq sodium diet, P113 had no effect upon supine blood pressure, but did cause a significant drop in systolic blood pressure during ambulation. Three of the six subjects had orthostatic symptoms. Of note is the failure of the pulse rate to rise further despite the fall in blood pressure.

In Figures 6 and 7 are shown the PRA and aldosterone results. In the supine subjects on a normal sodium diet, P113 infusion had no significant effect on PRA, but caused a slight increase in plasma aldosterone in three of six subjects.

During the ambulatory period, the rise in aldosterone which occurs with ambulation was not blocked by P113. During the ambulatory period in subjects on a low sodium diet, PRA increased significantly, possibly as a result of blockade of angiotensin II feedback inhibition of renin release by P113.

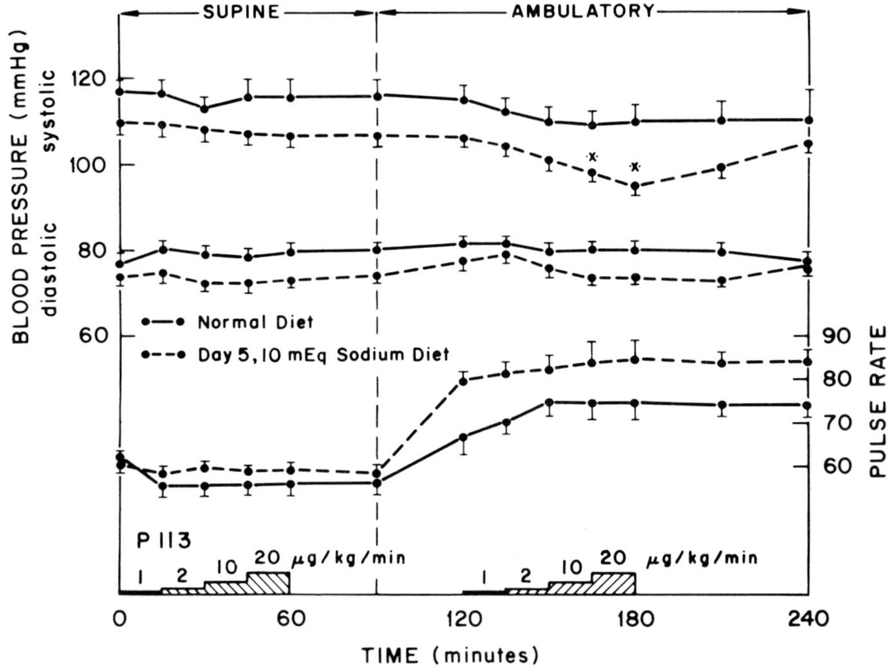

FIG. 5. Blood pressure and pulse rate of six normal subjects before, during and after 60-minute infusion of P113 at four different dose rates. Each rate was infused for 15 minutes. Supine indicates that the subjects were supine for at least one hour before, during and postinfusion. Ambulatory indicates the time period during which the subjects were in erect posture and walking intermittently. The solid line indicates the results from subjects on a normal sodium diet while the interrupted line shows the results in the subjects during the fifth day of a 10 mEq sodium diet. Means and S.E. are shown. -X- indicates orthostatic symptoms in three of six subjects.

Discussion

In normal supine man on a normal sodium intake, P113 has no effect on blood pressure or PRA, and an inconsistent effect upon plasma aldosterone levels; in fact, three of six subjects showed a slight increase.

In normal supine man on a low sodium diet, P113 had no effect upon blood pressure nor upon plasma aldosterone levels. Only after ambulation on a low sodium diet were we able to

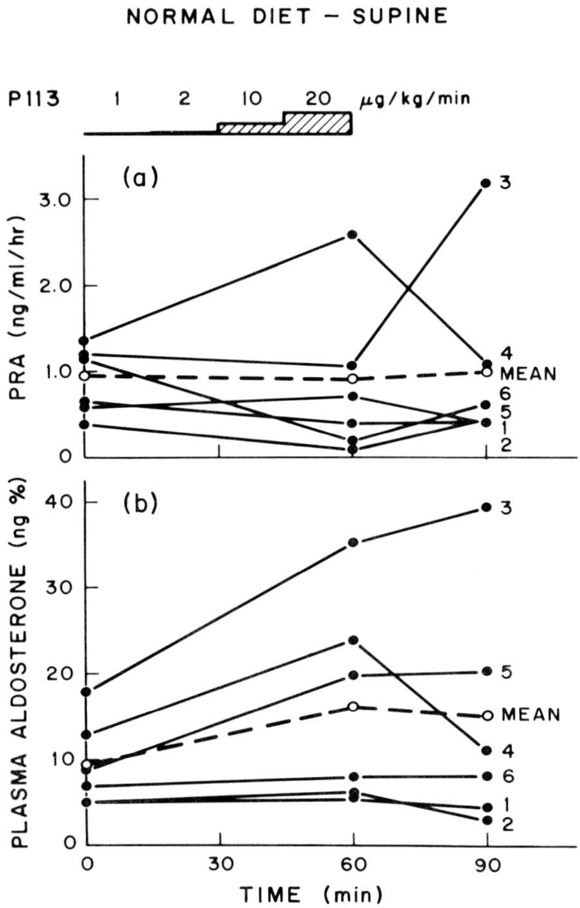

FIGS. 6 and 7. In these figures are shown the individual PRA and plasma aldosterone levels before, at the end of 60 minutes of P113 infusion and after 30 minutes postinfusion in the subjects supine (Fig. 6) and ambulatory (Fig. 7). The interrupted line represents the mean of the results. Numbers indicate results from an individual patient.

detect a physiological role for angiotensin II in blood pressure control. Surprisingly, P113 did not lower plasma aldosterone levels.

These data suggest either P113 has a mild agonistic effect upon aldosterone production, or that other factors were regulating aldosterone levels during the experiments.

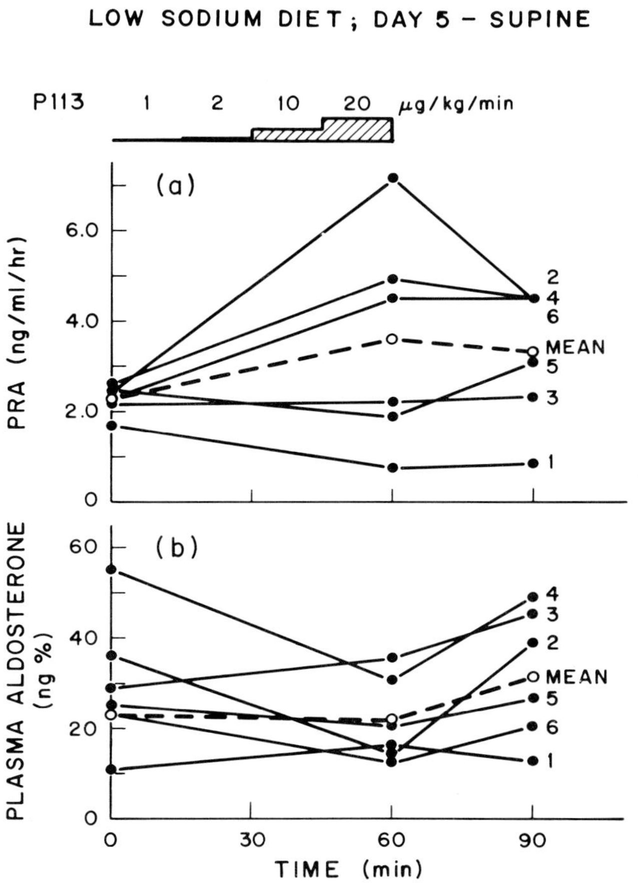

FIGURE 7.

The Effect of Aldactone upon Plasma Desoxycorticosterone Levels

In addition to its antimineralocorticoid effect, spironolactone may inhibit several adrenal enzyme systems including 11-Beta-hydroxylase [4-6]. In hypertensive patients on Aldactone therapy, we noted uniformly elevated plasma desoxycorticosterone (DOC) levels. Since Aldactone has been reported to interfere with some radioimmunoassays for digoxin and aldosterone [7, 8], we investigated whether the raised DOC levels were a consequence of 11-Beta-hydroxylase inhibition or interference by the drug in the assay system.

Blood specimens were obtained from seven hypertensive patients receiving 25-400 mg spironolactone per day. Plasma DOC was measured following Sephadex LH-20 chromatography by a previously described competitive-protein-binding (CPB) radioassay [9]. Also, radioimmunoassays utilizing three separate anti-DOC antibodies were performed on the LH-20 DOC eluate pooled from four patients on spironolactone. An aliquot was also acetylated and the acetylated DOC (DOCA) separated by chromatography from spironolactone and canrenone and then quantitated by CPB radioassay.

Results

Plasma DOC levels measured in normal subjects are shown in Figure 8. Hypertensive patients not receiving spironolactone

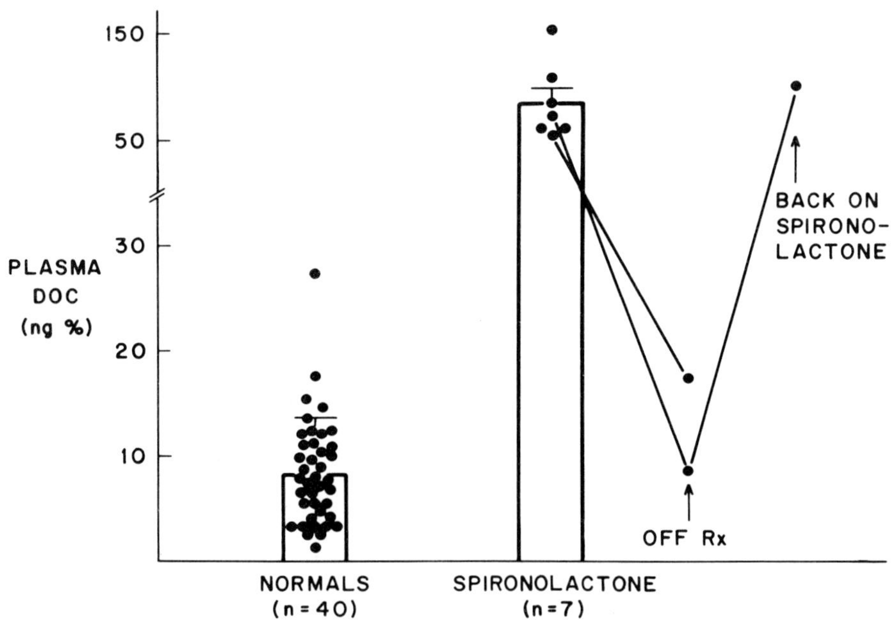

FIG. 8. Plasma DOC levels measured by competitive binding protein radioassay in patients receiving spironolactone.

had similar values. In contrast, all seven patients on spironolactone had elevated plasma DOC which returned to normal after stopping the drug.

In Table 2 are shown the values obtained in the four assay systems for the pooled DOC eluate from patients receiving spironolactone and the cross-reactivity of spironolactone and one of its metabolites, canrenone. A true plasma DOC level that was similar to the normal value of 10 ng% was obtained after acetylation, further chromatography and CPB radioassay of the DOCA. Antibody I had the least cross-reactivity with spironolactone or canrenone and gave a DOC level near the true value. The two drugs had similar Rf as DOC in a variety of chromatographic systems and therefore could not be separated prior to radioimmunoassay.

Discussion

We have shown that spironolactone and its major metabolite canrenone co-elute with DOC in several chromatographic systems and have significant affinity for several DOC-binding proteins. The elevated plasma DOC values in patients receiving spironolactone are, in fact, spuriously elevated. Although our results do not rule out an inhibition of 11-Beta-hydroxylase activity by spironolactone, they indicate that drug interference in the assay system accounts for the deviation in plasma DOC levels.

Table 2. DOC Eluate From Patients Receiving Spironolactone

	DOC Reading	*Cross-Interference*	
	ng%	S*	C**
CPB-Radioassay (Dog Transcortin)	100.0	0.05%	1.2%
Anti-DOC Antibody I (3-oxime)	13.5	0.05%	0.2%
Anti-DOC Antibody II (21-Hemisuc.)	200.0	24.00%	24.0%
Anti-DOC Antibody III	170.0	10.00%	12.0%

Following acetylation and TLC chromatography to remove canrenone, DOC level assayed by CPB-radioassay was 10 ng%.

*Spironolactone

**Canrenone

References

1. Pals, D.T. and Masucci, F.O.: Plasma renin and the antihypertensive effect of 1-Sar-8-Ala-angiotensin II. Europ. J. Pharm. 23:115-119, 1973.
2. Bumpus, F.M., Sen, S., Smeby, R. et al: Use of angiotensin II antagonists in experimental hypertension. Circ. Res. 32 (suppl. 1):1-150, 1973.
3. Peach, M.J. and Chiu, A.T.: Stimulation and inhibition of aldosterone biosynthesis in vitro by angiotensin II and analogs. Circ. Res. 35 (suppl. 1):1-7, 1974.
4. Erbler, H.C.: On the mechanism of the inhibitory action of the spirolactone SC 9376 (aldadiene) on the production of corticosteroids in rat adrenals in vitro. N.S. Arch. Pharmacol. 277:139-149, 1973.
5. Cheng, S.C., Sadee, W., Suzuki, K. et al: The Endocrine Society Abstracts 56th Annual Meeting, The Endrocrine Society, June 1974, pp. A-85.
6. Sundsfjord, J.A., Marton, P., Jorgensen, H. et al: Reduced aldosterone secretion during spironolactone treatment in primary aldosteronism: Report of a case. J. Clin. Endocrinol. Metab. 39:734-739, 1974.
7. Phillips, A.P.: The improvement of specificity in radioimmunoassays. Clin. Chem. Acta 44:333-340, 1973.
8. Sadee, W., Finn, A.M., Schmiedek, P. et al: Aldosterone plasma radioimmunoassay interference by a spirolactone metabolite. Steroids 25:301, 1975.
9. Tan, S.Y. and Mulrow, P.J.: A competitive protein binding radioassay for desoxycorticosterone in human plasma. Steroids 28:1-12, 1975.

Discussion

Moderator: Dr. J. Genest

Dr. Bumpus: I wanted to comment on Dr. Mulrow's paper. The use of angiotensin antagonists in studies on aldosterone release can certainly be misleading. For example, in sodium-depleted dogs Dr. Bravo has shown that both Sar^1, Ile^8 and Sar^1, Ala^8 angiotensin II are partial agonists and then act as antagonists. However, [Sar^1, Thr^8] angiotensin II acts as an antagonist immediately and the heptapeptide antagonists seem to be much more specific in blocking the release of aldosterone.

Dr. Vallotton: I just want to insist on what Dr. Mulrow just said about the importance of being aware that spironolactone interferes with the measurement of aldosterone by radioimmunoassay, not only in plasma but also in urine. Many people are not aware of that. In our laboratory, Dr. Anne Riondel compared the regression line of results of urinary aldosterone measurements comparing the double isotope dilution technique and the radioimmunoassay technique in patients having not received spironolactone and patients having received spironolactone. In the presence of spironolactone and its metabolites the regression line is shifted toward higher values obtained by radioimmunoassay though a significant correlation still obtained between the two methods.

Effects of Spironolactone and Hydrochlorothiazide on Blood Pressure and Plasma Renin Activity in Hypertension

Myron H. Weinberger, M.D. and Clarence E. Grim, M.D.

Introduction

Diuretics have long been advocated as efficacious, initial therapy in hypertension. A variety of mechanisms have been proposed for their antihypertensive effects. Recently it has been suggested that the antihypertensive efficacy of diuretic therapy may be related to the specific physiologic abnormality in hypertensive patients [1]. That is, it has been suggested that the hypertensive with low plasma renin activity (PRA) is more likely to respond to diuretic therapy. In addition, it has been suggested that spironolactone, by its action as a mineralocorticoid antagonist, is more effective in lowering blood pressure in the low renin hypertensive subgroup [2-5]. The current study was undertaken to examine the changes in PRA as a reflection of the therapeutic efficacy of such agents. The study was designed to compare the relative effects of hydrochlorothiazide with three doses of spironolactone alone and in combination with hydrochlorothiazide in patients with mild hypertension.

These studies were supported in part by USPHS grant HL 14159, Specialized Center of Research (SCOR)-Hypertension, and by a grant from Clinical Resources, Inc.

Myron H. Weinberger, M.D. and Clarence E. Grim, M.D., Specialized Center of Research in Hypertension and Department of Medicine, Indiana University School of Medicine, Indianapolis.

Methods

Hypertensive Patients

Sixty patients with diastolic blood pressure between 90 and 114 mm Hg were chosen for study. The group consisted of 32 males and 28 females and ranged in age from 24 to 63 years. None of the patients had known secondary forms of hypertension nor was there any evidence of cardiovascular or renal complications of hypertension. The study protocol was approved by the Indiana University Human Use Committee and informed consent was obtained from each patient after explanation of the study and duly documented.

The placebo-washout, double-blind study design consisted of patients being seen bi-weekly, as outlined in Table 1. A four-week wash-out period was instituted during which time the patient was given placebo capsules twice a day. At the end of this period, patients were randomly assigned to treatment groups for a period of eight weeks. The first group received hydrochlorothiazide 50 mg twice a day; the second group, spironolactone 50 mg twice a day; the third group, spironolactone 100 mg twice a day; and the fourth, spironolactone 200 mg twice a day. At the end of this eight-week treatment period, patients were continued on their previous medication and randomly subdivided into one of two additional treatment groups lasting four additional weeks. The first of these subdivided groups received hydrochlorothiazide 50 mg twice a day in addition to their previous treatment. The second group

Table 1. Study Design: 60 Hypertensives (32 Male, 28 Female)

A. Placebo bid:	4 weeks	
B. Random assignment into treatment groups:		8 weeks
1. Hydrochlorothiazide	50 mg bid	
2. Spironolactone	50 mg bid	
3. Spironolactone	100 mg bid	
4. Spironolactone	200 mg bid	
C. Additional randomization of each group:		4 weeks
1. Above treatment + Hydrochlorothiazide 50 mg bid		
2. Above treatment + Placebo bid		
D. Recovery:	4 weeks	

received placebo twice a day in addition to their previous treatment. Following this period of treatment all medications were stopped and the patient was followed for an additional four weeks. Patients were seen bi-weekly during the course of the study for measurement of blood pressure, pulse, weight, pill count and evaluation of side effects. At monthly intervals the patient had biochemical profiles obtained utilizing an SMA-12 automated analysis, serum electrolytes and BUN performed by standard analytical techniques and PRA measured by a radioimmunoassay technique [6]. In addition, a 24-hour urine sample was collected prior to the visit which was analyzed for sodium and potassium content and creatinine. Two such biochemical analyses were performed during the placebo period.

Normal Subjects

To provide a basis for categorization of hypertensive patients with respect to the appropriateness of their renin levels to urinary sodium excretion, 88 normal volunteer subjects were similarly studied. The subjects ranged in age from 15 to 80 years and were studied while ambulatory during both high and low sodium intake. In both hypertensive and normal subjects blood samples were obtained under appropriate conditions following two hours of ambulation between 8:00 A.M. and 10:00 A.M. Normal subjects also collected a 24-hour urine sample for estimation of electrolyte content.

Results

Figure 1 demonstrates the relationship between urinary sodium excretion and PRA among the normal subjects. These observations were analyzed by a polynomial regression technique. Ninety percent confidence limits are indicated by the solid lines. The formula derived from the second order polynomial regression analysis of the data for normal subjects is $Y = 7.779 - 0.02224x + 0.0000298x^2$.

Figure 2 demonstrates similar observations made in the hypertensive subjects during the placebo period. The majority of hypertensives fell within the 90% confidence limits established for the normal subjects. Three subjects had PRA above the 90% confidence limits for the level of sodium intake. Ten subjects had PRA below the 90% confidence limits for sodium

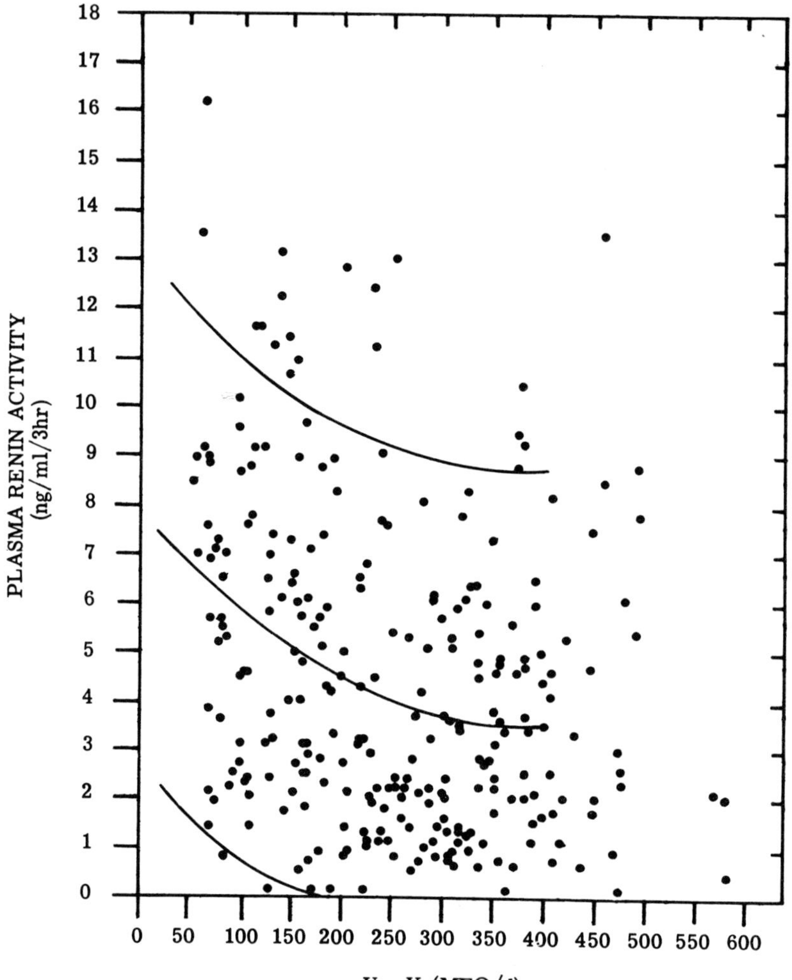

FIG. 1. Relationship between PRA and urinary sodium excretion among 88 normotensive subjects during high and low sodium intake. Ninety percent confidence limits are indicated by solid lines.

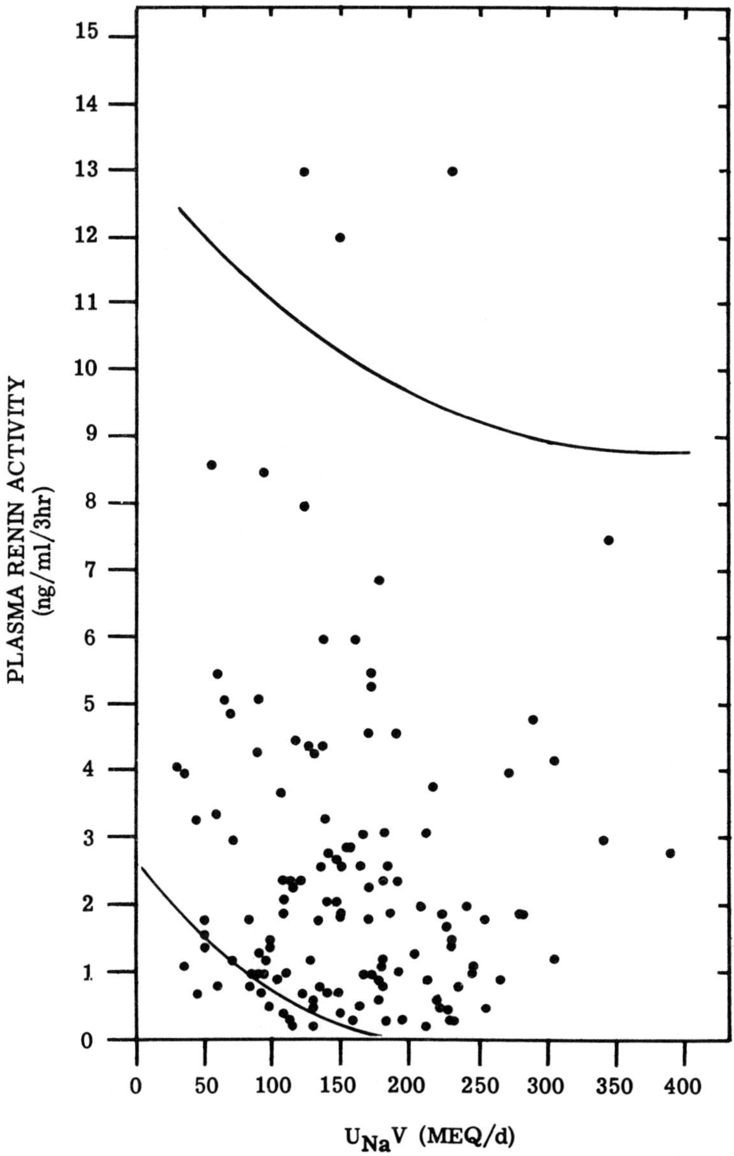

FIG. 2. Relationship between PRA and urinary sodium excretion among 60 hypertensive subjects studied during placebo period. Ninety percent confidence limits established for normal subjects are indicated by solid lines.

intake. In addition, 11 subjects had PRA less than 1.0 ng/ml/3 hr but had urinary sodium excretion greater than 150 mEq/d. At this level of sodium intake it is difficult to separate subnormal renin responsiveness from normal because of the low values of PRA observed among normal subjects at this level of sodium intake. For the purpose of this study, such hypertensives were classified as having probable renin suppression.

Table 2 outlines the distribution of hypertensive patients into the various treatment groups on the basis of the relation of the renin to urinary sodium excretion during the placebo period. Thirty-six patients had normal levels of PRA, 3 had high PRA, 10 had low PRA and 11 additional subjects had low PRA (< 1.0 ng/ml/3 hr) during periods of high sodium intake (> 150 mEq/d) who are classified as probable low renin hypertensives. These subjects were randomly distributed among the four treatment groups as indicated in Table 1.

The blood pressure responses in the various treatment groups are indicated in Table 3. Blood pressure measurements are indicated as average mean arterial blood pressure (diastolic + 1/3 pulse pressure) for the group during the placebo period and following 12 weeks of therapy. In addition, the number of subjects in each treatment group achieving mean arterial blood pressure at the 12th week of treatment less than 108 (< 140/90)mm Hg is also indicated. Fifty-five subjects completed the 12-week treatment period. There were no statistically significant differences between mean arterial blood pressure in the placebo period among the treatment groups. Following 12 weeks of therapy, mean arterial blood pressure declined in all groups. The greatest decrement in mean arterial pressure was seen in the high dose spironolactone group who had hydrochlorothiazide added during the final four weeks of therapy. Approximately 83% of the hypertensive patients studied had a mean arterial blood pressure less than 108 mm Hg at the end of the treatment period. There did not appear to be any differences in the degree of blood pressure responsiveness among the different treatment groups.

Figure 3 demonstrates the mean blood pressure measurements for the four treatment groups during the two placebo observations and at 4, 8 and 12 weeks of treatment as well as one month after cessation of therapy. The groups receiving the higher doses of spironolactone (100 or 200 mg bid) with

Table 2. Distribution and Blood Pressure Responses of Patients by Treatment Groups

	Hydrochlorothiazide 50 mg bid	*Spironolactone 50 mg bid*	*Spironolactone 100 mg bid*	*Spironolactone 200 mg bid*	*Total*
High PRA	0	1 (0)	0	2 (0)	3 (0)
Normal PRA	11 (8)	7 (5)	9 (8)	9 (7)	36 (28)
Low PRA	2 (1)	6 (4)	2 (1)	0	10 (6)
PRA < 1.0, $U_{Na}V > 150$	1 (1)	3 (2)	5 (3)	2 (2)	11 (8)
Total	14 (10)	17 (11)	16 (12)	13 (9)	60 (42)

Parentheses refer to patients achieving mean arterial blood pressure $\leqslant$ 107 mm Hg at the 12th treatment week.

Table 3. Blood Pressure Response to Treatment (12 Weeks)

	Con MABP	*Tx*	*MABP ≤ 107*	*Total*
Hydrochlorothiazide 50 mg bid	113.7	102.5	4	6
Hydrochlorothiazide + HCT 50 mg bid	112.3	103.0	6	8
Spironolactone 50 mg bid	120.1	104.1	6	8
Spironolactone + HCT 50 mg bid	116.3	100.7	5	6
Spironolactone 100 mg bid	114.4	101.7	7	9
Spironolactone + HCT 100 mg bid	110.1	101.7	5	6
Spironolactone 200 mg bid	118.5	104.2	4	6
Spironolactone + HCT 200 mg bid	113.6	96.5	5	6
			42	55

HCT = hydrochlorothiazide.
Con MABP = group mean arterial blood in placebo period.
Tx = group mean arterial blood pressure at 12th treatment week.

hydrochlorothiazide added during the last month of therapy had lower mean arterial blood pressure one month following cessation of therapy.

Mean PRA measurements for each treatment group are depicted in Figure 4. The two placebo observations are indicated as well as the mean PRA at the end of 4, 8 and 12 weeks of treatment and following 4 weeks cessation of antihypertensive therapy. Mean renin levels rose in all groups after therapy was initiated. At the end of two months a general, dose-related relationship with mean PRA was observed among the spironolactone-treated groups. During the final four weeks of therapy (12th week) hydrochlorothiazide or placebo was added to previous treatment regimens. No significant further increase in mean PRA was observed in the group receiving

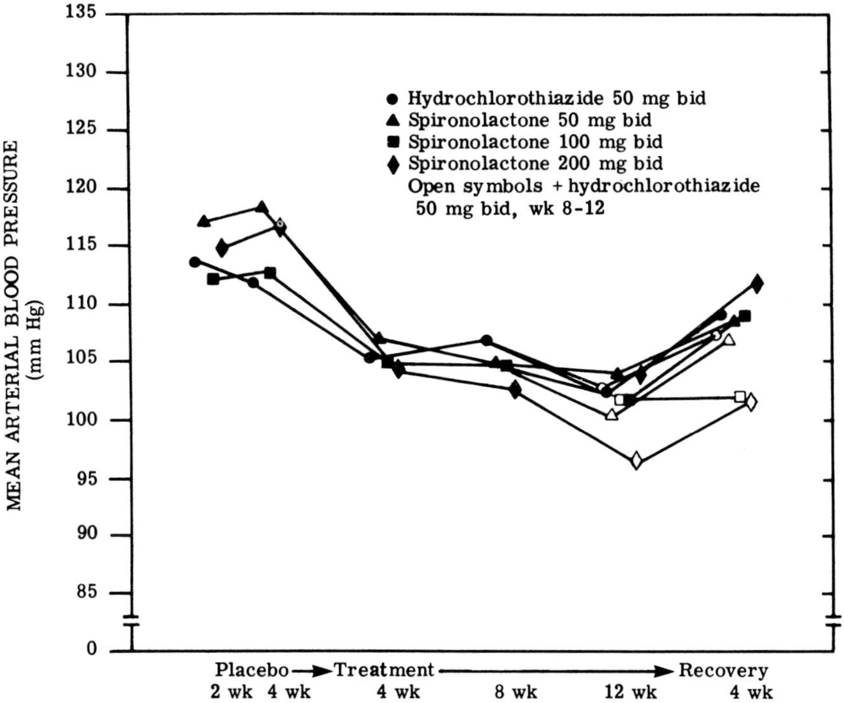

FIG. 3. Average mean arterial blood pressure for the treatment groups as indicated by the symbols in the key at 2 and 4 weeks of placebo, 4, 8 and 12 weeks of treatment and at 4 weeks after discontinuation of treatment (recovery). The group receiving hydrochlorothiazide 50 mg bid in addition to previous therapy during weeks 8-12 are indicated by open symbols at week 12 and recovery.

hydrochlorothiazide as initial treatment. However, in all three of the spironolactone-treated groups, a marked additional increment in mean PRA was observed with the addition of hydrochlorothiazide. The mean plasma renin levels in the recovery period also appeared to be higher in those patients receiving the higher doses of spironolactone and particularly those who received hydrochlorothiazide in addition to spironolactone during the last month of treatment.

Evaluation of the blood pressure responses to the various treatment regimens was performed on the basis of the renin

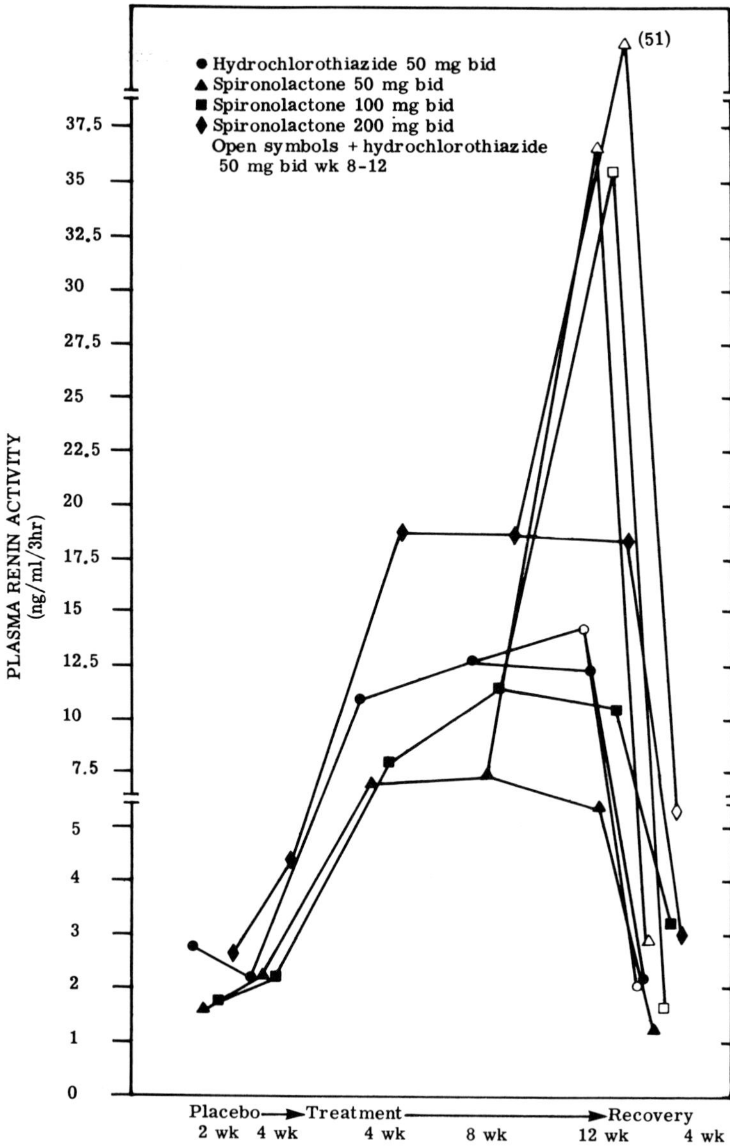

FIG. 4. Mean PRA for the treatment groups. Symbols and arrangements as for Figure 3.

profile. Patients were subdivided within each treatment group on the basis of the appropriateness of the PRA to urinary sodium excretion during the placebo period. Individuals in each renin category who demonstrated a decline in mean arterial blood pressure to less than 107 mm Hg at the 12th week of treatment are indicated by parentheses in Table 2.

When all patients were considered with respect to their blood pressure responses in relation to their placebo renin status, interesting patterns were observed. None of the three subjects with high PRA had a reduction of blood pressure into the normal range. Of the 34 patients with normal renin levels, 28 achieved normotensive levels during treatment. In the low renin group, six of nine, and in those classified as having "probable" renin suppression, ten of 11, demonstrated normal blood pressures during treatment. Although not shown in the data, there was no significant relationship between changes in PRA and blood pressure among any of the groups studied.

Discussion

The preliminary results of the present study have confirmed the observation that diuretic therapy is efficacious in the treatment of mild hypertension. In this study, 42 of 55 (76%) hypertensive subjects demonstrated a decline in mean arterial blood pressure to levels of less than 108 mm Hg following three months of diuretic treatment. There did not appear to be significant differences in the frequency of normotensive responses between those treated with hydrochlorothiazide alone or with the various doses of spironolactone. However, the range of blood pressure measurements among the individuals in each group may be too great to permit a demonstration of statistically significant differences in such responses. In all groups there was a consistent response of PRA to diuretic therapy. In general, a dose-relationship with spironolactone was evident.

From the mean renin observations (Fig. 4) among the various treatment groups it would appear that hydrochlorothiazide alone (50 mg bid) was a more potent stimulus to renin than spironolactone in a dose of 50 mg bid; roughly equipotent in stimulating renin as spironolactone 100 mg bid; and not as effective as the high-dose spironolactone. Evidence that thiazide diuretics differ in their mechanism of volume depletion from spironolactone can be presumed from the marked additional increase in PRA in the groups treated initially with spironolactone who had hydrochlorothiazide added during the last month of therapy. Furthermore, the effects of combined thiazide and spironolactone treatment on both PRA and mean arterial blood pressure appeared to be more long lasting following cessation of therapy than the utilization of either agent alone.

In an attempt to evaluate whether the renin profile provides a predictive basis for choosing antihypertensive therapy or the response to specific diuretic therapy, the data from this study, while preliminary, are of interest. Among the three patients studied with high PRA none had a reduction of blood pressure to less than 108 mm Hg despite treatment in two subjects with high doses of spironolactone and in one with the addition of hydrochlorothiazide during the final month of therapy. This observation suggests that in this group volume expansion is not the major hypertensive mechanism. Among the normal renin population approximately 85% (28/34) of the subjects studied had a reduction of blood pressure to normal levels with any of the therapeutic regimens. In the low renin category a comparable response was observed with six of nine patients with clear-cut suppression of PRA in the placebo period and ten of 11 of those classified as having probable low PRA demonstrating a reduction in blood pressure to normotensive levels following treatment. Again, this response was independent of the treatment group to which they were assigned. These observations confirm the usefulness of diuretic therapy in a majority of hypertensive patients.

In the small number of patients in the low and probable low renin classification in this study, it is not possible to obtain support for the greater efficacy of spironolactone over thiazide. However, the observations in the three high renin subjects would suggest that diuretic therapy may not be an approach of major efficacy. This observation confirms the contention of others [1] that these subjects have vasoconstriction as the primary component of their hypertension. Finally, there appears to be no discernible correlation between the magnitude of change in PRA and the magnitude of response of mean arterial blood pressure among any of the groups studied. These observations represent a preliminary evaluation of a larger sample a more detailed analysis of which may yield additional new information.

Acknowledgments

The authors wish to express gratitude to Drs. James T. Higgins, Jr., and Norman J. Kramer for the referral of and assistance with many of the patients studied. We are particularly indebted to Ms. Sherrill Adkins, R.N., and Ms. Mary Jo Herr, R.N., for their expert help in these studies. We also wish to thank Ms. Mary B. Wade for expert technical assistance and Mrs. Irene Rosevear and Ms. Gwendolyn Morgan for preparation of the manuscript.

References

1. Laragh, J.H.: Vasoconstriction-volume analysis for understanding and treating hypertension. Am. J. Med. 55:261, 1973.
2. Adlin, E.V., Marks, A.D. and Channick, B.J.: Spironolactone and hydrochlorothiazide in essential hypertension. Arch. Intern. Med. 130:855, 1972.
3. Carey, R.M., Douglas, J.G., Schweikert, J.R. et al: The syndrome of essential hypertension and suppressed plasma renin activity. Arch. Intern. Med. 130:849, 1972.
4. Crane, M.G. and Harris, J.G.: Effect of spironolactone in hypertensive patients. Am. J. Med. Sci. 260:311, 1970.
5. Spark, R.F. and Melby, J.C.: Hypertension and low plasma renin activity. Ann. Intern. Med. 75:831, 1971.
6. Weinberger, M.H., Ramsdell, J.W., Rosner, D.R. et al: Effect of chlorothiazide and sodium on vascular responsiveness to angiotensin II. Am. J. Physiol. 223:1049, 1972.

Discussion

Moderator: Dr. F. Gross

Dr. Kirkendall: I would like to ask Dr. Weinberger if he was able to identify any of their nonresponders to thiazide therapy on the basis of other hemodynamic characteristics, particularly pulse rate? Some patients who have a very rapid pulse rate do not respond well to thiazide diuretics. I wonder if, in more carefully controlled studies, such association was seen.

Dr. Weinberger: Is your question whether we may have had some evidence of sympathetic activity or some other hemodynamic compensatory mechanism which may be explicable in terms of the nonresponse to therapy?

Dr. Kirkendall: Was there a correlation between the plasma renin activity in nonresponders and the resting pulse rate during the placebo period?

Dr. Weinberger: I cannot recall offhand. It would be an easy matter to look at, as there were only three high renin patients. In all of the patients studied we have pulse rate measurements; however, I do not recall the data.

Dr. Luetscher: Dr. Weinberger, have you considered the possibility that potassium depletion might be a potent stimulator of renin activity in the patients who received chlorothiazide? Might the greater effect of the chlorothiazide in raising renin in your cases be related to the potassium loss produced by that diuretic, as opposed to potassium retention which might occur with spironolactone?

Dr. Weinberger: The potassium responses were much greater in the spironolactone-treated patients. When thiazides were added, there was not a significant decrease in serum potassium concentrations. However, in patients receiving hydrochlorothiazide alone, either 50 mg twice a day or in the double dose during their last month of treatment, there was a significant reduction in serum potassium.

IV

Effects of Acute Receptor Blockade

Effects of Infusing Angiotensin II Antagonist Saralasin on Arterial Blood Pressure and on Plasma Concentrations of Aldosterone, Renin and Angiotensin II in Normal Subjects and Selected Hypertensive Patients

J. J. Brown, B.Sc., F.R.C.P., W. C. B. Brown, F.I.S.T., R. Fraser, M.Sc., Ph.D., A. F. Lever, B.Sc., F.R.C.P., J. J. Morton, Ph.D., J. I. S. Robertson, B.Sc., F.R.C.P., E. Agabiti-Rosei, M.D.,* M. Tree, Ph.D. and P. M. Trust, M.B.B.S.

The role of the renin-angiotensin system in both physiological and pathological circumstances remains uncertain. However, the availability of substances which specifically block the actions of some component of the system provides a new approach to this problem [1]. Saralasin† is an analogue of angiotensin II (1-Sar, $_5$Va 1, 8-Ala), synthesized by Pals et al [2], a peptide which specifically blocks the actions of angiotensin II. We report here the effects observed across infusion of saralasin on the arterial blood pressure and on the plasma concentrations of renin, angiotensin II and aldosterone in two normal subjects and in patients with hypertension of varied etiology. In some instances the studies were performed twice, once when sodium intake was normal and again during sodium deprivation.

---

†Morton-Norwich Laboratories, Ltd.

J. J. Brown, B.Sc., F.R.C.P., W. C. B. Brown, F.I.S.T., R. Fraser, M.Sc., Ph.D., A. F. Lever, B.Sc., F.R.C.P., J. J. Morton, Ph.D., J. I. S. Robertson, B.Sc., F.R.C.P., E. Agabiti-Rosei, M.D., M. Tree, Ph.D. and P. M. Trust, M.B.B.S., Medical Research Council, Blood Pressure Unit, Western Infirmary, Glasgow, Scotland.

*British Council Scholar. Present address: Instituto di Semeiotica Medica-Policlinico Universitario, Perugia.

Methods

The protocol for the investigations is illustrated in Figure 1. Throughout the period of infusion and for at least the preceding 45 minutes, the subjects remained in the supine position. The infusions were given at a constant rate by an electrically driven pump* via a plastic cannula into a forearm vein. Blood samples were taken from a vein in the opposite forearm (Fig. 1) via an indwelling plastic cannula for measurements of plasma concentrations of renin [3], angiotensin II [4] and aldosterone [5]. No cross-reaction between angiotensin II and saralasin was

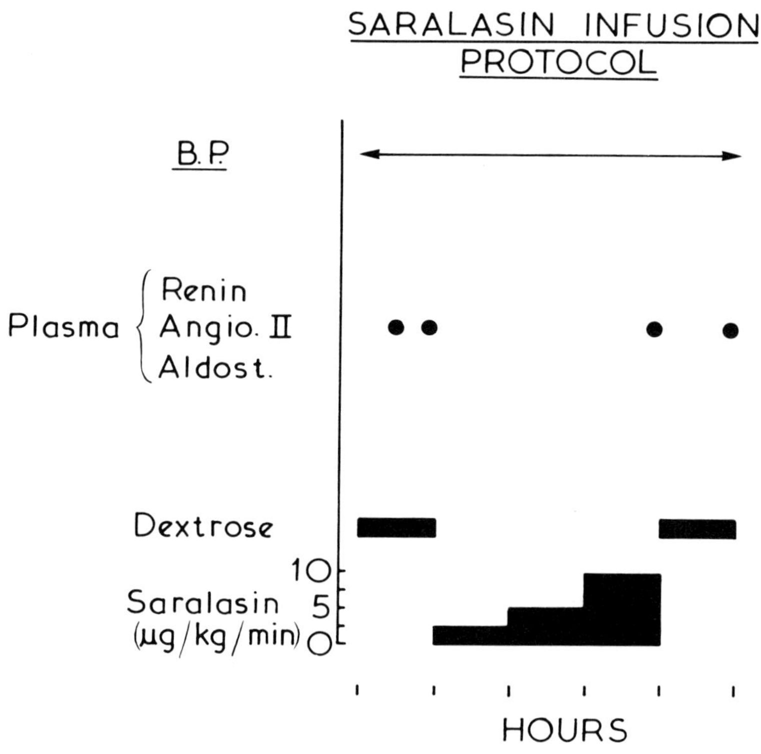

FIGURE 1.

*Dascon, Unden, Holland.

found in the assay system within the range 10-10,000 pg. Arterial blood pressure was measured indirectly every three to five minutes by a semi-automatic machine* checked at intervals by a traditional clinical sphygmomanometer applied to the opposite forearm. In most cases, the diet was fixed to contain known and normal amounts of sodium and potassium for at least three days before the infusions. Sodium depletion was produced by reducing sodium intake to 10 mEq/day for three days and by furosemide (40-80 mg) given by mouth once on the first day of the reduced intake. None of the patients had taken diuretics, potassium supplements, oral contraceptives or hypotensive drugs (other than bethanidine in a few instances) for at least four weeks before infusion. In the severely hypertensive patients treatment with bethanidine was continued until the day before infusion.

Results

Normal Subjects

Similar results were obtained in the two male subjects studied, aged 25 and 26 years. While the subjects ate a fixed diet providing a normal intake of sodium and potassium, infusion with saralasin produced no detectable change in arterial blood pressure or plasma aldosterone concentration. During sodium depletion (cumulative urine sodium loss minus sodium intake 207 and 143 mEq, respectively), infusion of saralasin led to a distinct fall in circulating aldosterone, despite an increase in plasma angiotensin II concentration, without change in blood pressure (Figs. 2A and 2B).

Hypertensive Patients

The results obtained during infusion of the angiotensin II antagonist in hypertensive patients with low, normal or raised levels of plasma renin and angiotensin II are illustrated in Figures 3 to 8. In the patient with low plasma concentrations of renin and angiotensin II, associated with raised plasma aldosterone (from whom an adrenocortical aldosterone secreting adenoma was removed subsequently), infusion of saralasin

*Elag — Koln

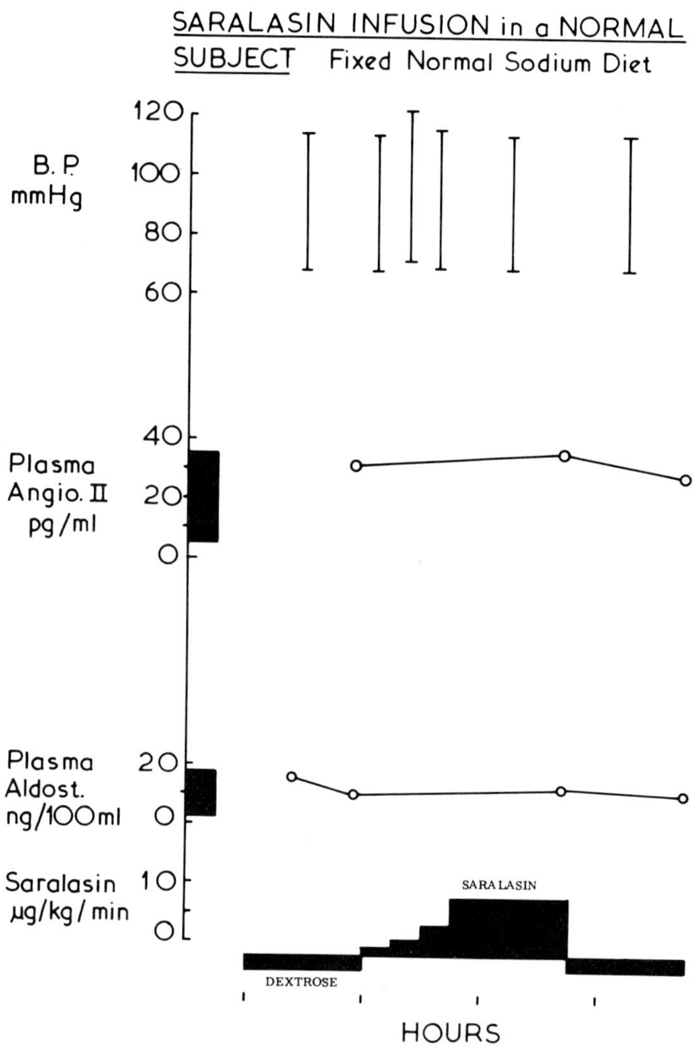
SARALASIN INFUSION in a NORMAL SUBJECT Fixed Normal Sodium Diet
B. P. mmHg
120
100
80
60
Plasma Angio. II pg/ml
40
20
0
Plasma Aldost. ng/100ml
20
0
Saralasin µg/kg/min
10
0
SARALASIN
DEXTROSE
HOURS

FIGURE 2A.

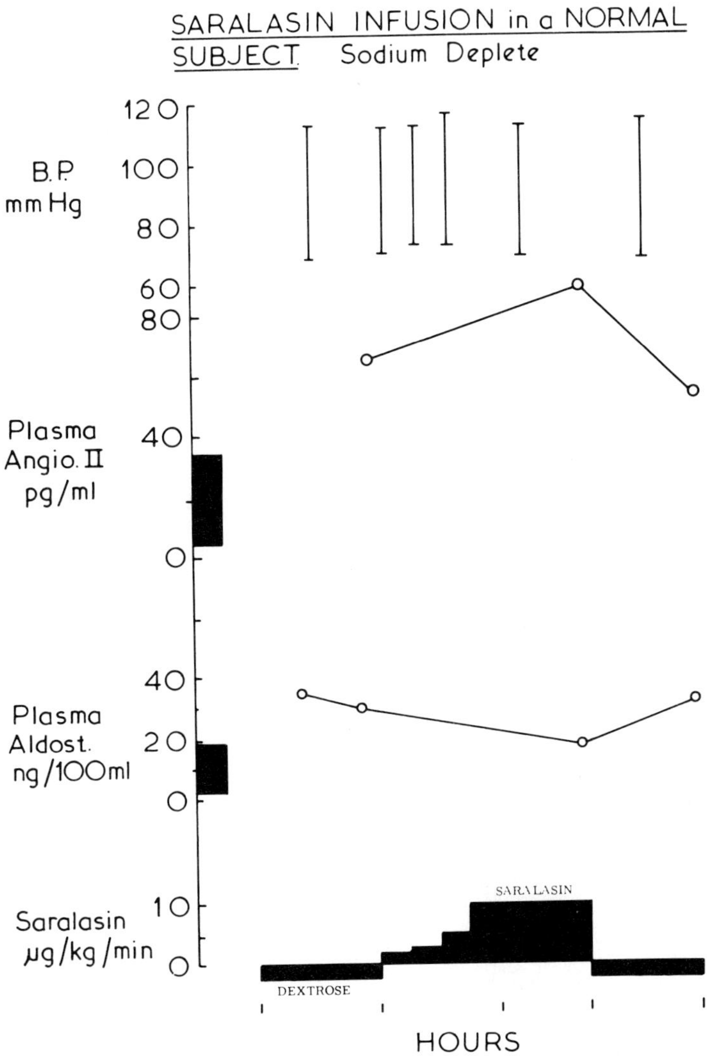
SARALASIN INFUSION in a NORMAL SUBJECT. Sodium Deplete
B.P. mmHg
120
100
80
60
80
Plasma Angio. II pg/ml
40
0
40
Plasma Aldost. ng/100ml
20
0
Saralasin µg/kg/min
10
0
SARALASIN
DEXTROSE
HOURS

FIGURE 2B.

produced a prolonged small increase in blood pressure unaccompanied by any marked changes in circulating renin, angiotensin II or aldosterone (Fig. 3).

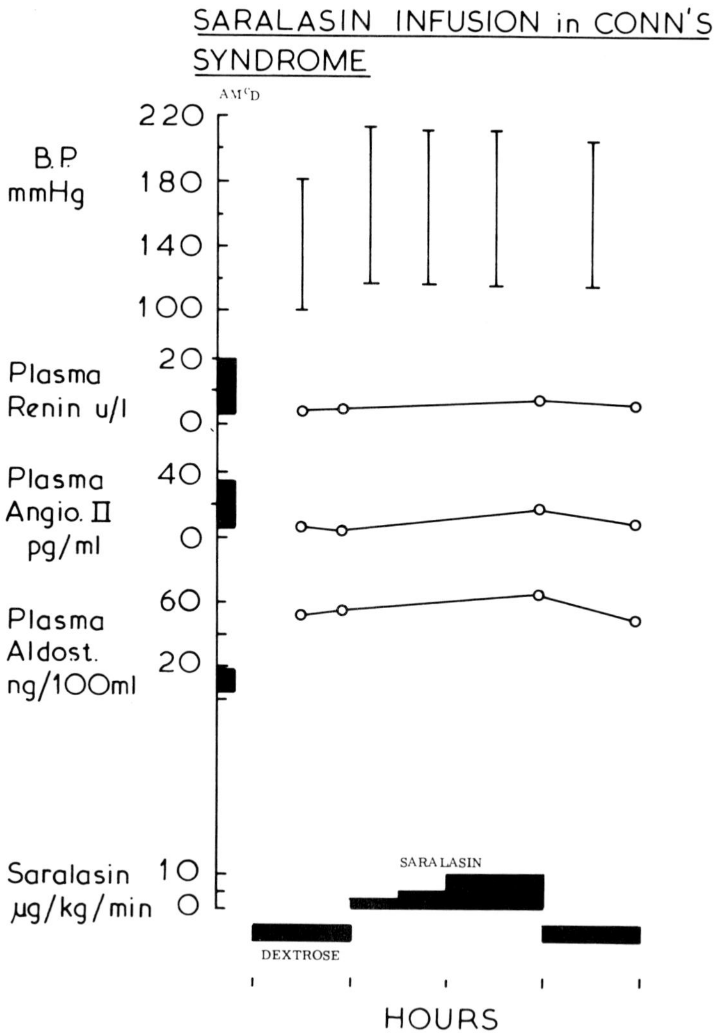

FIGURE 3.

No biochemical or arterial blood pressure changes were observed in patients with normal basal levels of renin and angiotensin II (Fig. 4).

However, during the infusion of saralasin into patients with raised renin and angiotensin II levels, blood pressure and plasma aldosterone concentrations fell while circulating renin and angiotensin II values increased. The changes in blood pressure were most distinct and consistent in patients with chronic renal failure who remained severely hypertensive despite regular

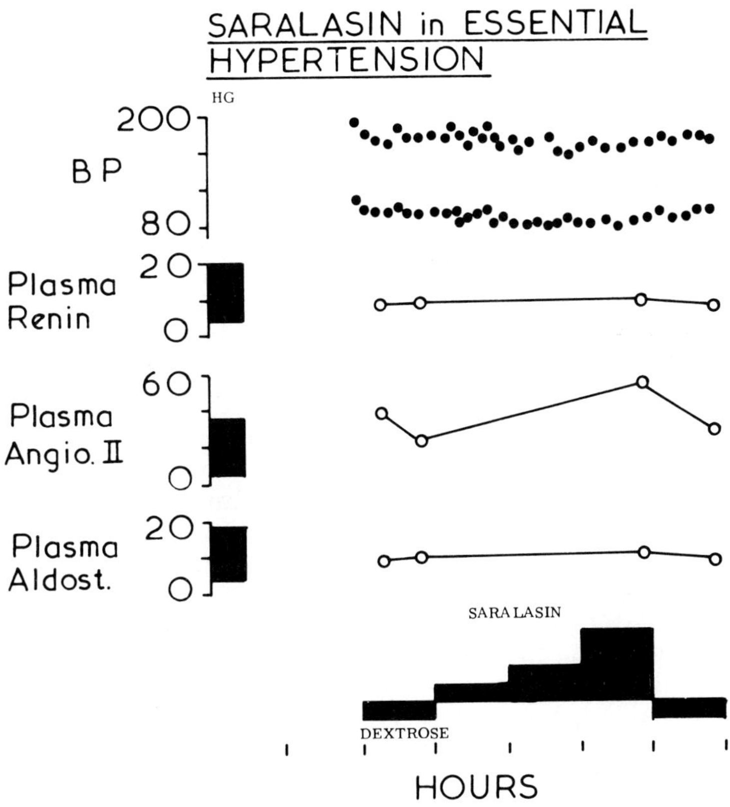

FIGURE 4.

dialysis therapy (Fig. 5). In the patients with unilateral renal artery stenosis (each with typical findings at urography, arteriography, ureteric catheterization, renin and angiotensin II measurements in bilateral renal vein plasma), less marked and less consistent changes were observed. Thus, in the 26-year-old male patient whose data are illustrated in Figure 6, saralasin infusion caused a moderate but distinct fall in blood pressure associated with a marked fall in plasma aldosterone and reciprocal alterations in both circulating renin and angiotensin II values. It is noteworthy that although the diastolic blood pressure did not fall below 120 mm Hg during this study (in which sodium intake remained normal), surgical reconstruction of the stenosed renal artery was followed by a return of arterial pressure to normal levels (122/80 eight months after operation).

The importance of sodium status in relation to the fall of blood pressure during saralasin infusion in patients with unilateral renal artery stenosis is illustrated in Figures 7 and 8. In a 45-year-old female patient (Fig. 7) infusion of saralasin during a period of normal sodium intake caused a symptomless fall of blood pressure to around 150/90 mm Hg. When the test was repeated four days later during sodium depletion, the saralasin infusion was stopped after nine minutes because of a precipitous fall of blood pressure (to 70/48 mm) with nausea, sweating, weakness and a sensation of impending loss of consciousness. The symptoms disappeared over the next ten minutes with a progressive increase of blood pressure back to basal values within 30 minutes. In the other patient, a 53-year-old male, infusion of saralasin during normal sodium intake did not cause a noteworthy change of blood pressure (Fig. 8). After three days of sodium depletion infusion of saralasin caused a small fall of blood pressure (200/123 to 188/109 mm Hg).

As illustrated in Figure 9, in the series as a whole, the fall of blood pressure during saralasin infusion was clearly related to the plasma angiotensin II concentrations during the initial control periods. The largest fall in blood pressure was observed in those patients with the highest basal plasma angiotensin II values.

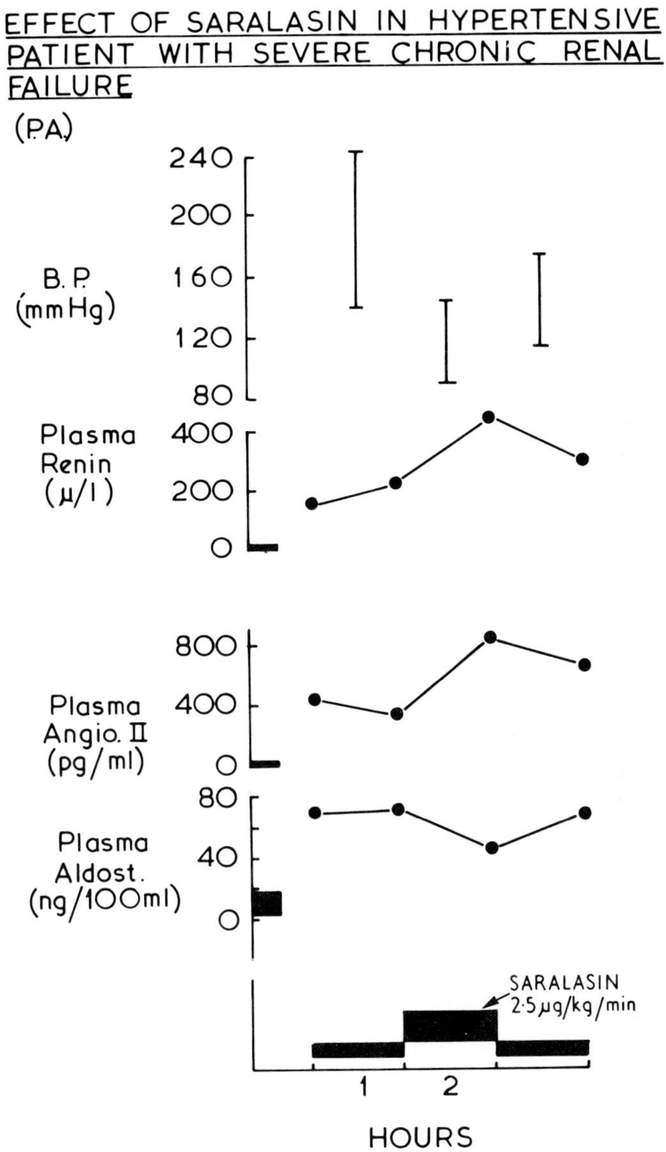
EFFECT OF SARALASIN IN HYPERTENSIVE PATIENT WITH SEVERE CHRONIC RENAL FAILURE
(P.A.)
B. P. (mm Hg)
240
200
160
120
80
Plasma Renin (μ/l)
400
200
0
800
Plasma Angio. II (pg/ml)
400
0
80
Plasma Aldost. (ng/100ml)
40
0
SARALASIN 2·5 μg/kg/min
1
2
HOURS

FIGURE 5.

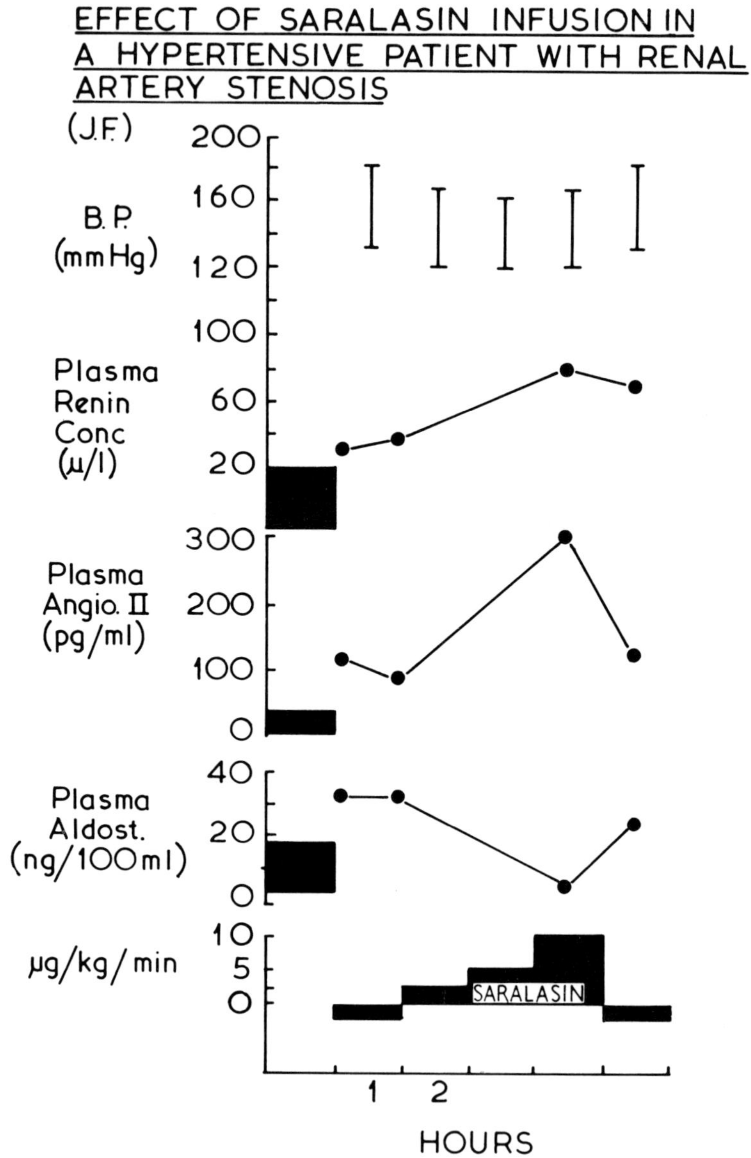
EFFECT OF SARALASIN INFUSION IN A HYPERTENSIVE PATIENT WITH RENAL ARTERY STENOSIS
(J.F.)
B.P. (mm Hg)
200
160
120
100
Plasma Renin Conc (μ/l)
60
20
300
Plasma Angio. II (pg/ml)
200
100
0
40
Plasma Aldost. (ng/100ml)
20
0
10
μg/kg/min
5
0
SARALASIN
1
2
HOURS

FIGURE 6.

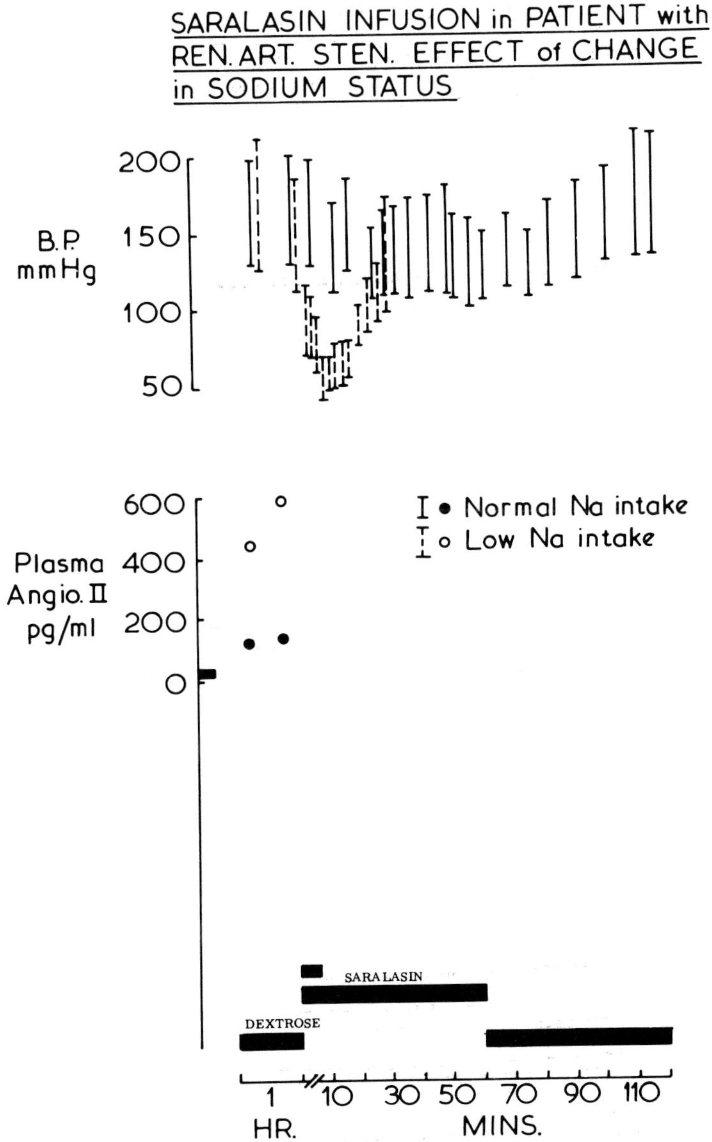
SARALASIN INFUSION in PATIENT with REN. ART. STEN. EFFECT of CHANGE in SODIUM STATUS
B.P. mmHg
200
150
100
50
Plasma Angio. II pg/ml
600
400
200
0
Normal Na intake
Low Na intake
SARALASIN
DEXTROSE
1
HR.
10 30 50 70 90 110
MINS.

FIGURE 7.

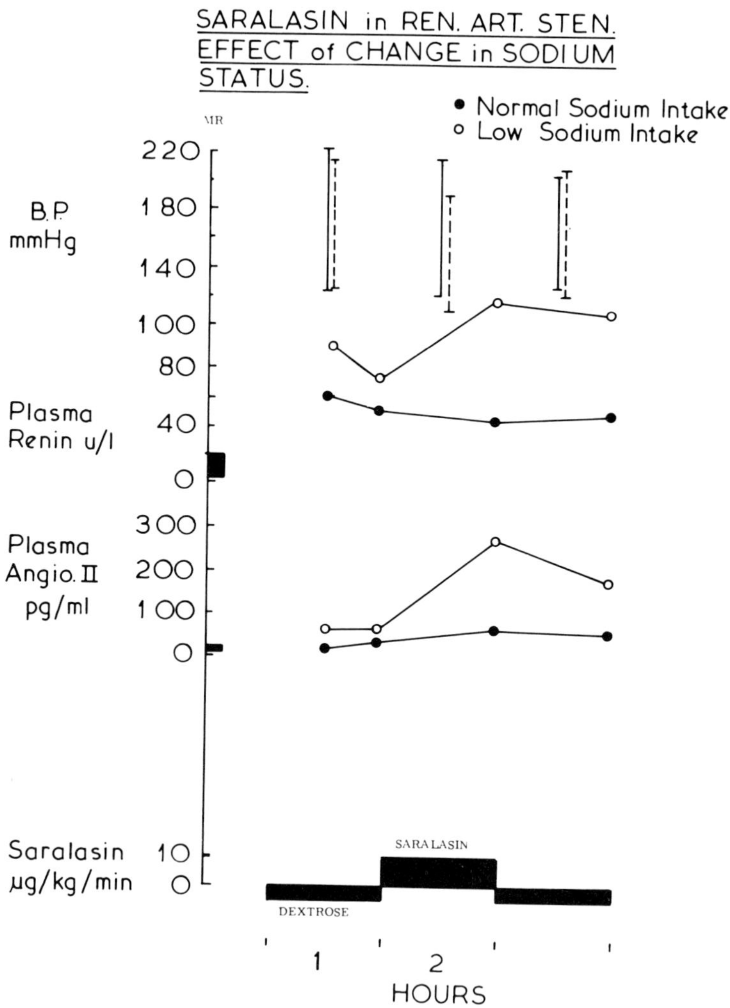
SARALASIN in REN. ART. STEN.
EFFECT of CHANGE in SODIUM STATUS.
• Normal Sodium Intake
○ Low Sodium Intake
MR
B.P mmHg
220
180
140
100
80
Plasma Renin u/l
40
0
300
Plasma Angio. II pg/ml
200
100
0
Saralasin µg/kg/min
10
0
SARALASIN
DEXTROSE
1
2
HOURS

FIGURE 8.

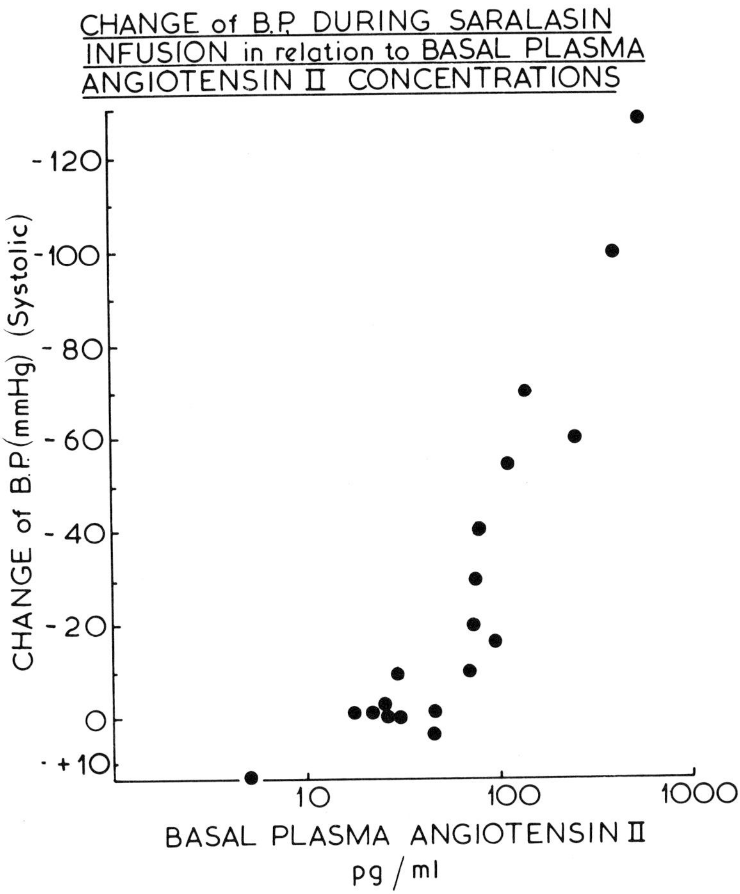
CHANGE of B.P. DURING SARALASIN INFUSION in relation to BASAL PLASMA ANGIOTENSIN II CONCENTRATIONS
CHANGE of B.P. (mmHg) (Systolic)
-120
-100
-80
-60
-40
-20
0
+10
10
100
1000
BASAL PLASMA ANGIOTENSIN II
pg/ml

FIGURE 9.

Conclusions

1. These results provide no evidence that renin and angiotensin are involved directly in the control of arterial blood pressure in normal supine subjects (whether sodium replete or deplete).
2. The renin-angiotensin system is directly involved in the pathogenesis of renal hypertension — at least in some circumstances.
3. The high plasma aldosterone values found in selected cases of renal hypertension, as well as in normal subjects during sodium depletion, are mediated, at least in part, by angiotensin II.
4. The effect of saralasin, on both blood pressure and plasma aldosterone concentration, can be more pronounced during sodium depletion.

Acknowledgments

We wish to thank Drs. R. Keenan, E. Harries and G. Hooper and Mrs. M. Vero of Eaton Laboratories Ltd. for generously supplying the saralasin, and Drs. A. Robertson and D. Barlow for their invaluable help with the studies in normal subjects.

References

1. Davis, J.O.: The use of blocking agents to define the functions of the renin-angiotensin system. Clin. Sci. Molec. Med. 48:1s, 1975.
2. Pals, D.T., Masucci, F.D., Denning, G.S. et al: Role of the pressor action of angiotensin II in experimental hypertension. Circ. Res. 29:673, 1971.
3. Brown, J.J., Davies, D.L., Lever, A.F. et al: The estimation of renin in human plasma. Biochem. J. 93:594, 1964.
4. Dusterdieck, G. and McElwee, G.: Estimation of angiotensin II concentration in human plasma by radioimmunoassay. Some applications to physiological and clinical states. Europ. J. Clin. Invest. 2:32-38, 1971.
5. Fraser, R., Guest, S. and Young, J.: A comparison of double isotope derivative and radioimmunological estimation of plasma aldosterone concentration in man. Clin. Sci. Molec. Med. 45:411, 1973.

Discussion

Moderator: Dr. F. M. Bumpus

Dr. Zanchetti: I think that the clear data by Dr. Brown leads us back to the argument of what is the meaning of using blocking agents to understand the mechanism of hypertension. In the previous discussion it has been said that it has very little meaning, because the mechanisms of hypertension are so complex, and if another factor is going to compensate the one that has been knocked down, then there is little hope of our gaining understanding. I certainly am not ready to dispute that hypertension mechanisms are very complicated, especially with Dr. Page being here. However, if compensation always and completely occurred, I think we would have lost the splendid opportunity of being here and discussing a treatment of hypertension because it would be thoroughly impossible to decrease blood pressure. I think the use of blocking agents is more or less rewarding according to the kinds of questions we are asking ourselves before making the observations. So if the question is: By using the blocking agent, am I going to understand if this particular mechanism is responsible for the hypertension? I think the observation is going to be misleading. I think that none of us would be ready to say that a given hypertension is due to overactivity of the sympathetic system because of blood pressure decrease with sympatho-inhibitory agents or that it is due to expansion of body fluid because of the favorable results of a diuretic. But if the question is: Does this particular mechanism play a role in the regulation of blood pressure in this particular subject? I think that particularly with blocking agents of short lasting action which, of course, are not so easily compensated, then the answer can be very useful and rewarding. I think that some of these agents can identify some patients in which renin is not necessarily the causative agent of hypertension but is really playing some pressor role, certainly more than it is in normotensive subjects.

Dr. Brown: I think I did not discuss the findings in relation to the etiology of hypertension. That was no accident. But if you push me, I think that I would suggest that in these particular circumstances, and I would not go beyond those, the results do suggest that the high levels of A II that we found in some of these patients were contributing to the level of blood pressure.

Dr. Williams: I have one question to ask Dr. Brown. I noticed that your A II levels went up during the course of the infusion. We saw the same thing, until someone had the brilliant idea that maybe we are cross-reacting with the P-113. The cross-reactivity was only about 1/100 of 1%. But at the doses that we were using, that is probably what we were measuring.

Dr. Brown: I can deal with that briefly. We have checked cross-reactions and, like you, we have found very little. However, I think we ought to extend this work to include higher concentrations of saralasin, in view of the high plasma concentrations recently reported by Pettinger during similar infusions. But in most of these patients in fact the change of angiotensin II was closely parallel to the change of renin. So that I do not think there is any major cross-reaction.

Dr. Mulrow: I have a question for Dr. Brown, specifically related to your slide showing the relationship between the depressor effect of P-113 and angiotensin II blood levels. I would like to ask how you think two kinds of patients would respond. One is the patient with renal artery stenosis who has normal levels of plasma renin activity and angiotensin II. From the slide you showed earlier, I would predict that there would not be much of a drop in blood pressure.

Second, if you had a patient who had essential hypertension, whom you volume depleted sufficiently, so you raise the A II levels into higher levels, would you expect that patient to have a depressor effect from P-113?

Dr. Brown: We have data on the first of those questions, that is, we have seen patients with renal artery stenosis with normal plasma levels of renin A II. When such patients were infused with saralasin, blood pressure did not fall. In fact, as I hope I said, in the whole series the response could be related, whatever the etiology, to the basal plasma levels of angiotensin II or renin. So we have evidence on that.

We have not yet done sodium depleting experiments in patients with essential hypertension, so I have no information to offer on that. I agree that it is something which we should do.

Dr. Doyle: I would like to ask Dr. Brown, in view of the relationship between the angiotensin levels and the fall in blood pressure which you showed, whether you have any data as to the amount of inhibitor that you have to give in relation to those alterations in plasma levels. Presumably, it is acting by competitive inhibition. One would anticipate that you would need a bigger dose to deal with the higher levels. Is that so?

Dr. Brown: We have not studied the effect of saralasin at doses less than 1μg/kg/min; perhaps we should in view of the results just reported by Dr. Williams. But what I can say is that the blood pressure in the patient with the highest levels of angiotensin II reaching 600 pg/ml, was reduced to near normal levels, as you saw, by saralasin given at 2.5 μg/kg/min. Whether we would have achieved the same response using a lower rate of infusion I cannot say because we did not try it. But it would seem from that evidence that we should get a maximum response unless there are marked changes in receptor avidity, with the 2.5 μg/kg/min infusions becuase we do often see levels of angiotensin II higher than that.

Dr. Gross: Dr. Brown, do you think that when you administer a low sodium diet or deprive the animals of sodium in cases of renal artery stenosis — as you have shown especially in the third case, the one with high angiotensin II levels and high renin activity — the renin-angiotensin system has some kind of emergency function to maintain blood pressure?

Dr. Brown: It would seem so. In the slide illustrating the data in the second case of renal artery stenosis, as you saw, there was no change in blood pressure in the basal state (while taking a normal fixed sodium intake), although that was associated with an increase in angiotensin II. When we then gave the antagonist after sodium depletion there was a major fall of blood pressure despite the further increase in plasma angiotensin II. So presumably in that circumstance the A II was helping to maintain the high blood pressure.

Dr. Streeten: I wanted to ask Dr. Brown, in the patients he has encountered with renal arterial stenosis and no response to saralasin (of whom we have quite a number, too), whether in fact the renal vein renin ratio was abnormal and/or whether the patients responded to surgery. Those are just the types of cases we are looking for, who may indicate that this procedure does let one down, but so far we have not found any like that.

Dr. Brown: We have only seen a couple of these. In these patients there were no marked differences in the plasma concentrations of renin or angiotensin II in left versus right renal vein plasma. Not surprisingly, we have not operated on these patients.

Dr. Coghlan: I have a comment for Dr. Brown. With the four papers concerning the effect of P-113 on aldosterone secretion in sodium-depleted normals, either man or sheep, there is reasonable concordance between all of us. Although both you and Dr. Williams got a fall, it was very modest. This might be largely due to reduced clearance rate. So it is possible that the actual secretion rate changes are very tiny.

Dr. Brown: I agree, that is possible. I hope I referred to changes in plasma aldosterone concentration only. I would not wish to infer that there was necessarily a similar alteration in aldosterone secretion. We need to check this by measurements of metabolic clearance rate of aldosterone during saralasin.

Dr. Coghlan: Is splanchnic flow increased or decreased? We simply do not know. One of the things that I did not mention earlier today is that the adrenal blood flow is normally extremely resistant to increased angiotensin II concentration. However, P-113 at the higher doses in the sodium-deficient sheep increased adrenal blood flow.

Dr. Brown: I have to accept that. I was very careful to use the term "plasma aldosterone concentration" and I am not necessarily extrapolating from that to aldosterone secretion.

The Therapeutic Potential of Angiotensin Antagonists

David H. P. Streeten, M.B., D. Phil.,
Gunnar H. Anderson, Jr., M.D.
Theodore G. Dalakos, M.D., J. Michael Freiberg, M.D.
and Edward T. Schroeder, M.D.

There is now compelling evidence that angiotensin II is the cause of hypertension in some patients who have high circulating and renal-vein levels of plasma renin activity (PRA) and angiotensin II, and in whom blood pressure returns to normal when (a) the release of excessive amounts of renin is prevented by arterial bypass surgery or nephrectomy; or (b) the formation of angiotensin II is prevented by the converting enzyme inhibitor SQ 20,881 [1]; or (c) the action of circulating angiotensin II is specifically antagonized by a chemical analogue such as saralasin, 1-sar-8-ala-angiotensin II [2-4]. Those patients, in whom hypertension is shown by evidence such as that cited to be "angiotensinogenic," can often be satisfactorily treated by corrective surgery. In many instances, however, surgery appears not to be necessary or advisable since the blood

---

Supported by a Graduate Training Grant in Endocrinology (AMO7146) from the National Institute of Arthritis, Metabolism and Digestive Diseases, A Clinical Research Center Grant (RR-00229) from the Division of Research Facilities and Resources; a grant from the Central New York Regional Medical Program and a grant from Eaton Laboratories, Norwich, N.Y.

David H. P. Streeten, M.B., D.Phil., F.R.C.P., Professor of Medicine and Head, Section of Endocrinology; Gunnar H. Anderson, Jr., M.D., Instructor in Medicine; Theodore G. Dalakos, M.D., Assistant Professor of Medicine; J. Michael Freiberg, M.D., Previously Research Fellow in Endocrinology; and Edward T. Schroeder, M.D., Associate Professor of Medicine, Department of Medicine, Section of Endocrinology, State University of New York, Upstate Medical Center, Syracuse.

pressure can be satisfactorily controlled by nonspecific antihypertensive therapy, or since a unilateral lesion which would be amenable to surgery may not be present. The questions which will be addressed in this paper are:

1. How commonly does angiotensin cause hypertension in the absence of an evident surgically correctable lesion?
2. What is the likelihood that prevention of angiotensin II formation or antagonism of its action might be more helpful than other available therapy in such cases of angiotensinogenic hypertension?

How Common Is Angiotensinogenic Hypertension Which Cannot Be Successfully Treated Surgically?

We are currently studying in hypertensive patients the blood pressure responses to infusions of saralasin (0.05-10.0 μg/kg/min) starting 3½ hours after intravenous injection of furosemide (40 mg) [5]. In 69 of 643 hypertensive patients (10.7%) who have been given saralasin infusions, the blood pressure fell to an extent greater than that seen in any of 29 normal subjects so treated (ie, by more than 10/8 mm Hg). Measurements of PRA in blood from both renal veins have been completed in 50 of these patients. A ratio greater than 1.5 between the PRA levels in the two renal veins, presumably signifying unilaterality of the lesion causing excessive renin release [6], was found in 23 of the 50 patients. Among these 23 patients arteriography disclosed a macroscopic renal arterial constriction on the side of the higher PRA level which was treated by renal arterial bypass surgery or nephrectomy in 12 patients. All 12 patients are alive more than six months after surgery, with diastolic blood pressures below 90 mm Hg in 11 and considerably reduced, from 132 to 92 mm Hg in the 12th patient. The remaining 38 patients were not operated upon either because no arteriographic evidence of renal arterial stenosis could be found or because such lesions were bilateral or considered inoperable in the presence of renal insufficiency.

It cannot be claimed that the 643 patients who were the subjects of this study were completely unselected, since it must be assumed that physicians would tend to refer their more severely ill hypertensive patients for study. The exact incidence of angiotensinogenic hypertension whether correctable by surgery or not cannot, therefore, be deduced from these findings or from any other observations in the literature. However, since these patients were virtually all derived from the Central New York area (total population 0.8 million) and seen within an 18-month period, the findings clearly indicate that surgically incorrectable angiotensinogenic hypertension is a fairly common disorder, comprising as it did at least 38 of 643, or 6% of the hypertensives studied.

Is "Specific" Better Than "Non-specific" Therapy of Angiotensinogenic Hypertension?

Patients with angiotensin-dependent hypertension may have three different types of responses to therapy:

1. The first type comprises a fall in blood pressure to normal in response to simple measures such as a small dose of chlorthalidone with or without methyldopa and without any noticeable side effects. At present there is no evidence that the prognosis in these patients might be improved by the use of therapy aimed specifically at reducing blood pressure via inhibition or antagonism of angiotensin II. However, it should be recognized that the treatment of these patients with diuretics would almost certainly raise their plasma angiotensin levels even further despite the blood pressure lowering effect of the drugs which must be brought about through another mechanism. The possibility that hyperangiotensinemia per se might have serious effects on the vasculature, even in the absence of hypertension, has to be considered in view of experimental evidence of endothelial damage resulting from angiotensin II in animals [7]. Although there is, as yet, no positive evidence to indicate that an angiotensin antagonist or an angiotensin lowering drug would be preferable to drugs which raise plasma angiotensin levels further in these patients, this possibility deserves serious consideration.

2. A second group of patients responds less satisfactorily to the usual mixtures of antihypertensive agents and appears to show a better response, frequently with a fall to normal blood pressure levels, when propranolol is used in their treatment.

Thus, in nine of our patients with surgically incorrectable angiotensinogenic hypertension, we have been able, in conjunction with the referring physicians, to substitute propranolol for all previous medications. On propranolol alone blood pressure has fallen to lower levels than on the various previous combinations of therapy in eight of the nine patients so treated, the mean diastolic pressure falling from 124 ± 7.7 (SEM) to 97 ± 5.3 mm Hg ($p < 0.02$). Although propranolol is known to lower blood pressure by mechanisms other than by reducing PRA, there is no doubt that it does lower PRA. Our limited observations indicate that in patients with angiotensinogenic hypertension its effects on blood pressure are seen only if and when PRA is reduced by this drug. Furthermore, there is in these patients an excellent correlation between the blood pressure response to propranolol and to saralasin ($r = +0.76$, $n = 8$, $p < 0.01$) as we have reported previously [3]. To the extent that its PRA-lowering action might reasonably be interpreted as a specific antihypertensive mechanism in patients with this type of angiotensinogenic hypertension [8], specific therapy appears to have advantages over nonspecific therapy.

3. The third type of therapeutic response seen in patients with angiotensinogenic hypertension is fortunately less common but much more serious than the other two types. In these patients, who often have some of the clinical features of malignant hypertension, blood pressure remains severely elevated despite large doses of propranolol and other antihypertensive agents in various combinations. The patients frequently have severe, progressive renal insufficiency and may require bilateral nephrectomy as a life-saving procedure [9, 10]. Some of them respond to minoxidil therapy [11], but this does not always avert a fatal outcome in our limited experience. When such patients have presented with acute features of malignant or advanced hypertension, it has been found that intravenous infusions of saralasin lowered the blood pressure in three of seven patients [2]. The three responders to saralasin had high PRA whereas the four who responded poorly or not at all had normal or low levels of PRA. Similarly, in four patients with malignant hypertension and high peripheral PRA levels to whom we have given saralasin infusions, the blood pressure fell somewhat in all cases, without side effects. Figure 1 shows the

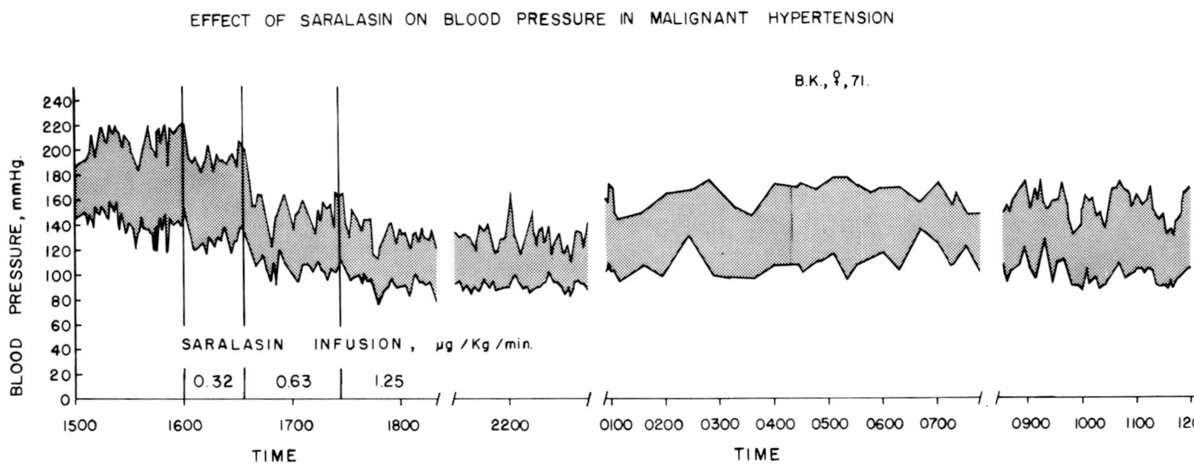

FIG. 1. BP measurements in a female with unilateral renal arterial occlusion, high peripheral PRA levels and malignant hypertension before and during an intravenous infusion of saralasin lasting 20 hours. At 1.25μg/kg/min, saralasin maintained greatly improved BP. BP measurements in this and subsequent figures were recorded automatically with an Arteriosonde (Roche).

reduction of blood pressure starting within a few minutes of the onset of a saralasin infusion at 0.32μg/kg/min, with a further fall when the infusion was accelerated to 0.63μg/kg/min and still a further fall to frequently normal levels of blood pressure (approximately 110-160/75-100 mm Hg) at an infusion rate of 1.25μg/kg/min in a woman with renal arterial occlusion and malignant hypertension. Good blood pressure control continued over a 20-hour period of saralasin infusion in this patient. Among our four patients with malignant hypertension, however, normal levels of blood pressure were reached in only two of the patients with saralasin alone. Nitroprusside was more effective than saralasin in two of these patients. Thus, the present inadequate evidence suggests that saralasin is an effective, safe hypotensive agent in malignant hypertension, but that it is not as consistently successful as nitroprusside in lowering the blood pressure. Furthermore, saralasin is frequently less effective in malignant hypertension, as indeed in all types of angiotensinogenic hypertension, when the patients are salt loaded and unless a diuretic is administered beforehand or concurrently. Figure 2 shows blood pressure falling inadequately (from 219/130 to 201/129) during saralasin infusion at 1 and 10μg/kg/min in a man of 54 with malignant hypertension and a more satisfactory fall (to 166/116) between one and five hours after furosemide administration (80 mg intravenously) during continuing infusion of saralasin at 1μg/kg/min. In view of its lack of toxicity and its failure to lower blood pressure below normal levels when administered alone or with a diuretic, saralasin might eventually become recognized as the best drug with which to initiate the treatment of patients with malignant hypertensive crises. When saralasin and furosemide fail to lower blood pressure adequately within 15 to 30 minutes in such patients, however, it would seem wise to rely instead on other forms of therapy, especially nitroprusside infusion or diazoxide injections.

Need for Angiotensin Antagonist in Chronic Therapy

A more difficult problem is posed by patients with angiotensinogenic hypertension which responds inadequately to the chronic use of propranolol therapy, with or without other

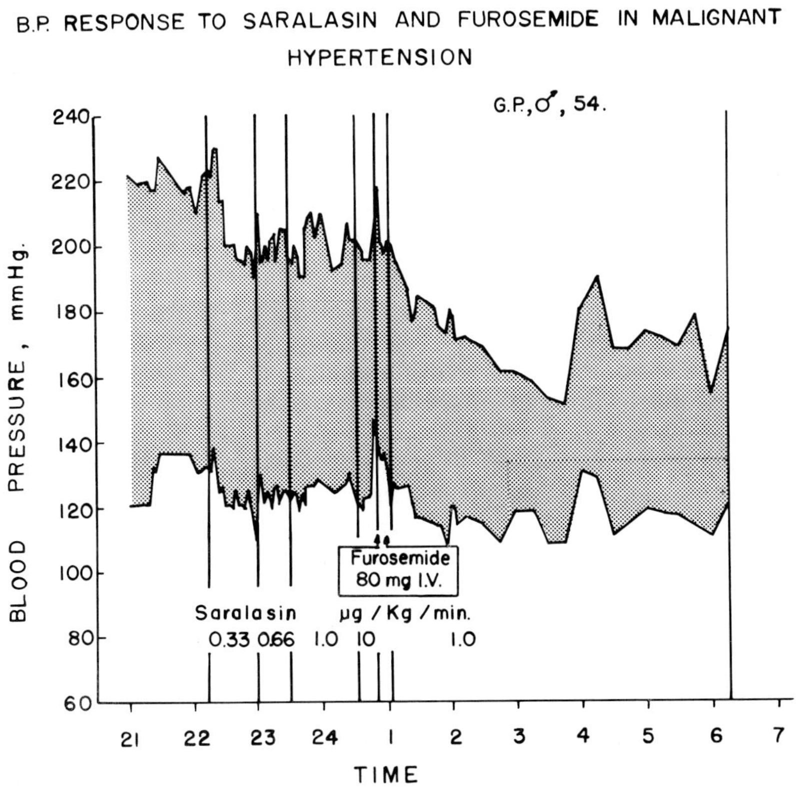

FIG. 2. BP measurements in a man of 54 with malignant hypertension, showing a poor response in BP to saralasin infusion alone (BP 219/130 — 201/129), with a better response to continuing saralasin infusion (to 166/116) after an intravenous injection of furosemide, 80 mg. From 0100 to 0625, saralasin was infused at 1.0μg/kg/min.

oral agents. The following case report exemplifies this predicament:

V.K. was first seen by our group in 1967 when she was 27 and had had hypertension and Raynaud's phenomenon in the fingers for a few months. Because of the severity of her hypertension (diastolic 110-120 mm Hg) and her young age, she was studied extensively and found to have normal physical findings (except for the hypertension), normal serum electrolytes, blood count, and urinalysis, normal creatinine clearance (100 ml/min), normal excretion of VMA, epinephrine (8.1μg) and norepinephrine (38.8μg/day), no response to phentolamine (5 mg intravenously), a normal PRA of 1600 ng/100 ml (by bioassay) after four hours in the upright posture on the fourth day of a 10 mEq Na diet (normal 500-2000 ng/100 ml), normal aldosterone excretion on a 200 mEq Na diet (17.2μg/day), a normal intravenous pyelogram and a normal aortogram. A needle biopsy of one kidney showed no abnormalities of the juxtaglomerular apparatus and only mild arteriolar nephrosclerosis. She left the Syracuse area shortly after these observations had been made and was treated vigorously with various drugs including guanethidine (up to 100 mg), methyldopa (2 gm), hydrochlorothiazide (100 mg) and spironolactone (100 mg) without improvement in her hypertension. In 1969, she was referred to another clinic where further studies, including another arteriogram and renin measurements, confirmed the normal observations made in 1967. Blood pressure remained refractory to therapy and she was seen again in our hospital for a few days in February 1974. Blood pressure was 240/150, the fundi contained some exudates and severe arteriolar narrowing, and there was cardiomegaly on x-ray. Urinalysis revealed 3+ proteinuria, without cells in the sediment, while the BUN was 36 mg%, serum creatinine 2.0 mg%, and an isotopic renal flow study and scan [12] revealed bilateral renal parenchymal disease. After adhering to a 10 mEq Na diet for three days she was found to show a striking fall in blood pressure to the normal range during an intravenous infusion of saralasin (Fig. 3). PRA was measured by radioimmunoassay of angiotensin I after standing for two hours and was very high: 51.3 ng/ml/hr (normal up to 14.6 ng/ml/hr). Renal vein PRA levels were approximately equal (rt 42.7, lt 35.1 ng/ml/hr) while the PRA in the inferior vena cava (below the renal veins) was 19.7 ng/ml/hr at the same time. It was evident that severe angiotensinogenic hypertension had developed between 1969 and 1974. The patient was given propranolol (200 mg/day) which caused the blood pressure to fall initially to 138/100. After a few weeks, however, the blood pressure again rose and propranolol therapy was discontinued. The patient was started on treatment with minoxidil at another Center but developed intractable congestive heart failure in spite of concomitant diuretic therapy. Renal insufficiency became rapidly progressive and she

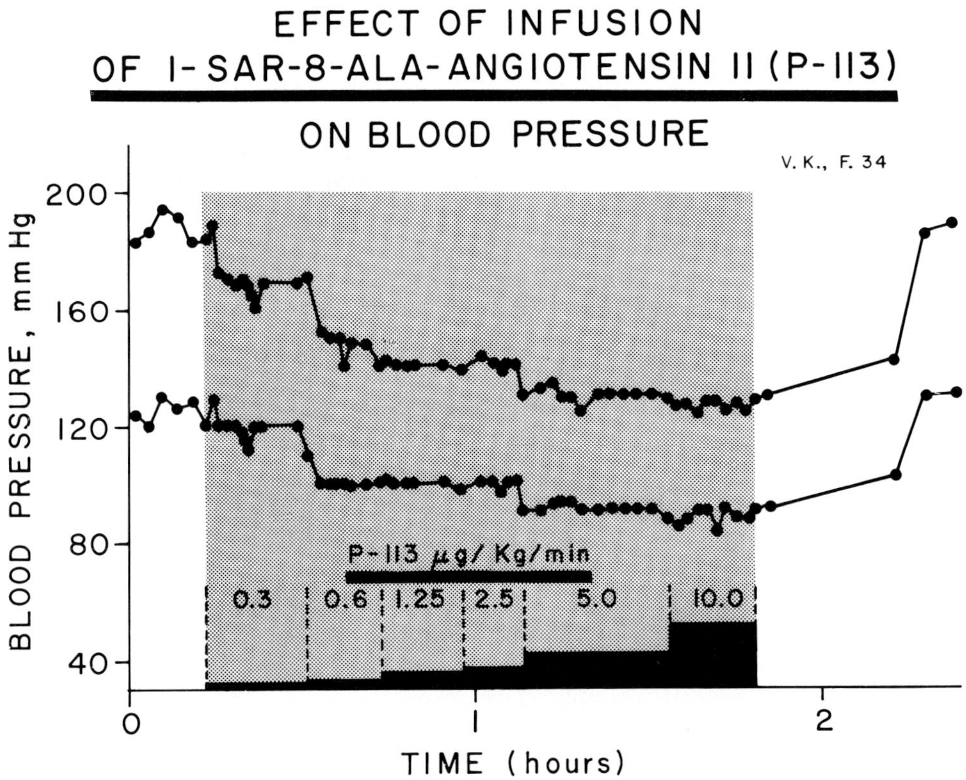

FIG. 3. Excellent BP response to increasing rates of infusion of saralasin in a female with severe angiotensinogenic hypertension of bilateral renal origin. The patient died five months later.

died in August 1974 while awaiting nephrectomy and renal transplantation. Thus, this patient had angiotensinogenic hypertension in February and March 1974 with an excellent blood pressure response to saralasin and relatively mild renal insufficiency. Five months later the renal lesion had progressed to severe renal insufficiency and she died.

Another patient has been studied with similar results and the same outcome. Initially she was found to have angiotensinogenic hypertension with bilaterally equal renal vein PRA levels (each slightly above 100 ng/ml/hr by radioimmunoassay of angiotensin I) and a good fall in blood pressure during saralasin infusion in December 1974. She was treated with large doses of propranolol (up to 1.6 gm/day) together with furosemide for several weeks in the hospital, but the blood pressure remained between 180/120 and 240/140. A trial of therapy with minoxidil was more successful, reducing her blood pressure initially to 140-180/80-110. This treatment was maintained for several weeks and the patient was discharged and seemed to improve. Later she developed congestive heart failure with increasing pedal edema despite diuretic therapy and the blood pressure rose to 200/130 in spite of minoxidil 30 mg, propranolol 160 mg and furosemide 120 mg per day. She was readmitted with abdominal pain which preceded rupture of an abdominal aneurysm and sudden death from exsanguination 80 days after the blood pressure had been shown still to fall to normal levels during an intravenous infusion of saralasin (Fig. 4).

Besides these two patients who have died, we have had six additional patients on chronic hemodialysis with severe hypertension who were usually initially responsive to propranolol with lowered PRA but who later became unresponsive to propranolol therapy with an associated rise in plasma renin. Uncontrollable hypertension led eventually to bilateral nephrectomy. In these individuals, with no exceptions, the nephrectomy has been followed by a gratifying fall in blood pressure and dramatic clinical improvement. None of the patients treated in this way has yet died. Each of three patients who were tested with saralasin infusion before nephrectomy showed a significant hypotensive response.

Of the 643 "unselected" patients who were given saralasin infusions, death, apparently attributable to hypertension, has occurred within 18 months in five patients with angiotensinogenic hypertension, one patient with normal renin essential hypertension and two patients with low renin hypertension. This strikingly higher incidence of rapid death in the small group of angiotensinogenic hypertensives (10% of the total) is in good agreement with the evidence of far more serious prognoses in the group of "high renin" hypertensives recorded in a similar prospective study [13]. Thus, there is a real need to find more effective methods of treating these patients, preferably before renal insufficiency becomes extreme and by methods short of bilateral nephrectomy.

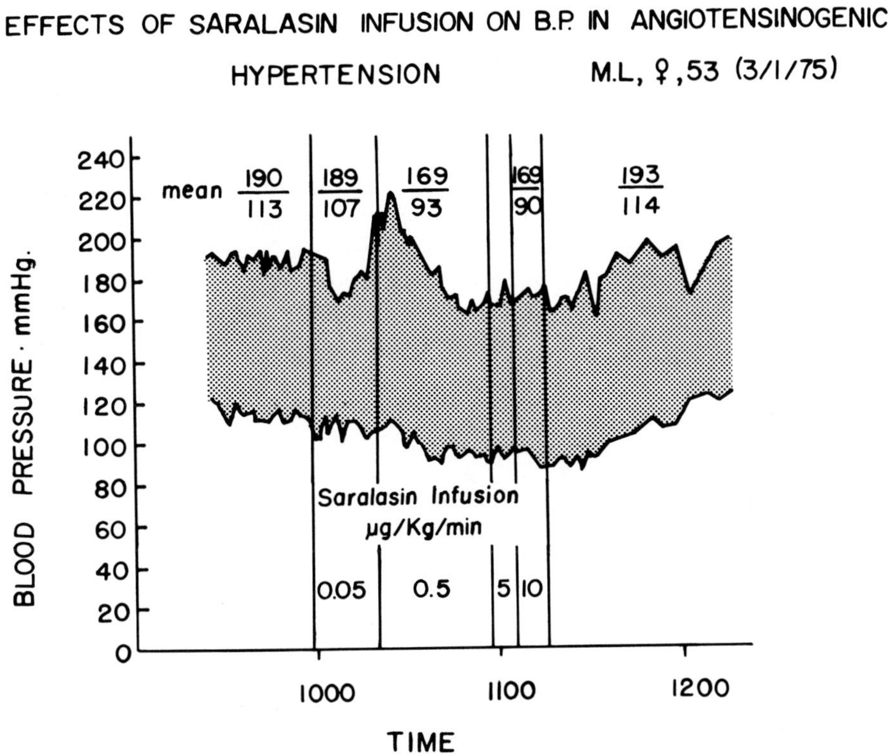

FIG. 4. Good BP response to saralasin infusion in a woman of 53 with severe angiotensinogenic hypertension resulting from bilateral elevation of renal renin production. The patient died 80 days later of a ruptured aortic aneurysm when her blood pressure rose in spite of continuing minoxidil therapy.

Since at least two of these patients with severe angiotensinogenic hypertension have remained responsive to saralasin until a few months before their demise, it becomes important to determine whether long-term antagonism of angiotensin II or prevention of its formation by a converting enzyme inhibitor might be effective and consequently life-saving. Unfortunately, saralasin has very short biochemical and pharmacological half-lives after its intravenous administration to rats (4.2 and 3.9 minutes, respectively) [14]. Subcutaneous injection in Pharmagel A has greatly prolonged these half-lives but not to an extent sufficient to give much hope that subcutaneous injections two or three times daily might control blood pressure in patients with angiotensinogenic hypertension. The far longer duration of action of the converting enzyme inhibitor SQ 20,881 suggests that this compound might well become an effective and valuable agent in the therapy of otherwise uncontrollable angiotensinogenic hypertension. A therapeutic trial of subcutaneously injected saralasin in Pharmagel A, or SQ 20,881, would be of great interest and well worth while.

References

1. Gavras, H., Brunner, H.R., Laragh, J.H. et al: An angiotensin converting-enzyme inhibitor to identify and treat vasoconstrictor and volume factors in hypertensive patients. N. Engl. J. Med. 291:817, 1974.
2. Brunner, H.R., Gavras, H., Laragh, J.H. et al: Angiotensin II blockade in man by sar^{1}-ala^{8}-angiotensin II for understanding and treatment of high blood-pressure. Lancet 2:1045, 1973.
3. Streeten, D.H.P., Anderson, G.H., Freiberg, J.M. et al: Use of an angiotensin II antagonist (saralasin) in the recognition of "angiotensinogenic" hypertension. N. Engl. J. Med. 292:657, 1975.
4. Streeten, D.H.P., Freiberg, J.M., Anderson, G.H. et al: Identification of angiotensinogenic hypertension in man using 1-sar-8-ala-angiotensin II (saralasin, P-113). Circ. Res. 36(suppl 1):1-125, 1975.
5. Freiberg, J.M., Anderson, G.H., Dalakos, T.G. et al: An 8-hour screening test for remediable hypertension. Clin. Res. 23:183A, 1975.
6. Vaughan, E.D., Jr., Bühler, F.R., Laragh, J.H. et al: Renovascular hypertension: Renin measurements to indicate hypersecretion and contralateral suppression, estimate renal plasma flow and score for surgical curability. Am. J. Med. 55:402, 1973.
7. Kincaid-Smith, P., Hobbs, J.B. and Friedman, A.: Structural and ultra-structural alterations in mesenteric and renal arterioles following infusion of vaso-active agents. *In* Genest, J. and Koiw, E. (eds.): Hypertension — 1972. 2nd International Symposium on the Renin-Angiotensin-Aldosterone-Sodium System. Berlin, Heidelberg and New York:Springer, 1972, p. 97.
8. Bühler, F.R., Laragh, J.H., Baer, L. et al: Propranolol inhibition of renin secretion: Specific approach to diagnosis and treatment of renin-dependent hypertensive diseases. N. Engl. J. Med. 287:1209, 1972.
9. Mahony, J.F., Gibson, G.R., Shiel, A.G.R. et al: Bilateral nephrectomy for malignant hypertension. Lancet 1:1036, 1972.
10. Vertes, V., Cangiano, J.L., Berman, L.B. et al: Hypertension in end-stage renal disease. N. Engl. J. Med. 280:978, 1969.

11. Pettinger, W.A. and Mitchell, H.C.: Minoxidil: An alternative to nephrectomy for refractory hypertension. N. Engl. J. Med. 289:167, 1973.
12. Bell, E.G., Sandler, M., O'Mara, R.E. et al: Use of ^{99m}Tc-iron ascorbate complex in the evaluation of diffuse renal parenchymal disease. J. Nucl. Med. 12:339, 1971.
13. Brunner, H.R., Laragh, J.H., Baer, L. et al: Essential hypertension: Renin and aldosterone, heart attack and stroke. N. Engl. J. Med. 286:441, 1972.
14. Pettinger, W.A., Keeton, K. and Tanaka, K.: Radioimmunoassay and pharmacokinetics of saralasin in the rat and hypertensive patients. Clin. Pharmacol. Ther. 17:146, 1975.

1-Sar, 8-Ala Angiotensin II's Effect on Renal, Adrenal and Vascular Receptors in Man

Its Usefulness in Screening for Renal and Adrenal Diseases

Gordon H. Williams, M.D. and
Norman K. Hollenberg, M.D., Ph.D.

Introduction

Recently, a series of analogues which act as antagonists to angiotensin II have been synthesized [1-4]. These agents have been useful in the characterization of angiotensin II receptors and in assessing its role in the pathogenesis of hypertension [5-10]. In this report, we have characterized the blockade of vascular and adrenal responses to angiotensin II in man produced by 1-Sar, 8-Ala angiotensin II (P113) [11]. It is not surprising that these studies also demonstrated that P113 acts as a partial agonist, ie, possesses intrinsic activity under certain conditions, since it was produced by a modification of the parent compound's structure. Thus, these studies provide

---

This work was supported by grants from NIH (HL14944, GM 18674, HE 05832), the John A. Hartford Foundation, Massachusetts Institute of Technology Health Science Fund, and the contract from U.S. Army R & D Command (DA-49-193-MD-2497).

Investigations were carried out in part in the Clinical Research Center of the Peter Bent Brigham Hospital, supported by NIH Grant (5-MO1-RR-31).

Gordon H. Williams, M.D. and Norman K. Hollenberg, M.D., Ph.D., Departments of Medicine and Radiology, Peter Bent Brigham Hospital and Harvard Medical School, Boston, Mass.

insight into the angiotensin II receptor mediating the renal, adrenal and vascular responses to angiotensin II and define P113's potential and limitations as a diagnostic and therapeutic agent.

Methods

These studies were carried out in 45 normal subjects, including 35 normal potential kidney donors, and in 65 subjects with hypertension. The normal subjects ranged in age from 22 to 58 years and the patients with hypertension from 21 to 66 years. Each received a careful evaluation with special emphasis on cardiovascular, renal and adrenal status, as described previously [12]. They were admitted to a metabolic ward and placed on a diet providing a constant dietary intake of 2500 ml of water, 100 mEq of potassium and 10 or 200 mEq of sodium for at least five days prior to study. Balance was assessed by measuring sodium and potassium excretion in 24-hour urine collections. Of the patients with hypertension, six were diagnosed as having primary aldosteronism confirmed by non-suppressible aldosterone secretion with sodium loading, low, unstimulatable renin activity, potassium wasting with sodium loading and demonstration of an adenoma at surgery with correction of blood pressure following its removal. Eight subjects were diagnosed as having renal hypertension on the basis of a renal arteriogram and bilateral renal vein renin estimations in a sodium-restricted state. The rest of the patients with hypertension had primary or essential hypertension or diffuse bilateral renal disease. Ten percent had low renin activity under the conditions of sodium restriction and upright posture.

Experimental Design

Two types of studies were carried out — those on the metabolic ward and those in the angiographic suite. Sixty percent of both the normotensive and hypertensive subjects had normal angiographic studies. The normal subjects who received arteriograms were those who were potential kidney donors, since a renal angiogram is part of their routine work-up in our hospital.

In subjects having a renal angiogram, the technique consists of a selective renal arterial catheterization, determination of renal blood flow with radioactive Xenon and external probe counting, and cardiovascular monitoring during the administration of vasoactive agents, as previously described [12]. In all subjects, at least 30 minutes were allowed to elapse between the arteriography and the initiation of the infusion of vasoactive materials. Studies on the metabolic ward were similar except only renin activity, blood pressure and aldosterone secretion were assessed in response to the infusion of the vasoactive material. All studies on the metabolic ward were performed after an overnight fast with patients supine for 12 to 24 hours. In both types of studies, after a 30 to 60 minute control period, a control sample was obtained for measurement of renin activity, aldosterone, cortisol, sodium and potassium. These determinations were repeated after the administration of the vasoactive material.

In the angiographic suite, arterial samples were used while venous samples were obtained in subjects studied on the metabolic ward. The dose of angiotensin II used in these studies was 10 ng/kg/min — a dose previously demonstrated to produce significant increments in aldosterone and blood pressure and decrements in renal blood flow. The dose of P113 utilized varied from 0.03μg/kg/min to 30μg/kg/min. In all studies, at least 30 minutes were allowed at a given dose prior to sampling. The vasoactive agents were infused intravenously in both sets of subjects using a constant infusion apparatus.*

Analytical Techniques

All blood samples were collected on ice, immediately spun and the plasma separated and frozen until the time of assay. Samples for plasma renin activity utilized EDTA as the anticoagulant; heparin was used in the samples for cortisol and aldosterone. Aldosterone and cortisol were measured by dis-

---

*The angiotensin II used was from CIBA Pharmaceutical Co., Summit, N.J., and the 1-Sar, 8-Ala angiotensin II (P113), saralasin acetate, was from Norwich Pharmaceutical Co., Norwich, N.Y.

placement analysis techniques, as previously described [13]. Plasma renin activity was measured by the radioimmunoassay of angiotensin I generated during a 30-minute incubation with endogenous substrate at 37°C [14]. No cross-reactivity was demonstrated between P113 and the angiotensin I antibody.

Mean renal blood flow was measured from the initial slope of 133 Xenon disappearance from the kidney, determined graphically with hematocrit corrected for tissue coefficient; compartmental analysis was also performed. Curves reanalyzed on a coded basis showed a coefficient of variation of 7%. Results are reported as mean ± standard error of the mean and they were evaluated statistically where appropriate with student *t* test or paired *t* test, otherwise the Wilcoxon Rank Sum (WRST) or Fisher Exact Test (FET) for nonparametric data was used [15]. The null hypothesis was rejected when the p value was less than 0.05.

The protocol was approved by the Human Experimental Committees of the Peter Bent Brigham Hospital and Harvard Medical School. Written permission for the procedure was obtained after careful description of the protocol.

Results

Normal Subjects

Effect of P113 on pressor and renal vascular responses. On a 200 mEq sodium intake, P113 induced a dose-related reduction in renal blood flow ($p < 0.01$) with a threshold dose between 0.1 and 0.3μg/kg/min (Fig. 1). In contrast to the dose response relationship between P113 and renal blood flow, there was no consistent relationship between the dose of P113 and the effect on blood pressure, although in most sodium-loaded subjects, P113 induced a rise in blood pressure in response to an infusion of 0.1μg/kg/min or greater (Fig. 1). P113's effect mimicked that of A II on these two systems except it possessed only 1/100th of A II's intrinsic activity.

In contrast, in states of high A II activity, induced, for example, by continuous infusion of 10 ng/kg/min of A II, P113 was an antagonist of the pressor and renal vascular responses at a dose of 0.1μg/kg/min (Fig. 2). Also, sodium restriction altered P113's effects. The sodium-restricted subject usually had a

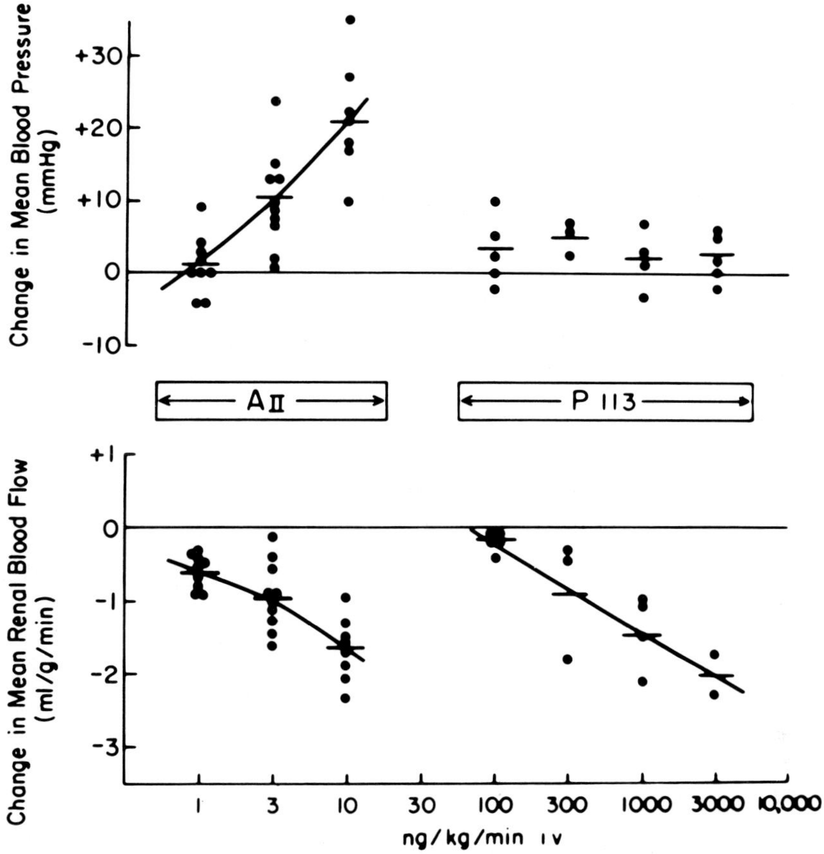

FIG. 1. Relationship between dose of agent infused (angiotensin II on the left and P113 on the right) and the pressor and renal vascular response in normal subjects. Endogenous renin was suppressed by a 200 mEq sodium, 100 mEq potassium diet. Note the similarity of the renal vascular responses to the two agents despite A II's 300-fold greater potency. Note also that unlike A II, P113 did not induce a dose-related pressor response. These observations suggest a difference in the vascular receptor mediating responses to A II in the renal and systemic circulation [11].

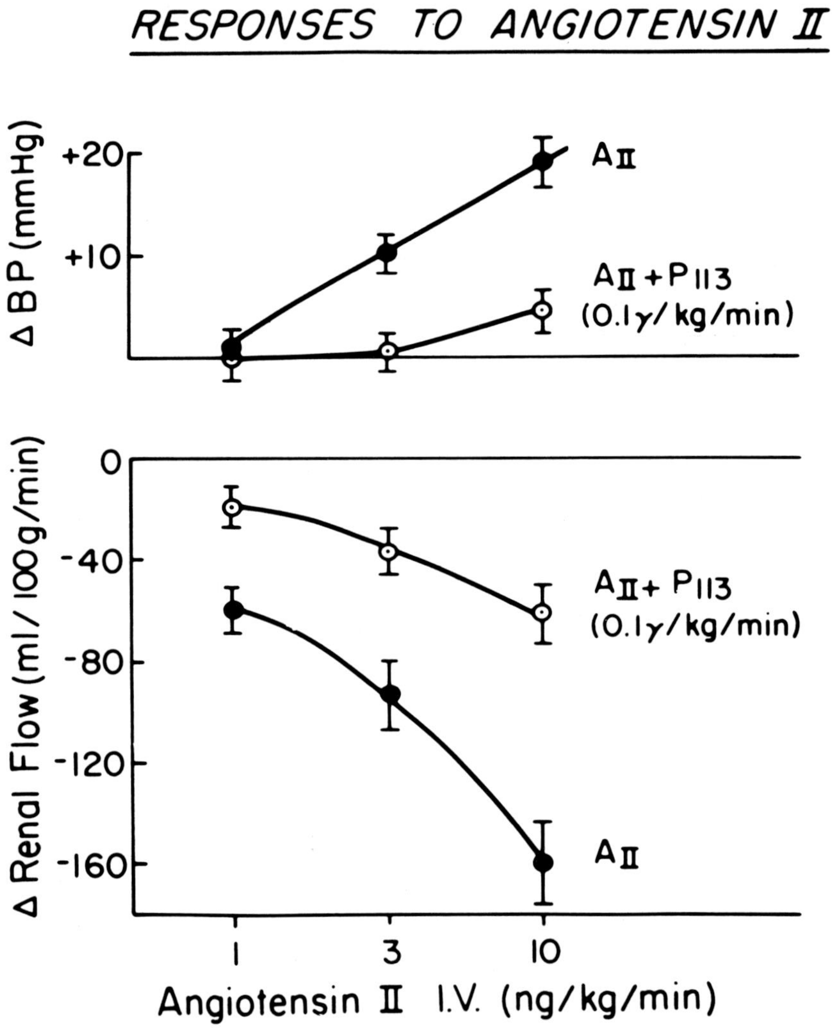

FIG. 2. P113 at its threshold dose for intrinsic activity, 0.1μg/kg/min administered intravenously, induced a significant reduction in both the pressor and renal vascular responses to A II. Larger doses of P113 totally obliterated pressor and renal vascular responses to these doses of angiotensin II [11].

modest reduction in blood pressure in response to P113 at a dose between 0.03 and 1μg/kg/min. Higher doses sometimes induced a mild pressor response consistent with the fact that this agent is a partial agonist.

P113's effects on plasma aldosterone levels and renin activity were also complicated by the fact that it is a partial agonist. Thus, P113 increased plasma aldosterone levels at doses ranging from 0.1 to 1μg/kg/min on a high sodium intake, although less so than 10 ng/kg/min of A II. Furthermore, P113 at a dose of 0.1μg/kg/min effectively blocked the aldosterone stimulating effect of A II, reducing the plasma levels to that achieved with P113 alone (Fig. 3). In contrast, in normal subjects on a 10 mEq sodium intake, P113 acted only as an antagonist at doses ranging from 0.1 to 30μg/kg/min (Fig. 4).

Similar effects were noted on plasma renin activity on a high sodium intake, ie, P113 produced a significant decrement

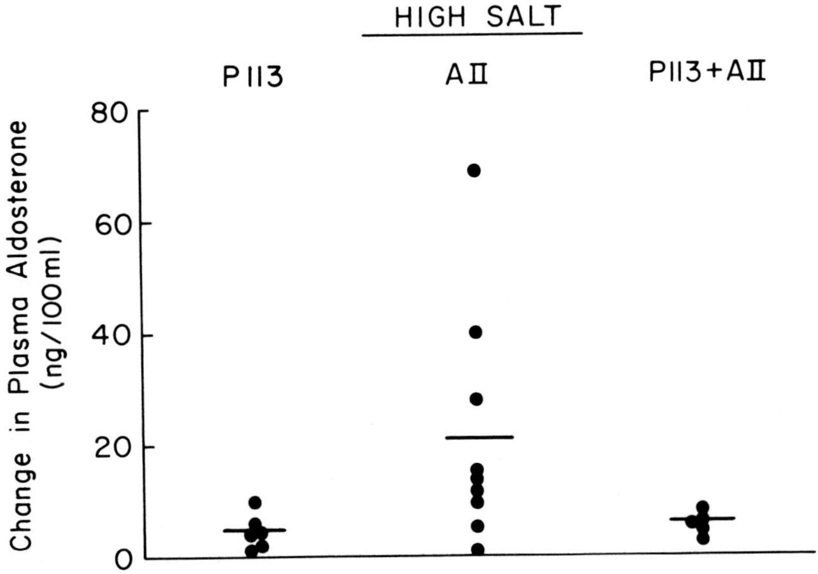

FIG. 3. Effect of P113 (0.1μg/kg/min), A II (10 ng/kg/min), either combined or separate on plasma aldosterone responses in normal subjects in balance on a 200 mEq sodium/100 mEq potassium diet.

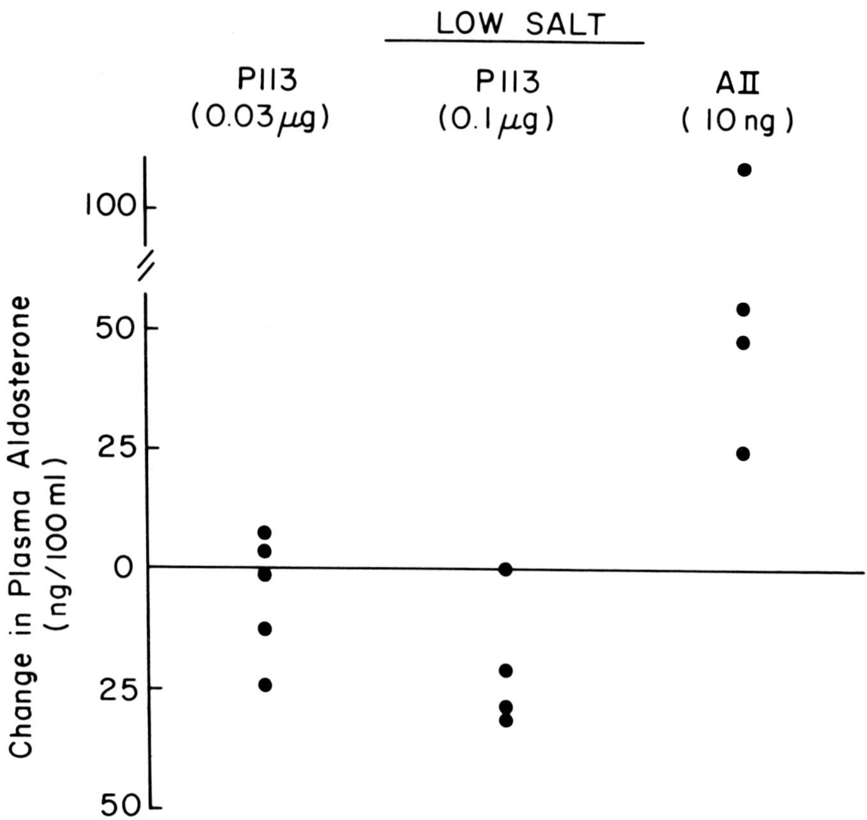

FIG. 4. Effect of P113 or A II on aldosterone levels in sodium-restricted normal subjects (infusion rates were mass/kg/min).

in renin activity at a dose of 0.1μg/kg/min, although not as great as 10 ng/kg/min of A II with reversal of the A II effect by simultaneous administration of 0.1μg/kg/min of P113 (Fig. 5). On the low sodium intake, there was a biphasic response. At a dose of 0.03μg/kg/min, there usually was an increment in renin activity (blockade), while at 0.1μg/kg/min P113 acted like A II and reduced renin activity (Fig. 6).

P113's effect on blood pressure in patients with hypertension. Eight patients were evaluated with significant renal stenosis demonstrable by renal angiogram and renal vein renins.

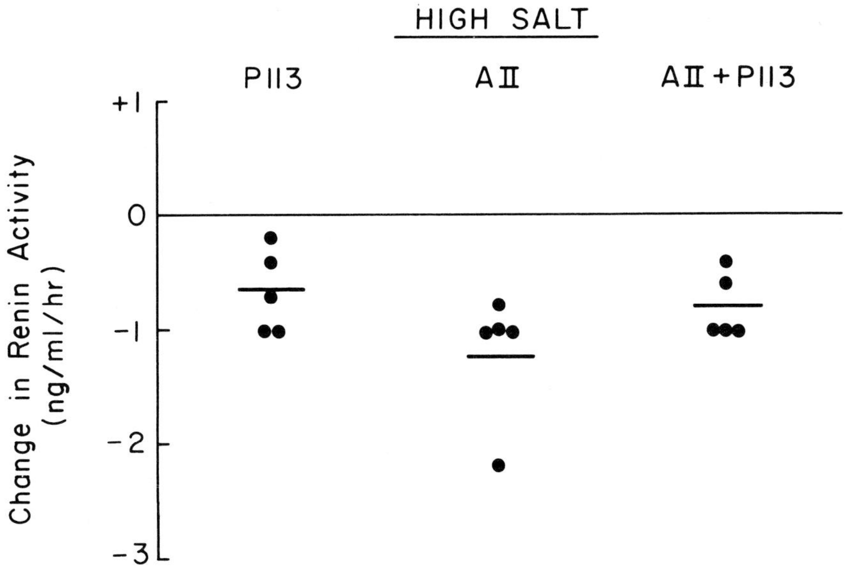

FIG. 5. Effect of P113 (0.1μg/kg/min), A II (10 ng/kg/min), either combined or separate on plasma renin activity in normal subjects on a high sodium intake.

Only four had significant decrements in blood pressure in response to P113. However, an additional two would also have been considered to be positive if dietary sodium intake was taken into consideration (Fig. 7). In two, P113 did not produce a significant decrement in blood pressure. One of these was studied on a sodium-restricted intake and had a normal blood pressure at the time of evaluation.

A total of 13 patients, or 22% of the subjects studied, showed a significant decrement in blood pressure in response to an infusion of P113 ranging from 1 to 30μg/kg/min (Fig. 8). Thus, more than half of the patients who showed a response did not have renal artery stenosis. Two of these had other forms of renal disease, ie, bilateral nephrosclerosis and bilateral pyelonephritis. The other subjects had no evidence of renal disease on the basis of routine laboratory studies, renal angiogram, hypertensive intravenous pyelogram, renalgram and renalscan.

There was also a significant number of false-negatives in individuals who had high renin hypertension. Of seven patients

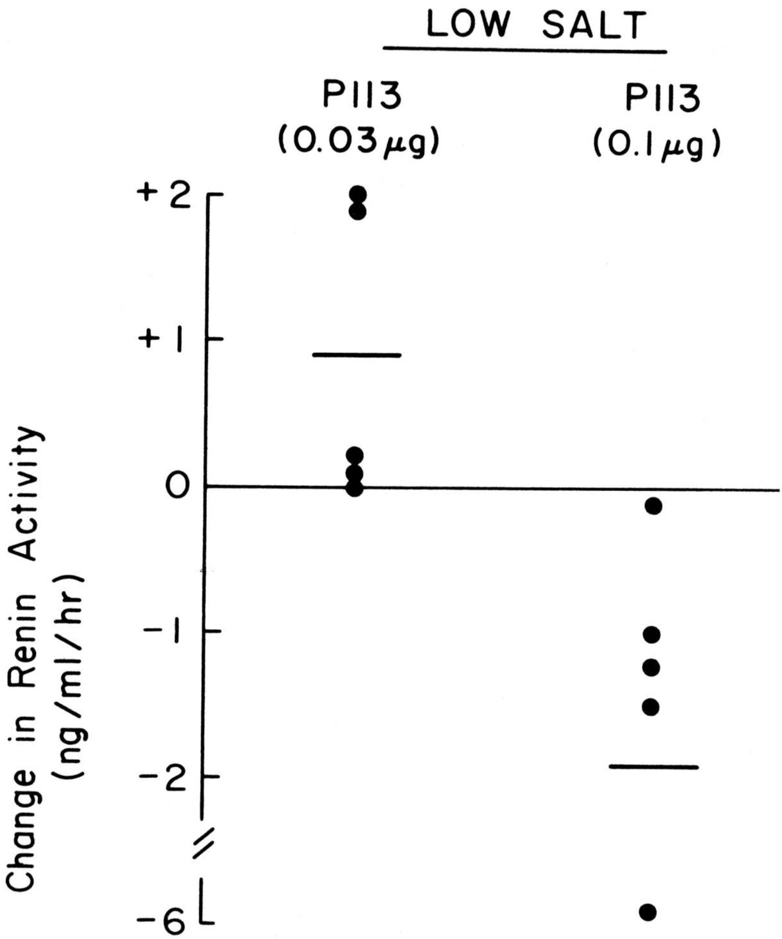

FIG. 6. Effect of P113 on plasma renin activity in sodium-restricted normal subjects.

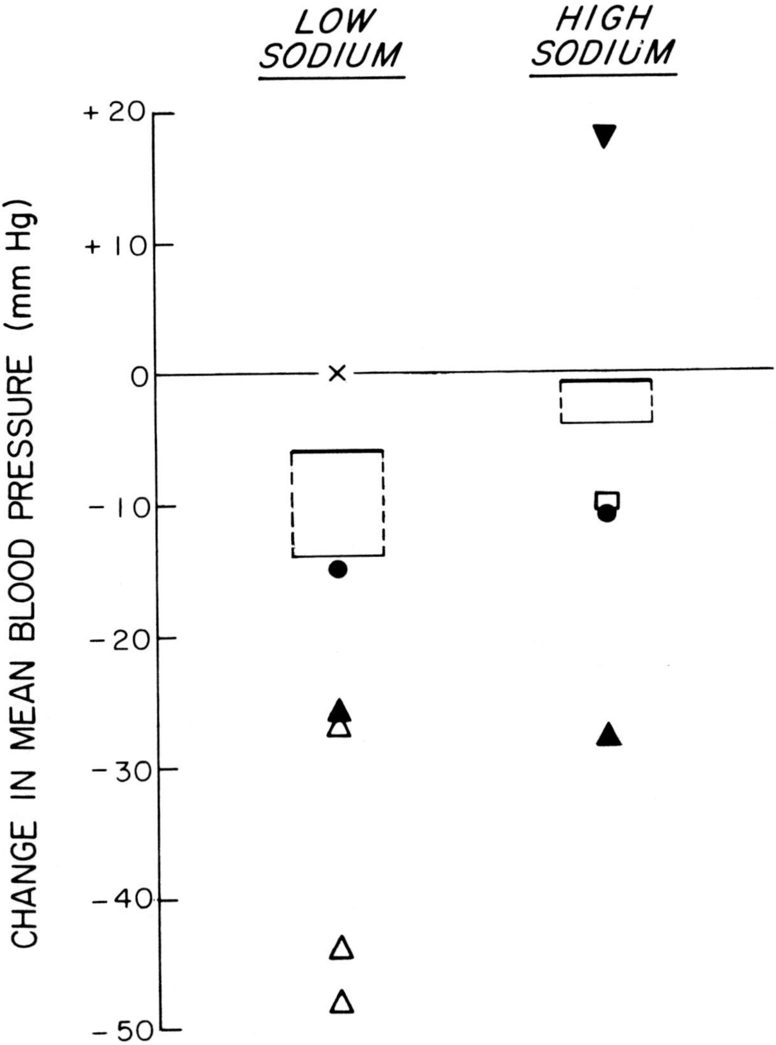

FIG. 7. Blood pressure response of patients with surgically proven renal vascular hypertension to P113 (1-30μg/kg/min). The normal mean decrement - 2 SD is outlined by a rectangle (X = patient normotensive at time of study; □, ● patients who would have been classified as non-responders if dietary sodium was not considered).

RENIN ACTIVITY	RENAL DISEASE: Present, correctable	Present, not correctable	Absent
Normal :	4	2	4
High :	2	0	1

FIG. 8. Characterization of patients with significant hypotensive responses to P113.

who fell into this category, only four showed a significant decrement in blood pressure in response to P113.

The ability of this drug to screen for low renin forms of hypertension was also assessed. Since P113 is a partial agonist, it would be assumed that patients with low levels of renin activity or A II would show a pressor response similar to what occurred in the normotensive subjects on a high sodium intake. Six patients showed a significant pressor response outside the normal range (Fig. 9). Of these patients, only one had primary aldosteronism. Two patients with primary aldosteronism did show borderline responses when dietary sodium intake was considered. However, an additional four patients who had primary aldosteronism did not show a significant pressor response. Only one of the six patients with low renin essential hypertension showed a significant pressor response to P113.

Discussion

A hormone requires two characteristics for activity: first, it must have affinity for a receptor; second, it must have intrinsic activity, ie, once combined with the receptor it must be capable of initiating the excitation process. According to this concept, a specific competitive antagonist has affinity for the same receptor as the agent being blocked and thus interferes with the agent's action by occupying the receptor without activating it.

There is an intermediate group of agents which are called partial agonists because they can block the action of the primary agent or mimic its response. In general, there are agents which have affinity for the same receptor as the primary agent but much less intrinsic activity. Thus, in the absence of the primary

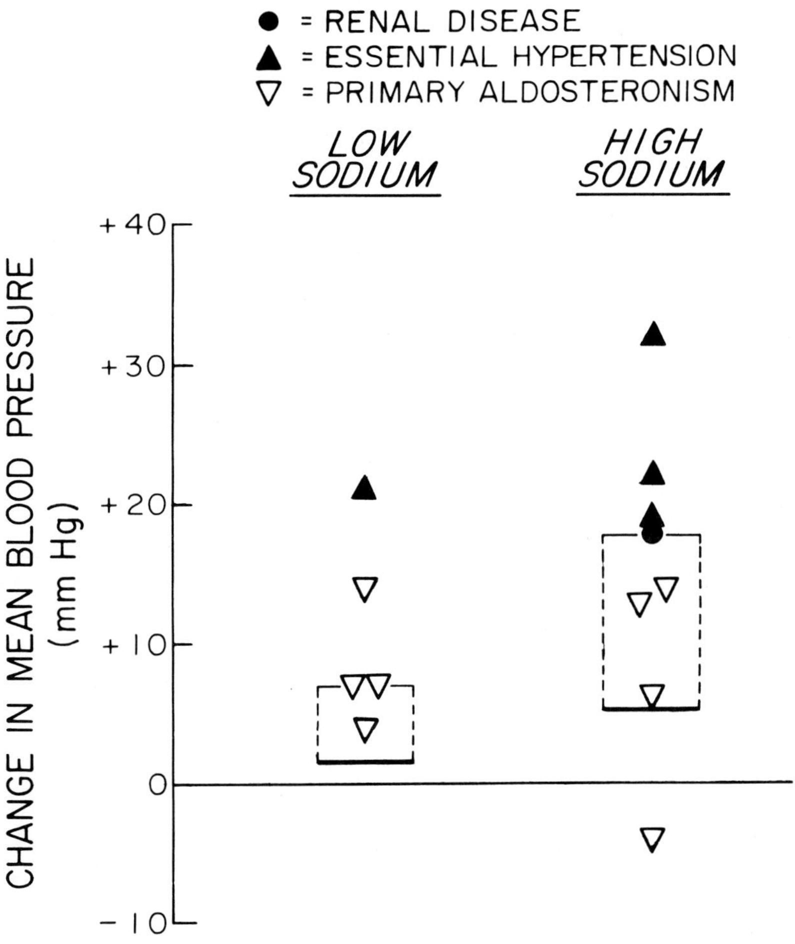

FIG. 9. Pressor effect of P113 in normal subjects (in rectangle mean + 2 SD) and patients with primary aldosteronism, renal hypertension and essential hypertension in relation to dietary sodium intake.

agonist, they will stimulate the system, although generally less effectively, but in its presence will induce competitive blockade [16]. P113 falls into this class of compounds in relationship to its interaction with A II receptors. In the normal subjects, four indices of A II activity were assessed, ie, blood pressure, aldosterone secretion, renin release and renal blood flow. All responded to P113 in a direction similar to their response to A II under the conditions of high sodium intake (low A II levels). However, under the conditions of high A II activity, either induced by sodium restriction or by infusion of A II, P113 induced striking blockade of the A II responses.

An assessment of P113's usefulness in screening of patients with hypertension [8-10] is immediately complicated by the fact that it is a partial agonist and its effect on at least four systems which may interact to regulate blood pressure is variable both as to dose and to the presence or absence of intrinsic activity. The need to assess sodium balance in order to interpret the responses properly is clearly illustrated by the studies in patients with proven renal vascular hypertension. If dietary sodium intake was not considered, the responses in two patients would not have been outside the normal range. From our studies, P113 will be most helpful if used in sodium-restricted subjects. Under these conditions, the renin-angiotensin system would be activated and P113 will for the most part act as an antagonist. Yet, sodium restriction might also increase the number of false-negative responses if the diet alone significantly reduces blood pressure. This is illustrated by one of our patients with surgically correctable hypertension whose P113 response was perfectly normal primarily because he was normotensive after five days of sodium restriction. Thus, as in pheochromocytoma, a negative response with a normal blood pressure is not evidence against the presence of the disease. Finally, even under conditions of sodium restriction, clearly 50% of the patients studied showed a false-positive response, ie, had a significant decrement in blood pressure without evidence of surgically correctable renal vascular disease. We would thus conclude that the usefulness of this test in screening for renal vascular hypertension is still limited and should be confirmed by more classical techniques of renal arteriogram and bilateral renal vein renins which also are more likely to provide useful information if performed on a sodium-restricted intake.

The study also provides useful information as to the interrelationship of A II with its vascular receptors in patients with hypertension. P113 in the normal subjects produced a significant effect on blood pressure, in the range of 0.1 to 3μg/kg/min. On the other hand, significant decrements in blood pressure were not produced even in patients with renal vascular hypertension until levels three to ten times higher. In fact, in one patient who had bilateral renal vascular disease, the previously standard infusion rate of 10μg/kg/min did not produce a significant decrement. It was only when the dose was increased to 30μg/kg/min that a significant fall occurred. Because of this, it is now our standard procedure to perform a P113 dose-response curve up to and including 30μg/kg/min before assuming a negative response.

P113's usefulness in screening for low renin hypertensive states is limited. Theoretically, it should be possible to screen for low renin hypertension by taking advantage of the fact that P113 is a partial agonist. Thus, in low renin states, P113 should act like A II, raising blood pressure. In our experience, this has not occurred. Only one patient with primary aldosteronism and one with low renin hypertension had values outside the normal range, suggesting that patients with low renin hypertension defined by sodium restriction and upright posture were not particularly responsive to P113. Finally, the infusion of P113 in a patient with primary aldosteronism might actually be dangerous. The one subject who showed a significant increment in blood pressure had a transient rise of 35 mm Hg (mean pressure) with accompanying chest pain.

In conclusion, 1-Sar, 8-Ala angiotensin II is a partial agonist of A II, having characteristics similar to A II in states where renin activity and A II levels are low (ie, high sodium intake) and acting as an antagonist when A II levels are high (ie, sodium restriction). These relationships were true for A II's effect on blood pressure, renal blood flow, renin activity and aldosterone secretion, although there were significant differences in the relative responses of these four sets of receptors. In patients with hypertension, when dietary intake, basal blood pressure and dose of P113 were appropriately adjusted, P113 induced significant decrements in blood pressure in seven out of eight patients with surgically correctable renal disease. However, an equal number of patients without surgically correctable renal disease also showed a positive response. On the other hand, blood pressure response to P113 was not an effective way to screen for low renin or low angiotensin II hypertensive states as a significant number of both false-positive and false-negative responses were observed.

References

1. Marshall, G.R., Vine, W. and Needleman, P.: A specific competitive inhibitor of angiotensin II. Proc. Nat. Acad. Sci., (U.S.) 67:1624, 1970.
2. Khairallah, P.A., Toth, A. and Bumpus, F.M.: Analogs of angiotensin II. II. Mechanism of receptor interactions. J. Med. Chem. 13:181, 1970.
3. Gagnon, D., Park, W.K. and Regoli, D.: Specific antagonists for the myotropic action of angiotensin II and angiotensin I on the isolated rat colon. Br. J. Pharmacol. 43:409, 1971.
4. Pals, D.T., Masucci, F.D., Denning, G.S., Jr. et al: Role of the pressor action of angiotensin II in experimental hypertension. Circ. Res. 29:673, 1971.
5. Freeman, R.H., Davis, J.O., Vitale, S.H. et al: Intrarenal role of angiotensin II: Homeostatic regulation of renal blood flow in the dog. Circ. Res. 32:692, 1973.
6. Brunner, H.R., Kirshman, J.D., Sealey, J.E. et al: Hypertension of renal origin: Evidence for two different mechanisms. Science 174:1344, 1971.
7. Williams, G.H., McDonnell, L.M., Raux, M.C. et al: Evidence for different angiotensin II receptors in rat adrenal glomerulosa and rabbit vascular smooth muscle cells: Studies with competitive antagonists. Circ. Res. 34:384, 1974.
8. Brunner, H.R., Gavras, H., Laragh, J.H. et al: Angiotensin II blockade in man by Sar^{1}-Ala^{8}-Angiotensin II for understanding and treatment of high blood pressure. Lancet 2:1045, 1973.
9. Ogihara, T., Yamamoto, T. and Kumahara, Y.: Clinical applications of synthetic angiotensin II analogue. Jap. Circ. J. 38:997, 1974.
10. Streeten, D.H.P., Anderson, G.H., Freiberg, J.M. et al: Use of an angiotensin II antagonist (saralasin) in the recognition of "angiotensinogenic" hypertension. N. Engl. J. Med. 292:657, 1975.
11. Hollenberg, N.K., Williams, G.H., Burger, B. et al: Blockade and stimulation of renal, adrenal and vascular angiotensin II receptors with 1-Sar, 8-Ala angiotensin II in normal man. J. Clin. Invest. 57:39, 1976.

12. Hollenberg, N.K., Chenitz, W.R., Adams, D.F. et al: Reciprocal influence of salt intake on adrenal glomerulosa and renal vascular responses to angiotensin II in normal man. J. Clin. Invest. 54:34, 1974.
13. Underwood, R.H. and Williams, G.H.: The simultaneous measurement of aldosterone, cortisol and corticosterone in human peripheral plasma by displacement analysis. J. Lab. Clin. Med. 79:848, 1972.
14. Emanuel, R.H. and Williams, G.H.: The simultaneous measurement of aldosterone, cortisol and corticosterone in human peripheral plasma by displacement analysis. J. Lab. Clin. Med. 79:848, 1972.
15. Snedecor, G.W. and Cochran, E.C.: Statistical methods. *In* The Iowa State University Press, ed. 6. Ames, Iowa, 1967.
16. Stephenson, R.P.: A modification of receptor theory. Br. J. Pharmacol. 11:379, 1956.

Discussion

Moderator: Dr. F. M. Bumpus

Dr. Weinberger: I would like to direct two questions and one comment to Dr. Streeten. I was very interested to know that you had five patients with estrogen-induced hypertension, all of whom had high renins. Did you evaluate their responses to saralasin?

Dr. Streeten: Yes, those five had elevated renin levels but no response to saralasin.

Dr. Weinberger: The second is a comment and a question. We would very strongly agree with you about the measurement of renal vein renins. Comparisons of renal vein renin concentrations that are extremely low are of very little practical value. For that reason, we utilize sodium restriction and tilting maneuvers to make sure that we have a well-stimulated sample with which to evaluate relative concentration. Do you use the same sort of procedure for renal vein measurement?

Dr. Streeten: Yes, our patients were all studied after sodium restriction or furosemide administration and after tilting for at least 15 minutes.

Dr. Tobian: I would like to ask either one of the panelists what the time course is on the rise in renin after P-113. I got the idea that renin went up a little bit at one-half hour and more at one and two hours. I would like to know just what the time course of that response is.

Dr. Williams: In normal subjects, if you take a person who is sodium restricted and you use the dose of 0.03, which we would presume to be a blocking dose, then there is a slight rise in plasma renin activity as early as about five minutes after starting the infusion. It tends to plateau somewhere between 10 and 20 minutes. On the other hand, if you use it as an agonist, that is, higher dose, the time course of response is considerably different. Within about 10 or 15 minutes, you bottom out.

Dr. Kincaid-Smith: I wonder if either of the speakers would comment on other forms of underlying renal disease other than renovascular disease. I am interested, of course, particularly in pyelonephritis, where high renins have been recorded on the side of the lesion. And I wonder also if the patients were screened for glomerulonephritis with such things as Addis counts, and whether they found any renal disease in these people.

Dr. Williams: I think that is a very good question because I forgot to mention that we had the one patient who had surgically correctable hypertension who showed, in effect, a pressor response to P-113. He actually had pyelonephritis on the same side he had the renal artery stenosis and high renins. The treatment was unilateral nephrectomy. So, maybe when you have pyelonephritis, that may alter the response.

Dr. Streeten: We, too, have found some patients with pyelonephritis, some with chronic glomerulonephritis, apparently, and some with renal disease of a type which we cannot characterize. I would like to say something too in response to my colleague Dr. Williams' comments on his false-positives. I think it is hard to be sure that all of those are actually false-positives just because the renal arteriograms are normal and because there is no other evidence of renal disease. The second to the last patient whom I discussed had a normal arteriogram, normal pyelogram and normal urinalysis until a few months before she died, when both renal vein renins rose. There was absolutely no evidence of any intrinsic renal disease of the conventional types until the last few months of her seven-year period of known hypertension.

Dr. Genest: I have a comment and maybe a little nasty question to you. Might not the absence of response to saralasin in women taking contraceptives be related to, not the high plasma renin activity, but, in fact, to the low renin concentration which these patients show with the high substrate? Have you measured angiotensin II levels?

The second point is: You showed a nice correlation between the response to P-113 and to propranolol in your patients. On the other hand, you also showed two patients seriously ill with hypertension resistant to therapy and who responded to P-113. You expressed the wish that this compound could have been given on a chronic basis. Why did you shift to propranolol?

Dr. Streeten: The first question is about the pill. I really do not know how the pill causes hypertension or whether it is the proximate cause of hypertension every time hypertension is discovered in a woman on the pill. Our conclusion from these five individuals was that they had hypertension which was discovered while they happened to be on the pill, but which did not result from the demonstrated elevation of PRA. Their renins returned to normal when the pill was stopped, but their blood pressures remained elevated. We have also had some women on the pill who did respond to saralasin, and in those circumstances, I believe that angiotensin was probably causing the hypertension.

Dr. Genest: The renin activities increase in those women but the renin concentration is lower.

Dr. Streeten: Yes.

Dr. Genest: The substrate is high.

Dr. Streeten: I do not think it really matters whether the renin concentration or the substrate level is higher or lower as long as the renin activity is elevated so that presumably the angiotensin II levels are elevated.

Question: You have not measured it?

Dr. Streeten: No, we have not, in those cases.

Dr. Williams: May I respond to the question about the A II levels, because we just finished a study with Norman Hollenberg on A II and the pill. The A II levels are significantly elevated in the people on the pill.

Dr. Streeten: Yes, but that still, of course, does not mean that elevated A II levels are causing the hypertension in all those cases.

In response to Dr. Genest's second question, I must have failed to make that clear. The patients had been on propranolol. One patient was on 1.6 gm of propranolol plus about 120 mg of furosemide daily and failed to respond to this or other combinations of drugs. I think it is well known that propranolol just simply does not always work and these are instances which exemplify that fact.

Dr. Brown: Could I ask Dr. Williams two questions? First, I think you talked of giving the saralasin over a very wide dose range. I was not clear how long you gave each of the various doses. As a sequel to that, at what stage do you take your blood sample for the measurement of plasma aldosterone?

Dr. Williams: In the studies that we did, you sort of have to separate how we do the blood pressure dose:response curve and how we do the measurements of either renal blood flow or renin or aldosterone. All of those studies were done on a fixed dose, whatever the dose was that we were using, either 0.03, 0.11, 10, 20 or 30 micrograms per kilogram per minute for at least 30 minutes. Then, we would have a very rapid dose: response curve in relationship to their blood pressure up to and including 30 mcg/kg/min.

Dr. Doyle: I just thought I might try to clear up some of the mystification that I have on this problem. It seems to me that if the renin angiotensin system is indeed one of the mechanisms which normally regulate blood pressure, and if we think back to yesterday and we were all agreed yesterday that the control of blood pressure was a very complicated affair and that all kinds of things seem to operate. And if we then think of the situation in which you sodium deplete patients, give them any anti-hypertensive drug you choose, they get an enormously enhanced response. I am really mystified as to how one can believe that giving an angiotensin antagonist is not, as a result of inhibiting one particular factor, going to set in train a whole series of compensatory mechanisms which will keep the blood pressure up. I am really not surprised to find that — I am not much of a statistician, but I think Dr. Williams' figures would suggest that if you were to toss a penny, you might get the same answer.

Dr. Williams: I think you are right, after you have a positive response. However, it is still valuable as a screening procedure. I am not sure that the false-positive, false-negative rate with this test is much different from Dr. Kaplan's A II infusion test.

Dr. Streeten: I would like to disagree with that view. Undoubtedly, hypertension is a very complicated issue, but I do not believe that it is always as complicated as all that. If you have a patient with primary aldosteronism and you remove the aldosterone-producing adenoma, the blood pressure comes down in most though not in all instances. If you have a patient with renal arterial stenosis or a pheochromocytoma, and that is the cause of the hypertension, the blood pressure comes down and normally stays down after surgical treatment. Now, there are many other types of hypertension in some of which the hypertension may result from a faulty bororeceptor control mechanism. In such situations, I agree with you entirely that lowering the blood pressure by knocking out one mechanism might well cause the blood pressure to rise by some other mechanism. But I think that where this agent saralasin is potentially useful, in our experience very useful, is exactly in those instances where the hypertension is relatively simple, due to angiotensin excess and nothing else. When the blood pressure has fallen under the conditions stated, as I say, we have almost always been able to find collateral evidence that it should have fallen since the plasma PRA or the renal vein PRA ratio was almost always above the normal range.

Dr. Sambhi: I have one question for Dr. Streeten and two for Dr. Williams. Dr. Streeten, that is the right time to ask you this question since you appear to be optimistic about the simplistic explanation of hypertension. Will you be willing to speculate on where do you think this antagonism by the antagonist occurs to bring the fall in blood pressure, as simple as in peripheral vasculature, for instance.

Dr. Streeten: Yes, in the absence of any real data, of course, our belief is that the A II antagonist lowers blood pressure by competitively inhibiting the constrictor action of endogenous A II on the arterioles.

Dr. Sambhi: Dr. Williams, since you and Dr. Hollenberg have been looking at regional blood flow in the kidney, have you had a chance yet to look at that in response to the antagonist? That is the first question. The second question is: Your elevated A II levels in women on the pill, maybe Dr. Catt would comment on this. Is this true in all of the women on the pill? Or just those who become hypertensive?

Dr. Williams: Let me answer the second question first. It is not in all women on the pill. It is a statistical analysis. It is only the sodium loaded supine A II levels of pill users that are statistically significantly higher. As regards the first question regarding the regional renal blood flow, we are yet in the process of analyzing that data.

Finally, the last thing is this: I did not mean to leave people with the impression about the use of P-113 as a screening test. Our own feeling is that it may be very useful from the point of view that it has a very low false-negative rate, if it is done in conjunction with arteriogram and renal vein renin determinations.

Dr. Stokes: Your comment, Dr. Williams, about the lady with the pain in her chest reminded me of the problem of side effects with this new preparation. I have already asked Dr. Streeten this question. Have you, like Dr. Pettinger reported earlier, struck any rebound hypertension? That is the first question. The second question is: This pain in the chest — was this associated with myocardial ischemia? I ask this because we have only just completed our second clinical study with P-113. We did both of them under EKG monitoring. During the second one, we discovered asymptomatic frequent ventricular ectopics in a patient who was not exceptional in any other way.

Dr. Williams: Yes, unfortunately, it was accompanied by ischemic EKG changes. We would assume that it is only ischemia and at least not transmural MI.

Dr. Hollifield: I have a couple of comments to make. First of all, we have done dose:response relationships, looking for the pressor effect of P-113 in salt-loaded, DOC-treated dogs. We find that in our 13 to 14 kg dogs that we get a fairly clearcut dose:response relationship from 0.1 ng to 1 mcg/kg/min. But beyond that level, we do not get additional pressor responses.

These are dogs which are not always hypertensive. They are certainly renin void, I guess. I have a comment about side effects.

We have done now between 140 and 160 patients. We have yet to see a single cardiovascular side effect, despite the fact that we have done the test in patients who have had known previous ischemic heart disease. We have done them all under EKG monitoring. We have not seen, I believe I am right when I say this, we have not seen any PVCs during the infusion, despite the fact that we have had some precipitous falls in blood pressure in some patients.

Dr. Streeten: After more than 600 of these studies, with electrocardiograms before and after every study, we also have found not a single instance of arrhythmia or myocardial ischemia. So we have been very impressed with the safety record of saralasin. I think that if you handle 600 hypertensives, each coming in and out of the hospital in one day, it might be considered fortunate and surprising that none of them have had serious hypertensive complications while they were there, unrelated to any drug effect. We have been very glad to find that saralasin has been very safe in our hands over the past 18 months.

Dr. Kaplan: Dr. Streeten's presentation brought a certain deja vu, recalling our work with the angiotensin infusion test. In response to Dr. Williams' comment, I'd like to make a few predictions: many others will use saralasin to identify angiotensinogenic hypertensives, but most will use different techniques, different end-points, etc. Thereby different results, at variance with Dr. Streeten's, will be reported, leading many to question the validity and usefulness of the procedure. At least that's what happened with the angiotensin infusion test. Some gave the drug by a single bolus; others measured blood pressure intra-arterially, others used different end-points, etc. Actually, the test didn't turn out too badly, with an overall 6% false-positive rate in all published series. But it soon became outdated with the availability of plasma renin measurements. My point, however, is not to defend that procedure, but rather to suggest an open mind about Dr. Streeten's procedure. Dr. Williams did it differently and got different results, but his purposes were more to elucidate underlying physiology than to verify the procedure as a clinical procedure. Hopefully, others will use Dr. Streeten's techniques — or equally valid ones — and we will soon have proof of the usefulness of this novel approach. At the moment, the least we can do is to keep an open mind.

Dr. Streeten: I would like to echo that opinion and would say that my interpretation of the beautiful data which we have had from Dr. Williams is just the reverse of his. In fact, he discovered seven out of eight of the patients he was looking for, and by his own admission he did not expect to discover evidence of angiotensin II action in the eighth case, and we would not either, since the blood pressure was normal when the saralasin was administered to the patient. He found four false-positives, but false-positives really do not bother one. The "false-positives" would be further investigated and one would presumably then find that they did not really have what one had thought they might have had. I think all of this goes to show that saralasin is a very useful agent in finding patients who can benefit from surgery.

Dr. Williams: I would not disagree with that.

Rapid Identification of Essential Hypertensive Patients Sensitive to Acebutolol (A New Cardioselective Beta-Blocker)

Joel Menard, M.D., Xavier Bertagna, M.D., Phan Tam N' Guyen, M.D., Marie-Blanche Ducrocq, M.D. and Pierre Corvol, M.D.

Since the observation by Prichard that pronethalol was able to decrease blood pressure in hypertensive patients with angina pectoris [1], numerous beta-blocking agents have been reported to have an antihypertensive action [2-7] despite differences in their other pharmacological characteristics. The present study has been undertaken to investigate in 44 hospitalized essential hypertensive patients the effects of a new cardioselective beta-blocking agent, acebutolol, on pulse rate, blood pressure and plasma renin activity (PRA).

It has been demonstrated that in less than 48 hours, a significant fall in blood pressure was obtained in recumbent and upright posture. The magnitude of the antihypertensive effect was correlated to the initial level of PRA in upright posture and to the importance of the decrease in PRA induced by the treatment.

Material and Methods

Patients

Subjects were 44 hypertensive patients: 26 male and 18 female. Mean body weight was 69.0 ± 12.5 kg (S.E.) and mean

---

Joel Menard, M.D. and Phan Tam N' Guyen, M.D., Service d'Hypertension Artérielle et de Médicine Interne, Hôpital Saint-Joseph, Paris; Xavier Bertagna, M.D. and Marie-Blanche Ducrocq, M.D., INSERM U 36; and Pierre Corvol, M.D., Clinique Médicale Propedeutique, Hôpital Broussais, Paris, France.

age was 44.6 ± 10.5 years. The diagnosis of essential hypertension was made after careful clinical evaluation, laboratory studies including serum electrolytes, serum creatinine, urinary excretion of vanyl mandelic acid, rapid sequence intravenous pyelogram and, when necessary, renal arteriogram. All patients had mild hypertension as judged by grade 0-11 fundi, normal serum creatinine and absence of left ventricular hypertrophy as estimated by x-ray and EKG. Patients either had never been treated or antihypertensive therapy had been withdrawn for at least one month before the study.

The study was performed under a constant sodium, potassium and caloric diet, each patient taking two pills three times a day from the second to the sixth hospital day. Placebo was given on the second, third and fourth day. Acebutolol was introduced on the fourth hospital day, 200 mg at 12 a.m. and 8 p.m., 400 mg three times on the fifth day and 400 mg at 8 a.m. on the sixth day. According to the same protocol eight other hypertensive subjects (six female and two male, mean age 44.1 years, mean body weight 60.3 kg) received placebo during the entire study.

Analytical Methods

Blood pressure was measured with mercury manometers attached to a 14 cm wide cuff in two positions: recumbent after ten minutes of rest, standing one minute after assumption of upright posture. Pulse rates were measured 30 seconds before blood pressure readings in the recumbent and upright positions. Two to four readings were made between 9 and 11 a.m. on day 4 (control) and day 6 (treatment). Mean blood pressure was calculated according to the formula: diastolic blood pressure + 1/3 pulse pressure. PRA was measured by radioimmunoassay of generated angiotensin I [8, 9] at 9 a.m., after one hour's ambulation. Normal values measured under the same conditions in 20 normal volunteers, aged 25 to 55, ranged from 0.7 to 3 ng/ml/hr with a mean natriuresis of 99.5 ± 21.8 mEq/24 hr.

Statistical Methods

Statistical methods included Student's test for group differences and paired data analysis, Wilcoxon's test and standard methods for calculation of correlation and regression coefficients [10].

Results

Effect of Acebutolol on Blood Pressure and Pulse Rate

All the blood pressure and pulse rate measurements are reported in Table 1. No significant change in blood pressure or in pulse rate was observed among the eight placebo-treated patients. In acebutolol-treated subjects, the decrease in systolic and diastolic blood pressure was highly significant ($p < 0.001$) in both positions. Resting pulse rate was decreased as was the acceleration which occurred on going from the recumbent to the upright posture (10.9 ± 10.2 before treatment, 4.36 ± 4.29 after treatment, $p < .001$). The antihypertensive effect was not accompanied by a change in body weight, or in natriuresis, which was 123 ± 34 mEq/day before acebutolol and 112 ± 38 mEq/day after acebutolol. The decrease in blood pressure was independent of age, initial blood pressure level, initial pulse rate in recumbent and upright posture. The decrease in blood pressure was not correlated to the slowing of pulse rate.

Effect of Acebutolol on PRA

In all cases but two, acebutolol lowered PRA. The mean change for the entire group was from 2.26 ± 2.11 ng/ml/hr to 0.87 ± 1.04 ng/ml/hr. In placebo-treated subjects, PRA was

Table 1. Influence of Two Days Acebutolol Treatment on Pulse Rate and Blood Pressure in Hospitalized Essential Hypertensive Patients

		Mean Arterial Blood Pressure mm Hg		*Pulse Rate min.*	
		Before	*After*	*Before*	*After*
Placebo	Recumbent	129 ± 19	129 ± 21	79 ± 13	71 ± 8
(8)	Upright	131 ± 23	132 ± 24	86 ± 12	81 ± 13
Acebutolol	Recumbent	127 ± 18	110 ± 20	82 ± 12	70 ± 7
(44)	Upright	128 ± 19	110 ± 19	93 ± 12	74 ± 9

unchanged from 1.75 ± 1.15 to 2.38 ± 2.24 ng/ml/hr. Initial PRA values were negatively correlated with age ($r = -0.417$, $p < 0.001$).

Relation of Changes in MABP to PRA

The decrease in MABP was significantly correlated with the initial PRA (Fig. 1) and with the decrease in PRA, both in recumbent ($r = 0.485$, $p < 0.001$) and upright posture ($r = 0.495$, $p < 0.001$).

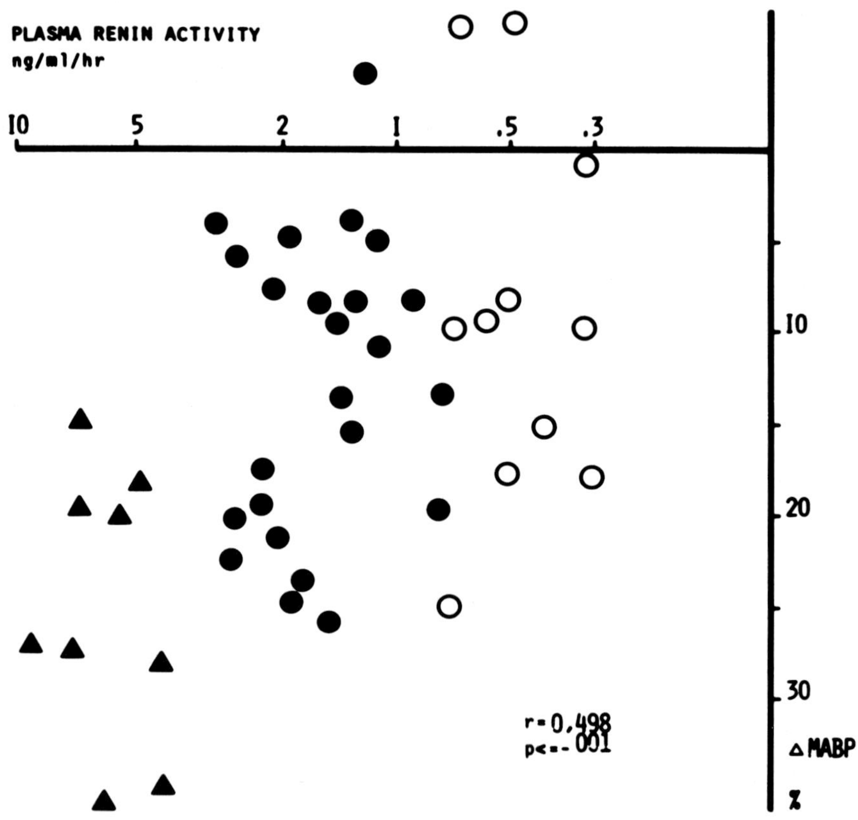

FIG. 1. Correlation between the initial PRA values in upright posture and the percentage of decrease in MABP in upright posture.

Classification of Patients

By comparison with the normal values, 11 patients exhibited a low PRA (less than 0.7 ng/ml/hr), 9 a high PRA (more than 3 ng/ml/hr) and 24 a normal PRA (Table 2). In the low renin patients, the decrease in MABP was not significant in both positions. In the high renin patients, the fall in MABP was much larger and statistically significant. Patients with a normal renin activity had a fall in blood pressure which was intermediary between the decrease observed in low and high renin patients (Fig. 2). Whereas blood pressure was identical in the three subgroups before treatment, after acebutolol administration, MABP was lower in high renin patients than in normal renin patients ($p < 0.01$), whose MABP was lower than in low renin subjects ($p < 0.05$). Pulse rate and body weight were identical in the three subgroups, but the high renin patients were younger than the others.

Discussion

These results clearly show that acebutolol, a new cardioselective β-blocker, exerts a clear-cut antihypertensive effect. The influence of acebutolol on the heart is shown in this study by the slowing of the heart rate and by the inhibition of tachycardia on standing. Acebutolol at the dosage used in this study is remarkable for its speed of action on the blood

Table 2. Influence of Acebutolol on Recumbent and Upright Mean Arterial Blood Pressure, According to Initial PRA Values

	Decrease in Mean Arterial Blood Pressure (mm Hg)			
	Recumbent	*t*	*Upright*	*t*
Low Renin (11)	- 6.8 ± 15.7	1.437	- 9.3 ± 16.3	1.888
Normal Renin (24)	-17.0 ± 12.0	6.983	-16.0 ± 11.1	7.123
High Renin (9)	-29.7 ± 10.0	8.889	-32.9 ± 14.0	7.023

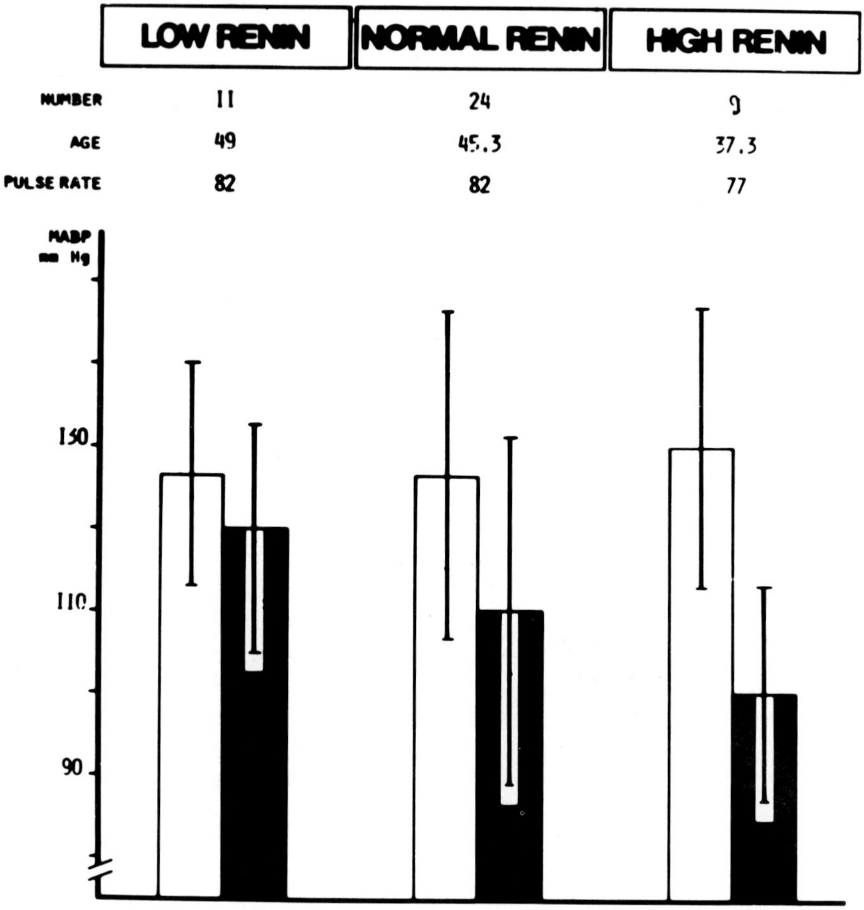

FIG. 2. Differences in the response to acebutolol treatment according to PRA.

pressure, which has been apparent in less than 48 hours. Bed rest in the hospital between the fourth and sixth days of the study could not account for the fall in blood pressure, since the eight hypertensive patients who received the placebo showed no change in their blood pressures. The speed of fall in the blood pressure contrasts with the long delay in effect which has been reported on several occasions with orally administered propranolol [2]. However, a rapid fall in blood pressure with propranolol has already been recorded by Waal [11], Hansson [12] and Buhler et al [13]. The delay in hypotensive effect of orally administered β-blockers is perhaps dependent upon the size of the initial dosage. These dosages are difficult to define, because the same dose of propranolol can vary in its β-blocking action from one individual to another [14] and it is equally difficult to make a comparison in dosage of two β-blockers. On the basis that a single oral dose of 300 mg of acebutolol is comparable to 40 mg of propranolol in the inhibition of isoprenaline-induced tachycardia [15], the average dosage of acebutolol used in this study would be equivalent to 2 mg/kg/day of propranolol. However, this dosage of acebutolol administered repeatedly is probably higher than the equivalent dosage of propranolol. The metabolism of the two products is quite different and the plasma half-life of acebutolol is approximately three times that of propranolol [16].

The effect on blood pressure varied from one patient to another. Nineteen of the 44 subjects showed either no fall in blood pressure or an average fall of below 10%; but on the other hand, 13 patients showed a considerable fall, more than 20% of the initial mean arterial pressure. This observation that variable results can be obtained in hypertensive subjects after only 48 hours on acebutolol may have important practical implications. It might be possible to select those who are sensitive or resistant to β-blockers on the basis of a simple and quick therapeutic test if the long-term results parallel those of the short-term, which has already been shown to be so with propranolol [13], but which has not yet been studied for acebutolol.

Simultaneous with its antihypertensive activity, acebutolol can lower PRA by 60% in 48 hours. In a recent study, two cardioselective beta-blockers, practolol and metoprolol, inhibited the chronotropic action of isoproterenol without preventing its stimulatory effect on PRA [17]. The marked influence of acebutolol on PRA can be interpreted in two different ways. Since evidence from animal work has suggested that acebutolol is cardioselective [18], the effect on PRA of β-blockers may not be dependent upon their affinity for beta-2 receptors. On the contrary, the effect of acebutolol on PRA may be another argument against its cardioselectivity, since in man acebutolol, unlike practolol, affects peripheral vasculature and airways as well as the heart [19].

What are the connecting links, if any, between the fall in blood pressure brought about by the β-blocker, the renin-angiotensin system and the effect of the β-blocker on the heart?

A number of clinical and laboratory measurements have been used to try to predict the antihypertensive action of β-blockers [7, 12, 13]. Buhler et al were the first to report that subjects with high PRA showed a greater fall in blood pressure after treatment with propranolol for a period averaging three to five months than subjects with a normal PRA who were themselves more responsive than those with a low PRA [13]. Hansson [12] using propranolol, Esler and Nestel with practolol [6] and Meekers et al with I.C.I. 66,082 [7] were unable to confirm these observations.

Our results agree with those of Buhler et al and the fall in blood pressure after 48 hours of treatment with acebutolol correlated in a very significant manner with the initial level of PRA measured after one hour in the upright position in subjects on a normal sodium intake. Among those treated with acebutolol, there was before treatment a very significant negative correlation between PRA and age as in normotensive subjects [20]. This observation increases interest in the correlation between PRA and the fall in blood pressure induced by acebutolol, since the hypotensive effect is independent of age. Furthermore, neither the initial level of blood pressure nor the initial heart rate can predict the hypotensive response.

When the results are expressed in the same way as those of Buhler et al [13] by distinguishing three groups of patients according to their PRA, our results can be seen to be very comparable to those of these authors. The number of cases in the three groups is also the same though the method of dosage and the conditions of the protocol were not identical. However, the limits of such a classification must be emphasized. In our study, the predictive value of PRA was not absolute, for one subject with a low renin level and six subjects with normal levels had falls in their blood pressures of over 20%. These divergences at the individual level could be interpreted in different ways.

1. Treatment had perhaps been for too short a period and a long-term treatment with acebutolol might not give the same results as in the short term.

2. The correlation between the initial PRA and the fall in blood pressure might be fortuitous.

3. Last, investigation of the renin-angiotensin system by measurement of PRA in subjects in the upright position and with a normal sodium intake might not always be sufficient to allow assessment of the degree of activity or inactivity of the renin-angiotensin system [21] which might be better explored by other tests which inhibit this system [22, 23].

There is one other correlation between the renin-angiotensin system and the fall in blood pressure induced by acebutolol: The greater the fall in renin, the greater the drop in blood pressure. Such a finding suggests that the slowing down of renin secretion might contribute to the fall in blood pressure induced by acebutolol, and this is in agreement with the results obtained by Buhler et al [13] with propranolol and against the findings of Leonetti et al [24] and Hansson [12], who found no relationship between the fall in blood pressure and that of renin. The slowing down of renin secretion is not, however, the only property of the β-blockers which could explain their hypotensive action, since under several circumstances, the two properties are clearly separated [25-27].

In conclusion, our results are in keeping with those of Laragh et al [28] and suggest that there is a parallel between the fall in blood pressure brought about by beta-blockade and the initial level and suppression of PRA. *However*, more direct evidence is necessary before we can assert that the early response of the blood pressure to treatment with acebutolol is characteristic of renin-dependent hypertension.

Summary

Acebutolol, a new cardioselective beta-blocking agent, was administered for 48 hours to 44 essential hypertensive patients at a total dosage of 2,000 mg. The slowing down of the pulse rate and the decrease in blood pressure were highly significant, whereas eight placebo-treated subjects had no change in pulse rate nor in blood pressure. Plasma renin activity decreased from 2.26 ± 2.11 ng/ml/hr to 0.87 ± 1.04 ng/ml/hr. The decrease in blood pressure was correlated with the initial PRA and with the decrease in PRA.

These results demonstrate that a rapid fall in blood pressure can be obtained in essential hypertensive patients treated with acebutolol and that the fall in blood pressure is related to the initial state of the renin angiotensin system.

References

1. Prichard, B.N.C.: Hypotensive action of pronethalol. Brit. Med. J. 1:1227, 1964.
2. Prichard, B.N.C. and Gillam, P.M.S.: Treatment of hypertension with propranolol. Brit. Med. J. 1:7, 1969.
3. Tibblin, G. and Ablad, B.: Antihypertensive therapy with alprenolol, a β-adrenergic receptor antagonist. Acta Med. Scand. 186:451, 1969.
4. Morgan, T.O., Louis, W.J., Dawborn, J.K. et al: The use of pindolol in the treatment of hypertension. Med. J. Aust. 2:309, 1972.
5. Lohmoller, G. and Frohlich, E.D.: A comparison of timolol and propranolol in essential hypertension. Am. Heart J. 89:437, 1975.
6. Esler, M.D. and Nestel, P.J.: Evaluation of practolol in hypertension — effects on sympathetic nervous system and renin responsiveness. Br. Heart J. 35:469, 1973.
7. Meekers, J., Missotten, A., Fagard, R. et al: Predictive value of various parameters for the antihypertensive effect of the beta blocker ICI 66,082. Arch. Int. Pharmacol. Ther. 213:294, 1975.
8. Menard, J., Corvol, P., Allegrini, J. et al: Mesure de l'activité Rénine-Plasmatique de l'homme par le dosage radioimmunologique de l'Angiotensine I. *In* Techniques Radioimmunologiques. Paris:INSERM Ed., 1972, p. 459.
9. Corvol, P., Rodbard, D., Drouet, J. et al: Monoiodinated angiotensins: Preparation and characterization by polyacrylamide gel electrophoresis and isoelectric focusing. Biochim. Biophys. Acta 251:254, 1971.
10. Armitage, P.: Statistical Methods in Medical Research. John Urley and Sons Ed., 1971.
11. Waal, H.J.: Hypotensive action of propranolol. Clin. Pharmacol. Ther. 7:588, 1966.
12. Hansson, L.: Beta-adrenergic blockade in essential hypertension: Effects of propranolol on hemodynamic parameters and plasma renin activity. Acta Med. Scand. 194 (Suppl. 550): 1973.
13. Buhler, F.R., Laragh, J.H., Baer, L. et al: Propranolol inhibition of renin secretion. A specific approach to diagnosis and treatment of renin-dependent hypertensive diseases. N. Engl. J. Med. 287:1209, 1972.
14. Nies, A.S., and Shand, D.G.: Clinical pharmacology of propranolol. Circulation 52:6, 1975.
15. Cuthbert, M.F. and Owusu-Ankomarch, K.: Effect of M. and B. 17,803 A, a new β adrenoceptor blocking agent on the cardiovascular

responses to tilting and to isoprenaline in man. Br. J. Pharmacol. 43:639, 1971.
16. Cuthbert, M.F. and Collins, R.F.: Plasma levels and β-adrenoceptor blockade with acebutolol, practolol and propranolol in man. Br. J. Clin. Pharmacol. 2:49, 1975.
17. Weber, M.A., Stokes, G.S. and Gain, J.M.: Comparison of the effects on renin release of beta adrenergic antagonists with differing properties. J. Clin. Invest. 54:1413, 1974.
18. Basil, B., Jordan, R., Loveless, A.H. et al: β-adrenoceptor blocking properties and cardioselectivity of M and B 17,803 A. Br. J. Pharmacol. 48:198, 1973.
19. Kumana, C.R., Kaye, C.M., Leighton, M. et al: Cardiac and pulmonary effects of acebutolol. Lancet 2:89, 1975.
20. Sambhi, M., Crane, M.G. and Genest, J.: Essential hypertension: New concepts about mechanisms. Ann. Intern. Med. 79:411, 1973.
21. Drayer, J.I.M., Kloppenborg, P.W.C. and Benraad, T.J.: Detection of low-renin hypertension; evaluation of outpatient renin-stimulating methods. Clin. Sci. Molec. Med. 48:91, 1975.
22. Gavras, G., Brunner, H.R., Laragh, J.H. et al: An angiotensin converting-enzyme inhibitor to identify and treat vasoconstrictor and volume factors in hypertensive patients. N. Engl. J. Med. 291:817, 1974.
23. Streeten, D.H.P., Anderson, G.H., Freiberg, M. et al: Use of an angiotensin II antagonist (Saralasin) in the recognition of angiotensinogenic hypertension. N. Engl. J. Med. 292:657, 1975.
24. Leonetti, G., Mayer, G., Morganti, A. et al: Hypotensive and renin-suppressing activities of propranolol in hypertensive patients. Clin. Sci. Molec. Med. 48:491, 1975.
25. Bravo, E.L., Tarazi, R.C., Dustan, H.P. et al: Dissociation between renin and arterial pressure responses to beta-adrenergic blockade in human essential hypertension. Circ. Res. 36 (suppl. 1):241, 1975.
26. Stokes, G.S., Weber, M.A. and Thornell, I.R.: Beta-blockers and plasma renin activity in hypertension. Br. Med. J. 1:60, 1974.
27. Menard, J., Corvol, P., Alexandre, J.M. et al: Equilibration du traitement des hypertensions artérielles sèvéres — Intérêt du d-1 propranolol. Nouv. Presse Med. 3:871, 1975.
28. Laragh, J.H., Sealey, J.E., Buhler, F.R. et al: The renin axis and vasoconstriction volume analysis for understanding and treating renovascular and renal hypertension. Amer. J. Med. 58:4-13, 1975.

Discussion

Moderator: Dr. A. E. Doyle

Dr. Stokes: Dr. Corvol, I think that you are unduly backward in claiming consistency between your results and those of Dr. Laragh. In fact, I would say that this was the type of study which a lot of us have been waiting to see, a substantial study which largely confirms what he claimed with regard to propranolol. It also concerns me a little, because it is so much in conflict with the findings of my own study, even making allowance for the fact that we were using different drugs and different protocols. So now I feel we must search for reasons for why these apparently inconsistent results from two groups can be explained. Groping at straws, it occurred to me first of all that your observations were made over fairly short periods of time, is that not right? That these were observations made after only a few days of treatment in the hospital. Therefore, the decrements in blood pressure you are working with were rather less than those that may have been observed in the same patient population over a longer period of time. One recalls at this time also the observations in the Nashville group which were annotated by Dr. Hollifield yesterday, showing that a dose relationship with propranolol effects, such that the first decrement in blood pressure at low doses (and could be that this applies also to the early effects of the drug?) are related to a fall in renin activity. But thereafter further decrements in blood pressure are unrelated to falls in plasma renin activity. It also brings to mind the first data we got in this area which were in a short-term study with propranolol, in which we did find a very low but nonetheless marginally significant correlation between blood pressure effects and renin levels in a study constructed in the same fashion as yours. That is, observing patients in hospital over just a few days in an open study. I would like your comment whether you feel that these were maximal blood pressure falls, whether you have outpatient follow-ups in these patients to define further falls that may have occurred.

Dr. Corvol: We don't believe very much in the ambulatory renin determinations because we have performed in all these patients an ambulatory renin determination and it did not correlate so well with the renin measurement we have made in the hospital. So that is why we decided to study these patients in the hospital. We have waited as you have seen for four days before giving the placebo or the treatment to be sure that there won't be any further decrease in blood pressure. Actually, in the placebo-treated patient there was no further decrease of blood pressure between the fourth day and the sixth hospital day. One of the main questions is: Will these patients who did respond well during hospitalization have the same response during the long-term treatment? We do not know yet. I hope to be able to give you the answer in perhaps one year. If we are obliged to increase the dosage of the drug, we might get a further decrease in blood pressure. However, this further decrease could be related to a central action of the drug.

Dr. Onesti: Our experience with acebutolol shows that in ambulatory patients treated for 30 days, the drug is quite effective in lowering the blood pressure. Our impression of the clinical effect of acebutolol is a good one. However, we have not shown any consistent effect on renin in ambulatory patients.

V

Epilogue

Closing Remarks

By all criteria, this Symposium on the Effects of Antihypertensive Therapy has been a great success. This is due in large part to the organizational ability of Dr. Sambhi, to his selection of key participants from many countries throughout the world and to the important help given by Mr. McGraw, President of the Pennwalt Prescription Products Co., and to his team.

The choice of the subject of the symposium was most appropriate, since any addition to our knowledge as to how antihypertensive drugs lower blood pressure in hypertensive patients may help greatly in our understanding of the basic mechanisms of essential hypertension.

In looking back over the past 15 years, we all owe a great deal for the elegant and efficient organization of these symposia to Dr. Franz Gross who was the first, I believe, to organize these small meetings of experts on hypertension from all over the world. After each one of these symposia, the published proceedings were used widely as sources of references by others working in the field and served as springboards for more research and more progress.

The mechanism of action of antihypertensive drugs is very ill-understood. As Dr. Grollman discussed, their use has been empirical and does not appear yet to correct the fundamental aspects involved in the mechanism of hypertension. We must not be swayed by the demonstration of an effect of these drugs either on renin, aldosterone, norepinephrine regulation, plasma or extracellular fluid volume, total body sodium or potassium as indicating that this is *the* way, or *the only* way, in which a certain drug exerts its blood pressure lowering action. This is a field where it is most dangerous to be dogmatic and many have learned it at their own expense.

We certainly have learned a great deal in this symposium, but the great lesson has been, at least for me, one of humility.

Its great value is that we have learned once more that we need to work harder and to have better ideas if we want to know more about the mechanisms of action of antihypertensive drugs. The assertion that beta-blockers, especially propranolol, exert their antihypertensive action by their supposedly suppressing effects on plasma renin activity has taken quite a beating, if not a funeral, as Dr. Kaplan put it. This seems true at least during chronic administration. In severe situations in patients with acutely high plasma renin activity levels, it is more likely that at least part of the blood pressure lowering effect of propranolol is due to the concomitant inhibition of the renin release, since this correlates very well with the findings obtained by others with the infusion of the angiotensin antagonist, saralasin.

A very pertinent question was raised concerning the reasons for the persistence of hypertension in a number of patients with primary aldosteronism, especially if due to bilateral hyperplasia. Some reasons were advanced, such as a poorer response to Aldactone administration and evidence of greater peripheral resistance, but definite data are still lacking at the present time.

The blood pressure lowering action of the thiazides, whether during acute or chronic administration, appears to be related in part at least to a decrease in plasma volume and extracellular fluid volume and also possibly through the stimulation of the kallikrein system and to the depletion of total body potassium.

In the past, the pharmaceutical industry has used normal or renal experimental hypertensive four-legged animals to detect the blood pressure lowering effect of new drugs. This procedure was cumbersome and not very specific. One example was guanethidine which was inactive in these preparations. Later, more attention was given to the effect of these drugs on catecholamine metabolism or on myocardial norepinephrine content. Now, plasma renin has taken the front page and I am not sure if it will fare better. Maybe the kallikrein system will come next!

What Dr. Page said in his opening remarks should be stressed again and this is the need for improvement in the teaching in medical schools of the physiopathology and pharmacology of hypertension and of the need of treating the atherosclerotic disease as well as hypertension.

Because of the pioneering work of Bumpus, there is a whole body of new and fascinating knowledge concerning the mode of action and the respective activities of angiotensin I, angiotensin II and angiotensin III (Des-Asp-1-Angiotensin II) thanks to the availability of new synthetic antagonists. It should not take very long before we know which of these three is the main stimulant of aldosterone production or whether the three may participate in various degrees, depending upon particular situations. A great benefit of this work has been the clinical application of one antagonist, saralasin, in the diagnosis of so-called angiotensinogenic hypertension and possibly in the treatment of acute hypertensive crises associated with high renin release.

One aspect has emerged in relation to the mechanism of action of antihypertensive drugs and it relates to the importance of measurements of plasma volume and extracellular fluid volume and the need for more accurate methods for their determination. These parameters should certainly be analyzed more frequently in parallel with changes in plasma renin, aldosterone, 18-hydroxy-DOC, norepinephrine, kallikrein excretion and other factors.

All in all, it was a very successful symposium, most informative and enriching thanks to the many occasions it permitted the participants to discuss and exchange views. I would like on your behalf to express our sincere thanks both to Mo and Minno Sambhi for the graciousness in which everything was organized and our gratitude also goes to Mr. and Mrs. McGraw and the Pennwalt team who made everything so pleasant and easy for each of us.

Jacques Genest, C.C., M.D., D.Sc.
Scientific Director, Clinical
Research Institute of Montreal, Canada

Hypertension: A Malady of Civilization?

Derek Denton, M.D.

At this meeting there has been a sophisticated experimental and clinical analysis of the established hypertensive state, and some interesting new aspects have emerged. However, there has been no discussion of the fact that there are some communities in the world where blood pressure does not rise with age. These communities warrant much closer study because they may (conceivably) provide fundamental insight into what goes wrong in our type of society. A singular issue for consideration in this regard is the very low salt content of diet of these communities.

Before following this theme, it needs to be stated at the outset that attempts to date to relate the incidence of hypertension in Western urban communities to the immediate salt intake of the individuals under study have been rather unsuccessful. The results are contradictory if one considers the results of Dahl and Love [1, 2] in the Brookhaven study, on the one hand, and those of Dawber et al [3] in the Framingham study and of Miall [4] in the Welsh mining communities, on the other. Individuals' statements on their own salt intake don't correspond with the concurrent evidence from urinary Na output. But, in any event, results on odd specimens of urine in a large population tell little in relation to the history of intake of the individual over decades which is the relevant issue. Further, if there be any parallel in the human situation to some data from animals [5], it may be that a measure of aversion to salt could develop with established high blood pressure. Salt

Derek Denton, M.D., Director, Howard Florey Institute of Experimental Physiology and Medicine, University of Melbourne, Parkville, Victoria, Australia.

restriction in the clinical context may ameliorate established hypertension but it must be severe to be effective.

A reading of some of the outstanding scholarly texts in this field [6] can give the impression that, as far as the author is concerned, the idea of excess salt intake as a major factor in the etiology of human hypertension is not worth too much consideration. Yet, at any international meeting analyzing and dissecting this issue at a clinical or experimental level, an ever-present and paramount feature of the discussion is the metabolism of Na and its protean influence on physiological processes. This centers on Na balance, its distribution within the organism with corresponding effect on volume of fluid compartments, the modulation of response characteristics of excitable tissue and the effects on hormone secretion — to name four important contexts.

Given the pivotal role of Na in the expression of the hypertensive process, a legitimate question follows. Can it be concluded that a high maternal salt intake, followed by a high intake during infancy and childhood, which then is sustained by induced hedonic preference through the next three to four decades of life is of little or no relevance to the basic genesis of hypertension in the Western urban community? Is it feasible that dietary Na loading over the early stages of differentiation and growth, and elaboration of response mechanisms of a diversity of tissues of the body may alter definitively, and perhaps irreversibly, the characteristics of the adult organism?

I would like to consider this question in a phylogenetic context on the basis that high salt intake is essentially a new nutritional situation of the past hundred years or so of civilization. This can be set against the fact that the physiological character of the appetite and regulatory metabolic systems of primates and man have evolved over millions of years under conditions where dietetic Na intake has been low and K^+ intake high.

One of the memorabilia of our Institute files is a letter from the Editor-in-Chief of a journal for publication of papers concerned with investigation of clinical relevance. He inquires whether we are aware that the sheep is a herbivore which has an adrenal gland which is constantly bombarded with K^+ and that, in this regard, it will differ as a species in its responses from, for example, man and the dog which are carnivores.

Two very interesting papers have come out recently on populations where no blood pressure rise occurs with age and hypertension is rare. The study of Oliver and colleagues [7] concerns the Yanomamo Indians of the tropical rain forests of Venezuela and Brazil. About 12,000 to 15,000 people are spread over about 100,000 square miles and have apparently lived in isolation for thousands of years. They eat banana, wild vegetables and occasional game and fish. The blood pressure of 506 members of the adult population of 16 villages showed no rise with age. Urinary Na excretion was about 1 mEq/day and urinary K, 150 mEq/day. Urinary aldosterone excretion was high relative to normal for Western urban man, as was plasma renin.

In the highlands of New Guinea at Tukisenta, Sinnett and Whyte [8] have studied a total population living in valleys between 6,000 and 8,500 feet. In a population of 779, no increase in blood pressure occurred with age. The maximum pressure in males was reached at the third decade and it then declined. Only 3% of males over 40 were hypertensive. Diet in the highlands consists of sweet potato, breadfruit, yams and bananas. Wildlife is scarce. Pig herding is practiced. Urinary Na^+ averaged 13 mEq/day in females and 6 mEq/day in males.

The Dutch anthropologists first pointed out a decade ago that the diet of feral man in New Guinea had a K:Na ratio of 100-200:1 and was very low in Na^+. Subsequently, in collaboration with Professor MacFarlane and Dr. Skinner, we have measured peripheral blood aldosterone of the Chimbu in the highlands of New Guinea and found the mean to be 28 ng/100 ml — four times that of Western urbanized man and urbanized New Guineans [9]. Urinary Na was very low and urinary K^+ high. Skinner found the plasma renin was not elevated.

In the populations cited above, salt was not available, and native salt is prepared from "wood ash." Transitional populations moving to Western style diet were found by MacFarlane et al [10] to have higher blood pressures than the highlanders living in traditional fashion.

Overall, this more recent data have elaborated on earlier observations on Cuna Indians, aboriginal populations in Australia and Sechwan, and some Melanesian and Polynesian Pacific island populations.

Though we have other primitive communities such as Eskimo and Masai with different dietetic habit, there are reasons, which I have considered in full elsewhere [11], for supposing that this metabolic pattern in relation to low sodium intake has been the prevalent circumstance of mineral nutrition during primate evolution.

It is interesting to consider and compare classical grazing herbivores to this situation. The sodium content of grass and browse will be predominantly determined by Na^+ content of rain. In general, grass tends to concentrate Na^+ more than fruits and many vegetables. Because of the decreasing Na content of rain water as we progress inland from the ocean, the Na^+ content of grass in continental interiors and in alpine regions falls, and the K^+:Na^+ ratio of grass can be as high as the food of feral man as cited above.

However, in large coastal areas of continents and in areas of continents of particular geographic shape or with volcanically derived sources of sodium, Na^+ content of soil will be quite high and K^+:Na^+ ratio of grass will be nearer 5-1:1. This would be the metabolic circumstance, for example, of millions of grazing animals on the Australian continent. On the other hand, we can recognize that feral human communities with fruit, seed and root tuber diet which supplement with hunting activities (see Clark's [12] emphasis that such hunting and gathering societies are often predominantly vegetarian), or for that matter with baboon or chimpanzee groups which occasionally eat meat, the K:Na ratio of mineral intake may be reduced also to 5-1:1 due to the Na content of meat. Thus, the idea that ruminant and other herbivores are in a radically different circumstance metabolically vis-à-vis K:Na intake, relative to the situation with feral man, is tenuous in large parts of the planet and probably invalid at a comparative level.

Looking at the prehistory of man, Dr. Oakley of the British Museum regards Proconsul, a herbivorous ape of the Miocene era 30 million years ago, as representative of a common ancestral stock. In the view of some workers the Prehominids (eg, Ramipithecus) of the late Miocene and Pliocene were graminiferous. The move from forest to savannah woodland involved change from lush fruit and leaf to stem, seed and rhizome diet which will be low also in Na^+. The distinguished American anthropologist Jolly [13] suggests the occupation of the seed-eating econiche by basal hominids — possibly parallel to the grassland baboon (Theropithicus) — was the genesis of many adaptations such as mobile tongue, large molars and incisor teeth reduction and forearm mobility.

Of the later representatives of the various prehominid lines in the late Pliocene-Pleistocene, it seems probable that Australopithicene robustus was vegetarian, whereas Australopithicene africanus included meat in their diet. Leakey [14] described the discovery of the skull of Zinjanthropus bosei in the upper part of the Villafrankian or Lower Pleistocene (Bed 1 — about 1.7 million years ago) at Olduvai Gorge. He suggests from the associated bones of small mammals, birds and the tools of the makers of this Oldowan culture that, although they were semicarnivorous, they were still not good hunters and had only just emerged from a purely vegetarian diet. The remains in the later Bed II indicated that Chellean man hunted the larger animals of Africa. Clark [12], in reviewing the lines of human evolution, discusses possible meat-eating further back in the emergent process, but emphasizes that with hunting and gathering societies, the total bulk of vegetable food consumed greatly exceeds that of meat eaten. Studies of contemporary groups such as the Kalahari Bushmen show 60%-80% of food supply of these hunting people is vegetable. He suggests that the hand tools of the Oldowan culture were used for preparing otherwise unpalatable parts of plants, breaking nuts, etc., as well as for breaking animal bones and cutting skin. Vegetable foods leave very little evidence in the archeological record.

Over the major period of evolution from the Miocene, the diet of prehominids, like that of contemporary apes, probably has been predominantly vegetarian with consequent stress on Na status. Carnivore diet insures Na^+ intake by virtue of the obligatory salt in tissue and viscera of prey. During the latter 2 million years, the facts are not known with certainty, but diet may have been intermediate between herbivore and pongid, on the one hand, and carnivore, on the other. The evidence of a substantially tropical mode of existence of man's ancestors also involves the perennial problem of temperature control with sweating and salt loss, and additional stress imposed episodically by reproduction and disease. Overall, during primate evolution, selection pressures favoring phylogenetic emergence of efficient behavioral and endocrinological mechanisms of sodium homeostasis probably would have operated at a high intensity.

Thus, the hedonic human liking or appetite for salt when it is available, and independent of any metabolic need, is an evolutionary legacy of behavior of considerable survival value.

In relation to possible genesis of hypertension, in contrast to the conditions over evolutionary time, the cheap and common availability of salt is a matter of the last 100 years or so. The gabelle and Gandhi's salt marches are events of recent history. For the large part of humanity there has been a quite recent and radical change in diet habit in this regard attributable to new technology and commerce. I appreciate that pickling activities have been going on for centuries. But for that matter, there is evidence which would indict this particular performance, with resulting very high salt intake, in the very high incidence of hypertension and death from cerebral hemorrhage in Akita and other provinces of Northern Honshu where daily Na intake averages approximately 500 mEq. This is rather than the high SO_4:CO_3 ratio in the water supply as a result of volcanic influences, or the high cadmium content in the kidneys of the local fish, being the operative factor.

In relation to the epidemiology of hypertension in our communities, and the question of why blood pressure does not rise with age in the population of the primitive communities instanced, there is the issue that there may be operative factors other than salt intake in the primitive communities. One possibility cited is that the conditions of life may be more tranquil and free of stress in the natural primitive community. Whereas this is feasible, the history of tribal warfare and also cannibalism until recent times does not give ready credence to the idea that for the population this is more tranquil stress-free life style than that of urban man.

Overall, it can be recognized that civilization and technology with greatly increased production of foodstuffs in affluent societies have introduced the issue of the subtle aggregate effects of long-term exposure to great excess of substances which are normal, indeed essential components of diet. There are good grounds, but by no means a proven case, for suspecting excess salt intake in the etiology of hypertension in Western communities. If not simply directly and commensurately causal, perhaps the high salt intake from infancy to middle age of a large segment of the population in Western communities is an important factor in the causal expression of other jointly sufficient and severally necessary factors which, in the long term, contrive the hypertensive state.

References

1. Dahl, L.K. and Love, R.A.: Evidence for relationship between sodium (chloride) intake and human essential hypertension. Arch. Intern. Med. 94:525, 1954.
2. Dahl, L.K. and Love, R.A.: Etiological role of sodium chloride intake in essential hypertension in humans. JAMA 164:397, 1957.
3. Dawber, T.R., Kannel, W.B., Kagan, A. et al: Environmental factors in hypertension. *In* Stamler, J., Stamler, R. and Pullman, T.N. (eds.): The Epidemiology of Hypertension: Proceedings of an International Symposium. New York:Grune and Stratton, 1967, p. 255.
4. Miall, W.E.: Follow-up study of arterial pressure in the population of a Welsh mining valley. Br. Med. J. 2:1205, 1959.
5. Toteson, D.C., DeFriez, A.I.C., Abrams, M. et al: Effects of adrenalectomy, desoxycorticosterone acetate and increased fluid intake on intake of sodium chloride and bicarbonate by hypertensive and normal rats. Am. J. Physiol. 164:369, 1951.
6. Pickering, G.: High Blood Pressure. London:J. & A. Churchill, Ltd., 1968.
7. Oliver, W.J., Cohen, E.L. and Neel, J.V.: Blood pressure, sodium intake and sodium related hormones in the Yanomamo Indians, a 'no-salt' culture. Circulation 2:146, 1975.
8. Sinnett, P.F. and Whyte, H.M.: Epidemiological studies in a total highland population, Tukisenta, New Guinea. Cardiovascular disease and relevant clinical, electrocardiographic, radiological and biochemical findings. J. Chron. Dis. 26:265, 1973.
9. Denton, D.A., Nelson, J.F., Orchard, E. et al: The role of adrenocortical hormone secretion in salt appetite. *In* Pfaffmann, C. (ed.): Olfaction and Taste, Rockefeller University Press, 1969, p. 535.
10. MacFarlane, W.V., Howard, B., Scoggins, B.A. et al: Water, electrolytes, hormones and blood pressure of Melanesians in relation to European contact. Proc. 24th Int. Congr. Physiol. Sci., Washington (1968), Vol. VII, 274, 1971.
11. Denton, D.A.: Sodium and hypertension. *In* Sambhi, M.P. (ed.): Mechanisms of Hypertension. ICS 302, Proc. Int. Workshop Conf., Excerpta Medica, 1973, p. 46.
12. Clark, J.D.: The Prehistory of Africa. New York:Praeger Publishers, 1970.
13. Jolly, C.J.: The seed-eaters: A new model of hominid differentiation based on a baboon analogy. Man 5:5, 1970.
14. Leakey, L.S.B.: The first men: Recent discovery in East Africa. Antiquity 33:285, 1959.

Summary of Round-Table Discussion on Antihypertensive Treatment

Franz Gross, M.D.

At some distance in time and place, it is much easier to summarize the gist of a round-table discussion than immediately afterwards. The opportunity for the leisurely reading of the Round-Table Discussion on Antihypertensive Therapy, of all that had to be squeezed into about two hours, compensated for my regret of not having been able to participate actively in the panel. In reviewing the discussion, several facts become obvious: (1) In the United States, the preference for the drugs with which to start and maintain the treatment of high blood pressure differs from that in various European countries and in Australia. (2) There is a trend to an increasing use of peripherally acting drugs, whereas drugs that affect alertness and mood are less frequently prescribed. (3) There is a growing reluctance to submit patients with uncomplicated primary hypertension too rapidly to an antihypertensive drug regimen; instead, blood pressure is watched for some time, particularly if it does not pass diastolic levels of 110 mm Hg. (4) The renin-angiotensin system is considered of minor significance for the selection of therapeutics.

As drugs of first choice, the *diuretics* are challenged by the *beta-adrenergic blockers* today, but the use of the latter is hampered in the United States by the fact that high blood

---

Panelists were A. E. Doyle, E. D. Freis, J. Genest, A. Grollman, N. M. Kaplan, P. Kincaid-Smith, P. J. Mulrow, G. Onesti, L. Tobian, A. Zanchetti; Chairman and Moderator: Mohinder P. Sambhi.

Franz Gross, M.D., Department of Pharmacology, University of Heidelberg, Federal Republic of Germany.

pressure is not yet an accepted indication for them and that only propranolol is available so far. In Australia, Great Britain and Sweden, the beta-adrenergic blockers have already replaced the diuretics, for the most part, as drugs to be given to a hypertensive first, and this trend may continue. In view of the lack of choice of beta-blockers in the United States, there was no need to discuss the advisability of using beta-blockers with or without intrinsic sympathetic activity or a cardioselective representative of this group, but sooner or later, specialists in the United States may be confronted with these problems, which doctors in Europe and Australia have had to face for several years already.

It is remarkable that none of the panelists felt it necessary to determine the activity of the renin-angiotensin system in order to decide whether treatment should be started with a beta-blocker or a diuretic. The oversimplified concept, according to which patients with high plasma renin concentration would best respond to beta-blockers, has not withstood critical scrutiny. Despite the continuously increasing share of beta-blockers in the drug treatment of hypertension, the *diuretics* still hold an important position as drugs of first choice. However, once again, a difference in national preferences of the favored diuretic is evident. From a pharmacokinetic point of view, chlorthalidone, with its long duration of action, seems to be the drug that comes nearest to the ideal of a mild and steady effect, allowing the administration of one dose every other day only. But neither in the United States nor in Great Britain or Australia has chlorthalidone gained the position it deserves. It remains to be demonstrated how Zaroxolyn (metolazone) will fit in with the row of the already existing diuretics. Despite a number of opinions expressed in favor of furosemide, it has to be stated once more that this powerful and short-acting drug is an excellent diuretic, but has no place in the long-term treatment of hypertension.

Assuming that beta-blockers and diuretics are similar in potency and comparable with respect to their tolerability, it is not indicated to campaign in favor of, or against, one or the other. In general, younger patients benefit more from beta-blockers, and in the elderly a first trial with a diuretic may give better results. Of course, beta-blockers alone are not recommendable in patients with marked bradycardia, but no principal differences with respect to their application have to be considered in most cases. There remains the question whether, instead of a plain thiazide diuretic or chlorthalidone, a combination with a potassium-sparing compound, such as triamterene, amiloride, or spironolactone, might be preferable. Again, in the elderly patient, such an alternative may be advisable, especially if he or she is simultaneously in need of cardiac glycosides. The fixed combination containing amiloride and hydrochlorothiazide (Moduretic) is accepted increasingly in Europe and Australia, whereas amiloride is not yet available in the United States. No potassium supplements have been considered necessary, but in practice, where it is not possible to have a rapid check of plasma potassium made, regular intake of potassium chloride, or at least a diet rich in potassium, may be advisable, provided that the kidney function is not impaired.

What next, if the blood pressure is not satisfactorily controlled by either a diuretic or a beta-blocker, or both? Following the trend toward peripherally acting drugs, *(di)hydralazine* would be the logical choice, but here the simultaneous administration of a beta-blocker, which prevents the increase in heart rate, is necessary. However, hydralazine is considered ineffective in Great Britain, and its dose is limited to 100 mg daily in other European countries. A legitimate successor of hydralazine seemed to be *minoxidil*, which is more powerful and longer acting, but too much time has already been spent on its clinical investigation. When it will be accepted eventually by drug control agencies, it may be limited to exceptional cases, which are not sufficiently controlled by "standard" drugs. *Prazosin* has been claimed to act directly on the smooth muscle and in this respect to be comparable to hydralazine or minoxidil, but the pharmacological data are more similar to those of an alpha-adrenergic blocking drug, and various observations of a dramatic fall in blood pressure after the first doses support such an assumption. Much more information is needed before prazosin may be recommended for wide use in the treatment of hypertension.

The centrally acting compounds, *reserpine*, *alpha-methyldopa* and *clonidine*, remain. Among these, reserpine still holds its position, provided the disease is not too far advanced, because its mild and sustained action and its relatively good tolerability — unless daily doses of 0.5 mg are exceeded — are definite advantages. This is especially the case if it is taken together with a diuretic and hydralazine, but much less so in combination with a beta-blocker, which may enhance the bradycardiac effect and also reduce stroke volume. The suspicion that the manifestation of mammary cancer may be favored by the administration of reserpine has not been confirmed in recent retrospective studies. *Methyldopa* still belongs to the standard antihypertensives, but the popularity it has gained in Great Britain has hardly been achieved in other countries, certainly not in Germany, where it is mostly given in too low dosages, nor in other countries, where the development of tolerance is considered a handicap. No doubt, methyldopa will retain a significant position as an antihypertensive, but its share is going to decline.

The opinion on *clonidine* is divided; it is considered tricky, and its side effects have prevented its wide acceptance. A strong sympathomimetic, which has to pass the blood-brain barrier in order to exert its antihypertensive effect, is difficult to handle, and therefore it ranks in the third rather than the second line of drugs. The rebound phenomenon after abrupt withdrawal is especially dangerous, and even though the administration of an antihypertensive should never be suddenly interrupted, such a procedure may have particular consequences in the case of clonidine. Hence, it is not surprising that some participants of the round table do not use it, and that others find it dispensable.

Guanethidine has maintained its role as drug of last choice, never alone, but always together with at least a diuretic or with other drugs, such as hydralazine, perhaps minoxidil, or a beta-adrenergic blocker. The irregular absorption, the tendency to orthostatic episodes and the occasionally insufficient lowering of pressure in supine position make its wider use problematic — interestingly enough, it has hardly been mentioned during the discussion.

Drug compliance of patients is a problem in all countries, and, if possible, one tablet a day is the preferred schedule. Among the available drugs, only chlorthalidone and reserpine (as well as guanethidine) correspond to such a duration of action; there is no long-acting beta-adrenergic blocker nor a vasodilator that is as long-acting as minoxidil. Administration of too many pills should be avoided, especially in elderly patients, who may need additional drugs and who quite frequently may forget to take the tablets. Consequently, fixed combinations may be the only way to escape an unsuitable number of tablets that may confuse the patient. We have to realize that we are still far from what might be considered a convenient treatment schedule. Of course, one should never try to exchange convenience for scientific reasoning or safety, but compromises between theoretical considerations and practical applications may become unavoidable.

In principle, the various stages of antihypertensive drug treatment may be classified as follows, although individual preference may result in some changes between 2 and 3:

1. diuretic or beta-adrenergic blocker
2. reserpine, hydralazine, alpha-methyldopa
3. clonidine, prazosin?, guanethidine.

Remarkable progress has been made since the ganglionic blocking drugs were launched as the first active antihypertensives, but much remains still to be done, and we have not at all reached the goal of an effective and well-tolerated treatment for all hypertensive patients. Research has to continue, and it is hoped that principally new drugs, which have definite advantages over the existing ones, will become available before long.

Subject Index